D1650745

The metric system

Weight (mass)

1 kilogram (kg)	= 1000 grams (g)
1 gram (g)	= 1000 milligrams (mg)
1 milligram (mg)	= 1000 micrograms (mcg)
1 microgram (mcg)	= 1000 nanograms (ng)

Volume

1 litre (l)	= 1000 millilitres (mL)
1 millilitre (mL)	= 1000 microlitres (µl)

When writing drug doses, the BNF recommends that micrograms is not abbreviated.

Intravenous drip flow rate

$$\text{Rate (drops/minute)} = \frac{\text{Vol. of solution (mL)} \times \text{no. of drops/mL}}{\text{time (minutes)}}$$

To calculate the volume in drops, you need to know how many drops of the find ordered are contained in 1 mL. You should find this information on the administration set.

Unless otherwise stated, use a drop factor of 20 drops/mL for clear fluids and 15 drops/mL for blood.

For example, 1 litre of saline in **6** hours:

$$\text{Rate} = \frac{1000 \text{ mL} \times 20}{6 \times 60}$$

Infusion pump rates

$$\text{Flow rate} = \frac{\text{Total volume (mL)}}{\text{Duration (hours)}}$$

For example, 1000 mL over 8 hours:

$$\text{Rate} = \frac{1000}{8} = 125 \text{ mL}.$$

(1 litre in 2 hours = 500; 1 litre in 4 hours = 150; l litre in 6 hours = 166; 1 litre in 12 hours = 83)

610.73/ OxF

Oxford Handbooks in Nursing

Oxford Handbook of Midwifery
Janet Medforth, Susan Battersby, Maggie Evans, Beverley Marsh,
and Angela Walker

Oxford Handbook of Mental Health Nursing
Edited by Patrick Callaghan and Helen Waldock

Oxford Handbook of Children's and Young People's Nursing
Edited by Edward Alan Glasper, Gillian McEwing, and Jim Richardson

Oxford Handbook of Nurse Prescribing
Sue Beckwith and Penny Franklin

Oxford Handbook of Cancer Nursing
Edited by Mike Tadman and Dave Roberts

Oxford Handbook of Cardiac Nursing
Edited by Kate Johnson and Karen Rawlings-Anderson

Oxford Handbook of Primary Care Nursing
Edited by Vari Drennan and Claire Goodman

Oxford Handbook of Gastrointestinal Nursing
Edited by Christine Norton, Julia Williams, Claire Taylor, Annmarie Nunwa,
and Kathy Whayman

Oxford Handbook of Respiratory Nursing
Terry Robinson and Jane Scullion

Oxford Handbook of Nursing Older People
Beverley Tabernacle, Marie Barnes, and Annette Jinks

Oxford Handbook of Clinical Skills in Adult Nursing
Jacqueline Randle, Frank Coffey, and Martyn Bradbury

Oxford Handbook of Emergency Nursing
Robert Crouch, Alan Charters, Mary Dawood, and Paula O'Gara

Oxford Handbook of Dental Nursing
K Seymour, DYD Samarawickrama, EC Boon, and RL Parr

Oxford Handbook of Diabetes Nursing
Lorraine Avery and Sue Beckwith

Oxford Handbook of Musculoskeletal Nursing
Susan Oliver

Oxford Handbook of Women's Health Nursing
Ali Kubba, Sunanda Gupta, and Debra Holloway

Oxford Handbook of Perioperative Practice
Suzanne Hughes and Andy Mardell

Oxford Handbook of Critical Care Nursing
Sheila Adam and Sue Osborne

Oxford Handbook of Neuroscience Nursing
Sue Woodward and Cath Waterhouse

Oxford Handbook of Adult Nursing
George Castledine and Ann Close

Oxford Handbook of
Adult Nursing

Edited by

George Castledine

Professor Sir George Castledine is Chief Executive of the
Institute of Ageing and Health and works as an external
nursing consultant both in the UK and in parts of the
developing world. He has strong academic links in
Birmingham and is a fellow of Glyndwr University in
North Wales. He still finds time despite his busy schedule
to work as a Bank Staff Nurse at Moseley Hall Hospital in
Birmingham.

Ann Close

Ann Close is a National Clinical Advisor, Care Quality
Commission, Fellow of the University of
Wolverhampton, and Visiting
Professor at Birmingham City University.

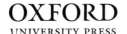

OXFORD
UNIVERSITY PRESS

OXFORD
UNIVERSITY PRESS

Great Clarendon Street, Oxford OX2 6DP

Oxford University Press is a department of the University of Oxford.
It furthers the University's objective of excellence in research, scholarship,
and education by publishing worldwide in

Oxford New York

Auckland Cape Town Dar es Salaam Hong Kong Karachi
Kuala Lumpur Madrid Melbourne Mexico City Nairobi
New Delhi Shanghai Taipei Toronto

With offices in

Argentina Austria Brazil Chile Czech Republic France Greece
Guatemala Hungary Italy Japan Poland Portugal Singapore
South Korea Switzerland Thailand Turkey Ukraine Vietnam

Oxford is a registered trade mark of Oxford University Press
in the UK and in certain other countries

Published in the United States
by Oxford University Press Inc., New York

© Oxford University Press, 2009

British Library Cataloguing in Publication Data
Data available

Library of Congress Cataloging in Publication Data
Data available

Typeset by Cepha Imaging Private Ltd., Bangalore, India
Printed in Italy
on acid-free paper by
L.E.G.O.S.p.A.

ISBN 978–0–19–923135–5

10 9 8 7 6 5 4 3 2 1

Contents

Section 1: Principles and practice of nursing

Section 2: Diagnosing nursing problems and implementing nursing care

Section 4: Emergencies

Section 5: Professional nursing practice

Preface

We have created this book to appeal to all pre-registration nurses studying adult nursing, and to those qualified nurses who work in a variety of specialist clinical areas. Such nurses often need a reliable source of information across a breadth of practice. In the past many of these nurses have been referred to as 'generalists' who have never become tied to a particular speciality.

This book is therefore intended for all those nurses who want a core nursing text not only to keep them up to date but also to keep them informed of the essentials underpinning the practice of nursing in other areas of adult nursing. We have designed the content of the book to include medical and nursing technical data, and some of the key clinical issues and emergencies which nurses may come across in the institutional setting.

It will be an invaluable text for all students of adult nursing as it covers the essentials and core of their curriculum and is small enough to carry around on placement. We are also confident that many qualified nurses will find it helpful, as it will serve as an essential reference point for queries and questions in their practice.

We have felt very strongly that this nursing handbook should not become too technical or full of medical jargon and that it should reflect the importance of the fundamentals of nursing care. That is why we have included such chapters as: defining nursing, individualizing nursing practice, nursing patients with intimate and sensitive care needs, and managing in the clinical environment. Nursing today despite all the advances in medical technology should still be delivered in a compassionate and personal way that preserves the dignity and individuality of the person receiving it.

The essential medical and nursing information which a general nurse needs to know has been provided by an expert group of contributors and we are indebted to them for all their help and hard work in producing the quality of information which we feel this text has achieved.

Finally, we hope that you the reader will find this book to be an indispensable help which you will have with you, whenever you need it in your clinical nursing practice. May we wish you success and happiness in your nursing career, and we hope we have provided a small but essential text to help you on your way.

George Castledine and Ann Close.

For

Patients we have nursed and influenced
And who have taught and influenced us,
For colleagues and students we have taught and supported
And who have taught and supported us,
For the staff at OUP who have kept faith in us,
And to our close family and friends for their love and patience
During those lost days and disrupted vacations.

Contributors

Dr Nick Allcock
Associate Professor,
The University of Nottingham
School of Nursing,
Queens Medical Centre
Nottingham, UK

Dr S Alusi
The Walton Centre for Neurology
and Neurosurgery,
Fazakerley, Liverpool, UK

Lorraine Avery
at the time of writing:
Diabetes Nurse Consultant,
Western Sussex PCT, Chichester,
West Sussex, UK

Julie Bloom
Royal Devon and Exeter NHS
Trust, Exeter, UK

Sue Beckwith
Consortium for Healthcare
Research, Doctoral Research
Fellow, Centre for Research
into Primary and Community
Care, Faculty of Health
and Human Sciences, University
of Hertfordshire, Hatfield,
Hertfordshire, UK

Sue Blyden
Senior Lecturer, Adult Branch
Nursing, Faculty of Health and Life
Sciences, Coventry University,
Coventry, UK

Angeline Boaden
Consultant Nurse, Colorectal
Services, Peterborough and
Stamford Hospitals NHS
Foundation Trust, UK

Mr A Brodbelt
The Walton Centre for Neurology
and Neurosurgery,
Fazakerley, Liverpool, UK

Jackie Brown
Team Leader, Sexual &
Reproductive Healthcare
Partnership,
Hull Primary Care Trust,
Conifer House,
Hull, UK

Helen Butterfield
Department of Dermatology,
Churchill Hospital,
Old Road, Headington,
Oxford, UK

Sharon Clovis
Prostate Clinical Nurse Specialist,
Guy's & St Thomas' NHS
Foundation Trust,
Guy's Hospital,
Urology Centre,
London, UK

Myra Cooper
Senior Reseach Tutor, Oxford
Doctoral Course in Clinical
Psychology, University of Oxford,
Warneford Hospital,
Oxford, UK

Sue Cox
Nurse Consultant – Pre-Dialysis
Management, 6th floor
New Guy's House,
Guy's Hospital,
St Thomas Street,
London, UK

Patricia Crofton
The Walton Centre for Neurology
and Neurosurgery,
Fazakerley, Liverpool, UK

Carolyn Dow
Nurse Consultant, Emergency
Department,
United Hospitals of Leicester
NHS Trust,
UK

Vari Drennan
Professor of Health Policy &
Service Delivery, Faculty of
Health and Social Care Sciences,
St George's, University of
London, & Kingston University,
London, UK

Tracey Galletly
Senior Infection Control Nurse,
Imperial College Healthcare NHS
Trust, Charing Cross Hospital,
London, UK

Bob Gates
Project Leader, Learning
Disabilities Workforce
Development,
NHS South Central, Newbury,
Berkshire, UK

Brian George
The Mortimer Market Centre,
Capper Street, London, UK

Claire Goodman
Professor of Health Care
Research, Centre for Research in
Primary and Community Care,
University of Hertfordshire,
Hatfield, UK

Jackie Green
Advanced Clinical Practice, Board
Director, Myeloma, UK

Tina O'Hara
Palliative Care Team Leader,
Oncology Department,
Addenbrooke's NHS Trust,
Cambridge, UK

Hilary Harkin
ENT Department, St Thomas'
Hospital, London, UK

Sanjeev Heemraz
Matron, Ophthalmology
Department, Guy's and
St Thomas' NHS Foundation
Trust, Lambeth Palace Road,
London, UK

Deborah Hofman
Department of Dermatology,
Churchill Hospital, Old Road,
Headington, Oxford, UK

Marie Honey
Nurse Consultant, Older People
Services, St Helens and Knowsley
Teaching Hospitals NHS Trust,
Liverpool, UK

Mr M Javadpour
The Walton Centre for Neurology
and Neurosurgery, Fazakerley,
Liverpool, UK

Kath Jones
Community midwife/lecturer,
Wrexham Maelor Hospital,
North Wales, UK

David Kelly
Senior Nurse, Liver Unit,
University Hospital of Birmingham
Foundation Trust, UK

Mourad Labib
Consultant Chemical Pathologist,
Dudley Group of Hospitals NHS
Foundation Trust, Dudley, West
Midlands, UK

Brian Lucas
Orthopaedic Advanced Practice
Nurse, Whipps Cross University
Hospital NHS Trust, London, UK

Dr T Nixon
The Walton Centre for Neurology
and Neurosurgery, Fazakerley,
Liverpool, UK

Jan Parsons
The Walton Centre for Neurology
and Neurosurgery, Fazakerley,
Liverpool, UK

Ron Pate
Secondary Care Pharmaceutical
Adviser, Department of Medicines
Management, Keele University,
UK

Glynis Pellatt
Senior Lecturer, University of
Bedfordshire, AVEC, Stoke
Mandeville Hospital,
Aylesbury, UK

Liz Plastow
at the time of writing:
Professional Advisor Specialist,
Community Public Health Nursing,
Nursing and Midwifery Council,
London, UK

June Poston
The Walton Centre for Neurology
and Neurosurgery, Fazakerley,
Liverpool, UK

Terry Robinson
Specialist Respiratory Nurse,
Harrogate and District NHS
Foundation Trust, UK

Sarah Ryan
Nurse Consultant Rheumatology,
Haywood Hospital, High Lane,
Burslem,
Stoke-on-Trent, UK

Dr N Silver
The Walton Centre for
Neurology and Neurosurgery,
Fazakerley,
Liverpool, UK

Graeme Smith
Nursing Studies, The University
of Edinburgh, Medical School,
Edinburgh, UK

Professor T Solomon
The Walton Centre for Neurology
and Neurosurgery, Fazakerley,
Liverpool, UK

Janet Sumner
The Oxford Centre for Diabetes,
Endocrinology and Metabolism,
Churchill Hospital, Old Road,
Headington, Oxford, UK

Mike Tadman
Ward Manager, Frank Ellis Unit,
Churchill Hospital, Oxford, and
Associate Lecturer, Oxford
Brookes University, Oxford, UK

Rose Thompson
Adult Branch Nursing,
Coventry University,
Coventry, UK

Vivien Thornton-Jones
The Oxford Centre for Diabetes
Endocrinology and Metabolism,
Churchill Hospital, Old Road,
Headington, Oxford, UK

Caroline Watkins
Professor of Stroke and Older
People's Care, Clinical Practice
Research Unit, School of Nursing
and Caring Sciences, University of
Central Lancashire, Preston, UK

Professor CA Young
The Walton Centre for Neurology
and Neurosurgery, Fazakerley,
Liverpool, UK

Reviewers

Dr Sani Aliyu
Consultant in Microbiology
and Infectious Diseases,
Addenbrooke's Hospital,
Cambridge, UK

Dr Sara Booth
Director Palliative Care Services,
Macmillan Consultant in Palliative
Medicine, Addenbrookes NHS
Trust, Cambridge, UK

Dr Lesley Bowker
Consultant Physician, Care of
the Elderly Department, Norfolk
and Norwich University Hospital;
and Clinical Skills Coordinator
and Hon. Senior Lecturer for the
School of Medicine, Health Policy
and Practice at the University of
East Anglia, Norwich, UK

Graham Brack
Associate Lecturer in
Pharmacology,
University of Plymouth; and
Pharmaceutical Adviser, Cornwall
and Isles of Scilly Primary Care
Trust, St Austell, UK

Dr Michael Brown
Nurse Consultant, Learning
Disability Services, NHS Lothian;
and Lecturer, School of Nursing,
Midwifery and Social Care,
Napier University,
Edinburgh, UK

Professor Patrick Callaghan
Professor of Mental Health
Nursing and Chartered Health
Psychologist, University of
Nottingham & Nottinghamshire
Healthcare NHS Trust,
Nottingham, UK

Rogan Corbridge
The ENT Department, West Wing,
John Radcliffe Hospital,
Oxford, UK

Dr Stuart Crisp
Consultant Paediatrician,
Orange, NSW, Australia

Dr Shreelatta Datta
Specialist Registrar in Obstetrics
and Gynaecology, Brighton, UK

Dr Richard Davies
General Practitioner,
The Ridgeway Surgery, Redditch,
Worcestershire, UK

Dr Alastair Denniston
MRC Clinical Research Fellow in
Ophthalmology, Academic Unit
of Ophthalmology, University of
Birmingham, UK

Dr Babikar Elawad
GU Consultant,
North Tyneside, UK

Matthew Fletcher
Consultant Orthopaedic Surgeon,
Head, NE Department of Surgical
Services, Dawson Creek & District
Hospital, Dawson Creek,
British Columbia, Canada

Dr John Hanley
Department of Haematology,
Royal Victoria Infirmary,
Newcastle upon Tyne, UK

Dr Inam Haq
Senior Lecturer in Rheumatology
and Medical Education,
Brighton and Sussex Medical
School, University of Brighton,
Falmer, Sussex, UK

Professor Peter Hoskin

Consultant in Clinical Oncology,
Mount Vernon Cancer Centre,
Professor in Clinical Oncology,
University College London;
and Honorary Consultant,
University College Hospitals
NHS Trust, London, UK

Dr Jason Jennings

Consultant Gastroenterologist,
Leeds General Infirmary,
Tadcaster,
North Yorkshire, UK

Professor Dora Kohen

Consultant Psychiatrist,
University of Central Lancashire,
Lancashire Postgraduate
School of Medicine,
London, UK

Dr Andrew Mitchell

Consultant Cardiologist,
Jersey Heart and Lung Unit,
General Hospital,
Gloucester Street,
St Helier, Jersey

Professor Kevin Moore

Centre for Hepatology,
Department of Medicine,
Hampstead Campus, University
College Medical School,
University College London, UK

Dr John Rees

Dean of Undergraduate Education,
King's College London School
of Medicine at Guy's,
King's College & St Thomas'
Hospitals, London, UK

Dr Sarah Smith

Consultant Geriatrician,
Department of Clinical Geratology,
John Radcliffe Hospital,
Headley Way, Oxford, UK

Dr Roger Smyth

Consultant Psychiatrist,
Department of Psychological
Medicine, Royal Infirmary of
Edinburgh, UK

Dr Cathy Stannard

Consultant in Pain Medicine, Pain
Clinic, Macmillan Centre, Frenchay
Hospital, Bristol, UK

Professor John Wass

Professor of Endocrinology,
Oxford University; Consultant
Endocrinologist, Churchill
Hospital, Oxford, UK

Rose Watson

Fellow of The Higher Education
Academy (2007), Medical
Education Facilitator, University
of Leeds, Medical Education
Department, UK

Symbols and abbreviations

−ve	negative
+ve	positive
<	less than
>	greater than
≥	equivalent to and greater than
≤	equivalent to and less than
±	plus or minus
↓	decreased
↑	increased
↔	normal
°	degrees
ABGs	arterial blood gases
ACE	angiotensin-converting enzyme
AF	atrial fibrillation
AIDS	acquired immunodeficiency syndrome
ARF	acute renal failure
AV	atrio-ventricular
Ba	barium
BD	twice daily
BLS	basic life support
BNF	British National Formulary
BP	blood pressure
Ca	carcinoma
CABG	coronary artery bypass graft
CAPD	continuous ambulatory peritoneal dialysis
CCF	congestive cardiac failure
CCU	coronary care unit
CD	controlled drug
CHB	complete heart block
CNS	central nervous system
COPD	chronic obstructive pulmonary disease
CPAP	continuous positive airway pressure
CPR	cardiopulmonary resuscitation
CRF	chronic renal failure
CSF	cerebrospinal fluid
CT	computed tomography

CVA	cerebrovascular accident
CVP	central venous pressure
CXR	chest X-ray
D&V	diarrhoea and vomiting
DVT	deep vein thrombosis
ECG	electrocardiograph
ED	emergency department
EDTA	ethylene diamine etetracetic acid
EEG	electroencephalogram
ENT	ear, nose, and throat
ESR	erythrocyte sedimentation rate
ET	endotracheal
FBC	full blood count
FVC	forced vital capacity
g	gram
GA	general anaesthetic
GFR	glomerular filtration rate
GP	general practitioner
GTN	glyceryl trinitrate
GU	genitourinary
GUM	genitourinary medicine
Hct	haematocrit
HIV	human immunodeficiency virus
HRT	hormone replacement therapy
ICP	integrated care pathway
ICU/ITU	intensive care/therapy unit
Ig	immunoglobulin
IM	intramuscularly
IV	intravenous/ly
IVI	intravenous infusion
JVP	jugular venous pressure
kg	kilogram
l	litre
LA	local anaesthetic
LFT	live function test
LP	lumbar puncture
LVF	left ventricular failure
mg	milligram
μg	microgram
LA	local anaesthetic

MCV	mean cell/corpuscular volume
MI	myocardial infarction
mL	millilitre
mmHg	millilitres of mercury
MRI	magnetic resonance imaging
MRSA	meticillin-resistant *Staphylococcus aureus*
MS	multiple sclerosis
MSU	mid-stream specimen of urine
NAD	nothing abnormal detected
NBM	nil by mouth
Neb	by nebulizer
NG tube	nasogastric tube
OD	once daily
OM	in the morning
ON	at night
OPD	outpatient department
$PaCO_2$	partial pressure of carbon dioxide in arterial blood
PaO_2	partial pressure of oxygen in arterial blood
PCV	packed cell volume
PE	pulmonary embolism
PEG	percutaneous endoscopic gastrostomy
PET	positron emission tomography
PMH	past medical history
PO	orally
POMS	prescription-only medicines
PR	rectally
PRN	as necessary
PT	prothrombin time
PUO	pyrexia of unknown origin
PV	vaginally
QDS, QUID	four times a day
RBC	red blood cell
Rh	rhesus
RTA	road traffic accident
RVF	right ventricular failure
SC	subcutaneous
SL	sublingual
SLE	systemic lupus erythematosus
Stat	immediate
T_3	triiodothyronine

T_4	thyroxine
Tb	tuberculosis
TDS/TID	three times a day
TIA	transient ischaemic attack
TPN	total parenteral nutrition
TPR	temperature, pulse, and respiration
TRH	thyrotropin-releasing hormone
TSH	thyroid-stimulating hormone
TURP	transurethral resection of prostate
U&E	urea and electrolytes
UTI	urinary tract infection
UV	ultraviolet
VC	vital capacity
VE	ventricular extrasystole
VF	ventricular fibrillation
VT	ventricular tachycardia
WBC	white blood cell
WCC	white cell count
WR	Wasserman reaction

Principles and practice of nursing

Defining nursing

Values and principles of nursing

Nursing has traditionally focused on providing a compassionate service to patients. The purpose of nursing as defined by Florence Nightingale in 1882 is to put the patient in the best condition for nature to act upon them. Nightingale emphasized that the nurse's role is to anticipate the patient's needs and to do things for patients even before they recognize their own needs. This type of anticipatory care forms the basis of nursing care in all clinical situations and is often regarded as the cornerstone of essential nursing care.

The nursing profession values the image of compassion. Unfortunately, nursing care receives the most attention when it is inadequate or absent. Patients who are deprived of compassionate nursing care voice dissatisfaction with nursing services. Therefore, compassionate care should always be a primary focus of patient-centred nursing care.

Nursing's contribution to society is partially influenced by the value that society places on health and health care. Society also determines the value of specific services rendered by nurses. Although nursing will continually evolve as a result of scientific advances and modernization, the fundamentals will always involve providing a compassionate service of helping and caring; promoting health; preventing illness; and assisting people in health-related activities that are normally performed unaided (i.e. self-care activities or daily living activities).

Definitions and properties of nursing

The International Council of Nurses (2002) defined nursing as follows: 'Nursing encompasses autonomous and collaborative care of individuals of all ages, families, groups and communities, sick or well and in all settings. Nursing includes the promotion of health, prevention of illness, and the care of ill, disabled, and dying people. Advocacy, promotion of a safe environment, research, participation in shaping health policy and in patient health systems, management, and education are also key nursing roles.'

The Royal College of Nursing UK (2002) defined nursing as the 'use of clinical judgment and the provision of care to enable people to promote, improve, maintain or recover health or, when death is inevitable, to die peacefully.'

Further information

RCN: www.rcn.org.uk

Role of nursing

1. Nursing is culturally and economically determined.
2. In a complex society nursing is divided into various specialist roles.
3. The fundamentals of nursing transcend all medical specialities.
4. At times there is a crossover into medical care and some nurses prescribe medical treatment.
5. Nursing is both an art and a science.
6. As nursing becomes acceptable in a society so it develops and seeks a knowledge base which eventually becomes more exclusive and concerned with professionalism.
7. The root meaning of the word 'nurse' is to nourish and a simple definition of nursing is closely related to nurturing.
8. Nursing is involved with meeting the problems and concerns relating to human bodily functioning.
9. Nursing is also concerned with mental and emotional health, social care, and spirituality.
10. One of the major goals of nursing is to enable adaptation and coping.
11. Nursing is about being 'there' (present), available, and perceptive.
12. Nursing is an interactive process emphasizing an interpersonal relationship and a shared experience in health-related matters.
13. Nursing has high moral and ethical standards of which accountability, autonomy, advocacy, collaboration, and duty of care are key elements.
14. Nurses are part of a wider health and social care team with the common goal of patient-centred personalized care. Working as a team, therefore, is an essential part of nursing.
15. Nursing aims to protect the public and respect the laws of the land.
16. There is a nursing role in educating for health, i.e. aiding health promotion and disease prevention.
17. Nursing is concerned with social policies and political decisions that may affect the health of those who are being cared for.
18. Nursing uses an eclectic approach to its understanding of its aims in society and its development as a service to people.
19. The contribution to health care by nurses is systematized by the role of the nursing process in which nursing needs are assessed and nursing care is prescribed, carried out, and evaluated.
20. Nurses work within the context of improving the public health and have a responsibility to see their actions within a wider context. This includes monitoring local health care practices, which leads to improving standards.

Fundamentals of general nursing practice

- Assist patients with their basic human needs or daily living functions.
- Convey through verbal and non-verbal behaviours and provide care that is nurturing, supportive, and guiding.
- Counsel patients, their friends, and their relatives when and where appropriate.
- Teach, coach, advise, and provide information so that patients and their significant others are able to understand and perform aspects of health and nursing care.
- Carry out medical and health care treatments as part of the clinical plan for patient care.
- Monitor and regularly review relevant information about patients and their situation through observing, questioning, assessing, and performing nursing care.
- Coordinate health and medical treatments delivered to patients, referring to other health and social care services where necessary.
- Collaborate with other health care professionals and service staff to ensure patients receive appropriate health care that fulfills their needs.
- Advocate and represent patients when appropriate and support vulnerable patients where needed.
- Collect information regarding patients' health and medical care in order to provide a high standard and quality of nursing care.
- Work within the parameters of the NMC Code.
- Provide fundamental aspects of nursing care as described above and by various nursing authors such as Florence Nightingale, Virginia Henderson, Nancy Roper, and George Castledine.
  - Nurses should link nursing with holistic care.
  - Nurses work in 'multidisciplinary' health care teams and often participate in 'crossover' working, where they take on medical tasks and other activities to help the team meet its targets and goals.
  - Nurses may perform 'interdependent' nursing actions, i.e. roles that overlap with roles of other health care professionals and are done collaboratively with other health care providers.
  - Nurses also perform 'independent' nursing actions, e.g. deciding what nursing actions should be provided to a particular patient in order to give comprehensive nursing care.

Further information

NMC (2008). *The Code*. www.nmc-uk.org

Domains of nursing practice[1]

1. Helping those with health care concerns and needs
2. Working with other professionals involved with health and social care
3. Assessing, diagnosing, and monitoring
4. Effectively managing rapidly changing situations
5. Administering and monitoring therapeutic interventions and regimens
6. Teaching and coaching
7. Monitoring and ensuring the quality of health care practices
8. Ensuring organizational and work-role competencies

1 Benner P (1984). *From novice to expert.* Addison-Wesley, Menlo-Park, CA

Differences between medicine and nursing

- The functions of health care professionals overlap in meeting the patient's needs, and health care in the 21st century depends on multidisciplinary teamwork.
- There are distinct differences between the medical and nursing role (See Table 1.1).
- The nurse has a colleague relationship with physicians and other health professionals.
- The nurse is responsible for promoting and maintaining daily living activities and carrying out fundamental aspects of nursing care. These activities form a background to all other health care activities. The nurse maintains the person while other health professionals intervene to diagnose and treat disease.
- The nurse performs a coordinating role, bringing order and continuity to care.
- The nurse cultivates an environment for the maintenance of life, which makes all other health functions possible. In a complex health system the nurse provides this essential and distinctive role alongside that of other health care workers.
- The nurse is the authority on the maintenance of daily living activities.
- The roles of the physician and nurse are complementary and so closely related as to prohibit an adversarial relationship.
- There is a great deal of reference and interaction between the physician and nurse in planning patient care and there is often overlap and interchangeability of roles.
- As nurses advance their skills, they will diagnose, plan, implement, and evaluate the care required to meet patients' needs.
- The nurse increasingly undertakes or requests diagnostic tests and therapeutic regimens. In some advanced practice roles the nurse undertakes medical treatments previously the domain of the physician. However, the nurse's major function is to maintain the overall care of the patients, ensuring they are able to meet daily living activities and their environmental needs, thus contributing to health and well-being.
- The contribution of one profession may predominate at one time; however, there may be a shift in the contribution required from other professions (e.g. physicians, nurses, social workers) at different times.
- While the interdependence of the health care professions is important, it is equally important that each profession develops and masters its own unique contribution.

Table 1.1 Differences between nursing and medical roles

	Primarily the general nursing role	Primarily medical–nursing teamwork, or medical role
Focus	To identify and monitor the patient's nursing and coping response to actual or potential health problems and concerns. (It may also identify the physiological and mental health issues involved.)	To identify and monitor pathophysiological and diagnostic responses to treatment and problems. It may also involve some of the caring issues.
Problem identification	To identify and confirm the nature of a given health care or social problem or concern, which is solely the responsibility of the nurse (some may have medical implications).	To identify and confirm the medical diagnosis. Some nurses may be qualified or trained to undertake this process but the final decision belongs to the physician or professional in charge.
Treatment and care	The nurse decides the most appropriate nursing interventions and care based on evidence and research. May also decide on some of the most appropriate medical treatment but would consult with a medical physician, or follow a protocol.	The physician decides on the most appropriate medical interventions and evaluates these together with the nurse and the rest of the multidisciplinary team.
Accountability	The nurse is accountable for all nursing treatment and care and those aspects of medical care and treatment they have incorporated into their role and clinical practice.	The doctor is accountable for all medical treatment and care which they give or direct others to give on their behalf.

Adapted with permission from Castledine G (1998). *Writing documentation and communication for nurses*. Quay Books, Mark Allen Publishing.

Scope of practice

The Scope of Professional Practice was introduced in 1992 to provide a means for nurses to expand the boundaries of practice and promote holistic care beyond the knowledge and skills gained for registration. The updated Nursing and Midwifery Council (NMC) Standards of Conduct, Performance and Ethics ('The Code') (2008) provides the guidance on expanding practice.

Principles for role expansion

- Nurses are accountable and responsible for gaining theoretical knowledge and practical skills to safeguard both patients and themselves and to ensure safe practice.
- Nurses must be aware of the boundaries of their own knowledge and skills and only undertake care for which they are prepared, competent, and confident.
- Patient care should be improved, e.g. more patient centred and holistic.
- Essential values and practices associated with caring should be preserved.
- The role expansion must be supported and agreed by the organization or clinical speciality in which the nurse works.
- The activity must be clearly defined including the circumstances and conditions under which it can occur and the procedures involved.
- The nurse must be appropriately prepared and the level of training/ education clearly set out.
- The nurse must be assessed as competent both in practice and underpinning knowledge. This may be by:
  - peer assessment by a proficient clinical expert willing to provide supervision and assessment; or
  - self-assessment to encourage self-reflection and role development.
- The nurse must be willing to take on the role.
- A system for ratification, cataloguing, and review of expanded (scope) practices should be in place. Where necessary, the nurse should refer to other health care professionals.

Further information

NMC (2008). *The Code*. www.nmc-uk.org

Evidence-based nursing practice

The NHS drive for providing more clinically effective and cost effective health care requires that nursing care decisions be based on explicit evidence-based information.

Sources for evidence-based practice

- Research—a systematic process of data collection that identifies new facts and relationships among facts for the purpose of prediction and explanation and adds to the body of knowledge in a particular area of practice.
- Experience—nurses reflecting on best practice from their experiences and using non-research publications to agree consensus view.
- Expert opinion—may be obtained through formal education, conference symposia, and journal publications.
- View and experiences of patients and their relatives—satisfaction or dissatisfaction with elements of care.
- Audit—a comparison of actual practice against preset standards.

Resources for developing evidence-based practice

Nurses can access systematic reviews, databases, and best practice guidelines from:

- The Cochrane Library which comprises the Cochrane Database of Systematic Reviews, the Cochrane Controlled Trials Register, and the Cochrane Review Methodology Database
- The Midwifery Information and Resource Service (MIDIRS)
- NHS Centre for Reviews and Dissemination and literature searching facilities such as Medline Psyclit and Cumulative Index of Nursing and Allied Health Literature (CINAHL)
- National Service Frameworks (NSFs)—this provides evidence-based national frameworks, outlining what patients can expect to receive
- National Institute for Clinical Excellence (NICE) (England and Wales)
- Scottish Intercollegiate Guidance Network (SIGN)
- Librarians from local organizations or from professional organizations.

Further information

National Electronic Library for Health www.nelh.nhs.uk
Department of Health www.dh.gov.uk
NHS Centre for Review and Dissemination www.york.ac.uk
NICE www.nice.org.uk

Standards of clinical nursing

Written standards provide explicit statements of the level of clinical nursing care expected to be delivered and are aimed at optimizing the quality of care to patients.

Clinical nursing practice is influenced by:
- National standards, e.g. NSFs, NICE, Department of Health guidelines and regulations, and Essence of Care.
- NMC requirements and guidelines, e.g. standards for education and practice, code of conduct, medicines management, and guidelines on documentation.
- Professional bodies, e.g. Royal College of Nursing (RCN) guidelines on best practice for manual handling, perioperative fasting, pain management, and tissue viability management.

Local standards are specifically developed to guide local practice and are derived from the above and adapted to the local context. Standards ensure all staff are aware of the methods of working agreed by the organization or a particular department or speciality. Standards should indicate the evidence base, e.g. research data, legislation or guidance produced if available, or the expert consensus opinion used.

Standards identify the purpose, method of patient assessment, details of interventions, expected outcomes, methods of evaluation, and audit. Standards should be regularly reviewed so that they are kept up to date. Clinical nursing standards help to identify:
- The scope of nursing practice.
- Possible complications and ways of overcoming these.
- Parameters of care and links with multidisciplinary care.
- The importance of patient's and relative's involvement.
- Criteria for evaluation, teaching, in-service review, and induction and orientation programmes.
- Objective criteria for self-evaluation, peer, and line manager review.
- Research needs.
- Areas that require improvement through audit.

Further information

DH: www.dh.gov.uk
NICE: www.nice.org.uk
NMC: www.nmc-uk.org
RCN: www.rcn.org.uk
Modernisation Agency (2003). *Essence of care. Patient-focused benchmark for clinical governance.* DH: London.
DH (2004). *National Standards Local Action.* DH: London.

Models for delivering nursing care

Key concepts of nursing care

These are the concepts that are the basis of nursing care models. Models are conceptual mental constructs of the essential factors in nursing care from which nursing methods are developed.

Comfort is providing someone with relief from their discomfort. It consists of physical, psychological, social, emotional, and environmental factors. Comfort is sometimes provided by carrying out regular comfort rounds, usually 2-hourly, that focus on the skin and pressure areas, personal grooming, giving and sharing of information, therapeutic touch, straightening the sheet under the patient, puffing up pillows, and any other nursing care that promotes patient comfort. This practice should not be restricted to 2-hourly rounds but should be offered to meet patients' needs.

Compassion relates to pity and is central to the approach nurses should show towards patients, especially when they are most vulnerable and distressed. Demonstrating a helpful or merciful sympathetic manner is often essential to establishing and maintaining the nurse–patient relationship.

Dignity is giving someone respect and a sense of self-worth and importance. It is achieved by nurturing a patient's self-respect and self-esteem, and by appreciating their individuality. Practically, this involves knocking on the door before entering a patient's room, pulling curtains around the bed, talking to the patient not over them, not exposing the patient's body unnecessarily, and viewing the patient as a person not just someone with a medical label. In the community, this involves recognizing that the nurse has been invited into the patient's home and understanding that the patient's wishes are paramount.

Empathy is to 'put yourself in the patient's shoes'; it is to imagine the psychological state and intrinsic feelings the patient may have. Practically, empathy involves perceiving emotional distress and demonstrating warmth, compassion, concern, and understanding. Therapeutic touch and making time to listen to the patient can be useful for demonstrating empathy.

Therapeutic touch is a basic fundamental nursing skill. Touch can be simply placing your hand on the patient's shoulder, holding their hand during an unpleasant procedure, or hugging them during severe distress or anxiety. Touch can give a patient a feeling of being cared for. It can also be used to demonstrate the nurse's presence. Nurses should be aware of the cultural differences and sensitivities of touch.

Care actions and activities are those performed by the nurse to assist and support patients during illness to lead them to a place of maximum independence. Practical applications of care and caring are displayed in the fundamental practices of nursing such as bathing, grooming, dressing, turning patients, and helping patients to mobilize.

Hope is multidimensional. To some hope may refer to 'having a positive outlook' and to others it may refer to 'having a deep inner faith'. This faith may not necessarily be in a divine being, but may be in themselves, the nurse, the physician, or the medical treatment. Patients sometimes say: 'I nearly lost all hope' after they come through a period of illness.

- Nurses should encourage hope during illness because patients can experience different degrees of mental stress.
- By encouraging and stirring inner hope in the patient, the nurse can help the patient achieve personal goals and recovery.
- It is important for nurses to have their own sense of hope as well.

Anticipation describes the ability of a nurse to foresee a need or problem which allows the nurse to act in advance of the patient. In practical terms this means the nurse carries out activities for the patient such as anticipating when they will want a drink, will need to be made comfortable in bed, and will require any other activities to ensure comfort. In the community this includes anticipating wider needs such as shopping, meals, cooking, and need for company.

Nursing presence describes the ability of a nurse to be available and of service to the patient and the family at the right time. It is the nurse's ability to recognize when a patient will need them the most. Presence also relates to a nurse's ability to present his or herself in a dignified manner, and to behave appropriately for a particular situation. For example, a nurse should develop the ability to act sensibly in a crisis or stressful situation. Presence, or opening oneself to another, is perhaps the highest level of human caring.

- Presence occurs when the nurse engages the patient in an empathetic, caring, and receptive interaction that is directed towards meeting all the patient's needs.
- Listening, interacting, and communicating are key.
- The appearance of a confident and professional nurse can help patients and their families cope with the stresses of ill health and disability.
- A professional nurse with a good demeanour, personality, poise, and self-assurance provides excellent company and companionship for the patient.

Advocacy can take many forms in health care and nursing. The term is used often in a legal context as someone who represents another (legal advocate, e.g. barrister). The term also is used to describe a person who publicly supports a cause or campaigns for change. In general nursing, the term describes a nurse who stands up for patients or represents them when they need help. An advocate:
- acts according to the patients' best interests
- acts as a patient's spokesperson to protect them from harm
- clarifies values and cultural needs
- represents patients at appropriate times in their health care journey
- promotes health, evidence-based decision making, patient involvement, and safety
- promotes the patient's wishes and freedom from suffering.

In practical terms advocacy may be nothing more than ensuring that patients receive sufficient pain medication, checking that patients clearly understand their treatment, or ensuring that patients know what to expect. Advocacy entails advising patients of their rights, providing information so they can make informed decisions, and then supporting those decisions.

Delivering clinical nursing care

Responsibility

Clinical nurses must make informed and mature judgements and perform nursing tasks based on an in-depth understanding of the sciences underlying nursing, the best possible evidence, and the interests of the patient.

To be responsible is to be obliged, either legally or morally, to take care of something or someone and to carry out a duty. A duty of care exists if one can see that one's actions are reasonably likely to cause harm to another person. Performing the role of a professional nurse demands a particular way of behaving or professional discipline. Nurses have an individual and collective responsibility as integral members of a multidisciplinary health care team to protect the patient and to be legally accountable for their actions.

Clinical accountability

- Nurses are liable to be called to account for their individual actions or omissions.
- Nurses must take reasonable care to avoid acts or omissions that they can reasonably foresee.
- Nurses must base their nursing care on evidence-based practice and reasonable standards of nursing.
- Nurses should question other professional health care colleagues (including physicians) about their actions and treatments if they, the patient, or the patient's close family member is concerned about the treatment, care, or outcomes.
- Nurses must protect and care for the vulnerable patient and act as a possible advocate for them.
- Nurses must help coordinate and encourage good multidisciplinary communication and working practices.
- Nurses must involve the patient and their family in decision-making and, where appropriate, aspects of nursing care and treatment.
- Nurses must be involved in providing appropriate information and education to patients and their family.
- Nurses must work within their own scope of personal skill and competence.
- Nurses should not delegate clinical nursing duties to others, including unqualified professional nurses, unless they are confident that the individual is competent to carry them out successfully.

Further information

NMC (2008). *The Code*. www.nmc-uk.org

The ten golden rules of clinical risk management
- Act within your own competence.
- Obtain informed consent from patients.
- Do no harm.
- Follow procedures.
- Report clinical incidents and near misses.
- Write full, legible, and signed notes.
- Maintain patient confidentiality at all times.
- Learn from failures.
- Ask if unsure of what you are doing.
- Always encourage good working practice.

Accountability

The nurse has accountability in five key areas: the patient, public, employer, profession, and self (See Fig. 2.1).

Accountability to the patient
- Involve patients in their care.
- Represent patients, if appropriate.
- Look after the patient's interests.
- Provide holistic individualized personal nursing care.
- Provide care based on the patient's wishes.
- Provide researched and evidence-based nursing care.

Accountability to the public
- Provide care that is in line with society's expectations.
- Perform duties in accordance with the law.
- Respect human rights and dignity, and provide ethical care to patients.
- Provide care that is in line with care provided in other countries around the world.
- Perform duties according to government regulations.
- Speak out against injustice, prejudice, and discrimination.

Accountability to employer
- Perform duties according to:
  - job description, expectations, scope of practice
  - local rules and regulations
  - local policies and procedures.
- Respect the organization.
- Maintain confidentiality of information.
- Give feedback about concerns.

Accountability to the profession
- Perform duties according to:
  - the expectations of the profession
  - the usual behaviour and conduct expected of the nurse
  - the Code of Conduct (NMC)
  - guidelines and advice from the NMC.
- Recognize and act on your duty to improve staff knowledge and skills.

Accountability to self
- Be honest and know yourself.
- Take personal responsibility for your actions.
- Be self-disciplined.
- Know your limitations.
- Be self-reflective.
- Be good to yourself and maintain your health.
- Enjoy life outside your job.

Further information
NMC (2008). *The Code.* www.nmc-uk.org

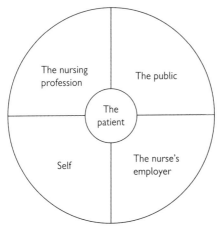

Fig. 2.1 The five key areas for which nurses are accountable.

Methods of nursing care delivery

There are several methods of delivering nursing care. These are often based on conceptual models (which are mental constructs of the essential factors in nursing care). Deciding on the method used is dependent on such factors as resources and ward or unit design.

Total patient care

- Nurses are allocated to patients and it is their responsibility to make sure that each patient receives all of the appropriate nursing care they require.
- Nurses have autonomy, authority, and accountability for 'their' group of patients.
- There should be a shared responsibility from all registered nurses towards all the patients in any setting.
- There is a designated registered nurse on each shift who has responsibility to coordinate and allocate nurses to patients according to each nurse's competency, ability, and work load.
- The designated registered nurse takes overall responsibility for patients in the care setting and ensures that the general management of the ward or unit continues. If there are problems, the designated registered nurse refers to the senior nurse or matron in charge of the wider clinical area.
- All staff should have an overview and summary of the key points and priorities for each patient in the care setting.
- Advantages of this system:
  - Each patient receives holistic non-fragmented care by one or two nurses.
  - Staff satisfaction is higher when the system is used appropriately.
- Disadvantages of this system:
  - Some nursing staff only concentrate on those patients allocated to them and ignore the needs of other patients in the same care environment.
  - Some nursing staff may not be prepared or may have insufficient knowledge, skill, and experience to take on this role.

Functional nursing care

- Nurses take responsibility for certain tasks that are assigned to them rather than caring for specific patients, i.e. one person takes specific responsibility for a task.
- Tasks are allocated according to the competencies and experience of the nurse or carer.
- Certain staff can be trained to do specific jobs or take on particular responsibilities.
- Care is given when the nurse or carer decides it is convenient.
- Most used when there are staff shortages and no time for holistic care.
- Works well in areas of care where there is a need for routine systematic or routinized working such as the operating room and emergency department.

- Advantages of this system:
  - Economical means of providing care.
  - Efficient and safe for tasks that must be completed in a short time span.
  - Allows more routine and unskilled tasks to be clearly identified from more complex activities of patient care.
  - Identifies tasks that can be performed by less skilled carers and frees up more qualified and professional nurses.
  - Every patient is more likely to receive a certain element of their prescribed care.
- Disadvantages of this system:
  - May lead to more fragmented care.
  - Very little opportunity for individualized care based on what or when the patient wants something.

Key points in selecting the appropriate method of nursing care

- What knowledge and skills are required for the patients you are caring for?
- What are the patients' individual needs and requirements?
- Who would be best suited to deliver the appropriate nursing care?
- Does your staff have the appropriate knowledge and skill?
- What mix of registered nurses and health care support workers is needed?
- What risks are involved in the chosen system?
- Is the chosen method of nursing organization understood in practical terms?
- Think carefully about the holistic quality issues, individualization, and patient involvement.
- Is the delivery/organization of nursing cost effective?
- Are patients, their families, and staff happy with the system?

Team approaches to care

Team nursing
- Nurses and health care support workers are allocated to a team that is responsible for a group of patients in a designated area or setting.
- Collaboration is critical with nurses and support workers working together under the direction of a team leader.
- The team leader's duties vary depending on the number and quality of workers in the team.
- Team nursing is usually associated with democratic leadership.
- Group members are given some autonomy, although the team shares overall responsibility and accountability for care. Final decisions and accountability rest with the team leader.
- Team nursing is a good system for encouraging staff participation and developing knowledge and skills.
- Time is needed to build a team that is cohesive and communicates effectively.
- There are many variations of team nursing.

Primary nursing
- The primary nurse takes responsibility and accountability for all nursing care delivered to a patient.
- Although the primary nurse is not always present, she or he has the principal role in making major decisions about nursing care, e.g. alterations in care plans and discharge planning.
- During work hours, the primary nurse provides total direction of the nursing care for the patient.
- When the primary nurse is not on duty, an associate or secondary nurse delivers patient care.
- Although designed for use in hospitals, this type of approach can be used in nursing homes, hospices, and the patient's own home.
- Primary nursing may be confused with the terms 'primary health care' and the 'primary care team' as used in the UK.
- Job satisfaction is high with primary nursing.
- It may be difficult to recruit competent and motivated staff.
- Relatives may get frustrated if the primary nurse is not on duty when they seek information.
- Registered nurses should still have an awareness of all the patients in any given setting.

Case management nursing
- The nurse is allocated a case on an individual basis, not on a group basis or part of a community population.
- The number of cases each nurse is assigned depends on the nurse's experience, knowledge, and skills.
- Case-load management is used in many settings, particularly the community and in mental health nursing.
- A collaborative approach is used with the case worker assessing, planning, implementing, coordinating, monitoring, and evaluating the case with some input by others.

Multidisciplinary team care

- Multidisciplinary team care is closely related to case management and involves all of the health care professions involved in a patient's case including physicians, nurses, social workers, and other voluntary community care providers.
- The case manager or coordinator is often selected by the patient or democratically by the team.
- This system can lead to improved communication and understanding of roles within the team.
- If several team members are from one particular profession, they may dominate the care and decision making.
- In some cases, members from a particular profession may be under-represented at team meetings.
- The patient and their key carer should be the focus of the team.
- This system encourages more 'crossover' working, i.e. one team member performs tasks that were previously the exclusive domain of another team member.
- This approach is encouraged by integration of records, multidisciplinary care plans, and care pathways.
- Team satisfaction is enhanced by holding specific team meetings to resolve any conflicts within the team.

Hospital–community links

Effective communication between the hospital team and the community health care team is vital for ensuring continuity and maximum effectiveness of care and for managing issues relating to discharge planning.

Discharging patients into the community

The fact that patients will eventually be discharged into the community is an important consideration beginning at the time the patient is admitted to the hospital. Throughout the patient's hospitalization, close liaison between the hospital and community is needed. The community nurse or another member of the community health and/or social care team should visit the patient before discharge and participate in the discharge planning. Equipment may need to be ordered, delivered, and set up prior to discharge. Special access to the patient's property such as the door key or keypad combination may be needed to enable community nurse admission. Planning for discharge takes time. Community services that the patient will need must be identified prior to the discharge date so that the necessary services can be assured, thus creating a safe and efficient discharge.

Community liaison nurses

Community liaison nurses work between the hospital and community setting. They visit the patient in their home and perform assessments and provide support to the patient and their family in the community.

Outreach nurses

Outreach nurses are nurses from the acute sector who provide care for patients living in the community. The patient remains the responsibility of the consultant, and nursing care is provided by nurses from the acute sector with the appropriate skills and knowledge. Some hospital trusts have developed special outreach services such as respiratory, heart failure, and anticoagulation teams. The nurses are based in the hospital and monitor the condition of the patients who live in the community, giving advice and education.

Clinical nurse specialists

Clinical nurse specialists have a particular expertise in an area of nursing such as pain control, wound care, stoma care, and respiratory nursing. They may work both in and out of the hospital setting, maintaining continuity of patient care and providing support for nurses. For example, a critical care specialist nurse may be asked to assess a patient on an acute medical ward, provide expert nursing care, and direct the general nurse in how best to nurse the patient. Specialist nurses are available to be consulted by generalist nurses; they are not intended to replace or de-skill the generalist, but to help them help their patients.

Rehabilitation nursing

Rehabilitation nursing is a speciality. Its principles underlie basic fundamental nursing practice with respect to helping an individual patient reach his or her potential. Rehabilitation nurses help disabled or chronically ill patients achieve or maintain their maximum functional independence, optimal health, and well-being. These nurses also help patients cope with life-altering changes that have resulted from an illness.

Rehabilitation can occur in the hospital setting, in an intermediate care setting (step down), in the patient's own home, or at a day centre. Whatever the setting the following are necessary.

- Perform a holistic assessment of the patient.
- Use good communication skills.
- Use good listening skills.
- Take a multidisciplinary approach to the individual's rehabilitation needs, e.g. involve physicians, nurses, physiotherapists, occupational therapists, speech and language therapists, social workers, and psychologists.
- Ensure an appropriate environment for rehabilitation, e.g. ensure that specialized equipment is available.
- Develop a therapeutic nurse–patient relationship that creates trust.
- Set patient-agreed short- and long-term goals that are realistic and achievable.
- Educate and teach patients and their families about the condition and ways of coping and adjusting to maximize independence.

In addition to the above, the rehabilitation nurse's role is to advocate on behalf of patients and sometimes on behalf of their families. The nurse should support and respect patients at all times. This includes providing emotional support to patients, encouraging them, and supporting them when difficult decisions must be made.

Following a period of rehabilitation in the hospital setting, patients are usually discharged to the community where further rehabilitation occurs. Patients may be placed in an intermediate care facility for up to 4 weeks, or may be placed in a 24-hour care facility. Patients discharged to their homes may undergo rehabilitation in the home or at a day centre.

Rehabilitation is not about making patients do everything for themselves. It is about providing expert help so that they gain maximum independence in as many activities of daily living as is possible.

Individualizing nursing care practice

The nursing process

The nursing process is an interactive problem-solving decision-making procedure for assessing, identifying, selecting, and implementing approaches, and evaluating results in relation to the nursing care of the ill or potentially ill person (See Fig. 3.1).

It is a functional process model that encourages the nurse to:
- Perform an *assessment* of the patient, which involves gathering information or relevant data.
- Interview the patient, their relatives, friends, and any other significant people or carers who know the patient.
- Perform a physical examination and take a health history.
- Identify specific nursing problems and any associated medical complaints (nursing diagnosis) by analysing the collected information.

Steps included in the process:
- Identify actual and potential problems.
- Determine what patients can and cannot do for themselves.
- Determine what the patient was like previous to their present problem.
- Identify the patient's priorities and concerns.
- Determine the nurse's view of the patient's problems which may differ from that of the patient (both are considered and priorities agreed).
- Determine the medical view of the patient's problems and their management—this also includes liaising with medics on the appropriate management of the patient.
- Identify any key risk factors affecting the patient, including their allergies.
- Identify key factors that may influence discharge and transfer to other services.
- Determine patient and family willingness to be involved in care and their teaching and health education needs.
- Identify any living wills or statements relating to the patient's treatment and resuscitation.

Planning nursing care
- Decide which core or standard care plans and care pathways to use.
- Individualize care plans (in consultation with the patient and other key carers or family members) to suit the patient and consider their personal needs.
- Decide which special nursing care charts to use, e.g. fluid balance, observation, pain, and diabetic monitoring.
- Decide how the patient's priorities should be met.
- Decide how the patient and/or their family can be involved and any teaching plans developed.
- Determine the appropriate nursing interventions and best evidence to address the patient's problems and outcomes.
- Make explicit the equipment required to carry out certain nursing actions.
- Identify the knowledge and skills to carry out the nursing actions and determine which nurse is best qualified to carry them out (or other health care professional, as appropriate).

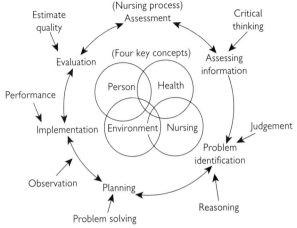

Fig. 3.1 Diagrammatic representation of the nursing process.

Implementing the nursing care plan (or pathway)

Key skills

Key skills involved in implementation are manipulation and safe handling of patients and equipment; communication; teaching; and coaching skills.
- Put the plans of nursing care into action.
- Think about the method or organization of care delivery (📖 Chapter 2, Methods of nursing care delivery, pp.20–21).
- Decide how best to monitor the patient's response.
- Report and record progress.
- Chart information for evaluation.
- Encourage the patient and their family to be involved and record their response.
- Know when to carry out and link together the variety of nursing actions to achieve holistic care and avoid fragmentation.
- Observe the patient's condition and reactions to interventions.
- Coordinate with the rest of the multidisciplinary team and attend relevant meetings and ward rounds.
- Ensure prescribed nursing actions are carried out with skill and competence.
- Adapt interventions as the situation develops.
- Teach patients and their families and check that key health information has been understood.

Evaluation of nursing care

This involves examining the effectiveness of the nursing interventions in resolving the patient's problems and meeting goals or outcomes of care. It is the final stage of the nursing process. Nursing care can be evaluated from a review of patient outcomes, nurse performance, and the organization or system of delivering the nursing care.

Evaluation demands good verbal and written communication skills. It examines:
- whether the patient is ready to manage their own care
- the effectiveness of patient and family education and teaching
- how satisfied and involved the patient was in their care
- whether the nursing care was too fragmented, poorly individualized, or not as comprehensive as it should have been.

Nurses develop their critical thinking and reasoning skills through experience. These skills help them to use the nursing process approach as a basis and then move on to more analytical methods of approaching nursing care.

The nursing history

This is divided into two parts: essential *general information* and *specific information*.

General information

- Name, address, and occupation
- Family background, social history, culture, next-of-kin, and telephone number
- General practitioner and emergency contact numbers
- Past medical history, chronic diseases, allergies, sensitivities, and current medical conditions
- Reason for admission to hospital or referral to a nurse
- Up-to-date medications and medical treatment

Specific information

The ability to obtain specific information commences with the patient's understanding of their illness, referral, or admission to hospital. A health history is used to gather subjective data about the patient and should be combined with a general physical examination which collects objective data.

First ask the patient about their general physical and emotional health and then take a basic patient history. There are a variety of different approaches. The Roper, Logan, and Tierney model is one model that is used by nurses to undertake a basic nursing history. This is a functional approach that assesses activities of daily living.

The accuracy and completeness of the patient's answers will largely depend on the nurse's communication skills. Find out what the patient's normal routine is and their style of living. Ask older people to describe a typical day. The nursing history should include an assessment of:

- Diet and nutritional intake, i.e. appetite, special diets, ability to eat and chew food, and difficulty in preparing or cooking a meal
- Fluid intake and alcohol consumption
- Bowel and bladder movements
- Personal hygiene and dressing difficulties
- Ability of patient to move and mobilize
- Breathing problems or use of any inhalers
- Smoking habits, e.g. how many years and how often
- Associated drug and alcohol use and abuse
- Allergies
- Difficulties in communicating, e.g. deafness, blindness, difficulty seeing or speaking and expressing themselves
- Rest and sleep patterns, including the use of sedatives
- Activities associated with occupation, leisure, or hobbies
- Religious or cultural beliefs and effects on diet, dress, or health practices

Throughout the interview maintain a professional neutral approach and do not offer advice at this stage. Use a combination of open-ended questions to elicit information about feelings, opinions, and ideas, and closed questions to elicit information about factual specific points. Nurses who practice at an advanced level would undertake a thorough medical history of a patient (from the patient and/or their family), before making a diagnosis and possibly prescribing for a patient. For more information the reader is advised to refer to literature on advanced nursing practice.

Further information

Roper N, Logan WW, and Tierney AJ (2000). *The Roper-Logan-Tierney model of nursing: based on activities of living*. Elsevier Health Sciences, Edinburgh.

Interviewing tips and communication skills

Preparing the environment

Choose and prepare an environment that is suitable for discussing personal information. The environment should be free from distractions. This is often very difficult in the hospital setting but is an important consideration.

Preparing the patient being interviewed

- Make sure the patient is comfortable.
- Reassure the patient of the confidential nature of the interview, but inform them that, with their permission, the information may be shared within the multidisciplinary team caring for them.
- Ask the patient their full name and the name that they prefer you to address them by. Do not assume you have the right to refer to the patient by their first name or given name.
- Determine whether there will be a language barrier or problems in communication. If necessary, seek the support of an interpreter or use cue cards.
- Encourage the patient to express themselves fully when talking about their health, social care, and nursing issues.

Self-awareness

- Be self-aware—you yourself may be a distraction, so check that you have no personal characteristic behaviours that are off-putting to the person.
- Introduce yourself, explain the purpose and content of the interview, and provide an estimate of the time it will take.
- Be wary of raising your voice too loudly and adapt your interview to the individual and the setting.
- Speak slowly and clearly.
- Observe non-verbal cues and be aware of your own body language and communication. (Nurses are often in a rush and may give the impression of being too busy to have time to care and listen.)
- Try to put the patient at ease whenever possible. Use communication strategies to facilitate this, e.g. silence, facilitation, confirmation, open-ended questions, or closed questions.
- Be aware that the patient may be embarrassed by the topic of conversation.

Non-verbal communication

- Use touch sparingly and only when you are certain that it is appropriate.
- Use reassuring nods and words of encouragement to show concern, empathy, and understanding.
- Use eye contact (if appropriate to the person's culture).

Verbal communication
- Listen actively. (📖 Chapter 21, Basic Counselling Tips, p.745.)
- Avoid using medical terms where possible and explain terminology, as necessary. Avoid jargon.
- If patients are having difficulty expressing their problems verbally, offer several possible answers for them to choose from or allow them to write down their thoughts, if required.
- Be aware that some patients will be wary about the questions you ask them and may rush their replies and try to agree too readily. Others may give short answers or become over-talkative.

Note taking
- Make key notes as you go along and explain to the patient the purpose of these notes.
- Write down any significant words or phrases the patient continually uses or feels are significant.

Concluding the interview
- At the end of the interview, sum up and clarify key points.
- Interviewing is an ongoing process and patients should be continually encouraged to express their feelings and concerns.

General mental/psychological assessment

Mental status examination is a systematic check of emotional and cognitive functioning. General nurses rarely need to assess a patient fully in this way but they must have some basic knowledge and skill in this type of examination.

Psychology is the study of how people behave, feel, and think. It explores people's motivation, personality traits, patterns of emotional response, and behaviours, both normal and abnormal. It can help give the nurse insight into how patients and their families are responding to an illness, disability, or death.

The main areas of psychological functioning are linked to the three main areas of mental status assessment:

- Feelings and emotional behaviour   Appearance, mood
- Interpersonal behaviour   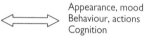   Behaviour, actions
- Intellectual activity   Cognition

Mental status assessment can easily be carried out at a basic level when the nurse interviews and examines the patient. Discuss with the patient their feelings and emotions. Ask about their social circumstances, family and friends, occupation, pastimes and hobbies, education, economic status, and responsibilities and roles in life. Use questions that are open-ended and encourage a good response. Remember, it takes time to establish a good working relationship with patients.

Ask about:

- Any previous emotional or mental health problems
- Usual reactions to stressful events and the methods they use to cope
- Any medical ill-health crises they have experienced in the past
- Recent changes to their lifestyle or any aspect of their usual routine
- Type and source of emotional support
- Effectiveness of emotional support they receive from their family and friends, and, if under the care of medical and nursing staff, effectiveness of their help and support

Recording, reporting, and documenting

It is a nurse's responsibility to observe and carefully record accurately behaviour and emotion. Ask questions, record what the patient says by quoting them, and describe behaviour.

A mnemonic for the parts of a mental status examination[1]

- **A**ppearance
- **B**ehaviour
- **E**motion (mood)
- **A**ffect
- **S**peech
- **T**houghts (delusional, suicidal, homicidal, violent)
- **P**erception (hallucinations)
- **R**easoning (including judgement and insight)
- **O**rientation
- **M**emory

1 Manos PJ and Braun J (2006). *Care of the difficult patient: a nurse's guide*. Routledge, London

Mental status assessment

A full mental status examination should be performed when the nurse discovers that the patient is behaving in an inappropriate manner or when there are signs and reports of severe emotional distress, lack of coping, and cognitive difficulties. General hospital nurses often lack confidence in their ability to care for patients with mental health problems and may need to seek advice and consultation with a liaison or specialist mental health nurse.

- Appearance
  - Facial expression
  - Posture and position
  - Physical features that characterize the person
  - Grooming and hygiene
  - Body movements
  - Dress
- Behaviour
  - Drowsy, alert, restless, agitated, aggressive
  - Level of consciousness
  - Facial expression
  - Speech
- Emotion
  - Mood and affect
  - Expression of feelings
  - Tone of voice, speech
  - Sadness, depression
  - Anxious, worried
- Speech
  - Loud, soft, normal
  - Fast, slow, logical, coherent
  - Slurred, stuttering
- Thoughts
  - Delusions, false beliefs
  - Ways of thinking and expressing
- Perception
- Hallucinations or perceiving things that do not exist—these can be visual, auditory (i.e. hearing voices), tactile, or olfactory. Delirium due to infection, surgery, drugs, etc. is the chief cause of hallucinations in the general hospital. Opioids may cause colourful cartoon-like hallucinations. *Note* that if a person has a hallucination but does not believe the object is real, the person is *not* delusional. When a person does believe it is real, then they may be.
- Reasoning
  - Cognitive ability
  - Attention span
  - Intelligence
  - Problem solving
  - Insight
  - Abstract thinking

- Orientation
  - Who they are
  - Where they are
  - What time it is
- Memory
  - Short- and long-term

Mental status assessment questions

Each question scores one mark

1. Age
2. Time (to nearest hour)
3. Address for recall at end (e.g. 42 West Street)
4. What year is it?
5. Name of institution
6. Recognition of two persons
7. Date of birth (day and month)
8. Year of First World War
9. Name of present monarch
10. Count backwards from 20 to 1

A score of 6 or below is likely to indicate impaired cognition.

Taken from Hodkinson HM (1972). 'Evaluation of a mental test score for assessment of mental impairment in the elderly'. *Age Ageing* **1**(4), 233–8, Table 1. Reproduced with permission from Oxford University Press and the Geriatric Society.

Performing a nursing physical examination: overview

Purpose is to identify and interpret potential and actual nursing problems and to evaluate the effectiveness of nursing care.

Sequence of assessment should be systematic. One method is to start with the patient's hands (See Fig. 3.2). This is a more holistic and sensitive opening assessment than focusing directly on the patient's anatomical problem. From the hands the nurse then follows a head-to-toe approach.

What to assess depends on the health of the individual, on their ability to care for themselves, and on their ability to express their health care concerns. Nursing assessment includes functional assessment and is the evaluation of a person's ability to carry out basic activities of daily living (ADLs). It includes obvious problems, such as pressure sores, but focuses on capabilities and deficiencies of the person at risk from consequences of ill health, disease, disability, and ageing (See Fig. 3.3).

Functional ability of a patient is the dynamic interaction of the physical state of the body with emotional, spiritual, psychological, environmental, and social factors.

Functional assessment establishes the patient's baseline abilities and nursing problems for future comparison. It helps determine which other health professionals and social services the patient may need, along with any special aids or mobility devices required. At the same time it can help in evaluating and confirming the patient's medical diagnosis, medical problems, deterioration due to disease processes, and the effects of medical interventions and treatments. Functional assessment identifies the physical strengths, weaknesses, and abilities that should be considered when formulating the patient's care plan. It is also useful when preparing the patient for health and medical or surgical interventions and for discharge or transfer to another care setting.

When performing a physical assessment, find out how the patient has changed because of their current ill health. Systematically reviewing the patient's body can help detect any other early or neglected signs and symptoms of an illness or disability. It can help in screening, risk assessment, health promotion, and disease prevention. Assessment should be carried out on admission to hospital, on transfer from one care facility to the next, and at regular intervals to determine the patient's progress.

The depth and detail of the assessment depends on the patient's health state and their potential and actual nursing problems. Other factors that may need to be considered are signs of self harm, neglect, or abuse; consent to care and treatment; who is present during the examination; and the environment where the examination is being carried out.

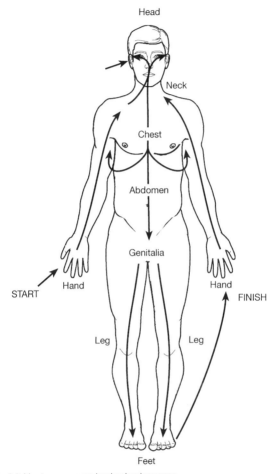

Fig. 3.2 Nursing assessment: hand-to-hand sequence.

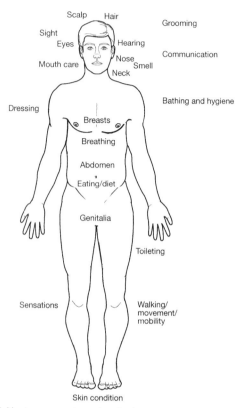

Fig. 3.3 Nursing assessment: overview of patient.

Performing a nursing physical examination: procedure

Overview of the patient

Throughout the examination, use your senses of touch, hearing, smell and, most important of all, observation. Commence the assessment as soon as you meet the patient. Assess general appearance, presentation, demeanour, eye contact, non-verbal communication, initial reactions, personal grooming, hygiene, state of clothing, body position, mobility, movement, and gait. Include pallor, jaundice, and asymmetry.

Introduce yourself and establish how the patient wishes to be addressed. Explain what you are going to do and why an examination is necessary. It is sometimes helpful to assess the vital signs before commencing the examination. Conduct the assessment in a suitable environment that promotes privacy and reduces disruptions. Wash hands before and after the procedure.

Starting with the hands

Note size, shape, colour, general condition, quality of the skin, tremor, muscle wasting, bony abnormalities, and temperature. Compare the hands and assess function. Test grip (See Fig. 3.4) and assess for tenderness and swelling. Note dexterity and range of finger movement (Fig. 3.5). Observe condition, shape, and colour of nails (See Fig. 3.6).

Arms

Observe size, shape, colour, general condition, quality of the skin, muscle mass, and any abnormalities. Ask patient to move their arms and note any difficulties. Compare both arms. Ask about any weakness, heaviness, pain in arms, or sensory loss. Assess joint movement and any signs of deformity and swelling (See Fig. 3.7).

Head examination

The patient should be sitting for ease of examination. Inspect and observe face for swelling, size, shape, symmetry, and evidence of trauma. Look at the patient's facial expression for evidence of anxiety, hostility, pain, depression, embarrassment, or fear. Confirm that mandible is in the midline, not shifted to the right or left. Look for signs of involuntary movements such as tics, tremors, spasms, frowns, or squints. Observe skin colour, pallor, flushing, yellowness, or blueness. Note any rashes, lesions, warts, moles, and abrasions. Feel texture of skin—smooth, thick, or coarse. Observe for signs of dehydration—dry, wrinkled skin, sunken eyes and cheeks. Note the distribution of facial hair (e.g., does the patient shave?). Note any headaches or injuries to the head.

Skull, scalp, and hair

If appropriate, examine the condition of the scalp and hair. Look for signs of infestation. Does the patient groom and wash their hair regularly? Note colour, texture, and distribution. If appropriate, palpate the scalp for tenderness, lesions, and crusts. Note any dandruff or sebaceous cysts.

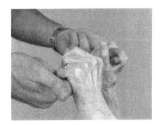

Fig. 3.4 Testing grip.

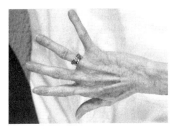

Fig. 3.5 Examination of hands.

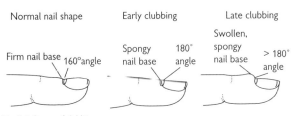

Fig. 3.6 Stages of clubbing.

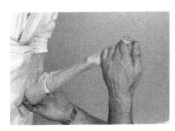

Fig. 3.7 Examination of arms.

Eyes, eyebrows, and eyelids

Note hair distribution—any cosmetic practices used? Note eyelids for colour, vascular problems, and oedema. Note any tremors or drooping eyelids. Observe the eyeballs—are they normal with no sunkenness or protrusion (exophthalmos)? Note the conjunctiva (deep pink colour) and sclera (smooth white). Are there adequate tears, with no dryness? Note any markings and colour of iris. Pupils should be round and equal, reacting equally to light. Does the patient wear spectacles, contact lenses, or do they have any difficulties with vision? (See Fig. 3.8).

Ears

Inspect the external ear for any deformities, lumps, lesions, and signs of inflammation. Note whether the patient moves their head to one side when trying to listen to what you say. Is there any history of deafness, ear problems, wax, or discharges? Note use of hearing aids and their cleanliness. Is there any loss of balance or ringing in the ears?

Nose

Inspect the nose for any abnormalities. Observe patency of the nasal passages and the presence of excessive mucus. Has the patient got a good sense of smell? Note any nasal problems, nosebleeds, breathing difficulties, or sinus trouble.

Mouth

Inspect the patient's lips for colour, moisture, lumps, ulcers, and cracking. Ask the patient to open their mouth wide. (A click as the mouth opens may indicate an improperly aligned jaw.) Use a torch and tongue depressor to examine the inside of the mouth and teeth. Does the patient wear dentures? Can they clean their teeth with a toothbrush? Note colour, pigmentation, and any ulcers or nodules. Inspect gums for inflammation, swelling, bleeding, and discoloration. Note colour of tongue. Are there any signs of infection and oral thrush (candidosis)? Note any history or presence of a sore throat, difficulty swallowing, speaking, or eating (chewing food). Note the patient's breath for any odours such as acetone (See Fig. 3.9).

Neck

Observe for symmetry, normal pulsations, pressure of lesions or tumours, and normal range of motion. Ask the patient whether they have any swelling, lack of movement, stiffness, or pain.

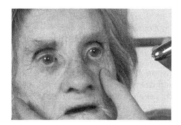

Fig. 3.8   Examination of eyes.

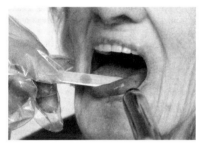

Fig. 3.9   Examination of mouth.

Chest

The chest is usually examined with the patient in a sitting position. Look at the shape and note any deformities. Note movement and breathing, particularly the rate and rhythm of respiration and difficulty in expectoration. Note whether trachea is central; note the respiratory rate, vocal resonance, and percussion. Use the diaphragm of the stethoscope to listen to the anterior and lateral chest areas for breath sounds. Encourage the patient to breathe deeply with their mouth open. Compare the sounds on both sides of the body. (Do not forget to allow time for the patient to breathe normally.) Move round to the patient's back and ask them to lean slightly forward, arms crossed at the waist. Again ask them to breathe deeply through their mouth. Using the stethoscope's diaphragm with light pressure, listen to both sides of the back of the chest. Allow the patient to breathe normally as they may become lightheaded and feel faint (See Fig. 3.10).

Normal breath sounds are produced by airflow through the respiratory passages and are classified according to frequency (pitch), amplitude or intensity (loudness), phase (inspiration or expiration), and location.

There are three types of normal breath sounds. Use these as a guide when hearing abnormalities (See Table 3.1).

Additional or adventitious sounds are rales, wheezing, and pleural friction rub. These are caused by movement of air through fluid, exudate, or swollen constricted airways, or by the rubbing together of two inflamed surfaces.

Breasts

Breast examination should not just be limited to women. Men develop breast problems such as gynaecomastia (enlargement due to hormone imbalance) and cancer. Observe the breasts for size, shape, colour, and contour. Compare one breast with the other for symmetry. Inspect the skin for cleanliness and any signs of breakdown. Check nipples for redness, discoloration, pigmentation, oedema, changes in texture, and signs of retraction. Ask the patient about any signs of lumps and whether they carry out their own breast self-examination and attend regular screening.

Table 3.1 Classification of normal breath sounds

Sound	Phase	Pitch	Amplitude
Vesicular	Inspiratory slightly longer and higher pitched than expiratory	Soft, low	Low
Broncho-vesicular	Inspiratory and expiratory	Medium	Medium
Tracheo-bronchial	Expiratory more than inspiratory	High	Loud

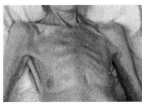

Fig. 3.10 Examination of chest.

Heart

Cardiac auscultation requires a methodical approach, good hearing, and a lot of practice. It may help to mentally visualize the underlying chambers and the great blood vessels of the cardiovascular system. Inspect the patient's neck to determine the condition of the pressure in the neck veins. Look for ankle and sacral oedema. Warm the stethoscope in your hands and then identify the sites where you will auscultate. Use the bell of the stethoscope to hear low-pitched sounds and the diaphragm to hear high-pitched sounds. Lie the patient on their back with the head of the bed raised 30–45°. Use a zigzag pattern over the area. Either start at the top of the heart and work down or at the base and work up. Concentrate and listen for the normal sounds; look and feel for the apical pulse with the palm of your hand. Ask the patient to roll over onto their left side if this is difficult to feel. Normal heart sounds are known as 'lub-dub'. Their duration and amplitude depend on the area being auscultated. If the patient has a suspected cardiovascular problem, it may be important to return to their neck and auscultate their carotid arteries. A bruit or sound may be heard which is the radiation of a systolic murmur from the aorta.

Back

Examine the back for shape, slope of the shoulders, and deformities of the thorax and spine. Check the condition of skin and any difficulties in maintaining hygiene (See Fig. 3.11).

Abdomen

Uncover the abdomen carefully in such a way as to maintain the patient's dignity at all times. The patient must be in a supine position with the head resting on a small pillow and arms at sides. Note the general contour, symmetry, and condition of the skin (See Fig. 3.12). Are there any abnormal masses? Does the patient have a stoma and do they care for it or have any problems associated with it? Is their abdomen swollen (e.g. due to ascites) and are there any lesions, scars, hernias, or cysts? It may be appropriate to listen for bowel sounds. These are usually high pitched and soft, and are identified as gurgles or clicks. Percussion over any solid firm mass or fluid accumulation will elicit dullness. If the patient is retaining urine, then the sound will be dull when distended with urine and tympanic when empty. Ask the patient about any abdominal pain, discomfort, or problems with their bladder function and bowels. Discuss their eating habits and nutritional intake, including fluid intake and output.

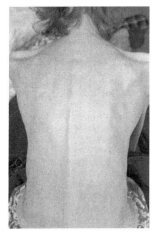

Fig. 3.11 Examination of back.

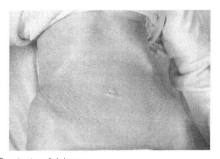

Fig. 3.12 Examination of abdomen.

Genitalia and anal area

Formal examination of this area of the body is often not carried out because of the potential embarrassment to both the patient and the nurse. However, because of the large number of nursing problems associated with this area (e.g. poor personal hygiene, infections, and skin problems), routine assessment should be carried out. Ask the patient about any specific difficulties or problems they have and explain the reasons for the examination. Put on disposable gloves and inspect carefully around the genitalia. Note any signs of skin breakdown, discoloration, tenderness, lesions, or discharges. Remove gloves and examine the buttocks, sacral area, and perineum. Look for discoloration, inflammation, skin lesions, scars, fissures, and fistulas. Note the size, shape, colour, consistency, and tenderness of any lesions. Expose the rectal area by gently pulling the buttocks apart and inspect the anal orifice for skin tags, haemorrhoids, and rectal prolapse. Discuss any functional problems relating to this area with the patient. Check with women for regular cervical screening and pap smears. Men should undertake regular testicular self-examination.

Legs and feet

When examining the lower limbs, maintain the patient's dignity by covering their genitalia. Remove any trousers, stockings, socks, or clothing obstructing a good view of both legs. Inspect and compare both legs. Note size, muscle mass, symmetry, colour, texture of the skin, signs of skin breakdown, previous or present ulcer formation, nail beds, and hair distribution on the lower legs, feet, and toes. Observe for pigmentation, rashes, scars as well as circulatory and venous enlargement and oedema. Inspect the feet and ankles for any deformity, nodules, swelling, calluses, corns, and bunions. Discuss foot hygiene and ability to walk, move, and mobilize. Test muscle strength and ability to maintain activity and exercises during illness. Discuss usual exercise routine, sports, and social activities.

Observe the patient when standing and walking and note any abnormality of gait. Also note the presence of hind foot deformity (valgus or arus), flattened foot (pes planus), or high (pes cavus) longitudinal arch, and any deformity of the toes (See Fig. 3.13 and Fig. 3.14).

Final physical overview of the patient

While examining the patient the nurse should observe the patient's skin, focusing on colour, texture, turgor, moisture, temperature, localized areas of bruising, cyanosis, pallor, erythema, and skin breakdown. Returning to the patient's hands and upper limbs, the nurse can repeat the patient's vital signs such as their pulse and blood pressure. It is also important to record the patient's height and weight. Carry out a routine urine dipstick and send off a midstream specimen of urine to the pathology laboratory if indicated.

When the assessment is completed, allow the patient to get dressed. Document your findings and include only essential information that communicates your overall impression of the patient and their nursing needs. The nurse can also use the physical examination as an opportune time to teach the patient about their health care state and the need to make any adjustments to their lifestyle and fitness. It is also an opportunity to put the building blocks in place for the development of a future therapeutic nurse–patient relationship.

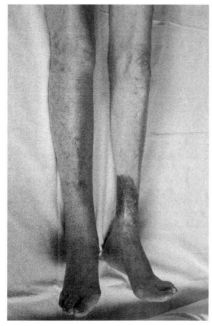

Fig. 3.13 Examination of legs and feet.

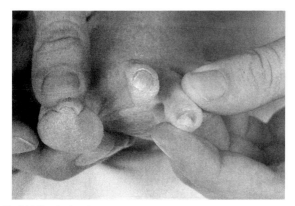

Fig. 3.14 Examination of toes.

Assessing spirituality

A difficult concept to understand, spirituality is often considered an essential part of the whole person. It is often an expression of something within the person that gives a sense of meaning, understanding, and purpose to life. This may or may not be linked to a belief or religious faith. It may be linked to an individual's psychological and emotional state. It can be seen as an inner strength, comfort, or peace that is realized when an individual comes into contact with an experience that leads them to question their life or events within it.

The spirit is what drives a person and forms part of their whole make-up. When in hospital or encountering a health crisis, patients can experience spiritual conflicts. These can be confused with mental health problems such as depression and anxiety. Spiritual conflict can occur because patients are separated from their usual support mechanisms such as personal belongings and familiar environment. They can wrestle with a variety of thoughts and feelings such as 'Why me?', 'How can this happen to me?', 'What next?', 'If there is a God, where is He now?' Such thoughts and questions occur in patients regardless of religious beliefs.

Nurses should understand their own spirituality as it will help them to understand their patients' spiritual feelings and issues.

The terms religion, religious, spirituality, and spiritual well-being are often used inconsistently and carelessly. Although related, they are not the same. Religion is derived from outside the self and is often a doctrine and guideline to follow. Spirituality is an inner experience and quest for meaning and understanding to life events. It gives meaning and purpose to our bodies and biological functions, our thoughts and feelings, and our relationships with other people and the rest of the world.

Although people may be becoming less religious, it would be a mistake to assume that they are becoming less spiritual or that they are no longer thinking or pursuing a sense of transcendence and spiritual fulfilment and achievement. 📖 Chapter 21, Nursing, religion, and spiritual needs, p.754.

Key practical points regarding spirituality

- Recognize the role of chaplains and other faith community leaders in our multi-faith society.
- Spirituality is what we all try to do to give expression to our lives and our world views.
- The world view and the values that a person chooses to live by illustrate the most 'inner' part of that person.
- Health care problems, hospitalization, and a whole host of personal and social problems can lead to people having spiritual, faith, and worship issues.
- Be sensitive and listen.
- Do not be judgemental.
- Be aware of your own spirituality.
- Explore with patients any help they may need with spiritual and religious issues.

Before you ask someone else, reflect over the following questions

- What 'switches you on' and makes life worthwhile?
- What gives you a sense of meaning and purpose in life?
- How do you cope in times of crisis and difficulty?
- How would a serious health problem affect your world view and lifestyle?

Identifying and prioritizing nursing problems

Nursing assessment is the collection of information about the patient. The nurse must carefully review and sift through those data to identify and prioritize problems for nursing intervention (See Fig. 3.15). A nursing problem is any condition or situation in which a patient requires nursing help to maintain or regain their state of health or to achieve a peaceful and dignified death. Examples of nursing problems in priority order include:
• Maintenance of a clear airway
• Observation of vital signs
• Problem (and potential problems) of pressure sores
• Maintenance of nutritional state
• Help with personal hygiene and comfort
• Emotional upset over loss of limb
• Information needs about their rehabilitation programme

Potential problems
These are situations that may occur if the nurse does not act.

Nursing problems versus medical problems
Nursing problems are specific to the patient and are the responsibility of the nurse for identification and action. Medical problems and medical diagnosis are the responsibility of the physician. However, there is increasing overlap between the two and many nurses undertake roles that were traditionally the remit of the medical profession. This leads to a truly holistic approach to care. Some nursing problems relate to the patient's medical diagnosis and treatment and also fall within the nurse's responsibility for identification and action, e.g. monitoring the patient's diabetes, hypertension, or other medical condition.

Nursing diagnosis
This was developed as a classification system during the 1980s and developed further by the North American Nursing Diagnosis Association (NANDA). Most of the nursing diagnostic labels on NANDA's list have three components: a label or title with a definition/description of the problem; a cluster of signs and symptoms associated with the problem; and factors that can cause or contribute to the problem.

Diagnostic reasoning
This is applying critical thinking to identify the actual and potential health and specific nursing care problems of the patient. It requires knowledge, skills, and experience. There are several principles involved in diagnostic reasoning:
• Analyze information.
• Identify specific nursing and health care implications.
• Create a list of possible problems.
• State the specific nursing and health care problems that may require nursing intervention or use of the NANDA list.
• Be systematic.
• Make judgements based on evidence.

- Reassess the patient's problem list and the consequences for the nursing care plan and nursing interventions on an ongoing basis.
- Refer to senior nurses and medical colleagues where unsure.

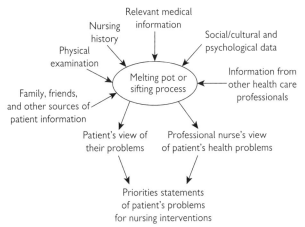

Fig. 3.15 Factors to consider when prioritizing the patient's problems.

Nursing care plans

At the end of a nursing assessment the nurse should have identified a list of problems currently experienced by the patient. The next stage involves making a nursing care plan that both the patient and the nurse use together to deal with the agreed problems.

Nursing care plans are created to provide individualized nursing care. Owing to staff shortages and time, they have become standardized and simplified and are now often combined with care pathways and designed for multidisciplinary use. Care plans should communicate the essential aspects of nursing care. They create a record that can later be used for evaluation, research, and legal reasons.

The nursing or health care plan is a formalized statement of goals and/or objectives of nursing action, together with how these goals can be achieved. Although care plans often tend to be preprinted because of time constraints, they should be individualized for each patient and, where necessary, completely rewritten. The care plan should include:

- The individual patient's problems
- Aims, objectives, or expected outcomes of nursing care for the individual
- The nursing action to be taken with methods and any special equipment needed
- Priorities for nursing interventions
- Who should carry out the plan
- The outcomes and evaluation of care as they occur

The care plan should be clear and easy to read so that objectives and goals can easily be identified. It should also be based upon best evidence available and the nurse's own clinical and professional judgement.

Skills needed in care planning

Cognitive
- Ability to analyse problems
- Ability to apply scientific knowledge relevant to the causation of problems
- Ability to state objectives
- Ability to identify methods and materials available for care

Management
- Ability to organize
- Ability to coordinate

Communication
- Ability to write clearly and concisely
- Ability to verbalize information accurately

Setting priorities in nursing care

- Assess the patient.
- Decide what problems to deal with first.
- Determine the urgent needs of the patient and any immediate medical interventions and emergency nursing care.
- If possible and appropriate, involve the patient and their family.
- Decide which problems can wait, which are priority nursing problems, and which should be referred to another member of the multidisciplinary team.
- Draw up an individualized care plan where possible using an existing template.
- Consider the patient's expected length of stay and preparations for discharge or transfer.

Components of nursing interventions

Best practice
This is the term used to refer to clinical practices, treatments, and nursing interventions that result in the best possible outcome for the patient and the multidisciplinary team.
- Evolved as a response to controlling costs and demonstrating statistical evidence of the effectiveness of medical treatment and nursing care.
- Involves a process of identifying high-quality nursing practices, analysing them, and applying them to local nursing practices.
- Uses information from a variety of sources, such as National Institute of Clinical Excellence (NICE), research and textbooks, the organization's quality/standard setting groups, colleagues, and other experts.
- Is usually a team effort organized within the organization to provide answers to clinical problems/questions.

Standards of care and benchmarks
Standards of care are statements based on research, where possible, describing an expected level of care or performance (📖 Chapter 1, Standards of clinical nursing, p.12). Benchmarks are a measure of performance that serves as a standard for evaluating other results. Benchmarks may be derived from standards of care, but in some situations where no evidence basis exists (in some nursing situations), these are locally set. The first step in benchmarking is for the team to identify clear, concrete, specific goals for patients and the service. Examples include decreased length of hospital stay, decreased complication rates, and increased patient and family satisfaction. Appropriate benchmarks can be found in research literature and internet sources. Benchmarks can be used to compare, measure, and evaluate clinical practice outcomes in evidence-based nursing practice. Evidence-based nursing practice is built on information obtained from research.

Procedures
These are sets of steps by which a desired outcome is accomplished. They are created to provide a safe and consistent course of action for health care workers in specific situations and to provide the best outcome for the patient.

Protocols
These are established sets of procedures for action in a given situation and circumstances. They outline the appropriate course or sequence of actions that a nurse should take to give a treatment or care for a specific patient.

Guidelines
These are general outlines for specific courses of action in response to a diagnosis or condition.

Patient and family education
It is essential to include this in all care plans. 📖 Chapter 5, Patient education, p.94.

Patient group direction

Patient group directions (PGDs) are specific written instructions for the supply or administration of a licensed named medicine including vaccines to specific groups of patients who may not be individually identified before presenting for treatment. A PGD provides a means for patients to access medicines without an individualized prescription and is useful in ensuring patients get relief from symptoms without delay.

Integrated care pathway

An integrated care pathway (ICP) is a multidisciplinary outline of antici-pated treatment and care that a patient requires for a specific condition based on knowledge and research. These pathways have been used to incorporate local and national guidelines into everyday practice. A time frame is used to move the patient through a clinical condition to positive outcomes. The time frame can vary according to the specific condition. This also acts as a guide for the patient, as they can see where they are on the pathway. Various members of the multidisciplinary team record information in them, keeping documentation in one place.

The clinical nurse's responsibility when using a pathway

- Have a good knowledge of the pathway and know how to use it, including how to complete it. Ensure that you are competent in using the pathway and that you have received the necessary training.
- Remember that the ICP is a guide and that patients are individuals and may deviate from the pathway.
- Continue to use your skills of observation and assessment.
- Document in the nursing sections of the pathway on a daily basis.
- Maintain communication with the patient and inform them of where they are on the pathway.
- Maintain communication with the multidisciplinary team and report any problems.
- Monitor variances to a particular ICP, assess if there is a trend, and discuss with the multidisciplinary team.

What should nurses do if a patient is not up to where the ICP says they should be?

- Evaluate the patient's condition, as they may be deteriorating.
- Speak to the patient to determine any other possible reasons.
- Document in the nursing records.
- Inform the multidisciplinary team.
- Consider changing the pathway and individualizing it to the patient.

Tips for nurses using ICPs

- Read and understand the ICP and what is required of you, the nurse.
- Ensure you have received adequate training in using ICPs.
- Remember ICPs are only a guide and should not replace nursing observation and clinical judgement.
- Maintain communication with the patient, e.g. ask them regularly how they feel they are getting on, or whether they have any problems.
- Remember each patient is an individual and therefore variations may occur from the ICP.

Implementing nursing care

This involves putting the plans of nursing care into action and carrying out nursing procedures. The method will depend on the way the nursing care is organized, managed, and delegated.

Getting a factual up-to-date report is important (📖 Chapter 3, The nursing handover, p.64). Use a special notebook or preprinted format to write down the key information you need to nurse your patients. In a hospital setting, once you are happy with the information you have received at handover, make a quick round of your patients, briefly checking the 'big picture' of how they are doing. This helps identify any issues not referred to during the handover report and helps you to relate to the actual patients mentioned in the report.

Check key equipment, intravenous lines, catheter drainage, and the need to carry out any immediate care to make patients comfortable. Attend to urgent problems and key monitoring of severely ill patients before commencing routine nursing care.

In the community you need to anticipate your patients' needs and ensure that you have the appropriate equipment and tools to meet their needs when you visit. Patients may live some distance apart and it is not possible to keep returning to base.

If working with an auxiliary or care assistant, delegate selected tasks you think are appropriate to their level of competence and for which they have been assessed as competent.

Do not delegate to unqualified staff if:
- complex assessment, thinking, and judgement are required
- the outcome of the task is unpredictable
- there is increased risk of harm to the patient
- complex problem solving will be needed
- the patient's problems and interventions require the expertise of a registered nurse.

Review care plans and charts of all your patients. Check medications, doses, and whether the patient has received them correctly. Decide whether there are any interventions outside your expertise and scope of practice; refer to other health care professionals, such as a physician, where necessary. Check the local procedures, protocols, guidelines, or standards for nursing interventions you are unsure of. Always be prepared to assess and reassess your patients during your shift. Write down nursing information on patients' charts and progress notes as you go along. Do not wait until the end of your shift. In the community you should write in the patient's held record to ensure the nurse visiting on the next occasion can maintain continuity of care. Involve the patient in their nursing care and record their responses. On individual assessment of your patients you should ensure that each patient is comfortable and that all their needs are met as individuals. Give an accurate, factual, and organized report at the end of your shift or within the community handover. Finally, reflect and evaluate your shift before leaving. In the community it is helpful to reflect on the care you have given as you travel from one patient to the next.

Patient comfort rounds

In the past these were referred to as 'back rounds' but due to shortages of staff and comments by patients there is now some evidence that such rounds should be implemented in some hospital wards. The nurse should refer to the patient's individual care plan as well as asking them if they require any comfort interventions.

It is essential that your patients are comfortable at all times on a busy ward. One of the ways of ensuring you achieve this is to undertake special 2-hourly rounds of patients on a ward or unit.

- Discuss with the patient and their family up-to-date concerns and progress.
- Give attention to daily living activities and bodily functions such as hand hygiene, toileting, and mouth care.
- Update bedside charting and nursing observations and documentation.
- Adjust the patient's position and check pressure area care and skin condition.
- Review and maintain the patient's privacy.
- Check comfort and pain control.
- Observe the patient's condition, appearance, clothing, bed linen, and pillows.
- Keep or tidy up the patient's immediate bedside environment— locker and bedside table.
- Check bedside medical equipment, e.g. oxygen and suction.
- Ensure patient's special daily living aids, such as spectacles, hearing aids, and walking frames, are being used correctly and are clean.
- Encourage patients to exercise, deep breathe, drink adequate fluids, maintain their dietary and nutritional needs, and mobilize.

Nurses should also attend the medical ward round to feed back to physicians as the patient's advocate and to understand the medical management plan. Where possible it is better to assess your patients individually and ensure that if they require any specific nursing intervention in between the 2-hour period, this is met. However, **all** patients should have been reviewed using the principles above **every** 2 hours as a minimum.

The nursing handover

This is a very important aspect of the nurse's duties. Adequate time should be allowed for one nurse to hand over to another and interruptions should be kept to a minimum to avoid important information being forgotten or misheard. Therefore it might be appropriate for the handover to take place away from the nursing station and away from the busy activities of the ward. In the community this should be at the base station or at an agreed venue where confidentiality can be protected with the whole nursing team. The nursing handover should be concise and follow a logical order.

- Patient's name and age
- Date of admission to hospital and details of where they were admitted from, e.g. home, work, GP, another ward, or hospital (where relevant if in the community)
- Reason for admission (and discharge if in the community)
- Medical diagnosis, if known, or suspected diagnosis
- Past medical history
- Current nursing problems, e.g. reduced mobility, continence problems, difficulty breathing, vomiting, diarrhoea
- Next-of-kin details—check that this is in the records and is accurate
- Details of the current plan of care and any specific orders, e.g. blood tests taken or to be taken and any specific requirements to be adhered to; x-rays; and other biological, histological or investigative tests completed or to be carried out
- Details of the current nursing plan of care, e.g. hourly catheter recordings, 2-hourly turns. Or if in the community, e.g. daily insulin, weekly dressings
- Details of the nursing goals, e.g. heal a pressure sore, promote independence
- Information regarding the current nursing care of the patient (e.g. nursed in bed, continuous intravenous fluids, or in the community, food supplements daily and weekly respite day care)

The handover should be based on what the receiving nurse needs to know. If the nurse already knows the patient, it would not be necessary to follow the above outline strictly but instead report on any changes relating to the patient. Auxiliary staff should be included in the handover and encouraged to contribute as they need to know information in order to carry out their duties.

Writing, recording, and documenting

The nursing contribution to care must be identified and emphasized in all aspects of written communication and recordkeeping. It is important to use the system for recordkeeping relevant to the area in which you practice. Documentation is used to communicate details of the nursing care provided and to inform others of any significant events. Communication is the cornerstone of effective documentation. It promotes continuity of care.

It is important to ensure proper balance between nursing care and documentation (do not neglect either). Each nurse's professional practice with respect to documentation should reflect safe, competent, and thoughtful nursing care. It is a nursing responsibility to document, and the nurse will be held accountable for what is written and recorded. Good recordkeeping not only protects patients but also supports the nurse when questions are asked about nursing care. It is often considered a reflection of the standard of nursing practice. When done well, therefore, it is a mark of the knowledge, skill, and behaviour of a safe nurse. Careless or incomplete recordkeeping often highlights wider problems with the individual's practice.

Legal issues

📖 Chapter 36, Legal issues, pp.1134–37.

Patient and client records are sometimes called as evidence to investigate a complaint at a local level, at the professional level with the NMC, and for criminal and other court proceedings.

General notes and observations made at the time of an incident, care plans, diaries, and any other source of record of nursing care of a patient can be used as evidence. The nurse should keep a copy of any entries or notes they make when an incident occurs that they feel may lead to questions about their behaviour and nursing care. Nursing records should demonstrate:

• The initial assessment made by the nurse on the patient's admission or first contact
• Relevant ongoing and updating of assessment information regarding the patient
• Care plans used to implement and guide nursing care
• A list of the patient's nursing problems and priorities for care
• Progress records that demonstrate a diary or history of the patient's progress
• Any relevant observation charts or instructions used to nurse the patient
• Evidence that the nursing care has been evaluated and outcomes met or changed
• That the patient has been involved where possible

NMC key principles

- Good recordkeeping is a mark of good practice.
- Records should not include abbreviations, jargon, meaningless phrases, irrelevant speculation, and offensive subjective statements.
- Records should be written in terms that the patient can easily understand.
- Records should be regularly audited.
- Any entry you make in a record should be easily identified.
- Patients have the right of access to records about them.
- All contributions should be seen as of equal importance.
- The confidentiality of the nursing record must be protected.
- Professional judgement must be used when recording.
- Entries should be written clearly in permanent black ink.
- Records should be factual and accurate.
- Entries should be written as soon as possible after an event.
- Date, time, and full signature are essential.
- Entries should be consecutive and follow a continuous sequence.
- Records should provide clear evidence of care assessed, planned, and evaluated.

Further information

NMC (2008). *The Code.* www.nmc-uk.org

Guidelines in writing nursing/medical notes

- Objectivity: Record acts, not subjective remarks.
- Relevant: Be precise, concise, and to the point.
- Plain English: Keep it simple, no jargon.
- Permanency: Use black ink.
- Errors: When correcting errors, do not try to cover up or use correction fluid. State the reason for error and date and sign.
- Accuracy: Never write about something you did not see, hear, or personally experience with the patient.
- Promptness: Try to chart as soon as possible after an observation, nursing intervention, or incident.
- Abbreviations: Use only those approved by your organization/ employer.
- Timing: Record time and date and use your full signature.
- Legibility: Use good grammar and make sure other members of the team can read your writing.
- Referrals: Include references to consultations with physicians and other members of the health care team.
- Access: Follow all appropriate legal constraints with regard to access to records.
- Destruction: A record must be kept for a specific time—check with your employer and legal advisory.
- Blank spaces: Do not leave blank spaces after the documentation is completed. Draw a line through the space at the end of a line.
- Accountability: Never document for someone else or sign for another person. Nurses have a duty of care to their patient's records and documentation.
- Involvement: Involve the patient in your documentation by recording their responses to health treatment, progress, and patient teaching and education. When you ask the patient questions, write down their exact words and enclose them in quotation marks.
- Source: Always note the source of any patient information, e.g. patient themselves, family, friend, physician, or other.
- Behaviour: Only describe the patient's behaviour, not your opinions on why the patient is behaving in a certain way.
- Legal: Keep in mind that the purpose of documentation is to create a sound legal document. The best defence that you did something, observed, or heard a key comment is the fact that you made a note of it.

Common deficiencies found in nursing records

- Too many subjective statements such as 'good day' and 'slept well'
- Illegibility, including illegibility of the signature
- Time and date of entries not included in documentation
- Poor evidence of patient involvement
- Lack of quotes from patients
- Failure to record an assessment on transfer from one clinical environment to the next
- Failure to document special needs of patients such as learning disability, deafness, blindness, difficulty in feeding self
- Failure to record key telephone messages
- Failure to record conversations and communications between health care professionals
- Often follow or duplicate what has been written or recorded previously
- Not enough information on the psychological and mental health aspects of the patient

Progress notes

These are ongoing notes made by nurses about specific patients they have been caring for. They function as an ongoing communication of what is happening to the patient, a diary of events, and a reflection of the patient's progress towards desired measurable outcomes. They describe incidents and events, emergency situations, patient's behaviour, and responses to nursing and medical care. They should contain direct quotations from patients and their significant others as is deemed appropriate by the nurse. They follow on from each other in a sequence, without breaks or gaps, and describe the progress that the patient is making.

- Progress notes must contain key information that is of importance to nurses coming on for the next shift or nurses visiting in the community. They are key in providing continuity of care.
- Nurses must ensure that all entries are written chronologically and in a timely manner. They should be written with reference to and in conjunction with the patient's care plan.
- Changes to the care plan must be referred to in the progress notes. All entries should be made as close as possible to the event or observation being noted.
- Sequential entries of developments must be made throughout the shift or, in the community, as soon as you can after visiting the patient.

Common methods of documenting progress notes

- Charting by exception: only significant findings or exceptions are recorded. This provides more time for individual nursing care by eliminating unnecessary and repetitive documentation.
- Problem-oriented documentation: notes are arranged according to a patient's problems or concerns. 'SOAP' is a common method used:
  - Subjective data (reports from patient, patient's relatives)
  - Objective data (nursing observations based on established criteria)
  - Assessment (decisions for actions based on data obtained)
  - Planning (summary of current patient problems and proposals for subsequent interventions)
- Integrated progress notes: in this system all the health care professionals use the same record and identify their entries by clearly stating which profession they are representing. They provide a common point of reference for everyone involved in the patient's care. These are frequently used in the community.

Patient drug record card (PDRC)

Following recommendations from the Shipman Inquiry a method of recording Schedule 2 injectable controlled drugs will be introduced. The PDRC will be initiated when the drug is first dispensed by the pharmacist. Each time the drug is administered by any health care professional or carer (in the community) they must complete the PDRC. Once the drug is no longer required, the remaining quantity must be sent back to pharmacy with the PDRC. The PDRC is currently being piloted. For the second pilot and beyond, this will be renamed the Controlled Drug Record Card (CDRC) as it is the drug that is recorded, not the patient.

Patient-centred case conferences

These are a method of evaluating the patient's progress, and in particular the nursing contribution. They can focus on:

- the patient's health history
- what has been achieved
- areas for improvement in nursing and the multidisciplinary team's patient care
- reviewing nursing care plans and plans of care that involve other health care professionals
- helping to plan the admission, transfer, or discharge of the patient to a hospital, another hospital, care facility, or home
- helping to evaluate the social aspects of the patient's condition, and future health care at home
- organizing home visits and services to support the patient at home
- helping the nursing team members develop a wider understanding of their patients
- evaluating evidence-based practice and a review of the research that underpins the nursing care
- giving members of the nursing team the opportunity to develop managerial and interpersonal communication skills.

The conference can be led by a registered nurse in charge from either the hospital or community setting as is relevant in each case. It is the responsibility of the leader to orient those present to the patient's history and current condition.

In all situations it is helpful if the nurse presenting the case is familiar and has nursed the patient. Other members of the team including the patient and/or their carers should join in and present their ideas and contribute to the holistic nature of the patient's case where relevant.

There is sometimes a danger that helpful comments may be seen as major criticisms and lapses in nursing care. Therefore it is important to ensure the aims of the meeting are clearly articulated and to encourage the case presenter and the nurses most closely involved in the case in a positive and supportive way.

The conference should be group-centred and not leader-centred. However, someone will need to organize the meeting, arrange the date and time, and schedule an appropriate room. Chairs should be arranged in a circle and as many staff as possible who have cared for the patient should be encouraged to attend.

Sometimes it is advisable to have some written guidelines and rules for the meeting. The leader should ensure that the presentation is not too long and the conference keeps to time, allowing for adequate evaluation and reflection of the nursing care of the case.

Medicines management

Note: This chapter provides a general overview of medicines management. Please refer to local medicines management policy for local details.

Supply and disposal of medicines

Supply of medicines

Pharmacy staff may only dispense medicines that comply with all legal requirements. Local formulary restrictions may also apply. The prescriptions may be for:

- Inpatients: including medicines charts, IV treatment cards, and anaesthetic record sheets
- Discharged patients: a TTO (to take out) prescription
- Outpatients: an outpatient prescription form
- Other patients: FP 10 prescriptions that may be dispensed at community pharmacies with NHS contracts

Pharmacy top-up

In many hospitals pharmacy technicians and assistants visit wards and departments to assess the need for stock items, to ensure stock items are replenished, and to ensure non-stock items are requisitioned on an individual basis.

Emergency supply

Many hospitals have a drug cupboard from which medicines may be obtained outside of normal pharmacy opening hours by designated members of staff. Most hospitals also have an on call pharmacist.

Delivery of medicines

- Medicines and requisition books should be transferred in tamper-evident containers or by an authorized person to wards, departments, and community bases.
- Controlled drugs (CDs) should be transported inside a locked container.
- Nursing staff are responsible for the security of the CD container in wards, departments, and community bases.
- Signatures of staff involved in transactions associated with the delivery of CDs (and sometimes other drugs) are required.
- All Trusts should have a written policy identifying staff authorized to handle CDs which should be adhered to.

Disposal of medicines

- Unwanted or out-of-date stock in acute hospitals should be returned to the pharmacy. Where this stock involves CDs, the ward/department pharmacist must be involved in this transaction.
- Patients' own medicines should only be returned for destruction if written approval has been given by the patient or their parent/guardian.
- In the patient's own home, written consent from the patient or authorized carer should be given for the nurse to remove the drugs.
- When a patient dies the family may dispose of the medicines by returning to the supplying pharmacy or dispensing physician, or by giving written permission for the nurse to do this.

Further information

NMC (2008). *Standards for medicines management.* Available at: www.nmc-uk.org

Storage and control of medicines

Registered nurse responsibilities
- The registered nurse in charge has overall responsibility for the storage and security of medicines in hospital wards and departments.
- Receiving and checking medicines, including CDs, must be performed by a registered nurse or under the direct supervision of a registered nurse.
- Medicine cupboard keys should be kept securely by the registered nurse on their person (but separately to other keys). CD cupboard keys must be kept separate to the key ring for other medicine cupboards. When drug cupboard keys are needed they should be directly handed to another RN. A senior nurse and the head of pharmacy should be notified of missing keys.

Security
- Medicines treatment charts, prescription pads, and pharmacy requisition forms should be kept in a secure area to prevent unauthorized access.
- Loss or theft should be reported to a senior nurse, the head of pharmacy, and in some cases the police.
- Most medicines should be kept in a locked cupboard. Exceptions include cardiac arrest boxes, ITU, and theatre medicine cupboards that are in constant use (not CDs). It is good practice to conduct a daily stock check of medicines that are not locked away. If cardiac arrest boxes are sealed, it is sufficient to verify that they are in place. If a ward temporarily closes, the medicines and keys should be returned to the pharmacy department until the ward reopens. The head of pharmacy will advise on the need to remove CDs to safe storage elsewhere.

Storage arrangements
Some medicines have special storage requirements.
- CDs must be kept in a double-locked cupboard used solely for that purpose.
- For medicines that require refrigeration, temperatures between 2 and 8°C are required (regular daily temperature monitoring should be in place).
- Separate storage is required for products for internal and external use, IV fluids, irrigation fluids, and medicines for parenteral use.
- Except for CDs, medicines required daily by patients are kept in the medicines trolley.
- Medicines brought into hospital by patients cannot be taken from them without their consent. They may be returned to the patient's home, may be stored in a locked cupboard until the patient is discharged, or may be used during a patient's stay, subject to local policy.
- In care homes providing nursing services, it is expected that competent patients who choose to self-medicate will have access to a lockable drawer or cupboard.

Stock balance

- Records of stocks should be maintained and checked on a regular basis, e.g. CDs checked daily and recorded in CD register.
- Stocks of medicines that go missing and cannot be accounted for must be reported to the senior nurse and head of pharmacy for investigation.
- Nurses should be familiar with their Trust's policy on the verification and recording of spillages, especially of controlled drugs.

In the community patients are responsible for the safe storage of drugs in their own home.

Further information

NMC (2008). *Standards for medicines management.* Available at: www.nmc-uk.org

Table 4.1 Common abbreviations used in prescribing medicines

PO	by mouth	mg	milligram
IM	intramuscular	g	gram
IV	intravenous	kg	kilogram
SC	subcutaneous	mL	millilitre
PR	rectally	l	litre
PV	vaginally	OD	once daily
SL	sublingual	BD	twice daily
Neb	by nebulizer	TDS	three times a day
		QDS	four times a day
		OM	in the morning
		ON	at night

Abbreviations should be written to ensure initials are clear, e.g. SL and SC. Directions in English are preferred to Latin abbreviations where space permits.

Table 4.2 Measures used in drug calculations

Weight or volume	Equivalent	Calculation
1 kilogram (kg)	1000 grams (g)	To convert kg to g multiply by 1000
1 gram (g)	1000 milligrams (mg)	To convert g to mg multiply by 1000
1 milligram (mg)	0.001 gram (g)	To convert mg to g divide by 1000
1 litre (l)	1000 millilitres (mL)	To convert l to mL multiply by 1000
1000 millilitres (mL)	1 litre (l)	To convert mL to l divide by 1000

Nurse prescribing

Mechanisms for nurse prescribing and supply of medicines

Independent prescribing by nurses

The prescribing nurse takes responsibility for the clinical assessment of the patient, diagnosis, and clinical management of the patient. The prescribing nurse also takes responsibility for prescribing where necessary and the appropriateness of any prescription. There are two types of independent nurse prescriber.

District nurse and health visitors

They may prescribe from a limited formulary of products, i.e. appliances, dressings, and some medicines.

Extended formulary nurse prescribers

All first-level registered nurses and midwives may now train to prescribe for the nurse prescribers' extended formulary (NEFP). This includes:
- All medicines in the district nurse/health visitor (DN/HV) formulary
- All licensed pharmacy (P) medicines and all general sales list (GSL)
- A range of almost 180 prescription-only medicines (POMS)

These medicines may only be prescribed for use in the specific medical conditions set out in Part XVIIB (ii) of the Drug Tariff and the British National Formulary (BNF). Nurses should not prescribe independently outside of these medical conditions.

Supplementary prescribing by nurses

Supplementary prescribing is a voluntary partnership between an independent prescriber and a supplementary prescriber. These partners implement an agreed patient-specific clinical management plan with the patient's agreement. There are no legal restrictions on the clinical condition to be treated. Supplementary prescribers are able to prescribe:
- All GSL medicines and all pharmacy medicines
- Appliances and devices prescribable by GPs
- Food and other borderline substances approved by the Advisory Committee on Borderline Substances
- All POMs
- Medicines for use outside their licensed indications (i.e. 'off label' prescribing), 'black triangle' drugs, and those marked 'less suitable' for prescribing in the BNF
- Unlicensed drugs provided they are part of a clinical trial that has a clinical trial certificate exemption

Nurse prescribing regulations are regularly reviewed and updated.

Legal and professional considerations of nurse prescribers

- Registered nurses are required to undertake additional training established by the NMC to become independent and supplementary prescribers. Updating is also required.
- Nurse prescribers:
  - are individually and professionally accountable to the NMC for this aspect of their practice
  - should only prescribe for patients in their areas of clinical responsibility and should only prescribe medicines that are within their sphere of competence—they are not entitled to prescribe for themselves, family, or friends
  - are required to keep contemporaneous records that are unambiguous and legible.
- Community-based non-medical prescribers must use approved FP 10 forms which must be annotated by the district nurse/health visitor, or extended formulary nurse prescribes (EFNP)/Nurse Supplementary Prescriber.
- Supplementary prescribers may only prescribe for patients for whom a clinical management plan exists, and only within the limits of that plan.
- Non-medical prescribers may not issue verbal prescriptions.

Further information

Beckwith S and Franklin P (2007). *Oxford handbook of nurse prescribing.* Oxford University Press, Oxford.

Safe practice in the administration of medicines

Minimizing errors

The prescription

- The patient should consent to the medications prescribed and understand their purpose.
- Check that the medicines chart:
  - is clearly written and includes the patient's full name, hospital, hospital number, ward, weight, sex, and lead clinician (the use of removable stickers is poor practice)
  - clearly specifies the substance to be given using the generic or brand name
  - clearly states the form, strength, dose, time, frequency, route, and start and finish dates
  - is signed and dated by the authorized prescriber
  - clearly identifies any medication allergies or intolerances—if unsure, contact the prescriber.

Administration

- Check that all medicines, equipment, formularies, and policies for administration are available.
- Organize workload and deployment of staff to reduce interruptions during medicine rounds. Ensure two nurses check CDs and this is recorded.
- Have a good working knowledge of the uses of the medicines to be administered, normal dosages, common side effects, precautions, and contraindications relative to the patient's treatment.
- Check:
  - the location of the patient before preparing medications
  - whether special observations are required before or after administration
  - that the medication on the medicines chart and the label on the medicine container or blister pack are the same
  - the expiry date, route, method of administration, timing, and that the patient has not previously received it
  - how much is needed to give the required dose
  - in the case of 'as required' medications, that the minimum interval since the last dose has elapsed
  - that the patient has no allergies and there are no contraindications to administering the medication
  - the patient's identity against the medicines chart.
- Administer the medication and provide the required instruction and support to the patient.
- Make a clear, accurate, and immediate record of the medicine administered with signature. If the patient refuses or is unable to take the medication, document that no medicine was administered and actions you have taken.

- Monitor the effects of the medication and document in the patient record. Report any abnormal effects or exceptions.
- Ask the patient about side effects and review all the drugs prescribed regularly.
- Where supervising a student in the administration of medicines, clearly countersign the signature of the student.

Formula used in oral drug calculation

Amount required =

$$\frac{\text{what you want (strength required)} \times \text{volume it is in (stock)}}{\text{what you have got (stock strength)}}$$

(e.g. if you need 1.2 mg of hyoscine and the stock you have is 0.4 mg/mL, what volume do you need?

Amount required = 1.2 × 1 mL / 0.4 = 3 mL)

Formula used in IM and IV drug calculations

$$\text{Volume required} = \frac{\text{what you want} \times \text{volume it is in (stock)}}{\text{what you have got}}$$

Formula used to calculate IV drip rates

To calculate the rate of infusion the following should be known:
- The number of drops per mL the giving set delivers (standard giving sets deliver 15 mL of blood or blood products per mL of solution and 20 drops of aqueous intravenous fluid per mL of solution)—check the giving set being used
- The volume to be administered
- The time period over which it should be administered

For manually controlled administration

$$\text{Infusion rate} = \frac{\text{volume of infusion in mL} \times \text{drop per mL of giving set}}{\text{time in minutes}}$$

For example:
The prescription requires 1 litre of normal saline to be given in 10 hours

$$\text{Infusion rate} = \frac{1000 \text{ mL (1 l)} \times 20 \text{ drops}}{10 \text{ hours} \times 60} = \frac{20\,000}{600} = 33.3 \text{ or } 33 \text{ drops/min}$$

(rounded down to nearest drop)

Further information

NMC (2008). *Standards for medicines management.* Available at: www.nmc-uk.org

Improving concordance with medicines

In keeping with the emphasis on partnership with patients, the term 'compliance' has been substantially replaced by 'concordance'.

Concordance sufficient to obtain therapeutic objectives is generally low and occurs about half the time in patients in the community. In hospital concordance is higher because of regular medicine rounds, closer supervision, and support by nursing staff.

Factors that influence concordance

Social and demographic factors

Old age, low socioeconomic status, little formal education, and a vulnerable family background reduce the likelihood of concordance. Inadequate language skills and other barriers to communication are also important inhibitors of concordance.

Impact and influence of health professionals

The degree of confidence the patient has in the health professionals will affect the degree of concordance.

Beliefs about health and the medication

The patient's view of their susceptibility to the effects of the condition, the perceived benefits of taking the medication, and the perceived consequences of not taking it will affect the degree of concordance.

Peer, social, and family pressure

Attitudes to taking medication are often learned from parents and may be influenced by peers at school or work.

Complexity of the medication regimen

Large numbers of medicines taken several times a day may reduce concordance, as will unpleasant side effects.

Self-administration

Is undertaken to:
- Improve concordance with prescribed medication requirements
- Reduce admission rates
- Help patients achieve greater independence
- Ensure medication is taken at the most appropriate times for each patient
- Rationalize medication regimens to support the above
- Improve patient's knowledge of prescribed medicines

Successful self-medication requires:
- *Proper patient selection* to ensure patient can benefit from the programme.
- *Patient consent*—the patient should fully understand what is involved.
- *Safe storage and supply of medicines* in a locked box easily accessible by the patient—in community practice, medicines should be safely stored out of the reach of children.
- *Preparation and education of the patient* including explanation of the programme and the requirements of the patient, a review of the medicines, explanation of what the medicines do, and common side effects—the patient's competence should be checked periodically.

- *Education of the family* to support the patient and maximize concordance.
- *Use of concordance aids* such as monitored dose containers and daily/weekly dosing aids may be helpful to some patients.
- *Keeping records* of the medication and preparation of the patient.
- *Monitoring* to check that the procedure is being followed.
- *Evaluation* to determine whether benefits have been achieved.

Further information

NMC (2008). *Standards for medicines management.* Available at: www.nmc-uk.org

Routes of administration

- Oral—tablets, capsules, linctus, mixtures
- Sublingual—drug administered under the tongue for rapid absorption
- Inhalation—absorption of the drug via the respiratory mucosa
- Topical—drugs are given as creams for local effect on the skin, drops on the mucous membranes of eyes and ears
- Rectal—drugs absorbed into rectal mucosa for systemic effect
- Transdermal—drugs absorbed into the blood stream via the skin, e.g. patches
- Injection
  - *Intradermal*—into the skin
  - *Subcutaneous*—under the skin
  - *Intravenous*—into the venous circulation
  - *Intramuscular*—into muscles, upper outer quadrant of buttocks, anterior lateral aspect of thigh, deltoid muscle of arm
  - *Intrathecal*—into spinal theca

Specific aspects of administration of medicines

Patient group directions

This is a written instruction for the supply or administration of medicines to a group of patients who may not be individually identified before presentation for treatment. A protocol is prepared locally by physicians, pharmacists, and other appropriate professionals and approved by the employer with advice from relevant professional bodies. The protocol must be signed by a physician or dentist and a pharmacist who was involved in writing the direction. It is not a form of prescribing and there is no specific statutory training registered nurses must undertake before supplying medicines this way.

Covert administration of medicines

This is the disguising of medicines in food and drink which, in the absence of informed consent, may be regarded as deception. It should only be considered if a patient is assessed not to have the mental capacity to consent to treatment and who actively refuses medication. A fully documented risk assessment should be undertaken incorporating the following principles:

- The treatment is in the best interest of the patient
- The treatment must be necessary to save life or prevent deterioration or for the safety of others
- Local policy is followed
- The views of the multidisciplinary team are considered
- The views of the family and carers are considered
- Existing living wills or advance statements are considered
- Advice of legal and professional advisors is considered
- Regular attempts to encourage the patient to take the medication are made

Prescribing of medical gases

Medical gases are regarded as drugs that must be prescribed. The prescription must identify:

- Medical gas required
- Delivery device, e.g. mask or nasal cannula
- Rate
- Other instructions

Oxygen may be administered in an emergency without a prescription, e.g. cardiac or respiratory arrest.

Further information

NMC (2008). *Standards for medicines management.* Available at: www.nmc-uk.org

Health promotion

Defining health promotion

Health promotion is a complex construct made up of many varied activities aimed at preventing disease, impairment, and disability, and promoting positive health by reducing health inequalities. It includes:

- *Creating a safe environment* in which to live and work through legislation and policies, e.g. health and safety at work, environmental health policies—these result in safe water supplies, safe sewage disposal, food hygiene, safe equipment, and machinery.
- *Implementing health-related public policies* that provide protection against ill health by banning certain products or practices (e.g. smoking in the workplace and some public places), requiring individuals to use certain equipment (e.g. wearing crash helmets and seat belts), or promoting healthy choices (e.g. taxing certain products, such as alcohol and cigarettes, and better food labeling).
- *Promoting community involvement* by encouraging communities to identify their health needs and supporting them in taking responsibility for their health by making healthy choices.
- *Fostering health education* by developing personal skills by raising awareness of health risks and positive health choices, providing information for individuals to make informed decisions, acquiring new skills, and developing positive attitudes and beliefs about health.
- *Re-focusing health services* to prevent ill health, in addition to cure and care, e.g. screening for disease, immunization, and identification of risks such as coronary heart disease.

Levels of health promotion

Three levels of prevention are:

- *Primary prevention:* focus is on healthy people to prevent ill health and to improve the quality of health through healthy lifestyle choices.
- *Secondary prevention:* focus is on detecting disease while it can be effectively cured, i.e. before it becomes problematic and irreversible (screening is performed to detect a disease, and then counselling, support, and advice are offered to encourage change in behaviour or compliance with treatment).
- *Tertiary prevention:* focus is on patients who have permanent disabilities or chronic diseases to help them modify their lifestyle and avoid restrictions on their life choices, i.e. preventing complications in those who are already symptomatic.

Factors that determine health

Many factors determine health and therefore also lead to health inequalities.

Genetics

Inherited factors determine physical characteristics (e.g. height and weight) and are responsible for some diseases (e.g. haemophilia and sickle cell disease). However, positive lifestyle choices may affect the course of genetic diseases and help people make the best of what their genes provide.

Lifestyle

Choices individuals make about the way they live can affect their health, e.g. smoking, physical activity, diet, alcohol intake, and sexual practices. These choices are influenced by education, poverty, culture, and social situation of the individual. For example, eating a balanced diet of fresh fruit, lowfat spreads, and lean meat is expensive and may be difficult for someone living in poverty. Eating habits are often passed down through family lines and are therefore affected by a person's culture. Peer group pressure is an example of a social factor that influences lifestyle choices, e.g. sexual practices or illicit drug use.

Environment

The environment in which a person lives can affect their health. Several environmental factors affect health:

- Air quality: Air pollution exacerbates asthma, respiratory infections, and lung cancer.
- Housing: Crowded, damp, cold, and rundown housing increases the likelihood of transmission of infections, increases exacerbation of asthma, and increases the incidence of accidents. High-rise blocks often lead to social segregation and subsequent anxiety, depression, and mental ill health.
- Water quality: Water should be free from pollutants and infectious diseases, e.g. cholera and typhoid, to prevent illness. Additions such as fluoride can positively affect the health of teeth.
- Food production: An imbalance in diet results in degrees of obesity or malnutrition. Food must be free from harmful bacteria, infectious organisms, and toxic substances. This requires healthy agricultural and food production, storage in proper conditions, cooking at adequate temperatures, a high standard of kitchen hygiene, and safe food-handling practices.

Education

Level of education influences attitudes and behaviour towards health. It may also affect employment potential which in turn influences earning potential.

Working environment

Health and safety legislation in the work place requires that hazards such as dangerous chemicals and machinery are identified and minimized to prevent accidents and industrial illnesses that were common in the past, e.g. asbestosis, pneumoconiosis.

Other factors such as social class, ethnic origins, poverty and employment also affect health.

Other factors determining health

- *Social class:* People from higher socioeconomic classes have a greater chance of avoiding illness and staying healthy than those in a lower class. This is partly due to the different lifestyle and living conditions experienced.
- *Ethnic differences:* Strokes and hypertension are more common in Afro-Caribbean communities. Heart disease, tuberculosis, and diabetes are more common in people who originate from the Indian subcontinent. A combination of lifestyle and genetic differences has some impact but evidence suggest these groups do not access health services as frequently as the indigenous community.
- *Poverty:* There is a strong association between low income and poor health. Poverty impairs the ability to obtain a healthy balanced diet. It may cause stress and anxiety leading to mental health problems and it reduces the lifestyle choices available. Low income may lead to inability to afford heating, which contributes to hypothermia and increased mortality of the elderly in winter.
- *Employment:* There is a strong association between unemployment and poor health for reasons similar to those described for poverty. Unemployed people are more likely to commit suicide and have chronic ill health as a result of their lifestyle and living conditions. Unemployment may lead to difficulty sleeping, which increases the likelihood of chronic chest conditions.

Health beliefs

Factors affecting health behaviours

Understanding factors that influence people's health behaviours will help the nurse plan health promotion and patient education activities (See Fig. 5.1).

- *Incentives:* such as absence of pain, better mobility, prevention of illness, and increased comfort will affect the degree to which the individual values the outcome and the extent to which they follow the course of treatment or preventive activity.
- *Expectation:* refers to the extent to which the individual believes the action they follow will result in the desired outcome.
- *Confidence:* refers to the self-confidence the individual has in undertaking the new behaviour or action required.
- *Opportunities for observation:* If the individual can see others undertaking the activity successfully then they are more likely to follow the same plan.
- *Previous experiences:* Individuals with a previous successful experience making a positive health choice are more likely to want to undertake and be confident about achieving another one.
- *Perceived risk:* is the extent to which the individual feels at risk of developing a disease or condition; the greater the risk the more likely the individual will be to follow the preventive behaviour.
- *Perceived severity of the condition:* The more the individual believes the condition is serious and the greater impact on their personal and working life, the more motivated they become to seek healthy behaviours.
- *Barriers:* refer to the extent to which the individual feels obstacles (e.g. the inconvenience, the effort, and the pain) are worth overcoming.
- *Influence of others:* Individuals who believe that health is determined by health care professionals, family members, or peers are more likely to follow their advice.
- *Chance:* refers to the extent to which the individual believes that health and illness are a matter of chance or whether they believe they can exert any influence or control over their health.

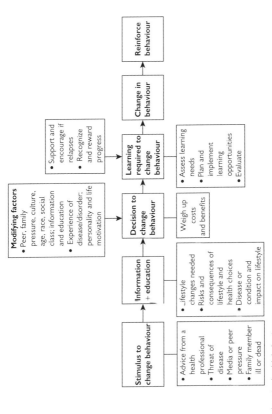

Fig. 5.1 Stages in changing health behaviours.

Role of the general nurse in health promotion

The general nurse may focus on diagnosis-related and non-diagnosis related health promotion.

Diagnosis-related health promotion

This is essential to help patients understand their illness and treatment, and participate in their care. The initial focus should be to help patients learn what they need to know about their current condition. They must then focus on their lifestyle that is relevant to the condition, e.g. smoking cessation for patients with peripheral vascular disease, balanced diet for obese patients following heart attack. Health promotion unrelated to their health problem may be confusing and unhelpful.

Non-diagnosis related health promotion

This may focus on patients, families, visitors, and staff and uses both planned and spontaneous opportunities.

- *Safe work practices* are implemented to help minimize the risks of infection, back and other injuries, and exposure to hazardous substances. Consider vaccinations and screening.
- *Environmentally friendly work practices* should be used to ensure the environment is not damaged, e.g. effective disposal of waste, effective use of all resources.
- *Policies to promote healthy lifestyles* should be implemented, e.g. smoke free environments, healthy eating opportunities.
- *Health information* should be readily available from leaflets and posters for both the patient and the carers.
- *Opportunities for staff* to promote their own health and act as positive role models should be available, e.g. exercise facilities on site or reduced membership costs at local gyms.
- *Patient and staff support groups* should be available, e.g. smoking cessation and support, exercise, and keep-fit groups.

Frequently the nurse will be able to combine the above (See Fig. 5.2).

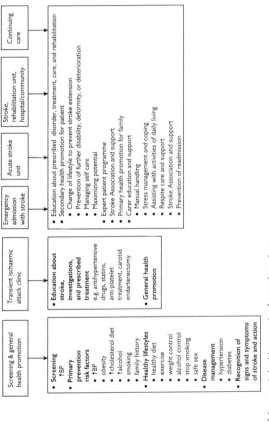

Fig. 5.2 Role of the nurse in health promotion for stroke pathway.

Patient education

Definition

This is a planned systematic process intended to influence the behaviour of others by producing changes in their knowledge, attitudes, and skills. It is part of health promotion and is concerned with educating and informing people who come into contact with health services.

Components

- *Information giving* refers to making information available to patients. However, passing on facts does not guarantee that the patient will learn or change their behaviour. Teaching and learning are required to achieve behavior change.
- *Learning* takes place when an individual is able to carry out specific actions and use the knowledge and skills appropriately.
- *Teaching* is a process of helping others to learn and incorporate new behaviour into everyday life. It involves informing, instructing, challenging, coaching, and guiding.

Patient education in practice

Patient education requires a systematic approach.

- Identify what the patient needs to know, including what they already know, what they want to know, how they like to learn, and their readiness to learn.
- Identify the patient's goals or desired outcomes—this includes clarifying the essential 'must know' skills and knowledge for safety and survival.
- Plan what the patient ideally needs to learn and how, i.e. the content, who will teach, and the methods.
- Implement the methods or strategies identified in the plan and overcome barriers such as lack of time, skill, knowledge, and other priorities.
- Measure the effectiveness of the process and decide what to do next.
- Record what has been undertaken, what information was imparted, and to what extent the patient has benefited by learning new knowledge and skills to enable them to improve their health.

Patient education materials

These can be used as a complement to teaching but should not be used as a substitute to teaching.

- *Written materials:* include leaflets, handouts, and booklets that should be kept simple and easy to read and understand so that they can be read by most people. They should be accurate, up-to-date, reflect current practices, and cover patients' major areas of concern.
- *Audiovisual materials:* include videos, posters, models, DVDs, and CDs. They can be used to:
  - Create interest and motivate patients
  - Explain how something works
  - Show what something looks like
  - Involve patients in learning
  - Help patients better retain what they have learned
  - Confirm what is being said verbally
  - Provide repeat demonstration or explanations for the patient in their own time

Diagnosing nursing problems and implementing nursing care

Nursing patients with respiratory problems

Nursing assessment of patients with respiratory problems

In addition to a general nursing assessment (□ Chapter 3, Individualizing nursing care practice, p.27) perform the following procedures.

- First establish whether the patient has a history of an acute or chronic respiratory problem.
- Determine the patient's chief complaint.
- Determine whether the patient requires immediate action, e.g. does the patient have a blocked airway or require oxygen therapy.
- Consider the effect of age, sex, and race on the physical and diagnostic findings.
- Evaluate the patient's cough: type, persistence over time (e.g. days, weeks, months), productive (i.e. with sputum), time of day, history, dry, tickling, or hacking.
- Evaluate the sputum: amount, colour, consistency, bloodstained (haemoptysis).
- Determine whether the patient is experiencing chest pain.
- Assess dyspnoea or breathlessness: time of day, duration, relieving factors, audible sounds (wheezing), cause, e.g. on exertion or type of precipitating factors.
- Obtain the patient's health history as well as that of their family members, e.g. is there any genetic predisposition to cystic fibrosis?
- Obtain a smoking history: cigarettes, marijuana, or other controlled substance? How long? Recently quit?
- Review childhood illnesses, e.g. asthma, pneumonia, infectious diseases, hay fever, allergies, eczema, frequent colds.
- Identify any allergies (e.g. pollen, dust, foods, grasses, medications, animals such as cats) and the patient's response to each allergy (e.g. wheezing).
- Review recent adult illnesses, especially related to breathing, e.g. pneumonia, tuberculosis, heart disease.
- Review employment history and environmental possibilities, e.g. pneumoconiosis (dust disease from working with coal and in the pottery industry).
- Assess the patient's home and living conditions.
- Determine whether the patient has recently undergone surgery.
- Obtain date of last chest x-ray.
- Assess presence of night sweats or sleep disturbances.
- Determine whether the patient has any problems when travelling and by what transport, e.g. aircraft.
- Identify any particular risk factors relating to their condition.
- Evaluate the patient's psychological state—signs of confusion, emotional upset, or distress.

Physical examination

- Perform overview from head to toe.
- Evaluate head—nasal flaring, colour—bluish-grey (cyanosis), tenderness in frontal and maxillary areas.
- Note condition of mouth—pursed-lip breathing.
- Note position of trachea for deviation and tenderness.
- Observe thorax for rate and pattern of breathing.
- Note symmetry of chest wall.
- Note chest wall deformities, discoloration, scars, lesions, masses and spinal deformities, such as kyphosis, scoliosis, and lordosis.
- Evaluate extremities—oedema, peripheral cyanosis, and clubbing.
- Perform general overview of patient—note body position, skin condition, muscle mass. In some situations the more experienced nurse would also assess chest sounds, assess use of accessory muscles to breathe, examine the lymph nodes, perform percussion of the chest, and listen for vocal fremitus.

Four keys to chest examination

- Inspection: Observe patient's chest, comparing one side with the other.
- Palpation: Touch the chest and observe movement, abnormalities, and vibrations.
- Percussion: Tap the chest wall for sounds of density.
- Auscultation: Listen for normal breath sounds (See Fig. 6.1).

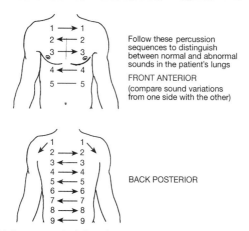

Fig. 6.1 Systematic method of auscultating all aspects of chest wall. Follow these percussion sequences to distinguish between normal and abnormal sounds in the patient's lungs. Although the diagram illustrates nine sequences, in the UK physicians ordinarily perform six. An increased number of sequences is usual in some countries and may be more helpful in patients with long torsos.

Common respiratory nursing problems

Difficulty in maintaining a clear airway

Maintaining a clear airway may be difficult due to excessive secretions from a variety of causes and conditions such as chronic obstructive pulmonary disease (COPD) and some neurological conditions such as multiple sclerosis and motor neurone disease. Several interventions can be used to aid clearance including:

- careful use of drugs combined with a controlled breathing technique
- postural drainage and the use of breathing devices
- good hydration.

The frequency of interventions to clear the airway depends on the thickness and volume of the sputum.

Postural drainage in combination with percussion or vibration may aid in loosening secretions. The patient is placed in a certain position (See Fig. 6.2) to drain the particular segment of the affected lung. The nurse and physiotherapist should work together on this technique.

Suctioning should be carefully performed when patients are unable to clear their own secretions.

- Apply oxygenation prior to suctioning.
- Monitor saturated oxygen levels constantly.
- Explain the procedure to the patient and agree to a signal that can be used if they want the suctioning stopped.
- Multiple tubes are often used; therefore use a single sterile glove with each sterile suction tube.
- Assess for dyspnoea and abnormal heart rates during the procedure.
- Ensure proper position and mobilization for effective ventilation.
- Ensure adequate hydration to help liquefy secretions.

Difficulty in maintaining an effective breathing pattern

- Identify the cause in conjunction with the multidisciplinary team.
- Implement suitable and appropriate breathing techniques, e.g. diaphragmatic or abdominal and pursed-lip breathing manoeuvres may be beneficial interventions for dyspnoeic episodes.
- Position patient upright.
- Exercise conditioning may be needed for patients with exercise-induced shortness of breath.

Shortness of breath when eating

A common complaint in acute and chronic lung disease is shortness of breath when eating. The patient may complain of food intolerance, nausea, and loss of appetite.

- Monitor the patient's diet and weight.
- Encourage the patient to rest before meals.
- Plan the biggest meal when the patient is most hungry or offer regular small meals.
- Suggest the patient try using a bronchodilator 30 minutes before a meal.

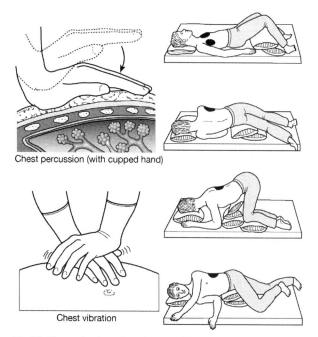

Chest percussion (with cupped hand)

Chest vibration

Fig. 6.2 Diagram showing positions for postural drainage and percussion.

Hypoxia and hypoxaemia

Hypoxia refers to a deficiency in the amount of oxygen reaching the tissues. Hypoxaemia refers to an abnormally low concentration of oxygen in the blood.

Oxygen therapy

Oxygen therapy requires a prescription by a physician, except in emergency situations. It is used in acute and chronic respiratory conditions. Pulse oximetry is commonly used to measure oxygen saturation levels (normal is 95–100%) and determine the need for oxygen therapy. However, arterial blood gas analysis is the best tool for determining the need for oxygen therapy and evaluating its effects.

Oxygen delivery systems

Numerous systems are available to deliver oxygen (See Table 6.1), and the type of system used is dependent on several factors:

- Oxygen concentration required
- Efficiency of the system to the patient
- Accuracy and control of the oxygen concentration
- Patient comfort
- Respiratory rate and depth
- Need for humidity
- Mobility of the patient

Low-flow delivery systems

- Low-flow delivery systems include the nasal cannula, simple face mask (See Fig. 6.3), partial rebreather masks, and non-rebreather masks (See Fig. 6.4).
- These systems may not provide enough oxygen to meet the patient's total inspiratory effort.
- The amount of oxygen delivered depends upon the patient's breathing pattern.
- Oxygen is diluted with room air (contains 21% oxygen) which lowers the amount the patient receives.
- Nasal cannulae (See Fig. 6.5) are used for patients with chronic lung disease and for patients who require long-term oxygen therapy. However, the percentage of oxygen from nasal cannulae is not reliable since it depends on the minute volume of the patient. Therefore, a venturi mask (high-flow delivery system) is the best treatment for acute exacerbations of COPD.
- Simple face masks are used to deliver oxygen concentrations of 40–60% for short-term therapy or in an emergency.

High-flow delivery systems

- High-flow delivery systems include the venturi systems (See Fig. 6.6) which are colour-coded and specify the flow of oxygen required to deliver 24%, 28%, 31%, 35%, 40%, or 60% oxygen.
- These systems provide a flow rate that is adequate to meet total inspiratory effort.
- These systems are used for acutely ill patients, when it is particularly important to know the precise concentration of oxygen being delivered.

There is a danger of carbon dioxide retention when oxygen therapy is administered. Therefore, the nurse must be aware that the use of oxygen treatment in COPD is one of the most important issues to cover in nursing and respiratory disease.

Key nursing points regarding oxygen therapy

- Except in an emergency, oxygen therapy requires a prescription.
- Carefully determine the most appropriate delivery system and mask to use.
- Explain the procedure to the patient and their family and visitors.
- A humidification system may be required if more than 24% oxygen is used for long periods.
- Position mask carefully after setting correct flow.
- Check comfort of the mask regularly.
- Observe the patient's colour, oxygen saturation, and breathing pattern.
- Offer drinks and mouth care.
- Provide ongoing teaching and reassurance to enhance patient concordance with therapy.
- Remember that while oxygen is inflammable it does support combustion. Health professionals and patients must be aware of the fire risks associated with oxygen use.
- Oxygen delivery equipment can harbour organisms that may cause infections.

Table 6.1 Types of oxygen flow mask

Type of mask	Flow of oxygen delivered
Nasal cannulae	24% at 1 l/min
	28% at 2 l/min
	32% at 3 l/min
	40% at 4 l/min
Simple face mask	40% at 5 l/min
	45–50% at 6 l/min
	55–60% at 8 l/min
Venturi masks	24–60% at 4–10 l/min

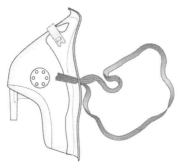

Fig. 6.3 Medium concentration mask. Courtesy of Intersurgical.

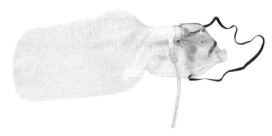

Fig. 6.4 Non-rebreathable device. Courtesy of Intersurgical.

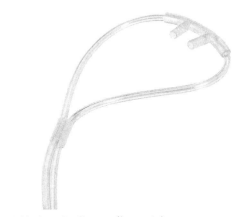

Fig. 6.5 Nasal cannulae. Courtesy of Intersurgical.

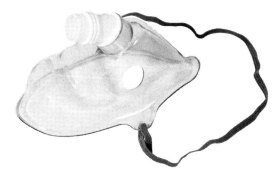

Fig. 6.6 Venturi mask. Courtesy of Intersurgical.

Tests and investigations

Various noninvasive methods are available for exploring the lungs, most of which involve measuring an individual's breathing and lung capacity. Prior to any test the patient should be provided with a full explanation to help alleviate anxiety.

Peak flow

Peak expiratory flow is the maximum rate of breathing out, after having taken a full breath in. The peak flow meter used for this test is a small tube with a mouthpiece and a gauge. Patients are instructed to take a full breath in, place their lips securely around the mouthpiece, and give a hard fast breath out. The rate is measured in litres per minute, and varies according to age, sex, height, and ethnicity. Peak expiratory flow is useful in the diagnosis of and monitoring of asthma.

Spirometry

Spirometry measures the rate of breathing out and lung capacity at the same time. Taken together these two measurements help distinguish between obstructive and restrictive lung disease. Patients are asked to take a full breath in, place their lips tightly around the mouthpiece, and then breathe out hard and in a controlled way (maximum expiration) until they have breathed out all their air. Two readings will be shown. The first is the volume of air breathed out in the first second (i.e. forced expiratory volume or FEV1), and the other is the amount of air breathed out in total (i.e. the vital capacity or VC). The ratio of one to the other defines the type of lung disease the patient has. A ratio of FEV1/VC of less than about 70–75% indicates airflow obstruction.

Carbon monoxide transfer

This test is usually done in the lung function laboratory and measures the amount of gas exchanging surface area of the lung.

Laboratory tests

📖 Chapter 39, Common laboratory tests and their interpretation, p.1167.
- Serum urea and electrolytes (U&E), FBC, clotting
- Serum total IgE and allergen-specific IgE antibodies, if indicated
- Blood gases to assess acid-base status
- Sputum for culture and sensitivity (for bacteria, fungi, and mycobacteria)
- Blood cultures prior to antimicrobial treatment

X-rays and scans
- Chest x-rays
- CT
- MRI

Specialist investigations aimed at getting tissue for histology
- Pleural biopsy
- Bronchoscopy
- CT guided biopsy

Respiratory infections

Influenza

Influenza is a viral infection that can be fatal in very young and elderly people and in those with certain chest diseases (e.g. COPD) or autoimmune diseases, which make them weaker and less likely to overcome the illness. Nurses should encourage such people to have annual influenza vaccine. Temperature and respiratory rate should be monitored; any fever should be treated with paracetamol and cool compresses; the patient should be encouraged to take oral fluids; and the patient's position should be changed regularly.

Acute exacerbations of chronic obstructive pulmonary disease (COPD)

An exacerbation of COPD (previously known as bronchitis) is a worsening of respiratory symptoms that is acute in onset and leads to an increase in the COPD patient's normal respiratory symptoms such as breathlessness and cough. Persistent coughing can tire patients; they may wheeze and need bronchodilator and corticosteroid medication. Patients may need assistance with coughing, remaining comfortable, and performing activities of daily living. Oxygen saturation and respiratory rate should be monitored regularly. Patients who smoke should be encouraged to stop.

Pneumonia

Pneumonia is an acute lower respiratory tract infection that is usually associated with fever, malaise, and laboured breathing. Patients should be cared for in a position that is comfortable to them; usually this is in a sitting position. Some patients may require nebulized bronchodilators and oxygen to maintain their oxygen saturation. Patients should be encouraged and assisted to cough up sputum, observe its colour, and collect it for culture, if necessary. Temperature, oxygen saturation, and respiratory rate should be monitored regularly. Temperature should be controlled with paracetamol and cool compresses. Treatment of pneumonia includes antibiotic therapy and analgesia. Pneumonia that is inadequately treated may progress to lung abscess or empyema.

Empyema

Empyema is a collection of pus that forms in the pleural space. This collection must be drained with a chest drain as antibiotic therapy alone is insufficient. Observations should be carried out at least every 4 hours, patients should be cared for in a comfortable position, and the chest drain should be monitored (📖 Chapter 6, Key points when caring for chest drains, p.121). Surgical intervention may be required.

Tuberculosis (TB)

Tuberculosis is a highly contagious infection caused by *Mycobacterium tuberculosis*. Cough and sputum are common symptoms of TB, but patients do not always exhibit these symptoms (known as silent TB). Other features associated with TB include night fever and sweats, anorexia and weight loss, and general malaise. Observations should be monitored depending on each individual case. The need for isolation should be clearly explained to the patient and family, and the patient should be monitored for signs of depression caused by isolation. The patient should be taught about their condition and anti-TB medication in order to help with concordance. Chest x-ray and sputum culture confirm the diagnosis of TB.

Lung abscess

Lung abscess can be caused by bacteria that reach the lung through aspiration or through the blood. The infected material lodges in the small bronchi and produces inflammation, which results in retention of secretions beyond the obstruction. Eventual necrosis of tissue ensues. Observations should be carried out according to each case. Patients should be cared for in a comfortable position and should be assisted in coughing up sputum and collecting it for culture. Postural drainage should be used. Lung abscess is treated with antibiotics and may require surgical drainage.

Chronic respiratory diseases: innate

Cor pulmonale

Cor pulmonale is right-sided ventricular heart failure caused by pulmonary disease with 90% of cases resulting from COPD. Chronic airflow limitation increases the workload on the right side of the heart. Blood vessels narrow as the disease progresses, leading to enlarged and thickened chambers. Signs and symptoms of cor pulmonale include dyspnoea, peripheral oedema, fatigue, syncope, tachycardia, cyanosis, and raised jugular venous pressure. Management includes monitoring vital signs, administering oxygen, assessing pain, and keeping the patient comfortable. Diuretics such as furosemide 40–160 mg may be prescribed. U&Es should be monitored.

Cystic fibrosis

Cystic fibrosis is one of the most common serious inherited diseases among white children and young people. It is a multisystem disease characterized by recurrent infections of the lower respiratory tract, inadequate functioning of the pancreas, high salt content of sweat, and male infertility. Abnormal viscid mucus is formed in the lungs, pancreas, and bowel. In the lungs this mucus allows bacteria to multiply causing infections. Symptoms typically include shortness of breath, dyspnoea, fatigue, cough, and wheezing. Chest infections are treated with IV antibiotics, indwelling IV lines, and nebulized antibiotics. IV therapy may be necessary at home, which requires the help of special teaching and the support of a specialist nurse. Depending upon how advanced the disease is, the patient may require continuous oxygen and must be educated how to use oxygen safely. Good nutrition is important, and referral to a dietitian is warranted. Patients undergo lengthy chest physiotherapy to help clear the mucus and some will eventually need a double lung transplant.

Chronic respiratory diseases: acquired

Asthma

Asthma is a chronic airway inflammatory disorder resulting from complex interactions between inflammatory cells, mediators, and airway cells. Airway hyperactivity caused by a variety of non-specific stimuli leads to variable degrees of airway obstruction. Asthma may become irreversible and chronic over many years. Peak flow tests are used to monitor the disease and should be explained to the patient. Management of asthma is through avoidance of triggers and the use of bronchodilator and steroid inhalers. There is a British Thoracic Society (BTS) standard plan, known as the 'asthma stepladder' used to treat patients with this condition. During an asthma attack patients can experience anxiety and should be taught relaxation techniques to keep them as calm as possible. It is very important that the patient receives a management plan when discharged home.

Chronic obstructive pulmonary disease (COPD)

COPD is the preferred term for a group of conditions previously known as chronic obstructive airways disease (COAD), chronic bronchitis (See Fig. 6.7) and emphysema (See Fig. 6.8). It is an irreversible, chronic progressive multisystem disorder that is characterized by airway obstruction. Individuals who smoke but have not developed COPD can prevent the disease by quitting. Those who smoke and have developed COPD can slow the progression of the disease by quitting. COPD is diagnosed by spirometry. The patient's breathing should be observed; details of the smoking history and any family history of COPD should be obtained; and respiratory rate, oxygen saturation, and pulse should be monitored. The amount of oxygen needed at home should be assessed. Arterial blood gases may be required to assess the need for ventilatory support. Destructive changes may take place in the alveoli and the patient may experience difficulty in expiration. Some patients experience 'purse-lipped' breathing and use accessory muscles, such as shoulders and abdomen, to breathe. COPD is treated by bronchodilators, inhaled steroids, and antibiotics (along with relevant health education, weight loss, diet, and exercise). Influenza and pneumonia vaccines are recommended. Patients should be referred to special respiratory nurses for monitoring and follow up.

Sarcoidosis

Sarcoidosis is a multisystem granulomatous disorder of unknown cause that affects adults aged 20–40 years. The lungs, as well as other organs, become scarred leading to difficulty in breathing. Symptoms of sarcoidosis include coughing, dyspnoea, and chest discomfort. The condition is diagnosed from chest x-ray, CT scan, lung function tests, and bronchoscopy. Symptom prevention and control is the goal of nursing. Steroids are often prescribed.

Pulmonary fibrosis

Pulmonary fibrosis is known to be caused by inhalation of particles. Smoking and exposure to metal dust and wood fibres are predictors of the disease. Pulmonary fibrosis is associated with connective tissue disease and may be an adverse effect of drugs commonly used to treat connective tissue diseases. Symptoms include dyspnoea and dry cough; cyanosis and heart failure can develop. The condition is diagnosed from chest x-ray, CT scan, and lung biopsy. A full respiratory assessment should be performed. The patient should be kept comfortable and informed about the disease process. Steroids are often prescribed, and many patients require home oxygen.

Occupational pulmonary disease

Exposure to occupational or environmental fumes such as dust, gases, or bacterial or fungal antigens can result in a variety of respiratory disorders.

Pneumoconiosis

Pneumoconiosis affects coal workers and is caused by inhaled coal dust lodging in the lungs. Symptoms are related to the amount and frequency of exposure to coal dust. Initial symptoms are similar to bronchitis. Pneumoconiosis can progress to emphysema and COPD.

Asbestosis

Asbestosis is a condition of diffuse fibrosis of the lungs caused by inhaling asbestos fibres. Patients can be exposed over many years (15–40) before symptoms appear. Asbestos was used in the production of paints, plastics, brake and clutch linings, and as insulation in buildings. Symptoms include breathlessness and cough. There is an increased risk of bronchial adeno-carcinoma.

Silicosis

Silicosis is a condition of chronic fibrosing of the lungs caused by inhalation of free crystalline silica dust, e.g. dust from potteries. Symptoms depend upon the length of exposure to the dust and range from mild breathing difficulties to significant dyspnoea and massive fibrosis that can be seen on chest x-ray and CT scan. Hypoxia, anorexia, and weight loss may occur.

For all of these conditions a full respiratory assessment is required. Administration of oxygen may be necessary and patients may require assistance to clear sputum, if present.

Lung cancer

Lung cancer is one of the leading causes of cancer-related deaths. Primary lung cancers, which arise from the bronchial epithelium, are called bronchogenic carcinomas. Symptoms can vary from mild breathlessness in early stages to pain, stridor, bloodstained sputum due to bronchial obstruction, dyspnoea, and hypoxia. Diagnosis requires a tissue specimen which can be obtained by bronchoscopy, CT-guided biopsy, pleural biopsy or a surgical operation such as mediastinoscopy or video-assisted thoracic surgery (VATS). Staging CT scans are performed to determine how advanced the disease is and what treatments are possible. Patients may have bloodstained pleural effusions requiring a chest drain. Once drained, pleural effusions can be treated with pleurodesis which involves inserting talc or a similar irritant into the pleural space to cause scarring which prevents the recurrence of the effusion. Some symptoms such as pain, breathlessness due to bronchial obstruction, and haemoptysis can be treated with palliative radiotherapy. Some patients receive chemotherapy. Regular observations and pain assessment are needed; oxygen may also be required. Prognosis is poor unless surgical resection can be accomplished.

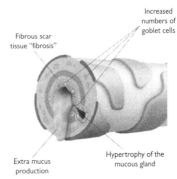

Fig. 6.7 Airway in chronic bronchitis.
Reproduced with permission from Boehringer Ingelheim.

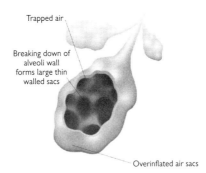

Fig. 6.8 Changes in emphysema.
Reproduced with permission from Boehringer Ingelheim.

Acute respiratory disease

Acute respiratory failure

Acute respiratory failure is categorized according to abnormal blood gases into two categories:

Type I
- Most common type of acute respiratory failure
- Classified as partial pressure of arterial oxygen (PaO_2) <8 kPa and arterial saturation (SaO_2) <92%
- Occurs in patients with severe acute asthma, pneumonia, pulmonary embolus, emphysema, fibrosing alveolitis, and acute respiratory distress syndrome (ARDS)

Type II
- Classified by a low PaO_2 (<8 kPa), a high partial pressure of carbon dioxide ($PaCO_2$) (>6.5 kPa) and blood pH that is normal or acidotic
- Occurs in patients with acute exacerbations of COPD or in neuromuscular disorders such as drug overdose (opiates/barbiturates), Guillain–Barré, polio, and myasthenia gravis
- Patients are hypoxic

Patients should be assessed for dyspnoea or changes in respiratory rate or pattern. Oxygen saturation, blood pressure, and pulse should be monitored regularly. Patients should be cared for in a comfortable position (usually sitting up). Anxiety should be monitored and interventions implemented to reduce anxiety.

Pulmonary embolism

A pulmonary embolism is a collection of particulate matters (gaseous substances, liquids, or solids) that become lodged in the pulmonary vascular system. A blood clot is the most common form and usually arises from a venous thrombosis in the pelvis or legs. Large emboli obstruct the pulmonary circulation causing a decrease in oxygen, hypoxia, and potential death. Symptoms vary from mild breathlessness to severe chest pain, haemoptysis, dyspnoea, and hypotension. The patient may be pale and clammy, with dizziness and confusion. Heparin therapy for 5–10 days is given to prevent further clotting. Following heparin therapy, oral anticoagulants (e.g. warfarin) are continued for up to 6 months.

Pneumothorax

Pneumothorax refers to the condition in which air in the pleural space causes the lung to collapse.
- Spontaneous pneumothoraces occur when there is no chest trauma, usually in fit young people, especially tall young men. There may be an underlying lung disease such as asthma.
- Traumatic pneumothoraces occur when chest trauma or surgery allow air in through the chest wall.

- Tension pneumothoraces occur when air is allowed into the pleural space during inspiration but does not exit during expiration. This causes pressure to build up in the chest and eventually decreases cardiac output. This is a medical emergency.

Pneumothoraces can be diagnosed clinically and on chest x-ray. Patients should be kept sitting and oxygen should be administered. Treatment by simple aspiration may be sufficient, or a chest drain may be required.

Haemothorax

Haemothorax refers to the presence of blood in the thoracic cavity and can occur following blunt chest trauma or a penetrating injury. A simple haemothorax is considered blood loss of <1500 mL into thoracic cavity; a massive haemothorax is considered blood loss >1500 mL. In a massive haemothorax, bleeding can be from the lung itself or from the heart. Chest x-ray can identify fluid in the cavity but an aspiration is required to identify the presence of blood. Chest tubes are inserted into the cavity to evacuate the blood. If blood evacuation exceeds 1500–2000 mL, an open thoracotomy may be considered. Vital signs, drainage volume, and site should be monitored. IV fluids and oxygen should be administered.

Pleural effusion

A pleural effusion describes the collection of fluid in the pleural cavity which compresses the lung, making breathing difficult. It can be caused by a chest infection, lung cancer, mesothelioma (primary cancer of the pleura), or any condition that causes fluid retention or low blood protein. A pleural effusion causes the area to sound 'dull' when percussed. A chest x-ray confirms diagnosis. Vital signs should be monitored and, if the patient is hypoxic, oxygen should be administered. Fluid withdrawn from the cavity through a needle should be sent for analysis. A chest drain may be used to drain the cavity.

Sleep apnoea

Sleep apnoea is defined as breathing disruption during sleep that occurs at least 5 times per hour and lasts at least 10 seconds. The most common cause of sleep apnoea is upper airway obstruction. A change in sleeping position or weight loss may resolve the apnoea. Other interventions include continuous positive airway pressure (CPAP) or devices to prevent obstruction of the tongue and neck structures. In severe cases surgical intervention may be attempted, but to date surgical results have been poor and unpredictable.

Common respiratory surgical interventions

Prior to surgical intervention, ensure that a respiratory assessment has taken place, informed consent has been obtained, and the patient has been given information about the procedure. Ensure that appropriate postoperative care is provided.

Thoracotomy
- Opening into the thoracic cavity to locate tumours, perform biopsies, or identify sites of bleeding or injury
- May be performed to remove the lung or a portion of the lung

Lobectomy
- Resection of a single pulmonary lobe
- Performed when a tumour is confined to one lobe
- After lobectomy the remaining lung tissue usually expands to fill previously occupied lung space

Pneumonectomy
- Removal of the entire lung
- Indications:
  - Large centrally located bronchogenic tumours
  - Involvement of a mainstem bronchus
  - Invasion of the main pulmonary artery

VATS (video-assisted thoracic surgery)
This is keyhole surgery used to look into the thoracic cavity.

Postoperative care for respiratory surgical interventions
- For thoracotomy and lobectomy the patient will have closed chest drainage to drain air and blood that may accumulate.
- For pneumonectomy the patient may initially have a clamped chest tube. Take care to ensure that the patient is not positioned on the affected side after a pneumonectomy as doing so can place pressure on bronchial stump incision line.
- Perform a full respiratory assessment 2-hourly.
- Provide care for the chest tube and drainage system.
- Perform a pain assessment.
- Reposition the patient 2-hourly to promote optimal comfort.
- Encourage deep breathing exercises 2-hourly.
- Assist with coughing and dispose of secretions.
- Assist with passive arm and shoulder movements on operative side twice every 4 hours in first 24 hours, then 10 times every 2 hours.
- Encourage expression of feelings and concerns and provide support.

Key points when caring for chest drains

- Regularly monitor and check that the patient is comfortable.
- Ensure that the chest tubes are not kinked or causing any unnecessary discomfort.
- Teach the patient about the care of the tubes and their purpose.
- Check that the tubes have not been trapped.
- Encourage mobilization, regular deep breathing, and coughing to promote pleural drainage.
- Clamp tubes only if the bottles need changing.
- The end of the longest tube in the bottle should be about 4–5 cm under water. Observe for bubbling.
- Check drainage carefully and accurately document the amount.
- Secure tubing and be careful that bottles are not damaged or knocked over.
- Check position of tubes by chest x-ray.
- The chest drains should always be kept below the level of the patient's chest to prevent siphoning.

Respiratory equipment

Inhalers

- *Metered-dose inhalers (MDI)* deliver drug directly into the lung when the device is activated on inspiration. Side effects are reduced as only a small amount of drug enters the general circulation.
- *Breath actuated inhalers (BAI)* are similar to MDIs but a slow inspiration triggers the device to release the drug. May be simpler to use than MDI.
- *Dry powder inhalers (DPI)* are activated by a deep breath. These were designed as an alternative to MDI.
- Spacers can be added to an MDI if possible. These are useful for patients who find it difficult to simultaneously press the device while inhaling. They may also be beneficial to those who find the propellant causes irritation or that the cold blast inhibits inhalation.

Humidifiers

A variety of humidifiers are available to prevent drying of the mucous membranes with oxygen therapy.

- Connect the humidifier to the oxygen flow meter according to the manufacturer's instructions. When flow is turned on it should produce a fine mist.
- Ensure the patient is comfortable and teach them about the system.
- Water often collects in the tubing and should be emptied regularly. Use only sterile water in the humidifier.
- Do not send the humidifying system home because of the concern of transporting highly resistant hospital organisms into the community.
- Establish a strict cleaning system.

Nebulizers

A nebulizer is a device for turning a drug solution into a mist of fine particles that may be inhaled by a patient directly into the lungs. It is driven either from an electronic compressor or from a flow meter that delivers high flow (>8 litres) oxygen or air. Patients experiencing an acute exacerbation of asthma should use oxygen-driven nebulizers. Patients with COPD should use air-driven nebulizers. The medication is added to the nebulizer pot. The face mask is placed on the patient after the base has been screwed back. Mouthpieces may be used. Drugs such as bronchodilators can be administered using a nebulizer.

Pulse oximetry

Pulse oximetry measures oxyhaemoglobin saturation. A sensor is placed on the patient's finger, toe, or ear lobe, and a beam of infrared light detects the level of saturation. Nail varnish, if present, should be removed prior to taking a measurement as this affects the reading displayed. Oximetry can detect desaturation before clinical signs are apparent. Conditions that affect the measurement include hypothermia, decreased peripheral circulation, and oedema. With some of these conditions a measurement may not be obtained. Normal pulse oximetry measurement is 95–100%; in elderly patients the measurement may be slightly lower.

How to use an MDI inhaler correctly

- Remove cap and shake the inhaler according to instructions.
- Tilt head slightly and breathe out fully.
- Place the mouthpiece into the mouth.
- On inspiration press down firmly on the canister to release a dose of medication.
- Breathe in slowly over 3–5 seconds.
- Hold breath for about 10 seconds allowing medication to be retained in the lungs, and then breathe out slowly.
- Wait at least 1 minute between puffs.
- Replace the cap.
- Clean the plastic mouthpiece regularly using warm water.
- Advise patient to rinse mouth after use of inhaler to prevent medication build-up on the tongue and soreness to the tongue and mouth.

How to use an inhaler with a spacer

- Remove cap and shake the inhaler according to instructions.
- Place the mouthpiece of the inhaler into the non-mouthpiece of the spacer.
- Place mouthpiece of spacer into the mouth.
- Press down firmly on the canister of the inhaler to release the medication into the spacer.
- Breathe using one of the following methods:
  - Breathe in slowly and deeply. Remove mouthpiece and hold breath for 10 seconds, and then breathe out slowly.
  - Breathe in and out slowly five times, keeping lips around mouthpiece of spacer.
- Wait at least 1 minute between puffs.
- Replace the cap on the inhaler.
- Clean both items regularly in the same way as above.

Respiratory nursing interventions

Early symptoms of respiratory disease may often be ignored by the public. Nurses should encourage individuals and families to seek proper medical attention if they have symptoms such as cough, difficulty in breathing, production of sputum, shortness of breath, and nose and throat problems that do not subside within 2–3 weeks.

Smoking cessation

Smoking cessation must be encouraged. Specialist counsellors and nurses are now available to help patients stop smoking. They assess the possible reasons why the individual is smoking and try to identify key factors which may help the patient stop. Promoting a healthy lifestyle is not easy, especially in some groups of young people such as teenage girls who see smoking as a way to stay slim and remain part of a specific group of friends.

Nicotine replacement therapy (NRT)

Nicotine replacement therapy allows short and medium-term nicotine withdrawal symptoms to be minimized by replacing the nicotine. Individuals who are still smoking should not use NRT as it is possible to overdose on nicotine. Possible symptoms of nicotine overdose include agitation, confusion, restlessness, palpitations, hypertension, dilated pupils, abdominal cramps, and vomiting.

Patches

Small amounts of nicotine can be administered via a transdermal patch that is applied to the patient's skin. Patches come in high and medium strength and nicotine is absorbed through the skin. They should be used for up to 8 weeks.

Chewing gum

Various strengths of nicotine chewing gum can be used depending upon individual need. When the mouth tingles and has a peppery taste, patients should stop chewing and 'park' the gum inside the cheek to allow absorption of the nicotine across the oral mucosa. Patients should be discouraged from drinking while chewing. Some patients may suffer from nausea.

Other forms of NRT and non-NRT therapies for smoking cessation

Other forms of NRT include sublingual tablets, lozenges, inhalers, and nasal sprays. Non-nicotine replacement includes drugs such as bupropion, hypnosis, and acupuncture/acupressure.

Useful contacts for smoking cessation

Action on Smoking and Health (ASH) 0207739 5902
NHS Smoking helpline 0800 169 0 169
Quit Helpline 0800 00 22 00

Nutrition and exercise

Patients should be encouraged to consume adequate amounts of fish oils, fresh fruit, and vegetables. Obese patients should be encouraged to lose weight and should be referred to a specialist obesity clinic. The nurse should support the patient's weight loss efforts. Those patients who are very underweight should be referred to a dietitian for assessment and dietary advice.

Keeping fit maintains muscle bulk and improves the efficiency of oxygen consumption. Exercise is critical to maintaining lung function. Many people stop exercising when they feel breathless, which leads to poorer fitness and increased energy to perform the same tasks. Thus a vicious cycle of breathlessness, lack of exercise, deconditioning, and demotivation continues. Whatever the person's age, exercise is essential.

Psychological considerations

Patients who experience breathlessness may have high levels of anxiety and depression. Moreover, patients may have low levels of self-esteem due to their poor fitness, inactivity, and demotivation. They may experience anger, guilt, and denial. Their quality of life may be poor and their relationships damaged. Family and friends may be unsympathetic to the difficulties experienced by the patient because they believe that the patient is responsible for their own problems. Therefore, many of the nurse's interventions are centred on psychosocial assessment and psychological help. Once adequate oxygenation is established, assessment of previous coping mechanisms is helpful in planning nursing care to alleviate anxiety or panic. Patients with a history of claustrophobia, panic disorder, bipolar disease, and depression have greater difficulty in tolerating the interventions commonly used in the treatment of acute respiratory failure, e.g. mechanical ventilation, suctioning, or oxygen masks.

Nursing patients with acute respiratory conditions

- Monitor vital signs, especially breathing pattern and respirations.
- Encourage oral fluid intake of 2–3 l/day with strict fluid balance monitoring.
- Encourage rest.
- If a bronchodilator is prescribed, teach the patient how to use an inhaler with a spacer. If a dry powder device is being used, check that the patient is using it correctly.
- If the patient is unable to clear their own airway, provide help if needed, e.g. suction.
- Assist with nebulizer therapy.
- Help the patient with prescribed therapy and medications.
- Recognize that antibiotics are usually not prescribed unless there is evidence of bacterial infection.
- Assist the patient to cough effectively.
- Help the patient with activities of daily living.
- Encourage good postural drainage and air intake by appropriate technique and positioning.
- Change the patient's position 2-hourly. Patients may find it helpful to put their head and arms on a pillow placed on an over-bed table.
- Some patients may breathe best when sitting up in a large armchair.
- Most patients prefer cool air that is not too humid.
- Inform patients that hand washing and the use of alcoholic gels are the most effective way to prevent spread of infections.
- Handle sputum carefully.
- Document and record nursing interventions and patient's progress.

Collaborative management in respiratory care
- Pulmonary health care teams consist of physicians, nurses, therapists, social workers, and psychologists working together across the continuum of care from home through outpatients, emergency situations, and the community.
- Treatment and nursing care are guided by the individual needs of the patient in consultation with the health care team.

Ventilated patients
- This is a specialist area of care usually on an ICU. For more information see the specialist nursing texts.
- If a patient has been ventilated because of a respiratory problem, they will need careful weaning. This can only be done with involvement of the patient, the respiratory therapist, a physician, and the nursing staff.
- The patient is particularly vulnerable in the first 48 hours after long-term ventilation. Weaning problems include respiratory muscle fatigue, laryngoedema, aspiration, and anxiety or panic.

Noninvasive ventilation
- This can be used on the hospital ward.
- Pressure support for ventilation is delivered through a tightly fitting facemask.
- Improves the clearance of carbon dioxide and respiratory acidosis.
- Can be claustrophobic and uncomfortable so patients may require a lot of reassurance and encouragement.
- Patients can have short breaks for eating and drinking but should sleep with the ventilator on.
- As the facemask must fit tightly, it can cause pressure areas on the nose.
- If the patient is vomiting, the face mask should be removed as there is a risk of aspiration.

Continuous positive airway pressure (CPAP)
- May be used as a treatment for sleep apnoea with simple air driven machines and a tightly fitting face mask or nasal mask.
- Should be worn for sleep as much as possible.
- These machines are not suitable for acutely ill patients as they do not allow adequate oxygen supplementation.
- High flow CPAP systems are available which are oxygen driven and are used to treat acute pulmonary oedema. These patients usually require a high dependency environment.

Nursing patients with chronic respiratory conditions

- Teach the patient to slow their respiratory rate and to breathe slowly and rhythmically.
- Patients with a 'purse-lipped' breathing pattern should not be discouraged from breathing like this.
- Discourage the patient from taking large gulps of air.
- Teach the patient to increase inspiratory/expiratory ratio so that expiration takes twice as long as inhalation.
- Teach pursed-lip breathing if necessary.
- Teach the forward-leaning position for exhalation.
- Teach abdominal breathing and leg-raising exercises.
- Administer oxygen therapy according to medical prescription and teach the patient about the system that will be used for self-administration at home.
- Monitor arterial blood gases.
- Encourage the patient to report signs and symptoms of hypoxaemia, respiratory problems, headache, irritability, confusion, and tachycardia. If hypercapnia is developing, patients may become confused and drowsy.
- Review the patient's medication concordance and evaluate their self-administration or their carer's concordance with timing and administration of medicines.
- Help with postural drainage and physiotherapy exercises where appropriate.
- Monitor and assess the patient's nutrition and dietary intake.
- Counsel the patient and/or carer to select foods that provide a high-protein high-calorie diet (keep in mind that weight may be a problem in chronic respiratory conditions—some COPD patients, and those with sleep apnoea).
- Consider financial status and ethnic background when planning meals.
- Encourage the patient to avoid readmissions for infections by avoiding large crowds in known cold and influenza periods.
- Encourage hand washing and general infection control.
- Teach the patient to identify early signs of any problems and the importance of contacting medical help or nursing advice.
- Encourage the patient to talk about anxiety and fears with nurse and family members.
- Encourage regular vaccination against influenza and pneumococcal infections (pneumococcal once only, influenza annual).

Home nursing and respiratory care

Because of the progressive nature of the disease, the aim of treatment and care is not curative, but a reduction in symptoms.

- Reassess the patient in their home setting as needs change over time.
- Encourage patient and carer/family involvement in their assessment.
- Continue empathetic approach to smoking cessation.
- Review medications, inhalers, spacers, and suitability for nebulizer use.
- Check any over-the-counter medications and effects on prescribed drugs.
- Continue to encourage vaccination against influenza and pneumococcal disease.
- Review tendency to osteoporosis and effective treatments.
- Perform pulse oximetry and review the amount of oxygen required at home.
- Continue to emphasize advice on oxygen safety, usage, and storage.
- Treat exacerbations of chronic respiratory disease at home, if possible.
- Treat breathlessness with relaxation and physiotherapy. Involve occupational therapists.
- Reassess patient for home aids and help with daily living activities.
- Counsel the patient and encourage them to express any anxiety and depression related to illness.
- Review nutrition and diet.
- Determine whether sexuality and relationships with their partner need to be discussed further with a specialist.
- Review the patient's social support networks and links into the local community.
- Recognize that palliative care eventually becomes important for patients with chronic respiratory disease.
- Criteria for referral of exacerbations of COPD to hospital are[1]:
  - Cyanosis
  - Severe peripheral oedema
  - Severe breathlessness
  - Impaired consciousness
  - Rapid deterioration
  - Inability to cope at home
  - Long-term oxygen therapy
  - Poor physical function
  - No carer or inability of carer to cope

---

1 Scullion J (2004). 'Nursing and respiratory care at home', in Garrod R (ed) *Pulmonary rehabilitation: an interdisciplinary approach*, p.102. Whurr, London.

Pulmonary rehabilitation

'...is a multidisciplinary continuum of services directed to persons with pulmonary disease and their families, usually by an interdisciplinary team of specialists, with the goal of achieving and maintaining the individual's maximum level of independence and functioning in the community.'[2] It consists of:

- reducing dyspnoea
- increasing exercise tolerance
- improving functional performance
- increasing muscle endurance (peripheral and respiratory)
- improving muscle strength (peripheral and respiratory)
- ensuring long-term commitment to exercise
- helping to allay patient fear and anxiety
- increasing knowledge of lung condition and promoting self-management
- patient education and self-care or care by an informed carer
- reducing the reliance on drugs such as steroids and oxygen therapy.

The team involved in this process includes specialist respiratory nurses who monitor the patient's progress at home and liaise with community staff. They may work to and adapt special respiratory care plans and pathways for patients and coordinate many of the aspects of multidisciplinary care. Community physiotherapists may visit the patients at home as may occupational therapists. Many GPs are now developing close links with local health and exercise gymnasiums to encourage people with respiratory problems to take supervised and monitored exercise. They are also encouraging such patients to keep up with regular health checks and immunizations. Special equipment and the use of oxygen at home can be provided as long as the person is taught how to use it and to follow the safety guidelines. Psychological, financial, and social help may be provided by clinical psychologists and social workers. There is also an ever-increasing number of voluntary groups concerned with people with respiratory problems.

2 Cole TM, Fishman AP (1994). 'Workshop on pulmonary rehabilitation research: a commentary'. *Am J Phys Med Rehab*, **73**, 132–133.

Common drugs used for respiratory disorders

Common drugs used for respiratory disorders are listed in Table 6.2. **All drug doses listed in this table are adult doses and not children's doses**. This table is only to be used as a guide and the current BNF should be consulted for further advice. Nurses should involve themselves only in the administration of medications which fall within their sphere of competence.

Table 6.2 Common drugs used for respiratory disorders

Cough suppressants	Dose	Common side effects
Codeine linctus BP (15 mg in 5 mL)	5–10 mL 3–4 times daily	Constipation; possible sputum retention; in high doses may cause dependence and respiratory depression; others noted with high dose include excitement, convulsions, drowsiness, confusion
Pholcodine linctus BP (5 mg in 5 mL)	5–10 mL 3–4 times daily	As above

Expectorants	Dose	Common side effects
Simple linctus	5 mL 3–4 times daily	

Systemic nasal decongestants: 🕮 Table 14.3 Common drugs used for nose, throat, and mouth conditions, p.548.

Adrenoreceptor agonists	NB all inhalers below refer to aerosol metered dose inhalers (MDI), not dry powder inhalers	
Salbutamol	Aerosol inhaler 100–200 mcg up to 4 times daily	Fine tremor (particularly hands), nervous tension, headache, muscle cramps, palpitations, tachycardia, arrhythmias, peripheral vasodilatation
	Oral 4 mg 3–4 times daily (elderly and sensitive patients initially 2 mg)	
Salmeterol	Asthma dose: aerosol inhaler 50–100 mcg twice daily	As above but with potential for paradoxical bronchospasm (calling for discontinuation and alternative therapy)
	Chronic obstructive pulmonary disease: inhaler 50 mcg twice daily	
Terbutaline	Dry powder inhaler 500 mcg up to 4 times daily	As for salbutamol
	Oral initially 2.5 mg 3 times daily for 1–2 weeks, then up to 5 mg 3 times daily	

Table 6.2 Common drugs used for respiratory disorders *(continued)*

Antimuscarinic bronchodilators	Dose	Common side effects
Ipratropium bromide	Inhaler 20–40 mcg 3–4 times daily	Dry mouth, nausea, constipation and headache; tachycardia and atrial fibrillation also reported

Theophyllines	Dose	Common side effects
Theophylline	Dose depends on the product used. It is important that the product used achieves a plasma concentration of 10–20 mg/l (55–110 µmol/l) since there is a narrow margin between therapeutic and toxic dose. Due to different bioavailability of different products patient must maintain the same brand	Tachycardia, palpitations, nausea and other gastrointestinal disturbances, headache, central nervous system stimulation, insomnia, arrhythmias, convulsions
Aminophylline	As for theophylline but dose in obese patients should be calculated on the basis of ideal weight for height	As for theophylline

Corticosteroids	Dose	Common side effects
Beclometasone	Inhaler—various doses used according to product selected and patient condition (See BNF for details) NB preparation must be used regularly	Hoarseness and candidiasis of the mouth and throat; high doses and long-term use have the potential to induce adrenal suppression, reduce bone mineral density, and increase risk of glaucoma; potential for paradoxical bronchospasm (calling for discontinuation and alternative therapy)
Budesonide	As above	As above
Fluticasone	Inhaler 100–250 mcg twice daily up to a maximum of 1 mg twice daily	As above

Antihistamines	Dose	Common side effects
Chlorphenamine	4 mg every 4–6 hours (orally)	Drowsiness, headache, psycho-motor impairment and antimuscarinic effects such as urinary retention, dry mouth, blurred vision, and gastrointestinal disturbances

Table 6.2 Common drugs used for respiratory disorders *(continued)*

Antihistamines	Dose	Common side effects
Cetirizine	10 mg daily or 5 mg twice daily	As above but incidence of sedation and antimuscarinic effects low
Loratadine	10 mg daily	As above but incidence of sedation and antimuscarinic effects low
Drugs used in cystic fibrosis	**Dose**	**Common side effects**
Pancreatin (various preparations)	Dosage adjusted according to size, number, and consistency of stools	Nausea, vomiting, and abdominal discomfort; can cause irritation of perioral skin, buccal mucosa, and perianal skin
Carbocisteine	Initially 750 mg 3 times daily, then 1.5 g daily in divided dose as condition improves	Occasional gastrointestinal irritation or bleeding, rashes
Dornase Alfa	By jet nebulizer—2500 units (2.5 mg) once daily (patients >21 may benefit from twice daily dosage)	Pharyngitis, voice changes, chest pain

Drugs for pulmonary embolism: 📖 Table 7.1, Common drugs used for cardiovascular disorders: anticoagulants, p.199–200.

Drugs for respiratory infections 📖 Table 20.1, Common drugs used for infectious diseases, p.728.

Drugs for lung cancer 📖 Table 25.6, Common drugs used for cancer care, p.854.

Drugs used for pleural effusion and pneumothorax: see local hospital guidelines.

Nursing patients with cardiovascular problems

Introduction

Heart and circulatory disease, known as cardiovascular disease, include disorders of the heart and blood vessels. All nurses, whether hospital or community based, are likely to encounter patients with cardiovascular disease. Cardiovascular symptoms account for a significant number of patient problems. With the increasing likelihood of patients having multiple pathologies, nurses working with *all* client groups must be able to accurately assess patients with potential cardiovascular symptoms and make appropriate decisions about their care.

Risk factors for cardiovascular disease

Risk factors are multifactorial. Widely accepted risk factors include:
- Male >45 years
- Female >55 years
- Cigarette smoking
- Raised serum LDL-C and/or low HDL-C (☐ Chapter 39, Cardiac tests, p.1178)
- Raised levels of plasma homocysteine (an amino acid which is influenced by diet and genetic factors)
- Hypertension
- Diabetes, metabolic syndrome
- Family history of premature cardiovascular disease
- Clotting abnormalities
- Lack of exercise/physical inactivity
- Diet high in saturated fat
- Obesity

Nursing assessment of patients with cardiovascular problems

The cardiovascular nursing assessment begins with an immediate overview of the patient's circulation and any significant factors that may be affecting the forces involved, i.e. the haemodynamic state. Urgent cardiovascular problems such as severe chest pain, breathing difficulties, cyanosis, or altered blood pressure and pulse due to significantly reduced cardiac output (arrhythmia, heart failure) must be identified. Much can be gained from focused questioning and informed observation, even before any tests are undertaken.

Immediate priorities

The order and content of immediate priorities will depend on the individual patient's clinical need. It is important to remember that effective treatment for an acute myocardial infarction (reperfusion therapy) is dependent on the treatment being initiated early, ideally within 60 minutes of the onset of symptoms. Therefore, the initial assessment should be brief and focused.

- Check the airway, breathing, and circulation. 📖 Chapter 33, Use of the ABCDE principles in the emergency department, p.1098.
- Assess for altered mental state (e.g. moribund, agitated), the presence of pain or discomfort, shortness of breath, and sweaty or clammy skin. Note, not all patients will have classic symptoms.
- Talk to the patient to evaluate their physical and emotional state. Focus initially on characteristics of the chief complaint (e.g. chest pain, palpitations, shortness of breath) including location, description, severity, time of onset, precipitating factors, relieving factors, time of onset, and previous experience of similar symptoms. Then move on to a detailed history.
- Assess the patient's response and coping style (e.g. anxiety, denial, anger).
- Ensure that the patient knows to report any new symptoms or worsening of existing symptoms.
- Assess and record the patient's vital signs (heart rate, respiratory rate, blood pressure, temperature) and note any recent changes. Changes may occur as a result of pain, anxiety, heart failure, anoxia, and certain medications.
  - Heart rate and rhythm – normal is a regular beat at a rate of 60–100 per minute.
  - Respiratory rate, rhythm, and quality – normal is the ability to hold a conversation without shortness of breath and to breathe comfortably at a rate of 14–20 times per minute. Observe for pain associated with breathing, productive sputum, cough, and wheezing.
  - Blood pressure – may be high if the patient is in pain, may be low if the patient has reduced cardiac output following myocardial infarction.
  - Temperature – a rise in temperature (pyrexia) usually indicates infection. Myocardial necrosis can produce low grade pyrexia in patients with myocardial infarction.
  - If the patient is acutely unwell or is haemodynamically unstable, consider cardiac monitoring to constantly record heart rate and rhythm. Establish venous access.

- Record a 12-lead ECG. 📖 Electrocardiogram (12-lead ECG), p.144.
- Undertake pulse oximetry to give an indication of the oxygen carrying capacity of the blood (i.e. percentage of haemoglobin saturated with oxygen). A saturation of over 95% corresponds to a normal PaO_2 of 60 mmHg.
- Manually assess the radial arterial pulse noting the regularity, rhythm, and rate. For patients with an irregular heart rate, auscultate the apical rate of the heart at the apex for a full minute while simultaneously palpating the radial pulse.
- Consider a central venous pressure (CVP) recording which is a direct measure of venous pressure and gives a guide to right heart function. Measurement is useful to estimate the patient's fluid status and act as a guide to fluid replacement and other treatment. The normal range is 4–10 cm H_2O or 0–8 mmHg. The CVP rises in fluid overload and falls in decreased circulatory volume.
- Consider a pulmonary artery catheter which is an invasive measure of the functioning of the left side of the heart used in acute and unstable patients.
- Refer to the section on vascular disorders for assessment of the systemic vascular system. 📖 Vascular disease: overview, p.176.

History taking

History is usually taken by a physician and supported by the nurse's observations and questions. More recently, specialist and advanced nurse practitioners have been involved.

- Do not overburden the patient who has just been admitted or is unwell; collect further information later.
- If the patient is unable to give a history, interview relatives, friends, and carers.
- Keep history taking precise, concise, and to the point.
- Establish details of past medical history (particularly cardiovascular history), family history, social factors, and medication history.
- Note any recent changes in symptoms, exercise capacity, or need for medication.
- Ask about chest pain, shortness of breath, anxiety, stress, vomiting, trauma, palpitations, and syncope.
- Assess risk factors for cardiovascular disease and the possible implications for the patient's treatment, recovery, and secondary prevention.
- Note which cardiovascular risk factors are modifiable (e.g. smoking, diet, exercise) and are non-modifiable (e.g. age, sex, ethnicity).
- Determine the patient's level of understanding of their health.
- Collect information from the patient while observing them and performing a physical examination.
- Consider a discussion on advanced directives to establish resuscitation status.
- Consider the nursing implications of the information collected.

Patient observation

- Observe for signs that the patient is experiencing pain or discomfort, e.g. body posture, facial expression.
- Observe for any breathlessness on talking and exertion. Dyspnoea is one of the most common and distressing symptoms of cardiovascular disease.
- Observe the patient's body build, skin condition, chest symmetry, and chest movement.
- Note any observable evidence of risk factors, e.g. obesity, stained fingers from smoking.
- Observe for xanthelasma (fatty deposits around the eyes) and corneal arcus (a white ring surrounding the cornea) which suggest hyperlipidaemia.
- Note any scars from previous cardiovascular surgery.
- Assess skin tightness, temperature, and colour including colour around the nail beds and mouth. Peripheral cyanosis is related to decreased perfusion and is seen in the cool exposed extremities, nail beds, and nose.
- Look for oedema in feet, legs, and sacral area. Oedema indicates poor circulation and fluid overload. Apply firm pressure with the ball of the thumb or index and middle finger for at least 5 seconds, release, and observe whether finger imprint remains for a short while – pitting oedema.
- Observe limbs for any signs of vascular disease or diabetic changes.
- Observe the ends of the fingers for a rounded and bulbous end which is known as clubbing. Finger clubbing indicates chronic hypoxia, possibly as a result of chronic heart disease.
- Observe for small tender nodules on finger or toe pads (Osler's nodes) which are indicative of congestive heart failure.
- Record height and weight in order to calculate the body mass index (BMI = weight in kg/height in m^2 – the patient is classed as obese if BMI >30 kg/m^2). Calculate the hip-to-waist ratio. The waist circumference is now considered a more accurate method of obesity than the BMI and should be measured between the lowest rib and the iliac crest while the patient is breathing out. If the waist in men is over 102 cm or 88 cm in women, the person is at risk for diabetes and CVD. It is recommended that individuals aim for a BMI of 20–25 kg/m^2 and avoid central obesity.
- Examine the lower limbs carefully for signs of swelling and skin breakdown.
- Perform urinalysis to evaluate renal impairment, infection, and diabetes.

Physical examination

Physical examination follows patient observation and is performed by those who are experienced in more advanced assessment skills.

- Inspect, palpate, and listen to the heart sounds (auscultation) (See Fig. 7.1). Heart sounds are produced by movement of the vascular walls, blood flow, heart muscle, and valves.

- Observe for distended external jugular veins in the neck. The jugular venous pressure gives some indication about the function of the right heart and is measured by observing the number of centimeters above the sternal angle that venous pulsations can be seen when the patient is lying supine at an angle of approximately 45°.
- Inspect, palpate, percuss, and auscultate the chest as cardiovascular disorders are often linked to respiratory problems.
- Measure the capillary refill time to assess fluid status. Refill times in excess of 3 seconds indicate a significant fluid deficit.
- If impaired peripheral circulation is suspected, evaluate the ulnar, brachial, femoral, popliteal, dorsalis pedis, and posterior tibial arterial pulses bilaterally for rate, rhythm, and volume (See Fig. 7.2).

   Peripheral venous disease, p.184 provides further details of specific peripheral vascular circulatory assessment.

Laboratory tests

Laboratory tests that are a useful component of the cardiac assessment include:

- Serum U&E (high/low potassium can lead to arrhythmias), liver function tests, and FBC
- Blood gases to assess acid-base status
- Biochemical cardiac markers (serum troponins) in suspected acute coronary syndrome
- Lipid profile (total cholesterol, triglycerides, and HDL-cholesterol)
- Plasma glucose
- D-dimer assay to screen for deep vein thrombosis

   Chapter 39, Cardiac tests, p.1178.

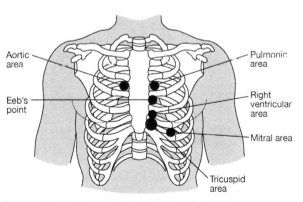

Fig. 7.1 Areas of myocardial inspection, palpation, and auscultation.

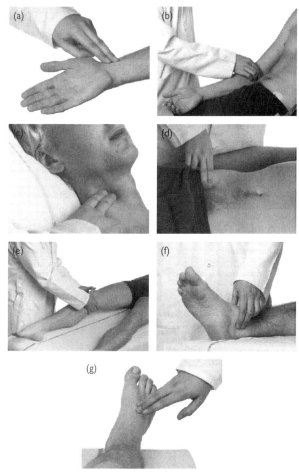

Fig. 7.2 Palpation of the peripheral pulses. (a) The radial pulse. (b) The brachial pulse. (c) The carotid pulse. (d) The femoral pulse. (e) The popliteal pulse. (f) The posterior tibial pulse. (g) The dorsalis pedis pulse. Taken from Thomas J and Monaghan T (2007). *Oxford Handbook of Clinical Examination and Practical Skills*, Oxford University Press. Reproduced with permission from Oxford University Press.

Investigations for diagnosing and monitoring cardiac conditions

📖 Vascular disease: overview, p.176 provides information regarding assessment of vascular disease.

Chest x-ray

A chest x-ray shows heart shape and size, lung vessel changes, and interstitial oedema. Radiographic findings usually correlate well with haemodynamic status although there may be a time lag because it takes some time for pulmonary oedema to accumulate to a level that can be seen on x-ray. Portable x-rays that are taken on unstable bedbound patients produce an anterior-posterior (front-to-back) view which tends to magnify thoracic structures. These x-rays are not as accurate as the posterior-anterior (back-to-front) film which allows better observation of the lung bases and provides a more accurate depiction of heart size.

Electrocardiography

Electrocardiogram (12-lead ECG)

A 12-lead ECG records the electrical activity that initiates myocardial contraction. The spread of electricity through the heart (conduction) is detected by small electrodes that are connected to each limb and across the chest. This electrical activity is then converted into a graphical representation that shows 12 electrical views (known as leads) of the heart on special paper (See Fig. 7.3). The ECG can identify a reduced blood supply to the myocardium (ischaemia) and myocardial necrosis (infarction) (See Fig. 7.4a). It can also identify rhythm, rate, and conduction disorders (See Fig. 7.4b, and Fig. 7.4c).

- Inform the patient of what to expect during the procedure.
- Reassure the patient of its safe and painless nature.

Cardiac monitoring

Self-adhesive electrodes (usually three) are fixed to the skin of the patient's chest to allow cardiac electrical activity from one lead (usually lead 1) to be detected and conveyed to a monitor for visual display. Continuous monitoring of cardiac rate and rhythm allows changes to be identified promptly, effects of therapy to be monitored, and problems to be anticipated. Monitors are now sophisticated and incorporate computers that detect and interpret arrhythmias and the shape of the ECG complex. Radiotelemetry, which allows patients more freedom of movement, is useful for patients who are able to mobilize.

- Ensure skin site is clean and dry before applying electrodes.
- Check frequently and ask patient to report any allergy to electrodes.
- Assist with activities as necessary if movement is restricted.

Stress testing—exercise tolerance testing (ETT)

Stress testing is commonly used to assess the heart's response to increased demand. It is used to diagnose coronary artery disease, determine functional capacity, and assess prognosis. The heart is monitored under increasing aerobic stress that is induced either pharmacologically or, more commonly, with exercise (exercise tolerance testing, ETT). During ETT, aerobic stress is induced by stair climbing, a treadmill, or bicycle. The patient's baseline ECG, blood pressure, and heart rate are compared before and fter graduated exercise. Ensure patient is wearing appropriate clothing and footwear to be able to undertake the ETT.

Ambulatory ECG monitoring

The patient wears an ECG recorder while carrying out usual activities for a period of 24 hours. Continuous ECG monitoring is used to record paroxysmal symptoms associated with arrhythmias and conduction defects that may not be picked up by a standard ECG. The patient keeps a diary and records any symptoms which are later matched with the ECG trace.

Implantable loop recorder (ILR)

A small recording playback device is used to monitor and record unexplained dizziness, syncope, and heart rhythm irregularities. It is introduced under the skin at the left side of the chest wall under local anaesthetic and can provide cardiac surveillance on a loop recording for up to one year or longer. The recording can be activated by the patient or by relatives using a hand-held activator. The ILR stores ECG recordings before, during, and after a cardiac event for later review.

Echocardiography

Echocardiography is a two-dimensional ultrasound picture of the heart. It is used to diagnose and monitor cardiac conditions and is particularly useful during rapid clinical deterioration in myocardial infarction. It is also useful for detecting defects in the septum. A hand-held transducer is placed on the patient's chest. The transducer picks up sound waves (echoes) that are reflected from various parts of the heart through electro-conductive jelly that is rubbed onto the skin. A recording device is connected to the transducer so that the reflected sound waves are converted into images and displayed on a screen (See Fig. 7.5). This test can detect conditions such as valve disease and heart failure.

Doppler echocardiography

Doppler echocardiography is used to evaluate the direction of blood flow, turbulence, and velocity by measuring echoes reflected from red blood cells as they move towards the transducer. It is useful for evaluating valvular stenosis or regurgitation and for measuring variation in flow and pressure (gradients) within the heart and great vessels.

Transoesophageal echocardiography (TOE)

This procedure uses a two-dimensional transducer on the end of a flexible endoscope, which is introduced into the oesophagus. The procedure can be performed with or without sedation. Because the oesophagus, and therefore the transducer, is close to the cardiac structures, superior images of the aorta, heart, and atria can be obtained.

- Help explain the procedure to the patient and ensure the physician has gained the patient's consent. The patient should be nil by mouth 4–6 hours prior to the procedure.
- During the TOE cardiac monitoring, ensure that oral suction, oxygen administration, and pulse oximetry are available.
- Following the procedure, sit the patient up or lie them on one side, encourage them to cough, slowly introduce drinks, and give sore throat lozenges, if required.
- Patients may be drowsy following the procedure and should be carefully monitored and observed to maintain a safe environment.

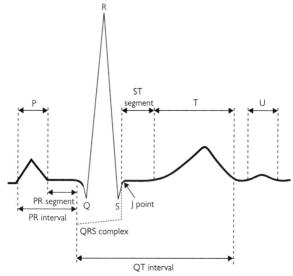

Fig. 7.3 Normal ECG pattern.

- P wave is associated with atrial electrical activation.
- PR interval is measured from the beginning of the P wave to the beginning of the QRS complex. This interval represents the spread of electrical conduction (depolarization) from the SA node, through the atrial muscle and the AV node. (Normally 0.12–0.2 s = 3–5 small squares.)
- QRS complex represents electrical activity of the ventricles. (Normally less than 0.12 s = 3 small squares.)
- ST segment represents the end of ventricular activity and the beginning of ventricular recovery or repolarization.
- T wave represents ventricular recovery/repolarization.
- QT interval represents ventricular depolarization and repolarization.
- U wave (not always seen) represents the recovery period of the Purkinje or ventricular fibres.

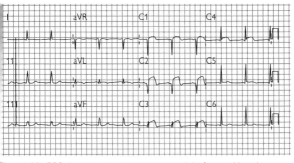

Fig. 7.4 (a) ECG showing an acute anterior myocardial infarction. Note the marked ST segment elevation and evolving Q waves in leads $V_1–V_4$. Taken from Longmore M and Wilkinson IB (2004). *Oxford Handbook of Clinical Medicine*, 6th edn, pp.102–4. Oxford University Press, Oxford. Reproduced with permission from Oxford University Press.

NB This patient would need to be assessed for appropriateness for reperfusion therapy as well as assessment for pain and haemodynamic stability.

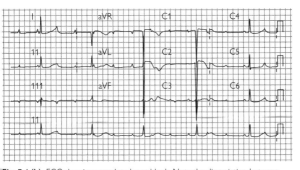

Fig. 7.4 (b) ECG showing complete heart block. Note the dissociation between the P waves and the QRS complexes. Taken from Longmore M and Wilkinson IB (2004). *Oxford Handbook of Clinical Medicine*, 6th edn, pp.102–4. Oxford University Press, Oxford. Reproduced with permission from Oxford University Press. The significance of complete heart block depends on the ventricular rate and resulting cardiac output. Monitor vital signs. Treatment, if required, involves increasing the ventricular rate through cardiac pacing.

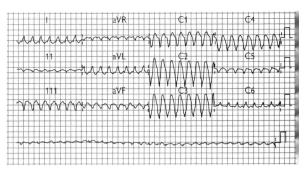

Fig. 7.4 (c) ECG showing ventricular tachycardia. Note the broad complexes.
NB The significance for the patient depends on the cardiac output. Monitor vital
signs. The patient may range from being haemodynamically stable to being in cardiac
arrest. In the cardiac arrest situation, perform airway, breathing, circulation check
(📖 Chapter 33, Use of the ABCDE principles in the emergency department, p.1080.)
Taken from Longmore M and Wilkinson IB (2004). *Oxford Handbook of Clinical
Medicine*, 6th edn, pp.102–4. Oxford University Press, Oxford. Reproduced with
permission from Oxford University Press.

Provocation tests

Provocation tests are used to identify arrhythmias thought to be produced
by problems with the electrical functioning of the conduction system. An
anti-arrhythmic drug (e.g. flecanide or adenosine) is given intravenously
under closely monitored conditions with resuscitation equipment nearby
as there is a risk of inducing potential life-threatening arrhythmia during
the procedure.

Cardiac catheterization

Cardiac catheterization is a generic term used to refer to percutaneous
insertion of a fine, flexible, radio-opaque catheter into one or more of the
heart chambers. The procedure can be used to visualize the heart chambers and valves by means of a radio-opaque substance under x-ray control
(referred to as **angiography**).

This invasive procedure usually requires sedation, requires a sterile
environment, and is usually performed in a catheterization laboratory.
The procedure can confirm the presence of a clinically suspected heart
condition, such as coronary artery disease, ventricular wall ischaemia
caused by infarction, or mitral and aortic valve incompetence/disease.
It can also identify abnormal cardiac anatomy and physiology and, in
appropriate cases, can be used to perform therapeutic procedures.
Cardiac catheterization is usually performed via the femoral artery,
although the radial and brachial approach can also be used. The test takes
about 30 minutes and is frequently carried out as a day case.
• The procedure can cause anxiety and mild sedatives may be prescribed
  for the patient. The patient and relatives should be fully informed of the
  procedure and informed consent should be obtained from the patient.

- Patients must be nil by mouth for at least 4 hours (except for prescribed medication as instructed by the clinician).
- Patients receiving anticoagulants, such as warfarin, may be instructed to discontinue these 1–3 days before the procedure.
- Intravenous hydration may be required before the procedure and continued afterward.
- When the catheters are removed, the arterial entry site must be sealed. This is either done by applying firm pressure to the site for about 15 minutes to allow the blood vessel to seal or by using self sealing vascular closure devices which remove the need for manual compression. The access site needs to be observed for haematoma, swelling, and pain.
- There will be an initial period of bed rest after the procedure followed by staged mobilization. The timing of mobilization post procedure depends on the method used to close the entry wound and local protocols. Therefore, the practitioner must be familiar with the protocol for their local area.
- Vital signs should be recorded according to the institutional protocol.
- Peripheral pulses below the access site should be monitored with observations of colour, sensation, and capillary refill.
- Where femoral access is used, patients should be reminded not to bend the limb to minimize bruising.
- For patients undergoing angiography, oral fluids should be encouraged to facilitate contrast dye excretion.

Electrophysiological studies (EPS)

EPS is a test that maps the electrical conduction system of the heart. Special wires are placed in the heart (via cardiac catheterization) to record electrical activity and to induce arrhythmias in a controlled situation. The test is used to assess arrhythmias, to identify abnormal patterns of conduction, and to monitor the effectiveness of treatments. The test takes 1–4 hours. Monitoring cardiac function via telemetry/cardiac monitor is advised post-procedure. The post-procedure management is similar to cardiac catheterization.

Radionuclide myocardial perfusion imaging

Radionuclide myocardial perfusion imaging is a noninvasive method of assessing myocardial perfusion by intravenous injection of a radioisotope (usually thallium or technetium). The isotope, which becomes distributed throughout the myocardium in proportion to blood flow, is observed through a gamma camera. The test can provide useful information on coronary artery blood flow, ventricular size, and ventricular wall movement.

Magnetic resonance imaging (MRI)

Magnetic resonance imaging uses powerful magnetic field and radiofrequency pulses to obtain images of internal structures. This test can be used to image various cardiac abnormalities. The patient will be expected to lie flat for about 60 minutes in a small tube-like structure. Advise patient to void before the test. MRI is not appropriate for patients with implanted cardiac pacemakers and defibrillators.

Positive emission tomography (PET)

Positive emission tomography is a scanning technique used to quantify cellular biological activity. It is useful for determining myocardial viability and for distinguishing among normal, infracted, and hibernating myocardium.

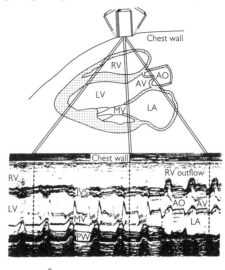

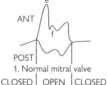

1. Normal mitral valve
CLOSED | OPEN | CLOSED

2. Mitral stenosis
• reduced e–f slope

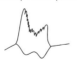

3. Aortic regurgitation
• fluttering of ant. leaflet

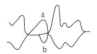

4. (a) Systolic anterior leaflet movement (SAM) in HOCM
(b) Mitral valve prolapse (late systole)

Fig. 7.5 Normal M-mode echocardiogram (RV = right ventricle; LV = left ventricle; AO = aorta; AV = aortic valve; LA = left atrium; MV = mitral valve; PW = posterior wall of LV; IVS = interventricular septum; HOCM = hypertrophic obstructive cardiomyopathy). Reproduced from Oxford Handbook of Clinical Medicine 7th edition, 2007. After R. Hall *Med International* **17**: 774.

Cardiac disorders

Acute coronary syndrome

Acute coronary syndrome is an umbrella term for a range of manifestations of coronary heart disease, all of which involve rupture of an atheromatous plaque within a coronary artery, followed by complete or partial blockage of that artery. The term covers unstable angina, non ST elevation myocardial infarction, and ST elevation myocardial infarction. 🔲 Myocardial infarction, below, includes an explanation of these terms.

Stable angina

Angina is chest pain or discomfort (e.g. pressure, heaviness, tightness, or squeezing) that occurs in patients with coronary heart disease. With stable angina the symptoms have a regular pattern and are relatively constant and are usually seen with exertion. The discomfort or pain experienced results from a transient, reversible episode of inadequate coronary circulation. This is caused by an imbalance between the amount of oxygen reaching the heart muscle/myocardium (i.e. supply) and the amount of oxygen the myocardial cells need to function (i.e. demand). A reduced blood supply usually results from arterial narrowing due to atherosclerosis (development of fatty streaks in the arterial wall followed by deposition of an atherosclerotic fibrous plaque which, as it grows, impedes blood flow). Increased demand is associated with physical or emotional exertion. An episode of angina typically lasts 2–5 minutes. Diagnosis is usually confirmed by ECG, exercise tolerance test, and cardiac catheterization. Treatment involves health education, support, and medication including nitrates (including glyceryl trinitrate, GTN), beta blockers, calcium channel blockers, statins, and antiplatelets (aspirin). 🔲 Medications commonly used in cardiovascular disorders, pp.192–201.

Unstable angina

In unstable angina there is often an unstable atheromatous plaque within a coronary artery. Patients experience increasing episodes of angina symptoms that may begin to occur while they are at rest. The symptoms are not relieved by usual amounts of GTN. Patients with unstable angina are potentially at risk of myocardial infarction if the artery blocks off completely. These patients must be medically assessed promptly. Distinguishing between unstable angina and myocardial infarction in the acute setting is often dependent on ECG changes and serum troponin levels. Management is based on the patient's risk of problems. Treatment includes symptom relief (🔲 Common cardiac conditions, p.168), anti-angina medication, and restoring adequate blood flow to the myocardium (i.e. revascularization), which may involve angioplasty, stenting, or coronary artery bypass grafting.

Myocardial infarction (MI)

The term myocardial infarction, also known as a heart attack or a coronary thrombosis, refers to necrosis of a portion of the myocardium. It is usually the result of a blood clot (thrombus) that blocks all or part of a coronary artery. Management options are now divided into two categories based on whether there is ST elevation on the ECG tracing (See Fig. 7.4a).

Management of both categories of MI should be undertaken in a specialized cardiac setting where patients can be closely monitored and life-threatening complications treated.

Immediate care includes:
- ECG monitoring (cardiac monitor and 12-lead ECG)
- Regular observations
- Bed rest

Management involves:
- Symptom relief (□ Common cardiac conditions, p.168)
- Reduction in oxygen demand by rest and beta blockers
- Alteration of early physiological changes using ACE inhibitors
- Secondary prevention involving aspirin, clopidogrel, and a statin (□ Medications commonly used in cardiovascular disorders, pp.192–201)

Long-term medical management includes:
- Education
- Psychological support
- Lifestyle moderation
- Referral to a cardiac rehabilitation programme

Non ST elevation MI (non STEMI) – Troponin testing is positive which indicates some myocardial damage.

ST elevation MI (STEMI, See Fig. 7.4a) – Total blockage of a coronary artery results in muscle damage to the myocardium, but in contrast to non-STEMI, ST is elevated on the ECG. Troponin testing is positive. Restoring blood flow to the damaged myocardium (reperfusion) is an important part of treatment but must be initiated as soon as possible for it to be effective. Patients therefore need to be in contact with health professionals and assessed early. Reperfusion can involve intravenous drug therapy (thrombolysis) which dissolves the blood clot to restore blood flow or angioplasty which mechanically widens the artery by pushing back the atherosclerotic deposits.

Arrhythmia: overview

Arrhythmia results from disorders of the heart's electrical conduction system. It may be caused by the electrical impulse starting somewhere other than the sinus node, which is the normal cardiac pacemaker, or by the electrical impulse following an abnormal route through the heart muscle. Arrhythmia can lead to significant alterations in the dynamics of the cardiac output and can also lead to clot (thrombus) formation. The patient with arrhythmia may experience a range of symptoms including chest pain, shortness of breath, lightheadedness, reduced exercise tolerance, and palpitations (an awareness of the heart beat). The diagnosis of arrhythmia is made from the patient history, physical symptoms and examination, and ECG.

The heart rate may be abnormally fast (tachycardia) or slow (bradycardia).

- *Bradycardia* – Heart rate is <60 bpm. This rate is normal for athletes and those on beta blocker therapy. If the individual has no symptoms, treatment is not indicated.
- *Tachycardia* – Heart rate is >100 bpm. This rate occurs with exercise, infection, pain, and blood loss. The urgency of treatment depends on the symptoms.

Significant disorders of impulse formation include atrial flutter, atrial fibrillation, and ventricular tachycardia (See Fig. 7.4c).

- *Atrial flutter* – Characterized by rapid but usually regular atrial contraction >200 bpm with a characteristic 'saw tooth' pattern. This is a stable rhythm that can progress to atrial fibrillation and should be reverted back to normal sinus rhythm by drug therapy or electrical cardioversion. 📖 Arrhythmia: treatment, p.156.
- *Atrial fibrillation* – Characterized by an irregular, often rapid, heart rate. There are no P waves on the ECG. This is the most common arrhythmia encountered in clinical practice. Many patients live with chronic atrial fibrillation. Treatment depends on the ventricular rate, haemodynamic state, and the risk of clot formation (thrombi).
- *Ventricular tachycardia* – Characterized by widened QRS complexes occurring at a (usually regular) rate between 120 and 250 bpm (See Fig. 7.4c). It is a potentially serious arrhythmia as it can produce shock, cardiac arrest, and can progress to ventricular fibrillation. Choice of treatment depends on the haemodynamic consequences for the patient.

Disturbances of impulse conduction are referred to as heart blocks (See Fig. 7.4b).

- *Heart block* – The most clinically relevant disruptions to conduction occur at the atrioventricular (AV) junction and the intraventricular conduction system (bundle branches) (See Fig. 7.6). Treatment is aimed at restoring normal rhythm. Compete heart block (See Fig. 7.4b) requires pacemaker insertion (📖 Arrhythmia: treatment, p.156) to increase ventricular rate and improve cardiac output.

(a)

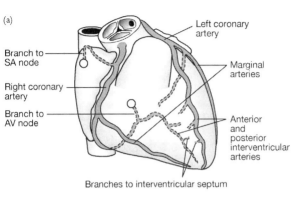

Left coronary artery

Branch to SA node

Right coronary artery

Branch to AV node

Marginal arteries

Anterior and posterior interventricular arteries

Branches to interventricular septum

(b)

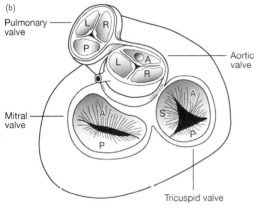

Pulmonary valve

Mitral valve

Aortic valve

Tricuspid valve

Fig. 7.6 Diagrams of heart showing (a) position of coronary arteries and (b) position of valves. Taken from Mackinnon P and Morris J (2005). *Oxford Textbook of Functional Anatomy*, vol 2, Fig 5.4.12, Fig 5.4.10, Oxford University Press, Oxford. Reproduced with permission from Oxford University Press.

Arrhythmia: treatment

Drug therapy

Aimed at reverting to normal sinus rhythm and/or maximizing cardiac output. 📖 Medications commonly used in cardiovascular disorders pp.192–201.

Cardioversion

Involves applying a predetermined energy current (electric shock) externally across the chest via pads or paddles. The energy current stimulates most of the cardiac cells, allowing an opportunity for the sinus node to resume its role as the pacemaker. Patients who are conscious should be lightly anaesthetized or sedated for this procedure.

Cardiac pacing

Involves placing a pulse generator either externally or internally. Internal pulse generators are implanted in a subcutaneous pocket between the skin and the chest muscles. Impulses from the pacemaker are generated at a set rate or at a rate that corresponds to the patient's own heart rhythm i.e. on demand. If pacing is necessary to manage an emergency or is necessary for only a short time (temporary pacing), an external power source is used to deliver electricity to the heart either through chest pads applied to the chest, through the venous system, or via the oesophagus.

Permanent pacemakers

Used when long-term control of the heart rhythm is necessary. This type of pacemaker is a small metal unit that weighs between 23 and 30 g and is implanted under local anaesthetic. Permanent pacemakers can have electrodes that stimulate the atrium, the ventricles, or both chambers of the heart (See Fig. 7.7).

Pre-procedure
• Perform clinical observations and possibly IV antibiotics.
• Discuss with the patient the need for the pacemaker, the type of device, and implications for after care and recovery.
• Ensure consent has been obtained.

Post-procedure
• Perform clinical observations (blood pressure, pulse, temperature, oxygen saturation). Cardiac monitoring will reveal whether the pacemaker is sensing the patient's own heart rhythm, generating an electrical impulse, and stimulating the myocardium.
• Perform wound check (for transvenous and permanent pacemakers). Observe for swelling, redness, and discharge.
• Administer IV antibiotics.
• Assess pain and give analgesics.

Pre-discharge
- Pacemaker check is carried out by a cardiology technician.
- Chest x-ray is obtained.
- Education and information about living with the device is provided to patient and family/carers. Patients should be taught how to take their own pulse and how to recognize signs of pacemaker malfunction, i.e. lethargy, faintness, chest pain, shortness of breath, sudden weight gain, or puffy ankles.
- Patients should carry pacemaker identity cards.
- Ensure that patients understand that pacemakers can trigger off alarms or metal detectors at airports.

Internal cardioverter defibrillator (ICD)

Used for patients who have survived, or who are at risk of, a life-threatening arrhythmic event. This battery operated device is implanted in the subcutaneous cavity of the chest. It monitors heart rate, initiates pacing and cardioversion/defibrillation, and records action taken. Patients selected for this treatment require thorough individualized preparation and ongoing psychological support and education.

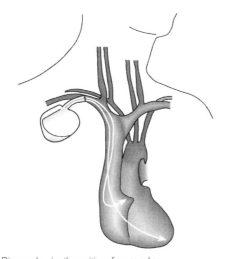

Fig. 7.7 Diagram showing the position of a pacemaker.

Catheter ablation therapy

This involves applying high radiofrequency energy via a temperature controlled cardiac catheter to concentrated areas of myocardium to cause localized cell damage and destroy the site of origin of the arrhythmia.

Heart failure: overview

Heart failure is the inability of the heart to pump enough blood through the venous and arterial circulation to meet the body's metabolic needs. The term congestive failure is sometimes used for ineffective heart pumping. Heart failure may involve the right or left ventricle either independently or together.

Left ventricle failure – Failure of the left heart (ventricle) causes an accumulation of blood in the left ventricle and atria causing congestion (pulmonary oedema) in the lungs.

Right ventricle failure – Failure of the right heart (ventricular) prevents deoxygenated blood from being transferred effectively to the pulmonary (lung) circulation. The deoxygenated blood accumulates in the body with corresponding systemic symptoms.

Causes
- Coronary heart disease
- Cardiac valve disease
- Arrhythmia
- Chronic hypertension
- Cardiac myopathy
- Certain drugs (beta blockers, anti-arrhythmics, and alcohol)

Symptoms
- Shortness of breath, particularly on exertion or when lying flat
- Exercise limitation
- Fatigue
- Ankle swelling, i.e. oedema
- Weight gain
- Palpitations

Investigations
- Clinical history
- Patient observation and physical assessment
- Echocardiogram
- Chest x-ray
- ECG
- Blood tests: U&E, LFTs, thyroid function tests and FBC
- Cardiopulmonary exercise testing

Treatment
Noninvasive treatments
- Oxygen therapy, to improve myocardial contractility
- Rest and activity management to reduce cardiac workload
- Medication to improve cardiac function and reduce accumulation of fluid

Invasive treatments
- Intra-aortic balloon pump
- Valve replacement or repair
- Revascularization
- Implantable cardiac defibrillator (ICD)
- Pacemaker (biventricular pacing)
- Cardiac transplantation

Lifestyle changes
- Smoking cessation
- Reduced alcohol intake
- Reduced salt and fat intake
- Exercise
- Flu jab
- Adherence to drug therapy
- Symptom monitoring

Heart failure: innate causes

Congenital heart defects in adults

Congenital heart defects are abnormalities of the heart or major blood vessels caused by abnormal development *in utero*. As more children with such problems are surviving into adulthood, it is becoming more common to see these defects in adults. Some of the commonest defects are a bicuspid aortic valve, coarctation of the aorta, atrial septal defect (ASD), ventricular septal defect (VSD), patent ductus arteriosus (PDA), and transposition of the great arteries (TGA). These patients require medical investigations, monitoring, and ongoing support. Some patients will require treatment for heart failure and arrhythmia. In some cases, patients will require invasive treatments, including surgery.

Coarctation of the aorta

This is narrowing of the descending aorta which can be severe. It can occur anywhere in the aorta but usually occurs just distal to the origin of the left subclavian artery. There is a significant obstruction of the blood flow from the heart, and blood pressure differs in upper limbs to lower. Sometimes this disorder is not diagnosed until adulthood. This defect is treated with balloon dilatation or stent insertion. Aneurysms at the site of the narrowing may require surgery.

Atrial septal defect (ASD)

ASD occurs when the septum between the right and left atria, which is normally open in the fetus, fails to close resulting in the recirculation of blood via the pulmonary circulation. Oxygenated blood in the left atrium passes into the right atrium. This defect is treated by closing the hole by a device or surgery.

Ventricular septal defect (VSD)

VSD is a hole in the septum between the ventricles that often closes spontaneously or closes during childhood. If the defect remains, it results in left to right shunting and pulmonary hypertension (Eisenmenger syndrome). This defect is treated by closing the hole by a device or surgery. Regular venesection may be required.

Patent ductus arteriosus (PDA)

PDA occurs when the fetal shunt fails to close after birth, resulting in recirculation of oxygenated blood through the lungs. This results in left ventricular hypertrophy and cardiac failure. This defect is treated by closing the duct by a device or surgery, and most patients will have been treated in childhood.

Transposition of the great arteries (TGA)

TGA occurs when the aorta branches off the right ventricle rather than the left and therefore pumps deoxygenated blood through the body. The pulmonary artery branches off the left ventricle rather than the right and returns oxygenated blood to the lungs. This results in severe cyanosis, congestive heart failure, and an enlarged heart. For survival, surgery (switch operation) must be performed in the first weeks of life to allow some oxygenated blood into the systemic circulation. Additional surgeries are required later.

Marfan syndrome

Marfan syndrome is an inherited multisystem disorder of the connective tissue that affects several parts of the body including the heart, heart valves, and aorta. Patients often present with aortic dissection or with aortic aneurism, valve disease, and heart failure. There are several implications of this syndrome including long-term management, psychological support, and future health of close relatives.

Heart failure: acquired causes

Cardiogenic shock

Cardiac output falls due to ineffective cardiac pumping. This is often the result of heart muscle damage following a heart attack. It can also occur with a ruptured mitral valve, ventricular aneurism, large pulmonary emboli, cardiac surgery, and cardiac tamponade (fluid in the pericardial sac pressing on the heart). Symptoms include low blood pressure, increased heart rate, reduced urine output, cold peripheries, and altered mental state. The patient may experience chest pain and shortness of breath. The prognosis is poor.

Treatment
Medical management focuses on improving ventricular function and limiting the size of heart muscle damage if the patient has had a heart attack. Echocardiography can show the cause of the problem. Intra-aortic balloon pumping, thrombolysis, and emergency cardiac catheterization and angioplasty are treatment options. Haemodynamic monitoring is useful to monitor the effects of therapy.

Nursing care
Patients in cardiogenic shock will require intense nursing care. They will require oxygen and may require intubation and positive pressure ventilation. Monitor vital signs, talk to patient and try to keep them calm, catheterize for accurate urine measurement, and administer intravenous inotropes (dopamine/adrenaline) as prescribed. Assist with activities of living and pressure area care. Keep relatives involved and informed.

Valve disorders

Valve disorders occur most often in the left-sided valves (aortic and mitral). These disorders are caused by degenerative changes, congenital problems, rheumatic fever, infective endocarditis, or inflammatory disorders. Symptoms include tiredness, dizziness, syncope, angina, and shortness of breath, and are managed by drug therapy. Patients require prophylactic antibiotic cover for dental and surgical procedures to prevent endocarditis, which will be defined by specialist nurses or medics.
Regurgitation occurs if the valve does not close sufficiently to prevent a backflow of blood from one chamber to the next. Surgery may be required to repair or replace the valve.
Stenosis is a narrowing of the valve orifice due to scar tissue formation. Aortic stenosis is the most common. Valvuloplasty, an invasive procedure, may be necessary to open up the stenotic valve. In some cases surgery is required to replace the valve.

Cardiomyopathy

This is a term that describes diseases of the myocardium associated with cardiac dysfunction. Cardiomyopathy is subdivided into three categories:
- *Dilated*—occasionally caused by inflammation of the myocardium (myocarditis)
- *Hypertrophic*—frequently inherited
- *Restrictive*—least common

Cardiomyopathy often results in left ventricular hypertrophy where the left ventricle becomes enlarged or abnormally thickened and is unable to contract efficiently to maintain cardiac output. It is also associated with conduction disturbances. Cardiomyopathy tends to progress to terminal heart failure. Because of its distressing impact on quality of life, patients and their families will need individual support. Depending on the type of cardiomyopathy, treatment is usually by anti-arrhythmics and anticoagulants.

Infective endocarditis

This occurs when blood-borne micro-organisms colonize the inner endocardial surface of the heart and valves causing tissue destruction. Micro-organisms adhere to the damaged endocardium (known as vegetation). Infective endocarditis can be caused by invasive dental treatment or intravenous drug use where the bacteria are introduced into the blood stream. Symptoms include fever, lethargy, and weight loss. Treatment includes prolonged antibiotic therapy and occasionally surgery.

Rheumatic fever

Rheumatic fever, an ailment most common in childhood, begins with a streptococcal throat infection and progresses to a systemic inflammatory disorder that affects the body's connective tissue. The heart muscle and valves may be affected. Stenosis or insufficiency (regurgitation) may develop in the valves, resulting in their failure to close properly. If not treated with antibiotics, heart failure may result. Nurse on bed rest and provide analgesia for carditis/arthritis. The incidence of rheumatic fever has decreased significantly over the past 50 years.

Pericarditis

Pericarditis is an inflammatory reaction involving the layers of the pericardium and is often viral in origin. The most common symptom is sharp chest pain that is made worse by inhaling deeply. Treatment includes rest, analgesia, and antipyretic drugs.

Further information

Johnson K and Rawlings-Anderson K (2007). *Oxford handbook of cardiac nursing*. Oxford University Press, Oxford

Cardiac surgery

There are several types of cardiac surgery which vary in severity and risk depending on the patients condition and symptoms. The list includes but is not exclusive to the following:

- *Coronary artery bypass graft (CABG)* – This is a surgical procedure where a graft is taken from the internal mammary artery or saphenous vein in the arm and/or leg and is used to bypass a blocked or narrowed coronary artery.
- *Correction of congenital abnormalities* (📖 Congenital heart defects in adults, p.160) – Congenital abnormalities present at birth, which can be serious and life-threatening, are corrected by a series of surgical operations over the period of the child's growth and development. Surgical correction may also be performed in adulthood, as some congenital conditions are diagnosed in adulthood.
- *Valve repair or replacement* – This is performed for congenital or acquired diseases of the cardiac valves. The diseased valve becomes stenotic or incompetent which directly affects cardiac function and output. If left untreated, the ventricles can become severely damaged and ventricular function impeded.
- *Heart transplant* – This is a major surgical intervention that has emerged as the therapeutic choice for carefully selected patients with chronic end-stage heart failure. The surgery is carried out in a highly specialized cardiac centre. The selection of potential transplant recipients is determined by a multidisciplinary committee to ensure equity, ethical objective, and medically justified allocation of the donor organs to the recipient patient.

Preoperative nursing interventions

- Provide educational and psychological support before surgical intervention. 📖 Education for cardiovascular patients and their families, p.190 and 📖 Psychosocial interventions for cardiovascular patients and their families, p.188.
- Ensure that informed consent is obtained, that the physical examination has been carried out by the cardiac surgical team, and that findings have been documented as the results can significantly influence the postoperative management.
- Perform basal blood tests: U&E, serum calcium, LFTs, plasma glucose, FBC, and coagulation screen. Some centres may request additional tests such as an observation for faecal occult blood so that gastric bleeding can be identified early, thereby limiting the risk of gastric intestinal bleeding postoperatively.
- Prior to surgery, record and document clinical observations to be used as a baseline to detect any deviation from the patient's normal recordings during the perioperative and postoperative phase.
- Omit medications such as anticoagulants and hypertensives only if directly instructed to do so by the cardiac physicians.
- Access the protocol for pre-surgery skin preparations such as the use of topical antibacterial/microbial agents such as chlorhexidine wash and removal of hair from the area of incision (i.e. shaving or using special clippers) as the skin preparation can vary between centres.

Postoperative care

The cardiac surgical patient is likely to initially be cared for in an ITU/HDU environment with support for ventilation and close haemodynamic monitoring. Multiple problems can occur in the postoperative cardiac patient and are best prevented by anticipating likely problems, close observation, and early intervention.

- Monitor vital signs – Blood pressure, pulse, and ECG monitoring and recording must be transitive in order to detect signs of haemodynamic instability/cardiovascular complications and to determine appropriate interventions. Arrhythmias are common in the recovery period. Some patients may require invasive haemodynamic monitoring with a pulmonary artery floatation catheter. Also, observe skin for colour (pallor, cyanosis), sweating, and temperature.
- Monitor for respiratory complications – Observe for rate, depth, ease of breathing, coughing, sputum, oxygen saturation, and changes in mental state.
- Perform wound checks – Observe for swelling at the suture site, redness, and discharge. If any discharge is present collect swabs for microbiology, culture, and sensitivity (MCS) where appropriate to ensure that the correct antibiotic medication is prescribed. Document and report findings. Record temperature regularly.
- Carefully monitor and manage fluid intake and output to prevent cardiac overload or dehydration and monitor diminished urine output for signs of acute renal complications. Where pericardial drains and urinary catheters are still *in situ*, record and document blood loss and urine output.
- Carry out comprehensive pain assessment regularly as uncontrolled pain will affect the patient's ability to deep breathe, expand their lungs, and cough to expectorate. Inability to perform these actives may lead to lung consolidation and chest infection, which will impact the patient's recovery.
- Give analgesics as prescribed and monitor their effects.
- Ensure patients receive appropriate psychological care. This is crucial in all cardiac surgical patients as they can suffer anxiety, depression, grief, and body image disturbance (Chapter 24, Nursing patients with body image problems, p.813). The latter is particularly true of some organ transplant recipients.
- Once the patient is haemodynamically stable, sit the patient out of bed. This can be as early as one day postoperative.
- In an immobile patient, skin breakdown may occur over pressure points. Employ appropriate pressure relieving devices.
- Monitor the patient's nutritional intake closely as this can affect wound healing and recovery. Inadequate nutrition impairs wound healing and postoperative recovery. Inactive or sluggish gut, although temporary, is common in cardiac patients.
- Consult with the dietetics department to ensure nutritional intake is adequate.
- Closely monitor and record elimination of urine and stools. Patients receiving opioids are prone to stool impaction.

- Start physiotherapy referral early to maintain mobility and to prevent and detect cardiovascular and respiratory dysfunction.
- Infection is a risk – make clinical and physical observations for signs of infection/fever and record findings. Maintain asepsis where appropriate. Give antibiotic medication as prescribed and monitor its effects.

Pre-discharge

- Take chest x-ray to ensure that the lungs have re-inflated and that there is no visible evidence of pnemo/haemothorax or ventricular hypertrophy as a postoperative complication. In the case of valve repair or replacement, echocardiogram (📖 Echocardiography, p.145) is required to review function and blood flow through the cardiac valves.
- Some patients may have pacing wires *in situ* postoperatively. Removal of pacing wires must be carried out only after INR and prothrombin time is established as normal to avoid initiation of a cardiac tamponade, which can be caused when removing the pacing wires.
- All sutures should be removed unless instructed otherwise by the surgeon. The patient may be asked to return to an outpatient clinic for removal of remaining sutures or a district nurse referral may be required for this purpose. In the presence of wound complications such as infection, a district nurse referral is essential.
- Ensure that cannula and other invasive lines are removed prior to discharge.
- Refer to cardiac rehabilitation.

Cardiac transplant recipient

- Transplant immunosuppressive drug therapy increases risk of in-hospital nosocomial (or health care acquired) infections. As these infections are complicated further by resistant organisms, most cardiac transplant recipients are discharged within 7–14 days.
- Outpatient follow up is carried out by an experienced transplant team who facilitates education and identifies early signs of rejection, opportunistic infections, patient non-concordance, and adverse reactions to the immunosuppressive therapy.
- The goal of immunosuppressive therapy is to modify the recipient's immune system response to the donor heart and prevent rejection of the transplanted organ. The management of immunosuppressive therapy is a fine balance between sparing the ability of the recipient's immune system to respond to infection and prevent rejection, while minimizing drug toxicity and neoplasms associated with immunosuppressive agents.
- Most centres use a triple-drug regimen consisting of ciclosporin, steroids, and azathioprine. However, this varies across centres.

Common cardiac conditions

Many cardiac disorders produce similar problems. The main ones are discussed below.

Chest pain

- Central chest pain accounts for 20–30% of emergency admissions.
- Cardiac ischaemic pain occurs as a result of an inadequate blood supply to the myocardium and is usually the result of atherosclerosis and blockage of the relevant coronary artery.
- The pain is often described as a band-like tightness around the chest with radiation down the left arm, into the jaw or into the centre of the back. Patients also describe the pain as 'indigestion' or a heavy pressure in the chest area. In fact, the presentation of cardiac chest pain is very individual and the severity of the pain bears little relationship to the underlying pathology.
- A proportion of patients will not experience any chest pain with cardiac ischaemia. This is more likely in elderly and diabetic patients.
- As many as two-thirds of patients with a suspected heart attack will ultimately have a different diagnosis. Differential diagnoses include pulmonary embolism, pneumothorax, chest infection, sternal costochondritis, aortic dissection, and herpes zoster.
- Ask the patient to describe the pain, its frequency, severity, location, radiation, duration, and relieving and aggravating factors.
- A comprehensive assessment of the pain and related symptoms will highlight whether the pain is cardiac or originating from another source. Some patients may experience pleuritic pain that is present on inspiration and/or expiration. This type of pain can be successfully managed with NSAID medication.
- Establish whether the patient has had similar pain and how it has been managed. Has the pattern of pain changed recently? Symptoms such as nausea and vomiting are fairly common in patients with cardiac disorders; anti-emetic medication is advised in managing these symptoms.
- Cardiac chest pain is often associated with shortness of breath, nausea, vomiting, and ashen, cold clammy skin.

Assessment of chest pain should be done as part of an overall cardiovascular assessment. 📖 Nursing assessment of patients with cardiovascular problems, pp.138–412.

Interventions for cardiac pain

- Administer GTN, anti-emetics, aspirin 300 mg and oxygen.
- Perform a 12-lead ECG.
- Talk to the patient and try to keep them calm.
- Sit patient upright.
- If the pain is persistent, inform the medical staff and repeat ECG, establish intravenous access, and prepare to administer morphine (with anti-emetic cover).
- Record vital signs every 15 minutes.
- Consider suitability for reperfusion therapy.

- Educate/support patient to manage chest pain after discharge from hospital.

Out of the hospital setting – If a patient experiences cardiac chest pain that is not relieved by rest and GTN after 15 minutes, advise them to call for an ambulance.

Shortness of breath

- Shortness of breath (dyspnoea) is a common presenting problem in cardiac patients.
- Left ventricular failure is the classic cardiac cause of acute shortness of breath. Pulmonary oedema causes lung rigidity and decreased oxygen transfer which makes breathing more difficult.
- Difficulty in breathing associated with angina may become worse in cold or windy weather.
- Shortness of breath may occur only on exertion or at rest – it may be brought on by the patient sliding down the bed, or not being in an upright position.
- Respiratory assessment is often neglected in cardiac patients. However, changes in respiration can be an early indicator of changes in the patient's condition.
- Assess for rate, rhythm, and ease of breathing. Note associated coughing, wheezing, and sputum production. Record pulse oximetry.

Assessment of respiration should be done as part of an overall cardiovascular assessment. 📖 Nursing assessment of patients with cardiovascular problems, pp.138–41.

Interventions

- Manage associated angina symptoms.
- Encourage patient to sit upright.
- Administer oxygen and diuretic therapy as prescribed.
- Monitor fluid balance and changes in weight.
- Encourage patient to stop smoking and to manage lifestyle within limitations of shortness of breath

Oedema

- Oedema is a relatively late manifestation of heart failure.
- Involves the abnormal accumulation of fluid in the interstitial tissues. The skin classically pits when pressure is applied.
- Oedema will collect preferentially in the tissues of the limb extremities; the distribution of fluid is determined by the mobility of the patient.
- In most patients fluid will collect in the legs and feet, but in bedbound patients it will collect over the sacrum. Greater degrees of oedema will gradually affect the whole of the lower extremities, the torso, and eventually the face.

Interventions

- Regularly assess the extent of oedema and condition of the skin.
- Use pressure relieving mattress and cushions, and give regular attention to pressure area care.
- Monitor fluid balance.

- Urinary catheterization may be necessary; obtain daily weights as this is considered a more accurate indication of a patient's fluid retention.
- Encourage concordance with drug therapy and fluid restriction.
- Monitor electrolytes.
- Elevate limbs.
- Assist with mobility and activities of living.

Reduced exercise capacity

Exercise capacity can be reduced for several reasons including reduced cardiac output, symptoms that limit exercise, and the patient's fear of exercise. Patients should be encouraged to exercise because the heart is a muscle and benefits from regular exercise.

Interventions

- Develop an individualized activity plan that gives the patient realistic targets and support.
- Refer the patient to a cardiac rehabilitation programme that addresses individual disease processes, lifestyle, and risk factors.
- Provide educational and psychosocial support, which is important for all cardiovascular patients. 📖 Education for cardiovascular patients and their families, p.190 and 📖 Psychosocial interventions for cardiovascular patients and their families, p.188.

Pleuritic pain

- Should be investigated as pleural effusions may occur in cardiac failure. O_2 should be provided and resuscitation as necessary, according to the underlying pathology.

Vomiting/nausea

- Is another common symptom which may occur in cardiovascular patients. Observe the amount, colour, old or recent, blood stained, 'coffee grounds', and relationship to eating and drugs. Report to doctor for further investigation and treatment.

Driving considerations for the cardiac patient

In the interests of road safety, those who suffer from a medical condition likely to cause a sudden disabling event at the wheel or who are unable to safely control their vehicle from any other cause should not drive. It is the duty of the licence holder to notify the Driver and Vehicle Licensing Agency (DVLA) of any condition that may affect safe driving.

The DVLA produces regularly updated medical guidelines on fitness to drive. This includes a comprehensive list of cardiovascular conditions indicating whether driving is permitted and whether the DVLA needs to be notified. They also provide guidelines for those that might drive as part of their employment (PSV, LGV, HGV). These guidelines, which only apply to the UK, are available on the DVLA website at www.dvla.gov.uk.

Once the DVLA has been notified, health care professionals must advise the patient about whether it is safe to drive until a full medical review has been considered. From a licensing point of view, drivers do not generally need to notify DVLA unless medical conditions persist for more than 3 months. Guidelines for specific conditions covered in this chapter in relation to entitlement to car driving include:

- Angina – Driving must cease when symptoms occur at rest or at the wheel. The DVLA need not be notified.
- Angioplasty (elective) – Driving must cease for at least 1 week. The DVLA need not be notified.
- CABG – Driving must cease for at least 4 weeks. The DVLA need not be notified.
- Angioplasty (emergency) with non ST elevation MI – Driving may recommence 1 week after successful angioplasty provided there are no other disqualifying conditions. The DVLA need not be notified.
- ST elevation MI – Driving must cease for at least 4 weeks. The DVLA need not be notified.
- Arrhythmia – Driving must cease if likely to cause incapacity and can restart when underlying cause is identified and arrhythmia is controlled for at least 4 weeks. The DVLA need not be notified.
- Heart transplant patients – Driving can continue provided there is no other disqualifying condition. The DVLA need not be notified.
- Thoracic/abdominal aneurysm – Licensing is subject to annual review of satisfactory blood pressure control and no evidence of further enlargement. Patients are disqualified from driving if the aortic diameter is ≥6.5 cm. The DVLA should be notified if the aneurysm is >6 cm.
- Peripheral arterial disease – Driving can continue provided there is no other disqualifying condition. The DVLA need not be notified.
- Syncope – With simple faint there is no restriction on driving. Otherwise notification is advised. Unexplained syncope with low risk of recurrence requires 4 weeks off driving. Syncope with high risk of recurrence requires 4 weeks off driving if the cause is identified and treated, otherwise 6 months off. Patients who have had a single episode of loss of consciousness (no cause found) still need to have at least 1 year off driving.

- Hypertension – Driving may continue unless treatment causes unacceptable side effects. DVLA need not be notified.

Drivers need to be advised to look at the wording of their insurance policies and consult their insurance companies for advice.

Hypertension

Hypertension is included in this section as it is a major risk factor for patients with vascular disease.

Definitions

Hypertension is defined as a consistent elevation of the blood pressure >140/90 mmHg. There are two main categories of hypertension:

- *Essential hypertension* accounts for >90% of cases and the cause is unknown.
- *Secondary hypertension* is caused by conditions such as renal disease, endocrine disease, and rare conditions such as coarctation of the aorta. It can also be raised in normal pregnancy.

Emergency hypertension is a term used to identify severe hypertension: 200 mmHg systolic or 130 mmHg diastolic. Hypertension is also associated with grade III–IV retinopathy.

Risk factors

- Age (primary risk as blood pressure can increase steadily with age)
- Race and culture (e.g. Afro-Caribbeans are more severely affected)
- Hereditary
- Obesity
- Atherosclerosis
- Smoking
- High salt intake
- Excess alcohol use
- Emotional stress

Signs and symptoms

These are usually subtle and only detected on screening or during routine check-ups.

- Headache
- Blurred vision
- Spontaneous nosebleeds

Diagnosis

Many factors can influence blood pressure, especially emotions and stress; therefore diagnosis is never made on a haphazard or single reading. The diagnosis should be based on at least two readings taken under the best conditions available on two subsequent clinic visits. The environment should be relaxed, warm, and quiet with the patient seated with their arm outstretched and supported. Recordings should be taken on both arms and the highest one taken. Record standing blood pressure if a patient reports symptoms of falls or postural dizziness.

If raised blood pressure persists and the patient does not have established cardiovascular disease, they should have their cardiovascular risk formally assessed.

- Blood tests: U&E, serum calcium, fasting lipid profile, thyroid function tests, plasma glucose, and FBC
- ECG
- Urinalysis for blood and protein

Management

Lifestyle interventions

Recommendations for lifestyle interventions should take into account patients' individual needs and preferences.

- Educate patients about their risk factors and encourage ways to help them follow a healthier lifestyle.
- Encourage cardiovascular exercise, such as gym work, sport activities, running, and walking.
- Encourage patients to monitor their pulse and its recovery when exercising.
- Suggest relaxation therapies to help reduce blood pressure.
- Encourage patients to stop smoking.
- Encourage patients to reduce intake of alcohol, caffeine, and salt.
- Suggest an annual review of care to monitor health, provide support, discuss lifestyle, symptoms, and medication.

Medical treatment

Consists of a variety of drugs depending upon the patient's condition.

- Calcium channel blocker or a thiazide type diuretic is usually the first treatment choice for patients >55 years.
- ACE inhibitors or angiotensin II receptor antagonists are used for hypertension.

Nursing interventions

- Monitor the patient's blood pressure.
- Promote lifestyle modifications, relaxation, and a healthy diet.
- Provide psychological support.
- Hypertensive patients may be asymptomatic, and experience side-effects from medications. It is therefore important that patients understand the need to take the medication, otherwise compliance will be poor. Blood pressure should be monitored regularly.

Vascular disease: overview

Vascular disease refers to a spectrum of conditions resulting from disease processes in the arteries, veins, or lymphatic system. Diseases of the arteries and veins can occur alone or together. They are frequently the result of impaired circulation and disturbed blood flow, which results in damage to the muscles and tissues of the extremities.

Risk factors
📖 Risk factors for cardiovascular disease, p.136.

Assessment
The assessment should be conducted with the patient at rest in a warm environment.
- Assess for the '5 Ps': pain, paraesthesia, pallor, paralysis and pulselessness.
- Assess arterial perfusion – compare bilateral brachial blood pressure, capillary refill, and the pulses (posterior tibial, popliteal, and femoral) for presence and volume.
- Assess and record signs of vascular disease in affected limb.
  - Skin colour of the extremities (i.e. red, blue, blotchy)
  - Temperature/coldness
  - Sensation
  - Presence of skin ulceration, hair loss, oedema
  - Severity of pain on walking and at rest
- Observe for evidence of tissue death (gangrene) or decay.
- Assess for pressure sore risk and implement prevention strategy. (These patients are susceptible and the preventive regimen must continue until the patient is sufficiently recovered to no longer be at risk.)
- Obtain height and weight; calculate BMI and hip-to-waist ratio.
- Obtain a detailed history. (📖 History taking, p.139.)
- Perform a cardiovascular risk factor assessment.

Diagnostic tests
- Ankle brachial pressure index (ABPI) – The ratio of the systolic ankle to brachial pressure is measured using a sphygmomanometer and helps differentiate whether the cause of the leg pain is due to arterial disease or other causes.
- Doppler assessment of both limbs.
- X-ray – may show calcification of the arterial walls.
- Hand held doppler ultrasound – Pulse volume recordings will be diminished in arterial occlusion or stenosis.
- Angiography (arteriography) – Radio-opaque dye is injected and x-rays are taken to show lumen of blood vessels.
- Magnetic resonance imaging – Useful for imaging aneurysms.
- Spiral (helical) computed tomography – Continuous rotation of gantry with patient moving through the x-ray beam.
- Colour duplex scanning – Ultrasound is used to show blood velocity in relation to tissue density and boundaries.

- Exercise testing – A treadmill test is used to assess the functional limitations of the limb and to differentiate between occlusive arterial disease and other causes of lower limb symptoms.
- Blood tests: U&E, plasma glucose, and FBC.
- Examination of cardiovascular system – ECG, echocardiogram, and isotope scan will provide evidence of existing CAD.
- Investigation should include assessment for presence of abdominal aortic aneurysm (with a stethoscope) as the cause.
- Coagulation screen and physical assessment of the limb to exclude deep vein thrombosis (DVT). Assessment for sciatica and muscle injury should be performed. Fibrin degradation product, d-Dimer, is used to diagnose DVT.

Vascular disease: types

Atherosclerosis

Definition
Atherosclerosis is a generalized, progressive disease process character-ized by complex changes in the artery wall (intima). An accumulation of fats (lipids), blood products, and fibrous tissue (atheroma) forms into a fibrous 'hardened' plaque that eventually obstructs arterial blood flow (See Fig. 7.8). Over time the atheromatous plaque reduces blood flow in the blood vessel. Sudden occlusion can arise where the plaque ruptures causing bleeding and thrombus formation. Inflammatory processes can mimic the symptoms of atherosclerosis and can be triggered by infective or immune response related processes.

Symptoms
- Lower extremity pain (i.e. pins and needles, sharp throbbing) that ranges from mild to significant and often occurs at rest
- Intermittent claudication (leg pain with physical activity) – pain can present at a fixed distance during walking and comes on more rapidly when walking up a hill than when walking on flat, even surface (the pain usually disappears when standing still)
- Pain in the buttocks or hip which may indicate the presence of disease in the aortic/iliac arteries
- Hair loss distal to occlusion
- Atrophy of skeletal muscle
- Thin, shiny, dry skin
- Skin cool to touch
- Painful ulcers between toes, upper surface of foot, bony prominences
- Weak or absent pulses
- Decreased sensation, particularly if diabetic
- Ischaemic tissue first appears pale, becomes mottled and then dark as the disease progresses
- Reduced muscle group function due to chronic compromised arterial blood supply – reduced ability to flex and extend toes

Acute arterial occlusion
Acute arterial thrombosis or emboli can result in the affected limb becoming acutely ischaemic due to sudden cessation of blood flow. In complete occlusion the skin will be white; however, the skin is more com-monly mottled in appearance. The patient experiences acute ischaemic pain at rest and often will hang the affected leg out of bed to get relief. Tissues will become necrotic if blood flow is not rapidly restored, leaving amputation as the only treatment option.

Peripheral arterial occlusive disease (PAOD)
This describes chronic occlusive atheroma of the large arteries supplying the lower limbs. Smaller arteries become affected as the disease pro-gresses. The condition is associated with intermittent claudication (leg pain with physical activity) that may progress to critical limb ischaemia (rest pain). It occurs in middle aged to elderly men. As blood flow to extremi-ties slows, and skin and muscle atrophy, there is a loss of subcutaneous fat

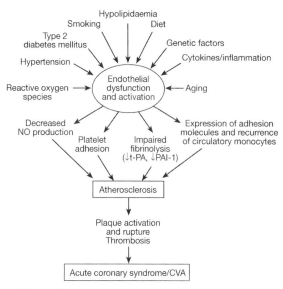

Fig. 7.8 Endothelial dysfunction is the underlying process in atherosclerosis, from lesion initiation, progression, through to acute cardiovascular events. Endothelial dysfunction is caused by a variety of genetic factors (and ageing) as well as environmental factors that can be modified. Taken from Ramrakha P and Hill J (2006). *Oxford Handbook of Cardiology*, Fig 4.1, Oxford University Press, Oxford. Reproduced with permission from Oxford University Press.

deposits, and ischaemic neuropathy and ulceration occur. Severe occlusion results in gangrene. Acute-on-chronic ischaemia can occur as a result of stenosis, occlusion, or worsening stenotic lesion, leading to critical limb ischaemia.

Buerger's disease (thromboangiitis obliterans)

Buerger's disease is an idiopathic chronic occlusive inflammatory disease resulting from acute inflammatory lesions and occlusive thrombosis of the veins and arteries. The disease affects the small and medium vessels, usually of the hands and feet. The presence of inflammation and/or thrombus impedes blood flow which results in ischaemic limb pain. Unlike atherosclerosis this disease is restricted to segments of the arteries and is seen in a younger population than atherosclerosis. It is strongly associated with cigarette smoking, although it is not clear how smoking influences the disease process.

Raynaud's disease

This is blanket terminology used interchangeably to describe episodic spasm or episodes of constriction of the small arteries and arterioles of the extremities such as the hands and feet, causing changes in colour and temperature of the skin in the extremities. The local changes are not necessarily related to the status of the peripheral vascular system as a whole. This disorder predominantly affects women.

Raynaud's phenomenon

Unlike Raynaud's disease, which is bilateral, Raynaud's phenomenon is unilateral and may affect only one or two digits of the extremities and may occur after trauma, e.g. after the use of high speed vibrating tools under conditions of cold. Pain may be present and in some cases function can be lost. Cyanosis may occur; however, the pulses are intact. In severe cases, ulceration and gangrene can occur.

Aneurysms

Aneurysms are localized dilation swelling or protrusion of the arterial wall and are classified according to location and shape. True aneurysms are the commonest and involve all three layers of arterial wall. They may be fusiform or sac-like (e.g. circle of Willis berry aneurysms). False aneurysms (pseudoaneurysms) are collections of blood around the vessel wall (e.g. after trauma) that communicate with the vessel lumen.

Aneurysms commonly occur in the aorta, but can present in any artery of the body. Acknowledged causes are atherosclerotic disease, degenerative processes, and coronary artery disease or vascular disease. Other causes include infection such as syphilis, congenital abnormalities of the vessel, connective tissue disorders such as Marfan's syndrome (📖 Marfan's syndrome, p.161), and iatrogenic (cause unknown) as in dissecting aneurysms, which can occur during pregnancy (although these are rare).

Complications of aneurysms include rupture, thrombosis, embolism, and pressure on other structures.

Aortic aneurysm

- A permanent localized swelling (dilatation) of the aorta (See Fig. 7.9).
- Strongly associated with atherosclerosis and made worse by hypertension.
- Patients may not have any symptoms but may experience shortness of breath, hoarseness, difficulty swallowing, a dry cough, haemoptysis, and pain.
- If the aneurysm splits (dissects) it is a life-threatening emergency characterized by sudden onset of searing pain radiating to the back, neck, and left chest.
- Managed medically with anticoagulation, antihypertensives, and regular check ups.
- Surgical repair is indicated if the aneurism is >5.5 cm.
- Various types of grafts can be used.
- Blood pressure must be lowered prior to surgical repair.
- Surgical intervention can be very successful and the patient's recovery uncomplicated.

- If the aneurism has ruptured, ITU care is required and recovery is longer.
- Death rates from ruptured aortic aneurysms rise with age; 75–95% of patients with ruptured aneurysms will die.

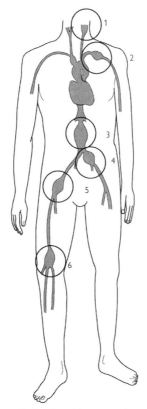

Fig. 7.9 Common anatomic sites of arterial aneurysms: 1 = carotid; 2 = subclavian; 3 = aortic-abdominal; 4 = bifurcation; 5 = femoral; 6 = popliteal. Taken from Al-Khaffaf H and Dorgans S (2005). *Vascular disease: a handbook for nurses*, Cambridge University Press, Cambridge. Copyright with permission from Cambridge University Press.

Vascular disease: management

The nurse must be aware of specific care pathways for each disease process. In general, management is aimed at:
- minimizing symptoms
- preventing vasoconstriction
- managing any other problems associated with underlying disease state, e.g. diabetes.

Medication
- Inter-arterial thrombolysis (clot breakdown)
- Anticoagulants
- Antiplatelet drugs such as clopidogrel as an alternative to aspirin
- Vasodilators
- Lipid lowering agents, e.g. statins
- Antihypertensives

📖 Common drugs used for cardiovascular disorders, pp.192–201.

Other measures
- Encourage and support the patient to stop smoking.
- Encourage exercise up to the limit of pain to maintain joint and muscle function and circulation.
- Provide appropriate pain management. The pain associated with vascular disease is of a chronic and continuous nature. For this reason the patient can become depressed and irritable. Pain should be monitored carefully and managed effectively if the patient is to rest and the symptoms improve.
- Provide patient education regarding the cause and management of their condition.
- Encourage strict control of all cardiovascular risk factors, i.e. managing diabetes, reducing cholesterol, lowering blood pressure, and reducing stress.

Surgical treatment and revascularization
- Percutaneous procedures
  - Percutaneous transluminal angioplasty (PTA)
  - Intraluminal stents
  - Atherectomy (catheter mounted device that rotates and cuts away atheroma from vessel wall)
- Surgical options
  - *Embolectomy/thrombectomy* – Emergency surgical procedure for acute critical limb ischaemia. Performed when thrombolysis is not an option. Thrombus is removed via femoral incision using a balloon catheter. Usually performed under general anaesthetic.
  - *Endarterectomy* – Opening blocked artery and excising atherosclerotic lesion on arterial wall. Risk of emboli breaking away from lesion and causing occlusion.
  - *Reconstructive bypass surgery* – Performed if patient has severe ischaemic rest pain/ulceration/gangrene and is unsuitable for angioplasty. Patient must be suitable for general anaesthetic. Can use vein grafts (saphenous/cephalic) or prosthetic grafts.

Potential complications include haemorrhage from site of anastomosis, wound bleeding, haematoma, graft occlusion, limb pain, reperfusion oedema of limb, chest infection, development of pressure sores, and other complications of reduced mobility.

Lower limb amputation

- Performed for those with irreversible tissue ischaemia.
- Patient and family must be physiologically and psychologically prepared (📖 Psychosocial interventions for cardiovascular patients and their families, p.188), which will involve the multidisciplinary team.
- The level of amputation needs to allow removal of dead tissue and provide a residual limb suitable for prosthesis.
- Postoperative care includes monitoring for haemodynamic stability (blood pressure, pulse, oxygen saturation, respiratory rate, fluid balance), diabetic control, wound care, wound pain management, psychological support, and rehabilitation (including support with mobility, e.g. transfer techniques, use of crutches, adaptation to prosthesis).
- Psychological support for patient and family is important. Patients need support to cope with altered body image.
- Patients need to be aware of the possibility of phantom limb pain and/ or sensation, which is described as crushing or tearing.

📖 Postoperative care, p.165.

Peripheral venous disease

Peripheral venous disease results from venous insufficiency due to an obstruction by a thrombus or thrombophlebitis, or incompetence of valves and veins. It can manifest as an acute or chronic condition.

Symptoms
- Tenderness along the course of an inflamed vein
- Chronic feeling of heaviness/fullness in the affected limb
- Pain that is relieved by limb elevation
- No associated hair loss
- Normal sensation
- Reddish brown skin colour (may be cyanotic)
- Skin mottling
- Warm to touch
- May have oedema (typically foot to calf)
- Normal pulses

Management
Management is disease specific, but options will involve the multidisciplinary team.
- Anticoagulation
- Limb elevation
- Support stockings/appropriate compression hosiery (check adequate arterial blood supply)
- Avoidance of prolonged standing, immobility, dehydration, and knocking limbs
- Pain relief
- Education to encourage control of cardiovascular risk factors, i.e. management of diabetes, reduce cholesterol, lower blood pressure, reduce weight, regular exercise, and healthy diet
- Revascularization
- Sclerotherapy for varicose veins (injecting special sealing fluid into vein emptied by elevation)
- Surgical repair, e.g. skin grafting for ulcers, stripping of veins for varicose veins
- Appropriate wound management
- Skin care strategies to limit damage, optimize healing, and prevent infection

Deep vein thrombosis (DVT)
DVT occurs in 25–50% of surgical patients but also occurs in non-surgical patients, many of whom are asymptomatic. Venous obstruction, reduced blood flow, increased blood viscosity, and endothelial damage predispose to clot formation. Features of DVT include patient immobility, recumbent position, and dehydration. The affected area will be tender, swollen, and hot, accompanied by mild fever and pitting oedema. Risk factors include age, pregnancy, oestrogen, surgery (especially pelvic/orthopaedic), past history of DVT, malignancy, obesity, immobility, recumbent position, dehydration, and thrombophilia. Before commencing anticoagulant therapy thrombophilia tests may be performed if there are no predisposing factors.

Chronic venous insufficiency

High pressure in the venous system as a result of valve failure and/or disease or vein blockage results in increased capillary pressure and chronic oedema develops. Oedema can result in malnutrition to subcutaneous tissue and fibrosis. Patients tend to have a history of DVTs. Blood stasis leads to trapping of red blood cells resulting in red pigmentation of the skin.

Venous ulcers

📖 Chapter 12, Leg ulcers, p.428 addresses arterial ulcers.

A venous ulcer may follow trauma or dermatitis of the affected area. It tends to occur in the lower third of the leg. Skin looks dry, discoloured and scaly. It may be associated with varicose eczema. Ulcers are prone to infection and need regular treatment.

Varicose veins

These are long and tortuously dilated veins. Patients complain of dull ache, cramps, itching, and tingling in legs. Family history is common. Incompetent valves fail to prevent backward flow (See Fig. 7.10). Effects of gravity exacerbate the problem and symptoms become worse after standing for prolonged periods. Predisposing factors include hormonal changes in pregnancy and obesity, smoking, and diet.

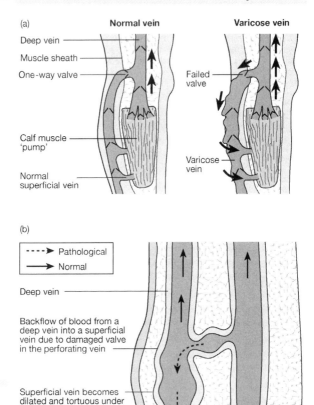

Fig. 7.10 (a) Flow in normal and varicose veins. (b) Homeodynamic changes in varicose veins.

Psychosocial interventions for cardiovascular patients and their families

Being diagnosed with a cardiovascular condition and coping with the consequences of symptoms and treatments can be difficult for many patients and their families. Many patients believe that the heart is the most important organ of the body. Therefore, cardiovascular disease can be a terrifying experience for them and their families, particularly if they must reduce their activities and perceive themselves as an invalid. Anxiety, depression, guilt, denial, anger, hostility, and grief may be experienced to varying degrees at various times. Developing open and trusting relationships with patients and their families will help support them. Referral to a cardiac rehabilitation service or specialist counselling services may be of help to some.

Nursing interventions should be directed toward helping the patient face the adaptive challenges of the illness and treatment, which may include anticipated loss of independence, financial security, or social support systems. Referral to other members of the multidisciplinary team may be necessary.

Pre-treatment period

- Waiting for cardiovascular treatment whether diagnostic, medical, or surgical is often characterized by high levels of anticipation and anxiety. This can be influenced by the seriousness of the diagnosis, treatment and/or pending surgery, pain, the appearance of incisions, and fears of dying.
- It is important to establish the cause of anxiety and discuss it with the patient. Explain the details of any planned tests and interventions including what they are for, alternatives, what is involved, and possible complications. Encourage patients and their family to ask questions.

In-hospital period

- This is a complex and critical period for the patient. The psychological state of the patient will be related to physical care procedures; dependence on others for care; anticipation of pain and discomfort caused by the underlying disorder and treatment; concern for family and work obligations; and fear for the future. Patients are also anxious on moving between clinical areas and on discharge home.
- It is important to encourage patients to express their feelings.
- The effects of sleep deprivation that result from sleeping in an unfamiliar surrounding, in an uncomfortable positioning or bed, and in a noisy environment can lead to dysphoric moods and feelings of depression. The care environment must be relaxed and designed to promote relaxation and sleep.
- Because unmanaged pain can increase levels of anxiety, effective pain management is essential. Denial, often the result of anxiety, can interfere with concordance with treatment.

- Partners and other family members must be included in the support given. It is important that information given to patients is reinforced to their families and friends.
- Misinformation about the patient's condition, overguarded statements, and vague advice about the patient's recovery can greatly contribute to patient and family stress. It can contribute to the fear of discharge and impact the patient and family's ability to rehabilitate following hospitalization. Providing appropriate information is reported to lower patient anxiety levels and enable the relatives and friends to provide greater support for the patient. It also facilitates an atmosphere and sense of trust between the health care professional, patient, and family.
- Worry about death of a partner, social functioning, role change, sexual activity, and quality of life are commonly reported causes of anxiety in partners of patients with cardiovascular disorders. It is important that the health care professionals provide timely information to the patient and partner about how and when to resume sexual activities, and include in the discussion any other significant changes to lifestyle activities including work and occupation.
- With shorter length of hospital stays resulting in patients being discharged with more complex conditions, it is important to perform an assessment of the patient's and family's social needs. Effective plans for discharge need to developed and implemented.

Patients may need advice in relation to returning to work including change in hours or job specifications, re-employment, and retirement options. If financial problems are identified, they should be discussed and the appropriate referral should be made to facilitate assistance and to reduce the patient's level of stress and anxiety.

Education for cardiovascular patients and their families

Educating patients about their illness or disease is a very important part of nursing and should not be rushed. It is helpful to break down the information into smaller more digestible parts to maximize retention of information. It is also important to assess the depth of information each individual patient needs and wants, and to alter the way the information is given accordingly. It may also be advantageous to encourage the patient to invite a relative to be present.

Medication
- Explain how each medication works and what it does.
- Explain when to take the medication.
- Explain special instructions that must be followed, e.g. taking medication with food.
- Describe side effects.

Disease/illness
- Explain what has happened to them.
- Explain what their disease or illness is.
- Explain likely reasons why this has occurred (risk factors).
- Explain any tests or examinations to be carried out while in hospital or as an outpatient.
- Inform the patient about the expected length of hospital stay and plans for follow up.
- Help patient and family sort through the available information about their condition and help them to make informed decisions.
- Explain the causes of body image changes and any phantom pain.
- Teach purpose of exercises and interventions.
- Provide guidelines for pre- and post-procedure care.
- Discuss plans for follow up.

Lifestyle (risk factors)
The original assessment should have identified each patient's individual risk factors.
- Provide education that focuses on identified risk factors, e.g. smoking, drinking, diet, and exercise. For example, explain why smoking has affected them, ask them if they have considered or attempted to stop smoking, and offer smoking cessation classes and support.
- Assess significance of loss to patient and family.
- Encourage patient to verbalize feelings.
- Explain the reasons for the necessary lifestyle changes, such as driving, which may be prohibited. 📖 Driving considerations for the cardiac patient, p.172.

- Provide patients with education, advice, and help that will help them adjust to:
  - Changes in physical ability and activity levels
  - Sexual activity
  - Returning to work
  - Diet and exercise
  - New medications
  - Managing symptoms

Educational material and delivery style (□ Chapter 5, pp.94–95).

- Use a mix of educational material which includes:
  - Leaflets and videos
  - Posters with diagrams
  - Visual aids, e.g. mould of heart showing coronary arteries
- Use simple language (e.g. avoid using medical jargon or complex explanations) or, where necessary, an interpreter to facilitate effective communication.
- Consider the patient's cultural needs and any specific personal factors that may affect their recovery.
- Check the patient's understanding by asking questions.
- Repeat and reinforce information given.

Common drugs used for cardiovascular disorders

Common drugs used for cardiovascular disorders are listed in Table 7.1. **All drug doses listed in this table are adult doses and not children's doses.** This table is only to be used as a guide and the current BNF should be consulted for further advice. Nurses should involve themselves only in the administration of medications which fall within their sphere of competence.

Table 7.1 Common drugs used for cardiovascular disorders

Diuretics	Dose	Common side effects
Bendroflumethiazide	Hypertension: 2.5 mg each morning Oedema: initially 5–10 mg each morning or on alternate days; maintenance dose 5–10 mg 1–3 times a week	Postural hypotension, mild gastrointestinal effects, hypokalaemia, hyponatraemia, hypomagnesaemia, hypercalcaemia, hypochloraemic alkalosis, impotence (reversible on withdrawal of treatment), hyperuricaemia, hyperglycaemia, gout, altered plasma lipid concentration
Metolazone	Hypertension: 5 mg each morning (maintenance 5 mg on alternate days) Oedema: 5–10 mg each morning (20 mg daily in resistant oedema to a maximum of 80 mg)	As above
Furosemide	Oedema: initially 40 mg in the morning; maintenance 20–40 mg daily, increased to 80 mg daily in resistant cases Oliguria: 250 mg daily (increased in steps of 250 mg every 4–6 hours if necessary to a maximum single dose of 2 g – this latter dose is rare)	Hyponatraemia, hypokalaemia, hypomagnesaemia, hypochloraemic alkalosis, increased calcium excretion, hypotension

Table 7.1 Common drugs used for cardiovascular disorders *(continued)*

Potassium-sparing diuretics	Dose	Common side effects
Bumetanide	1 mg each morning, repeated after 6–8 hours if necessary; severe cases 5 mg daily increased by 5 mg every 12–24 hours according to response; in elderly patients, 500 mcg daily may be sufficient	As above; also headache, dizziness, fatigue, gynaecomastia, myalgia
Amiloride	Used alone – 10 mg daily or 5 mg twice daily, adjusted according to response, maximum 20 mg With other diuretics – initially 5–10 mg daily	Gastrointestinal disturbances, dry mouth, rashes, confusion, postural hypotension, hyperkalaemia, hyponatraemia
Spironolactone (i.e. aldosterone antagonist)	100–200 mg daily, increased to 400 mg, if required Much lower doses are used as adjunctive treatment in heart failure (usually 25 mg daily)	Gastrointestinal disturbances, impotence, gynaecomastia, menstrual irregularities, lethargy, headache, confusion, rashes, hyperkalaemia (discontinue), hyponatraemia

Anti-arrhythmic drugs	Dose	Common side effects
Amiodarone	200 mg 3 times daily for 1 week, then 200 mg 2 times daily for 1 week, then 200 mg daily as maintenance or the minimum required to control the arrhythmia (should be initiated in hospital or under specialist supervision)	Nausea, vomiting, taste disturbances, raised serum transaminases (See BNF), jaundice, bradycardia, pulmonary toxicity, tremor, sleep disorders, hyper- or hypothyroidism, reversible corneal microdeposits, phototoxicity, slate-grey skin discoloration
Disopyramide	300–800 mg daily in divided doses	Ventricular tachycardia, ventricular fibrillation or torsades de pointes, myocardial depression, hypotension, AV block, dry mouth, blurred vision, urinary retention, gastrointestinal irritation, psychosis, cholestatic jaundice, hypoglycaemia

Table 7.1 Common drugs used for cardiovascular disorders *(continued)*

Beta-blocker drugs	Dose	Common side effects
Atenolol	Hypertension: 25–50 mg daily Angina: 100 mg daily in 1–2 doses Arrhythmias: 50–100 mg daily	Bradycardia, heart failure, hypotension, conduction disorders, bronchospasm, dyspnoea, headache, peripheral vasoconstriction, gastrointestinal disturbances, fatigue, sleep disturbances, sexual dysfunction
Bisoprolol	Hypertension and angina: 10 mg once daily (max 20 mg daily) As an adjunct in stable moderate to severe heart failure: 1.25 mg each morning for 1 week, then if well tolerated stepped increases up to 5 mg daily, then more slowly up to 10 mg daily	As above
Metoprolol	Hypertension: 100 mg increased if necessary to 200 mg daily in 1–2 divided doses, normal maximum 400 mg daily Angina: 50–100 mg 2–3 times a day Also used in arrhythmias and for migraine prophylaxis (See BNF for dosage schedules)	As above
Propranolol	Hypertension: initially 80 mg twice daily increased at weekly intervals as necessary to a maintenance of 160–320 mg daily Other indications: angina, arrhythmias, hypertrophic obstructive cardiomyopathy, anxiety, tachycardia, thyrotoxicosis, prophylaxis after myocardial infarction, migraine prophylaxis, sweating and tremor; all have doses which vary widely (See BNF)	As above

Table 7.1 Common drugs used for cardiovascular disorders *(continued)*

Alpha-blocker drugs	Dose	Common side effects
Doxazosin	Hypertension: 1 mg daily increased if necessary after 1–2 weeks to 2 mg daily and thereafter to 4 mg daily up to a maximum of 16 mg daily	Postural hypotension, dizziness, vertigo, headache, fatigue, asthenia oedema, sleep disturbance, nausea, rhinitis
Prazosin	Hypertension: 500 mcg 2–3 times a day for 3–7 days (initial dose taken **on retiring to bed,** increased to 1 mg 2–3 times a day for 3–7 days up to a maximum of 20 mg daily in divided doses) Other indications: congestive heart failure, Raynaud's syndrome, and benign prostatic hyperplasia (📖 Table 11.1: Benign prostate disease, p.393) for which varying dosage schedules are used (See BNF)	Postural hypotension, dizziness, weakness, drowsiness, lack of energy, headache, nausea, and palpitation; urinary frequency, incontinence, and priapism also reported

Vasodilator drugs	Dose	Common side effects
Hydralazine	Hypertension: 25–50 mg twice daily Heart failure: (initiated in hospital) 25 mg 3–4 times daily increased every 2 days if necessary to maintenance dose of 50–75 mg 3–4 times daily	Side effects few if dose kept below 100 mg daily but include tachycardia, palpitation, flushing, hypotension, fluid retention, gastrointestinal disturbances, headache, dizziness, systemic lupus erythematosus-like syndrome after long-term therapy with doses over 100 mg daily
Minoxidil	Reserved for severe hypertension; 5 mg (elderly 2.5 mg) daily in 1–2 doses, increased by 5–10 mg every 3 or more days to a maximum of 50 mg daily	Sodium and water retention, weight gain, peripheral oedema, tachycardia, hypertrichosis, reversible rise in creatinine and blood urea nitrogen

Table 7.1 Common drugs used for cardiovascular disorders *(continued)*

Angiotensin-converting enzyme inhibitors	Dose – may need adjustment if diuretic also given (See BNF)	Common side effects – NB Close observation of patient required if diuretic also given (See BNF)
Lisinopril	Hypertension: initially 10 mg daily (2.5–5 mg if used in addition to diuretic or in renal impairment) with usual maintenance dose 20 mg daily Heart failure and prophylaxis post-myocardial infarction: doses vary depending on blood pressure but start low (2.5–5 mg) and are increased gradually to a maintenance dose of 5–20 mg for heart failure and 5 mg for post-myocardial infarction prophylaxis	May cause rapid fall in blood pressure in patients taking diuretics; renal function (i.e. electrolytes) should be monitored before and during treatment; concomitant use of potassium-sparing diuretics increases the risk of hyperkalaemia; other side effects include profound hypotension, renal impairment, persistent dry cough, angioedema, rash, tachycardia, cerebrovascular accident, myocardial infarction, dry mouth, blurred vision, confusion, mood changes, asthenia, sweating, impotence, and alopecia
Ramipril	Hypertension and heart failure: 1.25 mg daily increased at intervals of 1–2 weeks, usual range 2.5–5 mg, maximum 10 mg Prophylaxis after myocardial infarction: started 3–10 days after infarction initially 2.5 mg twice daily increased after 2 days to a maintenance dose of 2.5–5 mg twice daily Prophylaxis of cardiovascular events or stroke: initially 2.5 mg once daily increased after 1 week to 5 mg once daily for 3 weeks, then 10 mg once daily	As above

Table 7.1 Common drugs used for cardiovascular disorders *(continued)*

Angiotensin-II receptor antagonists	Dose	Common side effects
Losartan	50 mg once daily (elderly over 75 years, moderate to severe renal impairment, intravascular volume depletion, initially 25 mg once daily); if necessary increase after several weeks to 100 mg daily	Symptomatic hypotension and dizziness (particularly in patients taking diuretics), hyperkalaemia, angioedema, diarrhoea, taste disturbance, cough, myalgia, asthenia, fatigue, migraine, vertigo, urticaria, pruritus, rash
Nitrates	**Dose**	**Common side effects**
Glyceryl trinitrate	Sublingually 300 µg–1 mg repeated as required	Throbbing headache, flushing, dizziness, postural hypotension, tachycardia (paradoxical bradycardia has also occurred)
Isosorbide mononitrate	Initially 20 mg 2–3 times daily or 40 mg twice daily (10 mg twice daily in those who have not previously received nitrates); up to 120 mg daily in divided doses	As above
Calcium channel blockers	**Dose – NB Different versions of modified-release preparations may not have the same clinical effect; therefore, patients should normally be retained on the same brand**	**Common side effects**
Amlodipine	Hypertension or angina: initially 5 mg once daily, maximum 10 mg once daily	Abdominal pain, nausea, palpitations, flushing, oedema, headache, dizziness, sleep disturbances, fatigue
Diltiazem	Angina: 60 mg 3 times daily (twice daily initially in the elderly) increased if necessary to 360 mg daily	Bradycardia, sino-atrial block, AV block, palpitation, dizziness, hypotension, malaise, asthenia, headache, hot flushes, gastrointestinal disturbances, oedema

Table 7.1 Common drugs used for cardiovascular disorders *(continued)*

Calcium channel blockers	Dose – NB Different versions of modified-release preparations may not have the same clinical effect; therefore, patients should normally be retained on the same brand	Common side effects
Nifedipine	Short-acting forms no longer recommended for angina prophylaxis or hypertension Long-acting preparations – see individual entry in BNF for details	Headache, flushing, dizziness, lethargy, tachycardia, palpitations; short-acting preparations may lead to exaggerated fall in blood pressure and reflex tachycardia which may lead to myocardial or cerebrovascular gravitational oedema ischaemia; many more side effects (See BNF)
Verapamil	By mouth Supraventricular arrhythmias: 40–120 mg 3 times daily Angina: 80–120 mg 3 times daily Hypertension: 240–480 mg daily in 2–3 divided doses NB It may be hazardous to give verapamil and a beta-blocker together by mouth unless myocardial function is known to be well preserved	Constipation, nausea, vomiting, flushing, headache, dizziness, fatigue, and ankle oedema
Peripheral vasodilators	**Dose**	**Common side effects**
Naftidrofuryl	Peripheral vascular disease: 100–200 mg 3 times daily Cerebral vascular disease: 100 mg 3 times daily	Nausea, epigastric pain, rash, hepatitis, and hepatic failure

Table 7.1 Common drugs used for cardiovascular disorders *(continued)*

Anticoagulants	Dose	Common side effects
Heparin (unfractionated)	Treatment of deep vein thrombosis or pulmonary embolism by IV injection: loading dose 5000 units (or 75 units/kg), 10,000 units in severe pulmonary embolism, followed by a continuous infusion of 18 units/kg/hour OR treatment of deep vein thrombosis by SC injection of 15,000 units every 12 hours with haematology monitoring (preferably daily and dose adjusted accordingly)	Haemorrhage, skin necrosis, thrombocytopenia, hyperkalaemia (in certain groups of patients), hypersensitivity reactions, osteoporosis after prolonged use
Low molecular weight (LMW) heparin, e.g. enoxaparin	For enoxaparin: prophylaxis of deep vein thrombosis in medical patients by SC injection 40 mg (4000 units) every 24 hours for at least 6 days until patient ambulant (maximum 14 days) Treatment of deep vein thrombosis or pulmonary embolism by SC injection: 1.5 mg/kg (150 units/kg) every 24 hours for at least 5 days and until oral anticoagulation established Unstable angina and non ST-segment-elevation myocardial infarction by SC injection: 1 mg/kg (100 units/kg) every 12 hours for 2–8 days (minimum 2 days) For other LMW heparins, see BNF	As above

Table 7.1 Common drugs used for cardiovascular disorders *(continued)*

Anticoagulants	Dose	Common side effects
Warfarin	Induction dose 10 mg (less if baseline prothrombin time is prolonged, if liver function tests abnormal, if patient is in cardiac failure, on parenteral feeding, less than average body weight, elderly, or receiving other drugs known to potentiate oral anticoagulants) daily for 2 days (See local protocol)	Haemorrhage, hypersensitivity, rash, alopecia, diarrhoea, drop in haematocrit, 'purple toes', skin necrosis, jaundice, hepatic dysfunction; also nausea, vomiting, and pancreatitis
	Maintenance dose dependent on prothrombin time (expressed as INR) and usually 3–9 mg taken at the same time each day	NB Many drugs interact with warfarin (See BNF Appendix 1)
	See current BNF for more details	

Antiplatelet drugs	Dose	Common side effects
Aspirin	150–300 mg as soon as possible after an ischaemic event preferably given in water or chewed, followed by maintenance of 75 mg daily	Bronchospasm, haemorrhage (mainly gastrointestinal but other also, e.g. subconjunctival)
Clopidogrel	Acute coronary syndrome: 12 months treatment only – initially 300 mg, then 75 mg daily; may also be given with aspirin if ST-segment elevation absent	Dyspepsia, abdominal pain, diarrhoea, bleeding disorders (including gastrointestinal and intracranial)
	Prevention of atherosclerotic events in peripheral arterial disease within 35 days of myocardial infarction or within 6 months of ischaemic stroke: 75 mg daily	

Table 7.1 Common drugs used for cardiovascular disorders *(continued)*

Antiplatelet	Dose	Common side effects
Dipyridamole	300–600 mg daily in 3–4 divided doses before food Secondary prevention of ischaemic stroke and transient ischaemic attacks (used alone or with aspirin), adjunct to oral anticoagulation for prophylaxis of thromboembolism associated with prosthetic heart valves: 200 mg of m/r formulation daily preferably with food	Gastrointestinal effects, dizziness, myalgia, headache, hypotension, hot flushes, tachycardia, worsening symptoms of coronary heart disease, hypersensitivity reactions, e.g. urticaria, bronchospasm, and angioedema; increased bleeding during or after surgery and thrombocytopenia

Thrombolytics	Dose	Common side effects
Streptokinase	Myocardial infarction: 1,500,000 units by IV infusion over 60 minutes; different schedules for other thromboembolic events (See BNF or product literature)	Nausea, vomiting, bleeding, reperfusion arrhythmias, and hypotension; allergic reactions may occur including rash, flushing, and uveitis; anaphylaxis has been reported
Reteplase	Myocardial infarction: IV injection of 10 units over not more than 2 minutes followed (after 30 minutes) by a further 10 units	Nausea, vomiting, bleeding, reperfusion arrhythmias, and hypotension

Lipid-regulating drugs—statins

Simvastatin	Dose range 10–80 mg daily at night (most patients 40 mg daily)	Reversible myositis is rare but significant side effect of 'statins'; myalgia, myopathy, and rhabdomyolysis have also been reported; other side effects include headache, altered liver function tests, peripheral neuropathy, alopecia, gastrointestinal effects, jaundice, dizziness, anaemia, hepatitis, and pancreatitis
Pravastatin	Prevention of cardiovascular events: 40 mg at night	As above
Atorvastatin	Dose 10 mg once daily; may be increased at intervals of at least 4 weeks to a maximum of 80 mg once daily	As above; also chest pain, angina, insomnia, dizziness, hypoaesthesia, arthralgia, and back pain

Nursing patients with nutritional and gastrointestinal problems

Nursing assessment of patients with GI disorders

Some patients are admitted as emergencies and it is important to stabilize their condition before taking a more detailed assessment. In addition to a general nursing assessment (□ Chapter 3, Individualizing nursing care practice, pp.32–3) perform the following procedures.

Observe the patient
- Signs of shock
- Haemorrhage
- Abdominal distension
- Pain
- Dehydration and thirst
- Cold clammy skin
- Sweating

Monitor temperature and blood pressure for tachycardia (low blood pressure, and shallow rapid respirations indicate emergencies such as GI bleeding, obstruction, peritonitis, perforation, and jaundice).

Ask the patient about
Nursing history
- Ability to manage self care and activities of living
- Social circumstances and housing (dependents at home, carers available, access to toilet)
- Misconceptions or lack of understanding about bodily functions, condition, care, and treatment
- Past and present nursing problems and issues
- Fears and anxieties about diagnosis, prognosis, treatment, and care, pain, ability to cope, effects on lifestyle, ability to support family, reactions from family, and body image, e.g. need for stoma

Past medical history
- Medications, e.g. laxatives, analgesics, antacids, anticholinergic drugs
- Pregnancy
- Past surgery
- Medical conditions, e.g. GI bleeding, inflammatory bowel conditions, malignancies, anaemia, diabetes, alcohol intake, infections, metabolic disease, family history of colorectal disease, and any allergies or recent travel

Current problems
- Oral care—caries, infections, dentures, and crowns; dryness and cleanliness of oral mucosa; normal care routine
- Gastric problems, e.g. dysphagia (difficulty in swallowing) and dyspepsia (heartburn, acidity)
- Nausea and vomiting—frequency, type (e.g. projectile), when or related circumstances (e.g. motion sickness), content (e.g. bile, digested/undigested food, blood), smell, volume, and eructation (belching)

- Altered bowel function—diarrhoea; constipation; normal pattern; nature of change, e.g. frequency, consistency, or appearance; presence of blood (melaena), mucus, or pus in stool; any pain; difficulty in defecation related to change in environment or lifestyle; increase, decrease, or absence of flatus; and incontinence
- Nutrition—weight changes, recent intake (e.g. if food poisoning is suspected), normal fluid intake. ▢ Nutritional assessment, p.242
- Pain—location, triggers, duration, character (sharp, dull, colicky), severity, association with guarding, exacerbating factors, methods of relief

Nursing problems for patients with GI disorders

Oral care—self-care deficit is the inability to carry out normal care routine to keep mouth clean and moist.

Nausea and vomiting usually occur with pain in GI conditions. Nausea is the feeling of wanting to vomit. Vomiting is the reflex action of emptying the stomach contents via the mouth.

Anorexia is the loss of appetite and desire to eat. It may be accompanied by weight loss and lead to malnutrition.

Dysphagia is difficulty in swallowing.

Dyspepsia is indigestion, acidity, heartburn (caused by acid reflux), and pain.

Dehydration is the loss of water from the body's cells and tissues. It may be due to reduced fluid intake or increased loss through vomiting and diarrhoea.

Fatigue describes feelings of weariness, tiredness, and malaise. It may be due to anaemia (blood loss or vitamin deficiency), infection, inflammation, or general condition.

Pain may be acute or chronic. Two types of GI pain include:
- *Epigastric:* over the stomach area. It may range from dull ache to tenderness to acute.
- *Abdominal:* over the abdominal area. It may be generalized or localized and may range from being tender, achy, or colicky to being excruciating or severe. It may be accompanied by muscle guarding.

Changes in bowel habits
- *Diarrhoea:* passage of loose, semi-solid, or liquid stools at more frequent intervals than is normal for the patient.
- *Constipation:* infrequent passage of hard stools with straining and difficulty. May lead to impaction and overflow—the faeces accumulate in the rectum and overflow incontinence of loose faecal matter may occur.
- *Faecal incontinence:* may occur in some bowel disorders, particularly with diarrhoea.
- *Melaena:* (blood in the stool) may also occur.

Fear and anxiety may be due to possible long-term prognosis, effects on future lifestyle and relationships, and planned treatments.

Changed self-image may be due to surgery, stoma, or medical condition.

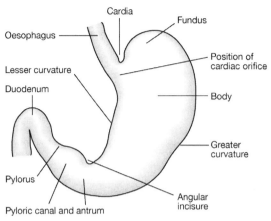

Fig. 8.1 Parts of the stomach. Taken from Mackinnon P and Morris J (2005). *Oxford Textbook of Functional Anatomy*, vol 2, Fig 6.4.7, Oxford University Press, Oxford. Reproduced with permission from Oxford University Press.

GI tests and investigations

Parts of the stomach are shown in Fig. 8.1 and the GI system is shown in Fig. 8.2.

Laboratory tests

- FBC, ESR, U&E, and liver function tests
- Serum CRP to assess inflammation; amylase if abdominal pain; pregnancy test, if suspected
- Serum iron, folate, and B$_{12}$ to characterize anaemia
- Tumour markers (CEA, AFP, Ca19-9), if indicated (📖 Chapter 39, Tumour markers, p.1183)
- Random blood glucose, calcium, magnesium, phosphate and possibly trace elements, if malnourished

📖 Chapter 39, Common laboratory tests and their interpretation, p.1167.

Proctoscopy and rigid sigmoidoscopy

These are examinations of the rectum and sigmoid colon to view the mucosa to detect haemorrhoids, anal fissures, rectal carcinomas, and diverticulitis.

Endoscopy

This is an examination of the GI tract. An endoscope can be inserted through the mouth to view the oesophagus, stomach, and duodenum, or through the anus and the rectum and colon (📖 Flexible sigmoidoscopy, below) The state of the mucosa is seen and biopsies can be taken.

Colonoscopy

This is an examination of the large bowel including the caecum. Bowel preparation and sedation are usually required. Diverticular disease, polyps, tumours, and ulceration may be detected. Biopsy may be taken and polypectomy can be performed.

Flexible sigmoidoscopy

This is an examination of the rectum, sigmoid, and descending colon and may detect the same pathology as colonoscopy. Preparation is with enema. Therapies include polypectomy, balloon dilatation, endoscopic mucosal resection (EMR), and stenting.

Rectal examination

A digital rectal examination can be undertaken to determine the presence, type, and volume of faeces; to identify defective sphincter control; or to identify the presence of carcinoma, haemorrhoids, and fissures. This examination can also be used to assess the prostate in male patients and the cervix in female patients if a vaginal exam is contraindicated.

Faecal examination

This examination involves collection of faeces to identify the presence of occult blood, ova cysts, parasites, pus and mucus, and bacterial infection, e.g. *Salmonella*, *Clostridium difficile*.

Radiological investigations

- *Abdominal x-rays* may show fluid level and gas collection indicating obstruction and perforation. May also show gallstones and renal calculi.
- *Barium swallow and follow-through* shows the upper GI anatomy and may detect reflux and small bowel disease. It is less sensitive than endoscopy.
- *Small bowel enema* achieves same as a barium swallow and follow-through but in a shorter time. Barium is introduced through a nasoduodenal tube. This is much less comfortable.
- *Barium enema* may be able to detect abnormalities such as megacolon, megarectum, volvulus, intussusception, diverticular disease, polyps and tumours.
- *CT scan* is used to stage a tumour preoperatively and to determine whether any metastatic disease is present in the lymph nodes or distant organs. It is also used as a surveillance investigation following surgery for colorectal cancer.
- *MRI scan* is used to stage rectal cancers and assist in the decision to offer preoperative radiotherapy to either downstage tumour before surgery or prevent recurrence. MR enterography is increasingly used to assess small bowel cancer in Crohn's disease.
- *Ultrasound* is used for investigation of GI pain and may indicate calculi or fluid collection or detect metastatic disease. It is a good screening modality for liver, biliary, and renal pathology.

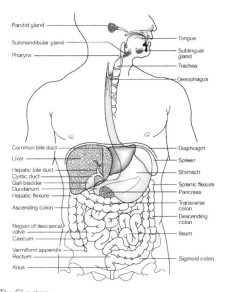

Fig. 8.2 The GI system.

Disorders of the mouth

Dental disorders

Dental caries (decay) and periodontal disease are the most common dental disorders. They are caused by bacteria and result in pain and problems with eating and speaking. Cavity formation, nerve damage, and abscess are complications. Prevention is by good oral hygiene, regular dental checks, and restricted intake of sugary foods and drink. Wearing ill-fitting dentures can cause mouth ulcers, frictional keratoses, and yeast infections, e.g. *Candida*.

Gingivitis

This is inflammation at the gum–tooth margin causing redness, swelling, and bleeding of the gums when brushing. Complications include periodontitis, pain, tooth loss, unpleasant tastes, halitosis, and problems with eating. It may affect general well-being. Prevention is as above but especially good tooth brushing at gum margins.

Glossitis

The tongue is smooth, sore, sensitive, and erythematous due to the atrophy of the papillae. It is usually caused by nutritional deficit.

Stomatitis

This is inflammation of the mouth and can be infective or non-infective.

- *Non-infective stomatitis:* often has an unknown cause but may be part of other GI problems, e.g. Crohn's disease due to vitamin deficiency. It is a feature of iron deficiency, vitamin B_2 deficiency, drug reactions, and Behcets (a multi-organ disease with unknown cause). Painful ulcers lasting up to 2 weeks are common.
- *Bacterial stomatitis:* may be associated with streptococcal sore throat. Rare causes are Vincent's angina (pharyngeal infection with ulcerative gingivitis), tuberculosis, and syphilis.
- *Fungal stomatitis:* usual cause is *Candida*. It may also affect the pharynx and oesophagus causing dysphagia. It occurs in patients who are immunosuppressed or who have severe illnesses (e.g. cancer), and also occurs as a result of broad-spectrum antibiotics.
- *Viral stomatitis:* may be caused by herpes simplex (cold sores); hand, foot, and mouth disease; herpes zoster (shingles); and glandular fever.
- *Angular stomatitis:* is inflammation at the angles of the mouth. It is common in older people and may be due to allergy, vitamin B deficiency, and iron deficiency.

Xerostomia

This is a dry mouth, commonly caused by medication and often multiple drugs. It is also caused by salivary gland hypofunction in Sjögren's syndrome.

Mouth cancer

The incidence of mouth cancer is rising. It presents with a sore or ulcer that is slow to heal; warty lumps or nodules; or white, speckled, or pigmented patches on the mucosa. Patients have difficulty speaking and swallowing. Treatment is by surgery, chemotherapy, and radiotherapy, alone or in combination.

Nurse's role in the prevention and early detection of oral cancer

- Ensure people are aware of the risk factors and support them in changing lifestyles and self-care habits. Common risk factors are:
  - Advanced age. More common in people >40 but can occur in younger people.
  - Use of tobacco (cigars, cigarettes, pipes, and chewing tobacco). Provide support in smoking cessation.
  - Alcohol, especially if in association with tobacco use. Encourage patients to limit intake. 📖 Chapter 31, Nursing alcohol and substance misuse problems, p.994.
  - Chewing betel nuts (common in Asian women).
  - Infection, e.g. herpes simplex, syphilis.
  - Dental caries and poor oral hygiene. Encourage use of dental services. 📖 Oral care, p.212.
  - Occupational risks, e.g. exposure to nickel, coal products, cement, wood, and organic chemicals.
- Work with community leaders to ensure information is provided in culturally sensitive ways.
- Explain that early detection and treatment is important in producing a better prognosis.
  - Take note of and report persistent mouth ulcers or red/white patches on the mucosa that last >3 weeks, whether painful or not.
  - Advise patients to attend dental checks on a regular basis for thorough inspection of the mucosa.
  - Provide information materials for future reference.
- Ensure health care professionals are up-to-date with information on oral cancer and are able to undertake oral assessments as part of overall holistic assessment.
- Ensure patients are referred to specialists for investigation, advice, and treatment.
- Provide support, advice, and information to patients and their families on treatment, side effects, complications, and prognosis.

Oral care

Prevention of disorders in the mouth
- Schedule regular check-ups with dentist.
- Brush teeth with fluoride-based toothpaste at least twice a day, including last thing at night; concentrate on the gums as well as the teeth. Seek advice from dentist or hygienist for correct technique.
- Ensure the toothbrush is right for the purpose and change it at least every 3 months.
- Avoid sugary sweet foods, e.g. sweets, cake, and biscuits.
- Avoid sweet sugary drinks. Only water should be drunk through the night.
- Ensure adequate fluid intake.
- Maintain good nutritional diet with vitamins.
- Take advice if dentures become loose.

Oral hygiene for patients unable to self-care
The aim is to keep the oral mucosa and lips clean and moist, prevent infection, remove food debris, and ensure the patient's mouth feels fresh and clean.
- Examine and assess the patient's mouth (Examination and assessment of the mouth, p.213) and check the patient's normal routine. Wear gloves to prevent cross-infection.
- Check for dehydration and ability/willingness to take oral fluids and plan to ensure patient is adequately hydrated (encourage fluid intake, nasogastric tube, IV).
- Check the patient's nutritional status and ability/willingness to take food orally and plan to ensure appropriate diet (seek advice on diet, parental feeding, nasogastric feeding, or PEG feeding).
- Avoid giving sugary drinks.
- If possible, follow the patient's daily oral hygiene routine.
- Ensure dentures are removed, cleaned, and replaced.
- Ensure that food is not lodged or retained in the gums or cheeks.
- Use a soft toothbrush with fluoride toothpaste on all surfaces of the tooth and brush the tongue and other tissues gently. Avoid the posterior third of the tongue as this will cause retching. Edentulous patients also benefit from this, but care should be taken in cases of stomatitis, when swabs wrapped round a gloved finger or sponge stick should be used.
- Consider use of chlorhexidine mouthwashes as they will help to prevent plaque. Water mouthwashes can also be used. Hydrogen peroxide mouthwashes should not be used.
- Use soft paraffin to prevent dry lips (lemon and glycerine swabs are contraindicated).
- Follow local oral hygiene protocols.

Examination and assessment of the mouth

- Gather equipment including gloves, a torch or light source, and a tongue depressor.
- Ensure patient is in a comfortable position.
- Explain the procedure and the purpose, and seek the patient's verbal consent.
- Examine systematically (See Fig. 8.3).
  - Lips: check for dryness, cuts, sores (particularly at the margins), and colour (pallor, cyanosis)
  - Mucous membrane including cheeks: note colour, whether moist or dry, lesions or ulcers (location, size, characteristics)
  - Gums: note bleeding, inflammation, and soreness
  - Teeth: note plaque, caries and periodontal disease, dentures, and crowns
  - Hard and soft palates: assess for lesions and ulcers, colour, and whether moist or dry
  - Tongue: note dryness, colour, smoothness, and coating
  - Roof and floor of mouth: note colour, lesions, and ulcers
- Record findings and use assessment to plan care to meet needs.
  📖 Chapter 3, Individualizing nursing care practice, p.46.

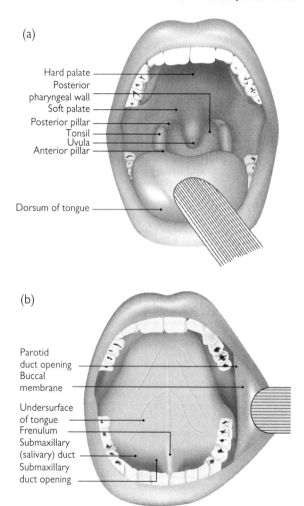

Fig. 8.3 Mouth and throat structures. Main anatomical areas of the inside of the mouth to be observed when assessing the patient. a) with the tongue forward and down to see the back and sides of the buccal cavity. b) tongue raised so as to see the floor and sides of the buccal cavity. In both cases looking for signs of abnormality, inflammation, infection, colour abnormal lesions, plaque and condition of gums and teeth. Taken from Mackinnon P and Morris J (2005). *Oxford Textbook of Functional Anatomy*, vol 2, Fig 6.5.9, Oxford University Press, Oxford. Reproduced with permission from Oxford University Press.

Oesophageal and gastric conditions

Oesophageal varices

These are varicosities of the veins of the lower oesophagus due to non-cirrhotic portal hypertension, e.g. in portal vein thrombosis. These can bleed profusely and this is an acute emergency. The preferred treatment is endoscopy with ligation of vessels or sclerotherapy and vasoactive drugs, e.g. terlipressin IV and oral propranolol for secondary prevention. It is important to protect the airway, give fluids, transfuse if necessary, observe, and catheterize as required.

Hiatus hernia

This is an oesophageal hernia. It is common but not necessarily pathological or symptomatic. Symptoms are due to oesophagitis or dysmotility provoked by reflux. Rarely gastric volvulus may occur. It may cause dysphagia, peptic ulcer, and possible regurgitation of food at night with the risk of aspiration pneumonia. It is more common in those >40 and in women. Conservative management includes advising small meals, not lying down before or after meals, not eating immediately before bed, sleeping elevated on pillows, losing weight, and stopping smoking. Surgery may be necessary.

Oesophageal reflux

This occurs when gastric content enters the oesophagus due to relaxation of the lower oesophageal sphincter. It causes heartburn and acid taste. It may cause oesophagitis with or without inflammation and erosions. Treatment includes antacids and alginates and H_2 receptor blockers, e.g. ranitidine to reduce acid secretion over long periods. A small number of people develop strictures (Oesophageal strictures, below). Diet and lifestyle changes are needed, e.g. reduction in smoking and alcohol intake. Advise on taking small regular meals and avoiding hot drinks. A change in medications that exacerbate symptoms may be necessary.

Oesophageal strictures

These are benign strictures, i.e. peptic strictures are caused by oesophageal reflux and subsequent scarring. Long history of reflux followed by dysphagia and heartburn with little weight loss is common. Regurgitation of food is common if the stricture is severe. Controlled radial expansion (CRE) balloon dilatation is the standard therapy plus proton pump inhibitors. Stricture may also be malignant.

Peptic ulcers

- *Gastric ulcer:* usually occurs in the antrum area of the stomach in middle age, and has a higher mortality than duodenal ulcers. Risk factors include *Helicobacter pylori* (60% are associated with this bacteria), NSAIDs, smoking, and steroids. Patients with these ulcers present with epigastric pain, especially after food, and are helped by lying flat or taking antacids.
- *Duodenal ulcer:* usually occurs in upper duodenal bulb in middle-aged men. These ulcers are 4 times more common than gastric ulcers in patients <40 years of age. The overall incidence in the UK is falling due to treatment of *Helicobacter*. More than 95% of non-drug related

duodenal ulcers are due to *Helicobacter*. The other main risk is use of NSAIDs. Patients with these ulcers present with epigastric pain that is often worse at night and increased weight. These ulcers are rarely malignant. Perforation may occur.

- *Other management:* focuses on lifestyle changes to reduce symptoms (e.g. eating little but often, smoking cessation), eliminating *H. pylori* by proton pump inhibitors and antibiotics, and discontinuing NSAID drugs. Surgery may be indicated, but this is rare. 📖 Nursing care of patients having oesophageal and gastric surgery, p.220.

Oesophageal and stomach cancer

Oesophageal cancer

Oesophageal cancers are most commonly squamous cell carcinoma with a small percentage of adenocarcinoma in the distal end. The incidence is increasing and it has a poor prognosis because of the tumour's rapid growth, early invasion, and late diagnosis. Risk factors include reflux (adenocarcinoma), smoking, excess alcohol consumption, corrosive injury, achalasia, geographic (common in Iran and China), and post-cricoids web. Patients may feel unwell for a period, have progressive dysphagia firstly with food then with liquids, regurgitation, and weight loss. Hoarseness and cough may occur if the upper third of the oesophagus is affected.

Investigations
- Endoscopy and biopsy
- Chest x-ray
- Barium swallow to assess the size of the tumour
- CT scan to estimate the spread to lymph nodes and operability
- Ultrasound scan of liver to determine metastases
- Endoscopic ultrasound for staging

Treatment
Tumour node metastasis (TNM) classification is used to determine the appropriate course of treatment. Radical resection of the tumour is done only if cure is possible and reconstruction of the oesophagus is required; this carries risk of anastomotic leakage and stenosis. Radiotherapy may be done to shrink the tumour before surgery for squamous upper tumours or for palliation. Insertion of mesh stents via endoscopy can be used to relieve obstruction. The value of chemotherapy is uncertain.

Stomach cancer

The incidence is declining for tumours in the antrum and body, but is rising for tumours in the caria. There is still a poor prognosis; cancers are usually adenocarcinomas. It may be associated with blood group A or *H. pylori* infection. Other risk factors include genetics, pernicious anaemia, low socioeconomic status, and previous gastric surgery. Patients often present late and complain of feeling unwell, fatigue, weight loss, dyspepsia, pain, and vomiting; anaemia and melaena may occur.

Investigations
- Gastroscopy to view the lesion
- Tissue biopsy for histological examination
- Barium studies to show mucosal irregularities
- CT, MRI scan, or staging laparoscopy to determine prognosis and treatment options

Treatment
Treatment includes surgery (partial or total gastrectomy depending on size and location of tumour). Radiotherapy and chemotherapy may be given with or without surgery. Nutritional support is required. The prognosis is poor with 5 year overall survival of 10%.

Nursing care of patients having oesophageal and gastric surgery

Information and education

These are major operations that will affect the patients and their families' lifestyle significantly.

- Ensure that the patient understands:
  - What the surgery involves in detail and the likely prognosis.
  - What type of preparation will be required for surgery.
  - What to expect during the postoperative period, e.g. recovery, HDU/ITU, then ward; discomfort caused by tubes and pain relief; and how they will participate in care.
  - The impact of the surgery on their lifestyle, e.g. regurgitation may occur initially after a meal. Dumping syndrome—advise to eat small meals slowly and chew thoroughly, use of high protein and vitamin supplements (B_{12} and possibly iron), possibly reduce carbohydrate intake, and rest after meals.
- Ensure patient sees dietitian during the preoperative and postoperative periods to discuss nutrition.
- Prepare family for the possibility of an inoperable tumour and inform them of whether radiotherapy and/or chemotherapy is planned.

Preoperative care

- Many patients are malnourished and a detailed nutritional assessment is required, preferably prior to admission.
- High-protein high-calorie intake with vitamin supplements is essential to maximize healing and the function of the immune system and to reduce oedema and tiredness.
- Preoperative fasting is necessary to reduce the risk of aspiration.
- Bowel preparation is necessary to reduce postoperative complications and to improve patient comfort. Follow local guidelines.
- Skin preparation is required to prevent infection. Follow local guidelines.

Postoperative care

- Respiratory support may be required including a period of ventilation; therefore a stay in an HDU is likely.
- Fasting for several days will be required to enable healing of the anastamosis.
- Fluids and nutrition will be managed via IV and central venous lines until oral intake is tolerated; jejunostomy feeding may be needed.
- Wound care including care of surgical drains is required and management of a urinary catheter if *in situ*.
- Drainage tubes will be required for several days postoperatively, e.g. nasogastric tube on free drainage (to promote healing of the anastamosis), gastrostomy tube, wound or chest drain. Ensure tubes are secure and patent, and monitor amount and type of drainage and report immediately any fresh blood or haemorrhage. Tubes are removed when drainage is minimal and normal bowel sounds have returned. Gastric aspiration, p.223.

- Sufficient pain relief must be provided; patient controlled analgesia may be useful.
- Fluids and diet are reintroduced slowly, beginning with small amounts of water, then free fluids, and progressing on to light diet.
- Discharge depends on the patient's condition, but usually after 1 week follow-up care will be as an outpatient via GP and primary care nurses.

Surgical operations of the oesophagus and stomach

Oesophageal surgery

Operations are usually performed either to attempt cure of cancer or for palliation and relief of dysphagia. Oesophageal resection may be done to remove a tumour or oesophagogastrectomy where there is a partial or total gastrectomy with an anastamosis to the remaining part of the oesophagus. These are highly risky operations because of the position and possible infiltration of the tumours.

Gastric surgery

May be carried out as an emergency, e.g. in uncontrollable haemorrhage or because of perforation. Alternatively it is done for gastric cancer or chronic ulceration.

Partial gastrectomy

Performed when the tumour is limited to one area. About two-thirds of the distal part of the stomach is resected and the rest anastamosed to the duodenum or the jejunum.

Total gastrectomy

Performed when the lesion is in the body of the stomach and lymph nodes are involved. The entire stomach and some of the oesophagus and duodenum are removed. A gastric reservoir is created from segments of the jejunum.

Side effects of total and partial gastrectomy:
- Reduced gastric capacity
- Dumping syndrome: rapid emptying of the stomach contents into the small intestine, causing transient hypovolaemia, weakness, faintness, palpitations, and nausea
- Diarrhoea due to intestinal hurry
- Vitamin B_{12} deficiency resulting in anaemia due to lack of intrinsic factor in the stomach
- Iron deficiency

Vagotomy

The vagus nerve is isolated and divided to reduce gastric acid secretion and slow gastric motility and emptying. As a result a pyloroplasty is done which enlarges the exit of the stomach to ensure gastric drainage. A highly selective vagotomy is intended to retain the nerves supplying the pyloric sphincter intact, and pyloroplasty should not be necessary.

Nursing care of patients with gastric problems

Nausea and vomiting

- Support the patient during vomiting; remove used vomit bowls and provide clean ones immediately. Give mouth washes or oral care to keep mouth fresh. Change clothing or bedding as necessary.
- Observe and record the characteristics, amount, and type of vomit.
- Observe for signs of dehydration and electrolyte imbalance (dry furred tongue, decreased urine output, inelastic skin) and highlight need for fluid replacement by IV if necessary.
- Give prescribed anti-emetics, e.g. metoclopramide, cyclizine.
- Monitor for signs of malnutrition if nausea and vomiting is prolonged, e.g. weight loss, food intake. Reduce risks of possible complications, e.g. support wounds when vomiting to reduce pain and wound dehiscence, position patient to prevent risk of aspiration.

Anorexia

- Undertake nutritional assessment. 📖 Nutritional assessment, p.242.
- Encourage small nutritious meals, often of favourite food if tolerated.
- Make sure the environment is clean and tidy and that the patient is positioned comfortably.
- Administer prescribed anti-emetics before meals.

Dyspepsia

Advise not to lie down before or after meals, to have small light meals, to sleep with head elevated on pillows, and to stop smoking.

Pain

- Reassure the patient by touch, presence, and good communication of information to reduce anxiety.
- Assess pain using an appropriate tool and administer prescribed analgesic, anti-inflammatory, and antacid drugs.
- Handle the patient carefully when moving and repositioning.
- Use massage and encourage relaxation.
- Evaluate the effectiveness of analgesia with the patient and change as necessary.

Anxiety

Take time to listen and encourage patients to discuss their fears and provide information as appropriate. Encourage them to discuss with family and friends and give advice on how they can be supportive.

Education and information

- Ensure the patient understands their condition, treatment, care plan, and prognosis. Encourage them to be involved in decisions.
- Ensure they are aware of the investigations and what will happen during them.

Gastric aspiration

Follow local policy and procedures.

A nasogastric tube is passed into the stomach and suction is applied in order to keep the stomach empty of its contents.

Indications

- Bowel obstruction
- Paralytic ileus
- Pre- and postoperatively for some gastric and abdominal surgery

Principles of management

- Follow local procedures for insertion of tube.
- Check whether the patient has any nasal defect or tenderness that might interfere with the insertion of the tube. Ensure each nostril is cleaned before insertion.
- Explain the procedure and its purpose to the patient and seek verbal consent. Inform the patient that the presence of the tube may cause:
  - Difficulty breathing—mouth breathing may be necessary
  - Dryness and irritation of the throat
  - Discomfort
  - Difficulty speaking
- Make sure the patient is comfortable (sitting upright is usually best) and relaxed, and privacy is ensured.
- A clean procedure is required and disposable gloves should be worn.
- The size of the tube depends on the size and age of the patient. An average adult requires GG 14–16. Measure the correct length of the tube required from nose to earlobe to bottom of xiphisternum; keep a record and mark the tube.
- Encourage the patient to participate and swallow when the tube reaches the pharynx.
- Observe the patient for signs of distress, breathing difficulties, and cyanosis.
- Test that the tube is in position by using a 50 mL syringe and gently withdrawing some gastric fluid to test on pH paper; aspirate should be pH 5.5 or below. (May not work if patient is on acid suppressing medication, e.g. proton-pump inhibitors or H_2-receptor antagonists.) Check the external marking to see if the tube has moved. Radiography should not be routinely used to check the position, but may be required for fine bore NG tube.
- Ensure the tube is securely taped and out of the patient's way, and a clean spigot is used or the tube is attached to a drainage system.
- Perform either continuous or intermittent aspiration, as indicated.
- Document the procedure and ensure the patient is comfortable.
- Provide frequent oral care.
- Record fluid balance chart.

Constipation

This is the passage of hard stools with diminished frequency, often with straining discomfort and difficulty.

Causes

- Dietary factors, e.g. lack of fibre and fluids
- Immobility (of patient and/or the bowel due to anaesthetic post-surgery)
- Diseases of the colon, e.g. irritable bowel disease, cancer, diverticular disease
- Anorectal disease, e.g. anal fissure, mucosal prolapse
- Neurological conditions, e.g. multiple sclerosis, Parkinson's disease
- Metabolic diseases, e.g. hypothyroidism, hypercalcaemia
- Perianal conditions, e.g. anal fissure, haemorrhoids
- Pregnancy
- Age (increased risk in those >45 years)
- Drugs, e.g. opioids, antacids, anticholingeric drugs, antihistamines, iron supplements, and diuretics

Assessment

Determine whether the patient:
- is at risk (📖 Causes, above.)
- has mild constipation—normal routine with some straining; stool is drier and harder than normal
- has moderate constipation—as above plus diminished frequency (1–3 days), mild distension, bloating, and feeling of fullness
- has severe constipation—as above plus diminished frequency (>3 days), painful evacuation, laxative/enema is needed, loss of appetite, and rectal bleeding
- has faecal impaction and spurious diarrhoea.

Obtain bowel, dietary, and exercise history; record the time and frequency of bowel movements; and measure intake and output of fluid. Some organizations may use assessment tools, e.g. Bristol stool chart (📖 Appendices, The Bristol stool form scale, p.1205). Also look for weight loss or rectal bleeding which could suggest colorectal cancer. Perform rectal examination according to local guidelines.

Faecal impaction

The rectum becomes impacted with a hard faecal mass that becomes too large to pass, the rectum over-distends, and faeces liquefy and leak as spurious or overflow diarrhoea. Treatment is aimed at clearing the rectum with suppositories, enemas, or manual removal. Surgery is indicated in rare circumstances.

Nursing management of primary constipation

- Educate and encourage the patient to consume a high-fibre diet with adequate fluids and exercise.
- Encourage the patient to respond to the urge to defecate. Ensure access to and cleanliness of toilet/commode bedpan, and privacy and comfort.

- Discuss any concerns, provide reassurance, and aim to reduce any embarrassment.
- Encourage the patient to be as mobile as possible.
- Administer prescribed treatment and monitor effect.
  - Oral laxatives: bulk-forming drugs (e.g. methylcellulose, ispaghula husk), stimulant laxatives (e.g. senna, bisacodyl), osmotic laxatives (e.g. lactulose) faecal softeners and lubricants (e.g. liquid paraffin), and strong laxatives in operative bowel preparation (e.g. Picolax®)
  - Local laxatives: glycerol suppositories, stimulant suppositories (e.g. bisacodyl), or micro-enemas (e.g. phosphate enemas)

Common bowel disorders

Inflammatory bowel disease

Crohn's disease

This is an inflammatory chronic incurable condition that follows a relapsing remitting course. It can affect any part of the GI tract but usually affects the terminal ileum, the ileo-caecal area, or the colon. It affects the full thickness of the bowel. It is common in Western, developed countries, affects 20–40 year-olds, and has a genetic link. Diet, smoking, stress, and infections (e.g. measles virus) may contribute. Patients have diarrhoea, abdominal pain, rectal bleeding, anorexia, and weight loss, and are susceptible to other inflammatory conditions of joints (arthralgia), skin (erythema nodosum), and eyes (uveitis, conjunctivitis). Complications include strictures, colorectal cancer, and fistulae.

Investigations

- Stool examination for blood, mucus, consistency, and steatorrhoea
- Blood for ESR, FBC, albumin, and C-reactive protein
- LFTs and UEs prior to commencing treatment
- Colonoscopy, MRI, and CT scan

Treatment

- Corticosteroids, aminosalicylates, antibiotics, immunosuppressive therapy including biological agents (e.g. infliximab), anti-diarrhoeal agents
- Diet 📖 High-fibre diet, p.248
- Surgical treatment—resection of the affected area of bowel

Ulcerative colitis

The symptoms and predisposing factors of ulcerative colitis are similar to Crohn's disease. The main differences are that it affects the mucous membrane of the rectum and spreads proximally to involve the colon. Mucosal disease is limited to the rectum and colon. Diarrhoea and bleeding are more frequent; abdominal pain and tenderness can be severe in toxic megacolon. Treatment is similar to above.

Diverticular disease

A diverticulum is a herniation in the mucosa of the bowel wall. Faeces become trapped and ferment, leading to altered bowel habits, abdominal pain, diverticulitis and infection, inflammation, abscess, fever, and peritonitis. Contributory factors include diet (high in refined carbohydrates and fast foods) and increased age, and it is more common among lower-income groups.

Investigations

- Sigmoidsocopy, barium enema, colonoscopy, and CT scan

Treatment

- High-fibre diet and increased fluids as maintenance
- Analgesia, antibiotics, rest, and fluids for diverticulitis
- Surgery for complications, i.e. abscess, perforation, fistula, and obstruction

Coeliac disease

This is an incurable condition where gluten induces an immunological driven damage of the small bowel mucosa. Features include atrophy of the villi. Gluten is a component of wheat, barley, and rye but not rice or maize. Patients are most commonly asymptomatic but may have IBS type symptoms. Investigations include jejunal biopsy and blood tests for serum IgA tissue transglutaminase antibodies – this is the standard antibody assay. Strict concordance with diet is necessary (📖 Gluten-free diet, p.249). Non-concordance may result in general ill health, growth retardation, and reproductive problems; bone, calcium, and neurological disorders; depression; and small bowel lymphoma. Stress seems to be a common causative agent in adults.

Nursing care of patients with common bowel disorders

Patients with bowel disorders are anxious and concerned about the uncertain nature of the disease, long-term treatment and medication, prognosis, effects on lifestyle, and whether surgery will be necessary. Care may be carried out by the GP and primary care team in the community, as an outpatient, or as an inpatient; therefore good communication is essential to ensure continuity of care. Many patients are embarrassed by the nature of the disorder and find it difficult to discuss bodily functions.

The role of the nurse is to:
- Ensure the patient's privacy and dignity when discussing and carrying out care, especially when the patient is using the toilet, commode, or bedpan.
- Ensure patients and their families understand the nature of the condition and are kept informed of care, treatment, progress, and future plans.
- Encourage patients to make decisions about their care and where possible give self care.
- Ensure they know how to administer medications, plan diet, monitor fluid intake and output, and keep a stool chart.
- Provide information and support, and prepare patients undergoing investigations, e.g. with bowel preparation prior to barium x-rays.
- Monitor the patient's condition including vital signs, intake and output, weight changes, diet, and stool (frequency, characteristics, and amount).
- Make referrals to the multidisciplinary team for specialist support and advice, e.g. stoma care specialist, cancer nurse specialist, dietitian, social worker.
- Provide support, advice, and encouragement with diet and ensure patients understand what is most appropriate for their condition. Help with choice of menu. Family members should also be involved in order to plan diets following discharge. Small frequent meals may be better than fewer large meals. Nutritional supplements may be necessary.
- Administer artificial feeding, if prescribed. 🕮 Artificial feeding, p.250.
- Support the patient with activities of living if unable to self care. Hygiene and skin care are particularly important as the patient is at risk of skin excoriation with frequent episodes of diarrhoea.
- Provide mouth care if the patient is fasting or on restricted fluids.
- Assess the frequency, location, characteristics, and duration of pain together with any precipitating events and ensure patient has appropriate pain relief.
- Observe the patient for complications (e.g. abdominal distension, fever, rectal bleeding) or side effects from medication (e.g. weight gain from steroids).
- Provide opportunities to discuss concerns such as possibility of surgery, effects on self-esteem, impact on sexual functioning and reproduction, changes in body image, and feelings of isolation.
- Encourage the patient to rest if lethargic but also encourage some activity to prevent boredom and frustration and distract attention from the illness.

Colorectal cancer

This is the second most common cancer; it affects both sexes and risk increases with age. Risk factors include diet (red meat, animal fat, and low intake of fibre, fruit, and vegetables) and genetic factors (risk is 5 times greater if there is family history) particularly hereditary non-polyposis colorectal cancer and familial adenomatous polyposis. Other possible risk factors include smoking, alcohol abuse, and lack of exercise. There is also an increased risk with inflammatory bowel disease.

Presentation
This depends on the tumour site. Patients often experience vague symptoms, changes in bowel habit, constipation, diarrhoea, rectal bleeding, blood in the faeces, anaemia, lethargy, weight loss, abdominal distension, increased flatulence, tenesmus, and, in the late stages, bowel obstruction or abdominal mass.

Investigations
• Faeces for occult blood
• MRI scan to stage preoperatively and to decide upon neo-adjuvant chemotherapy or radiotherapy
• Blood tests (such as LFTs or FBC for anaemia) and bone profile to detect metastases
• Barium enema, endoscopy, proctoscopy, sigmoidoscopy, colonoscopy, biopsy CT scan to determine extent of tumour and spread
• Chest x-ray (pulmonary metastases)

Staging of tumours
Different systems are used to describe the extent of the disease and likely survival. The TNM classification system describes size of the primary tumour (T), lymph node involvement (N), and metastasis (M).
• **T1–2, N0, M0:** limited to bowel wall, no lymph node involvement, no metastasis, 95–100% survival at 5 years
• **T3–4, N0, M0:** all layers of the bowel wall involved, no lymph node involvement, no metastasis, 65–70% survival at 5 years
• **T$_{(any)}$, N1, M0:** regional lymph nodes involved, no metastasis, 30–40% survival at 5 years
• **T$_{(any)}$, Neither, M1:** distant metastases survival, <5% at 5 years

Treatment
Includes surgery, radiotherapy, chemotherapy, or a combination of these.

Surgery – depends on the site. A wide excision of bowel is made proximal and distal to the tumour. An anastamosis (joining the ends) of the remaining bowel saving the anal sphincter muscle is done for tumours of the colon and upper two-thirds of the rectum. An abdominal perineal resection resulting in a permanent colostomy is done for tumours of the lower rectum.

Radiotherapy – preoperatively reduces rate of local recurrence and may improve overall survival by 10%.

Chemotherapy – used pre- or postoperatively or as an adjuvant therapy to surgery to reduce the risk of recurrence, and in later stages it can be used palliatively to improve symptoms. Palliative therapy also includes radiotherapy, chemotherapy, and stents.

Complications

These may include impotence and ejaculatory difficulties; urinary problems (e.g. incontinence, dysuria); body image and self-esteem concerns; bowel problems (e.g. faecal incontinence); and effects of radiotherapy including diarrhoea, fatigue, and sore skin. Stomatitis occurs in patients undergoing chemotherapy.

Nursing role in relation to colorectal cancer

Prevention

- Encourage patients to overcome their fears and embarrassment when talking about bodily functions.
- Explain that early detection with treatment will significantly increase the chance of survival and will reduce the treatment required.
- Raise awareness of the risk factors (📖 Health education for the prevention of GI disorders, p.258) and discuss with the patient any risk factors in their lifestyle, including family history.
- Identify patient's motivation for change in behaviour that will reduce risk of bowel cancer.
- Provide information on what comprises a high-fibre and healthy diet; how to stop smoking and where to get help; safe levels of alcohol consumption; and how to increase activity levels.
- Provide information on the symptoms of colorectal cancer and encourage attendance at the GP's surgery.
- Encourage patients with family history to request screening.

Screening

- Currently the UK has a screening programme.
- The following tests are the current methods available: faecal occult blood, digital rectal examination and sigmoidoscopy to detect distal lesions, and colonoscopy to examine the whole colon.
- The British Society of Gastroenterology guidelines recommend that screening be offered to at-risk genetic groups.
- Ensure patients understand the purpose of the test and what it involves. Many patients will find these embarrassing and the nurse should be sensitive, reassure the patient, and ensure privacy and dignity. Provide facilities to ensure the patient is clean and comfortable after the test.

Following diagnosis

- Develop an effective relationship with the patient by being present and supportive, actively listening, and empathizing.
- Ensure that an individualized assessment and plan of care is developed and implemented.
- Have an understanding of the staging process, forms of treatment, and after-care so that patients' questions can be answered.
- Encourage patients to express their feelings which may include anger, sadness, anxiety, and fear.

- Encourage patients to talk to their family and friends, who can offer support.
- Make sure patients have written information on colorectal cancer (📖 Health education for the prevention of GI disorders, p.258).
- Ensure patients have access to relevant members of the multidisciplinary team, in particular the colorectal nurse, counsellor or clinical psychologist, stoma nurse, and cancer nurse specialist. Ensure that care is coordinated.

Nursing care of patients having bowel surgery

Preoperative care

Bowel preparation
- It is important to decrease the incidence of spillage of faecal content into the peritoneal cavity which causes infection. This will also ensure the bowel is easier to handle and to help prevent constipation postoperatively.
- Aperients, e.g. Picolax® enemas, and distal washouts, may be given. However, this is not always the case with enhanced recovery programmes.

Fluids and diet
- Solid diet is usually restricted but nourishing fluids are allowed.
- If the patient is malnourished, artificial feeding may be required.
- Careful monitoring is necessary to prevent dehydration and electrolyte imbalance. IV hydration may be indicated.
- A nasogastric tube may be passed prior to surgery or when the patient is in theatre.
- 📖 Chapter 22, Preoperative fasting, p.764.

Skin preparation
This is necessary to prevent postoperative complications.
- Encourage patient to shower using an antiseptic lotion.
- Provide a clean gown and bed linen.

Information and psychological care
- Provide an opportunity for patients to discuss and understand the operation before they consent to surgery, including:
  - Risks and benefits
  - Postoperative treatment and care plan
  - Prognosis and complications
- Ensure patients understand:
  - Where they will be cared for
  - Preoperative and postoperative processes
  - Whether a drain, infusion, catheter, or stoma will be in place (📖 Stoma care, p.238).

Other
Administer prescribed antibiotics given as a prophylaxis measure to prevent infection and anti-thrombosis prophylaxis, e.g. subcutaneous heparin and compression stockings.

Postoperative care

Diet and fluids
These are usually restricted until bowel sounds return. A nasogastric tube may be *in situ* on continuous drainage, then spigoted and aspirated at 4–6 hour intervals, and an IV infusion. Sips of water are given and these are increased until the patient is having soft diet and then full diet (high in calories and protein). Nutritional supplements may be required if the patient is not eating. Monitoring of fluid and electrolyte balance is essential.

Pain relief
Administer either as patient-controlled analgesia or regularly by the nurse.

Wound care
Discharge from drains is monitored and drains are removed when the output has diminished. Clips and stitches are removed after 7–10 days when the wound has healed.

Undertake catheter care

Mobilization
Should commence as early as the patient can tolerate; support from a physiotherapist is helpful. TEDS (compression) stockings may be used.

Information and psychological care
Involves listening to the patient, providing information, encouraging them to ask questions, and ensuring they have access to members of the multi-disciplinary team including the MacMillan nurses where needed.

Bowel operations

Abdomino-perineal excision of rectum
This is for low rectal cancers involving the sphincters.

Sub-total colectomy and ileo-anal pouch or pan-proctocolectomy
These are for ulcerative colitis.

Colectomy
This is the resection of part of the colon, e.g. for complete or partial obstruction or disease (See Fig. 8.4).
- Right hemicolectomy, e.g. for cancer of the caecum and ascending colon (1)
- Transverse colectomy, e.g. for cancer of transverse colon (2)
- Left hemicolectomy, e.g. for cancer of the descending and sigmoid colon (3)
- Sigmoid colectomy, a less extensive procedure for cancer of the sigmoid colon (4)

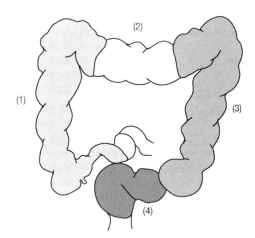

Fig. 8.4 Colectomy

Appendicectomy
Removal of the appendix for acute inflammation (appendicitis) with or without peritonitis.

Abdominal hernia repair
A hernia is a protrusion of an organ, e.g. bowel, through an opening in the cavity in which it is normally contained.
• Herniorrhaphy: repair by suturing the weakened muscle layers
• Herniotomy: excision of the sac and suturing the muscle layers
• Hernioplasty: refashioning and strengthening the muscle layers

Stoma care

A surgically created stoma is an opening of the bowel or urinary system into the abdomen.

Colostomy: This is formed from the colon and is usually sited in the left iliac fossa. If created from the sigmoid or descending colon faecal output is formed with normal odour; if created from the transverse or ascending colon faeces may be loose with a strong odour. Indications include bowel cancer, diverticulitis, Crohn's disease, volvulus, trauma, congenital abnormalities, faecal incontinence, and bowel ischaemia.

Ileostomy: This is formed from the small bowel and usually raised in the right iliac fossa. The faecal output is very soft and fluid, e.g. 1.5 l/day settling to 600–800 mL. Fluid and salt loss are a problem initially. Indications include Crohn's disease, ulcerative colitis, familial polyposis, irradiation damage, cancer, and trauma.

Urostomy (ileal conduit): This is formed in the urinary tract using a section of the ileum and is located in the right iliac fossa. Indications include bladder carcinoma, cystectomy, interstitial cystitis, disorders of the spinal column (e.g. spina bifida), and trauma.

Types of stoma: End stomas are the simplest to create; the divided bowel is brought to the abdominal wall and anastamosed to the skin. Loop stomas are temporary and created from a loop of ileum or colon.

Appliances

A wide range of appliances are available and a nurse specialist should guide the patient to choose the most suitable based on the patient's ability to cope (dexterity, eyesight); lifestyle; physical activity; mental and emotional state; culture; preferred site for stoma; shape and size of stoma; body contours; type of stoma and output; allergies; and patient preference (security, comfort, and discretion). Types of stoma bags include:

- Drainable bags—secured at the bottom for removal of liquid faeces.
- Closed-end bags—have no drainage facility. Removed when full.
- Urostomy bags—are drainable but have a non-return film to prevent backflow and a drainage tap at the bottom for emptying.
- One-piece appliances—have a skin protecting film and bag all-in-one that can be cut to fit individual stomas; they are slim fitting and flexible.
- Two-piece bags—have a separate base plate and bag; they are less fitting but provide good visibility and the bag is changed without disturbing the peristomal area.
- Accessories are available, including skin barriers (sprays, wipes, and gels), protective wafers (hypoallergenic for extra skin protection), powders to absorb moisture on excoriated skin, filler paste to fill creases in body contours to produce a flat surface, deodorizers; and flatus filters.

The nurse should observe the patient and their stoma for any of the following complications.

- *Anxiety and fear* can be reduced by careful preparation of the patient prior to surgery and is essential by both ward and specialist nurses. Teach patients how to care for the stoma and reassure them about concerns such as smell and how to dispose of contents. Continue to provide support postoperatively. It is essential to help patients cope with changes in body image.
- *Stoma ischaemia and necrosis* is caused by inadequate blood supply to the portion of the bowel. Observe the stoma colour in the early postoperative period—a purple dusky colour indicates ischaemia and a black odorous bowel suggest necrosis. Requires urgent surgical assessment.
- *Non-functioning stoma* may be caused by paralytic ileus postoperatively due to bowel handling. The bowel needs to be rested. Fluid and food intake is restricted and gastric aspiration implemented. At a later stage blockages may occur with specific foods, e.g. nuts and raw fruits, which should be avoided; fluids may need to be increased. Adhesions may occur requiring surgical interventions.
- *Prolapse* can result from inefficient fixing of the bowel onto the abdominal surface. Reassure the patient and try a larger appliance applied to the prolapsed bowel to reduce trauma caused by friction. Surgical repair may be necessary.
- *Sensitivity to the skin.* Inflamed or broken skin will compromise the adhesions and security of the appliance. Preoperative testing for allergies (if possible), use of barriers, and careful measuring of the stoma and selection of the appropriate size will help prevent effluent coming into contact with the skin.
- *Herniation* occurs in 25% of patients, usually with end colostomies. Patients should be checked to rule out obstruction; a change of appliance may be necessary together with a support garment for cases of slight herniation. Surgical revision may be necessary.
- *Bleeding.* Spotting of blood during cleaning is common and the patient should be reassured. Checks should be made to rule out serious conditions. Check that the stoma bag is of the correct size and is not causing trauma.
- *Retraction* occurs when the stoma recedes into the abdominal wall and does not protrude above the skin level. It may be due to poor surgical technique or weight gain, and may require surgical repair.
- *Stenosis* occurs when the lumen of the stoma narrows. Colostomy patients should maintain a soft stool to minimize pain and the risk of obstruction. The patient can be taught digital dilation by the nurse specialist.
- *Problems with faecal output*, e.g. constipation, fluid loss, odour, and flatus. Patients should be advised on diet, e.g. have high-fibre diet (porridge oats, Shredded Wheat, root vegetables, and bananas). Foods that help thicken output include white rice, stewed apple, and jelly. Ileostomy patients should avoid food that causes blockage, e.g. mushrooms, nuts, tough fruit skin, and dried fruits. Patients will gradually find which foods they can and cannot tolerate.

Perianal conditions

Haemorrhoids (piles)

These are locally dilated or engorged rectal veins resulting in anal pain, pruritis ani (itching), a mucus discharge, faecal soiling, and bright red rectal bleeding after defecation. They may be external or internal and are divided into four grades:

- *Grade I* do not prolapse out of anal canal.
- *Grade II* prolapse on defecation but reduce spontaneously.
- *Grade III* require manual reduction.
- *Grade IV* are permanently prolapsed. Infarction of the veins may occur (strangulated haemorrhoids) and are extremely painful.

Diagnosis

- Digital examination
- Proctoscopy
- Sigmoidoscopy

Treatment

- Hygiene measures to keep the perineum clean and dry after defecation
- Digital replacement of prolapsed haemorrhoids
- Local anaesthetic cream, topical glyceryl trinitrate
- Sclerotherapy injections (an irritant solution causes a fibrotic reaction which leads to atrophy of the haemorrhoid) or banding of the haemorrhoid (a tight rubber band constricts the vessels and the haemorrhoid shrivels)
- Haemorrhoidectomy if sclerotherapy and banding fail
  - The haemorrhoid plus surrounding skin tags are excised.
  - Postoperatively a rectal pack is in position for 24–36 hours.
  - Removal is painful and the patient should be given pain relief, e.g. IM pethidine; soaking in a warm bath will help.
  - Support and reassurance is necessary and the patient should be told to expect some rectal bleeding.
  - An aperient should be given to promote a soft stool and reduce further pain, together with a high-fibre diet.

Anal fissure

This is a split in the mucosa and skin of the anal canal, often following constipation or inflammatory bowel disease. The patient experiences pain on defecation, spasm of the anal sphincter, and fresh rectal bleeding. Management includes a high-fibre diet, glyceryl trinitrate, or diltiazem topically.

Anal fistula

This is an abnormal track between the perianal skin and the anal canal that may occur following an abscess. The patient has perianal discomfort with discharge and irritation. Treatment requires surgery to open the fistula and dressings to promote healing.

Perianal abscess

These abscesses cause perianal pain and swelling. Defecation and sitting are painful. A swab should be taken for culture and sensitivity, followed by antibiotics, incision, and drainage, if necessary.

Nutritional assessment

Nutritional assessment is important to identify patients with, or at risk of, malnutrition and to enable appropriate interventions to be introduced.

Contributors to malnourishment

Patient factors

- Lack of appetite
- Nausea, vomiting, or feeling unwell
- Pain or breathlessness
- Nil by mouth or fluids only required
- Nutritional losses (e.g. burns, malabsorption, dysphagia)

Nursing factors

- Failure to identify patients at risk
- Failure to take appropriate actions
- Failure to spend time helping patients make food choices and feeding patients
- Failure to ensure that meals are within reach and that patient can manage
- Failure to monitor intake
- Poor organization (drug and ward rounds when meals are served)
- Poor knowledge about nutrition
- Considering nutrition as a low priority

Other factors

- Food poorly prepared and presented
- Lack of choice
- Delivering wrong meal to patient
- Meals taken by bedside rather than at a table
- Awaiting assessment for swallowing
- Odours

Assessment

- Use a nutritional assessment tool/checklist to identify at-risk patients. 📖 Nutritional assessment, above.
- Note the patient's general appearance—presence of pressure sores, weight loss, muscle wasting, whether clothes and rings fit, oral problems, oedema, and self-neglect.
- Assess for any problems with feeding—assessment of mouth (📖 Examination and assessment of the mouth, p.213), dysphagia, difficulty in feeding self, problems with chewing, anorexia, and pain.
- Assess general condition—alertness, specific medical or surgical conditions.
- Evaluate patient's normal dietary intake and patterns and note whether these have changed; include alcohol consumption.
- Note normal levels of activity and exercise and any recent changes.
- Ask patient about recent changes in weight loss or gain.
- Measure patient's weight and height and calculate body mass index (BMI) (See Table 8.1); note method and conditions. Also measure skinfold thickness and serum proteins, if appropriate.

- Involve the dietitian or nutritional nurse specialist as appropriate in the assessment.

Body mass index (BMI)

$$\frac{\text{weight (kg)}}{\text{height (m}^2)} = \text{BMI}$$

Table 8.1 WHO classification of body mass index (BMI) in adults and the risk of developing health problems (BMI = weight in kg/height in m^2)

Classification	BMI* category	Risk of developing health problems
Underweight	<18.5	Increased
Normal weight	18.5–24.9	Least
Overweight	25.0–29.9	Increased
Obese	≥30.0	
Class I	30.0–34.9	High
Class II	35.0–39.9	Very high
Class III	≥40.0	Extremely high

*BMI cut-off values may not be appropriate for all ethnic populations.

Reproduced with permission of the World Health Organization (WHO). © 2004.
http://apps.who.int/bmi/index.jsp?intropage=intro_3.html

Nutritional problems and nursing care

Loss of appetite

Loss of appetite may be due to the patient's medical condition, anxiety, nausea and vomiting, sore mouth, psychological status (e.g. recent bereavement), prescribed medication, alterations in taste sensation, and food aversion.

- Present food in small attractive meals, served frequently, and take account of the patient's likes and dislikes.
- Spend time with the patient choosing from the menu and seeking alternatives when necessary, e.g. high-protein and high-energy diet if condition permits. Snacks and nutritious drinks may be good alternatives.
- Consider administering anti-emetics prior to eating, which may be helpful for patients with nausea.
- Ensure the mouth is clean before eating.
- Consider the use of an appetite stimulant such as a small glass of sherry in some circumstances.

Feeding difficulties

These may include problems with chewing food due to a sore mouth, dental problems or ill-fitting dentures, inability to manipulate cutlery or feed themselves, dislike of being fed, food being placed beyond reach, or patient's position at mealtimes. The patient's medical condition may also cause problems, e.g. dysphagia in neurological causes such as stroke.

- Ensure oral hygiene and dental care.
- Reorganize ward routines to free up nursing time to support patients (protected mealtimes).
- Use specially trained volunteers to help feed patients.
- Ensure adaptive cutlery is available.
- Use of 'red tray' system to identify patients who need help with feeding.
- Ensure that early swallowing assessment is done for stroke patients and others with dysphagia.

Lack of knowledge about nutritious diets and benefits to health

Both patients and staff must understand what a nutritious diet is and its impact on the patient's health. The prevalence of malnutrition in hospital patients is estimated to be 20–53%. Food can create an interest for patients as well as promote wound healing. It is necessary for the immune system and to prevent infection and muscle wasting. Patients with poor nutrition are at higher risk of developing major complications, experiencing readmission, and having extended stays in hospital. The dietitian and nutritional nurse specialist play a significant part in providing education. They also help distinguish between general malnutrition and deficiency of specific nutrients.

Lack of availability of a suitable diet

This may occur when the patient is on a restricted diet due to their condition or may be on fluids only or nil by mouth. Some patients may not have access to food that meets their cultural and religious needs or they are uncertain of the source and reliability. The implementation of the principles of 'Better Hospital Food' and monitoring process has improved the quality of food available to patients in hospital (See www.betterhospitalfood.com). Table 8.2 summarizes the essence of care benchmarks for food and nutrition.

Table 8.2 Essence of care benchmarks for food and nutrition[1]

Factors	Benchmark of best practice
1. Screening and assessment to identify patient's nutritional needs	Nutritional screening progresses to further assessment for all patients identified as 'at risk'
2. Planning, implementation, and evaluation of care for those patients who required nutritional assessment	Plans of care based on ongoing nutritional assessment are devised, implemented, and evaluated
3. A conducive environment (acceptable sights, smells, and sounds)	The environment is conducive to enabling the individual patients to eat
4. Assistance to eat and drink	Patients receive the care and assistance they require with eating and drinking
5. Obtaining food	Patient and/or carers, whatever their communication needs, have sufficient information to enable them to obtain their food
6. Food provided	Food that is provided by the services meets the needs of individual patients
7. Food availability	Patients have set meal times, are offered a replacement meal if a meal is missed, and can access snacks at any time
8. Food presentation	Food is presented to patients in a way that takes into account what appeals to them as individuals
9. Monitoring	The amount of food patients actually eat is monitored and recorded, and leads to action when cause for concern
10. Eating to promote health	All opportunities are used to encourage patients to eat to promote their own health

[1] The Modernisation Agency (2003). *The essence of care: guidance and benchmarks April 2003.* Department of Health, London.

Obesity

Obesity and being overweight are conditions in which weight gain has reached a point that endangers health, e.g. 20% above ideal weight or BMI=25–30 (overweight), 31–40 (obese), or >40 (morbidly obese). The prevalence of obesity is rising. In 2001, 8.5% of 6 year-olds, 15% of 15 year-olds, 67% of men, and 50% of women were either overweight or obese.

Causes of obesity

The most common cause is an excess of energy intake over energy expenditure. Less common factors are genetic factors, endocrine causes, and drugs. Contributory factors for weight increase include age, lower socioeconomic status, lower income, and certain ethnic groups, e.g. Afro-Caribbean and Pakistani women.

Health risks

- *Greatly increased risk* of type II diabetes, gall bladder disease, breathlessness, sleep apnoea, and fatty liver
- *Moderately increased risk* of coronary heart disease, immobility, osteoarthritis, gastro-oesophageal reflux, and gout
- *Slightly increased risk* of cancer (breast, endometrial, and colon), polycystic ovaries, infertility, low back pain, fetal defects, risks during general anaesthetic, anxiety, and depression
- *Mortality:* BMI >27 and weight gain of 10 kg over time are associated with an increase in mortality

Management of obesity

- *Dietary changes:* Low-calorie diets, 1000–1500 kilocalories per day, over a long-term period are effective; very low calorie diets, 400–500 kilocalories per day, are effective for acute weight loss but effectiveness over long term is not as conclusive. A low-fat diet in conjunction with a low-calorie diet is effective.
- *Physical activity* alone produces modest weight loss but is more effective when combined with diet.
- *Behaviour and cognitive therapy* is effective when used in combination with the above.
- *Pharmacological therapy:* Refer to current NICE guidelines.
- *Surgery:* Patients must be attending specialist clinics, have tried non-surgical treatment, and be psychologically assessed and fit for surgery. Gastrojejunal bypass (rarely done) or vertical banded gastroscopy (to reduce stomach capacity; is more common) may be performed.
- *Prevention and maintenance of weight loss:* 📖 Prevention of obesity/Maintenance of weight loss, p.247.

Prevention of obesity

This should include:
- Education for the parents during pregnancy on the importance of a healthy diet, what this consists of, and how it will impact on the baby.
  - Adjust energy intake to maintain ideal body weight.
  - Reduce the percentage of energy derived from fat.
  - Increase consumption of dietary fibre.
  - Increase consumption of complex carbohydrates.
- Practical advice on food shopping and menus. Ensure the information is culturally appropriate.
- Continuing parent education during early developmental years and explaining the benefits of exercise.
- School-based health promotion programmes for children that include nutrition advice and healthy eating.
- Availability of healthy eating options in school and restrictions on the selling of high-calorie sweets and snacks in school.
- School-based physical activity programmes and reduction in sedentary lifestyles.
- Practical sessions in school on learning how to plan and cook a healthy diet.
- Family-based health promotion that focuses on nutrition, what to cook and how to cook, and benefits of activity.
- Information materials on the benefits of healthy diet and exercise.

Maintenance of weight loss

In addition to above:
- Identifying motivating factors for losing weight and reinforcing these.
- Charting weight may be helpful to some.
- Training in dietary and exercise behaviours.
- Obtaining help and advice from support/self-help groups, e.g. Weight Watchers®.

Special GI diets

Postoperative diet
Following the initial postoperative period, fluids and diet are introduced.

Post-colostomy
- Generally patient may eat what they like.
- High-fibre content will help (e.g. porridge, wholemeal bread, root vegetables, bananas).
- Incorporate foods to thicken the stool (e.g. white rice, stewed apple, jelly).

Post-ileostomy
- Initially a soft diet should be consumed.
- A natural high-fibre diet and 'thickening' foods are required as above but avoid mushrooms, nuts, skins, seeds, coconut, celery, tough fruit skins, dried fruits, and raw vegetables.
- At least 2 litres of fluid a day should be consumed.
- Salt should be added to the diet to prevent loss.

Post-gastrectomy
- Encourage high protein intake.
- Reduce sugar and salt.
- Avoid high levels of carbohydrates.
- Take small meals frequently.
- Rest after meals.

Low-fibre diet
The diet is low in whole grains, cereals, nuts, fruit, and vegetables. Alternative sources of vitamin C and folic acid will need to be consumed or supplements taken. This diet may be prescribed in Crohn's disease if there is a history of stricture or obstruction, or in mild or moderate ulcerative colitis.

High-fibre diet
- Often prescribed for diverticular disease.
- Also prescribed for patients with Crohn's disease or ulcerative colitis with constipation.
- Fibre plus increasing fluid intake helps prevent constipation.
- Soluble fibre is found in fruit, vegetables, pulses, and cereals.
- Insoluble fibre is found in vegetables with edible skins (e.g. apples, peaches), whole grains (e.g. All Bran®, porridge, Weetabix®), nuts, and wholemeal bread.
- A sudden increase of fibre may result in flatulence, bloating, and diarrhoea.
- Advise the patient to increase intake slowly over 6–8 weeks.

Low-fat diet
Fat restriction may be needed in steatorrhoea. The diet will need to be supplemented with vitamins A, D, E, and K, calcium, magnesium, and zinc.

Gluten-free diet

- Gluten damages the lining of the small intestine in coeliac disease.
- Gluten is found in wheat, rye, and barley and should be avoided completely for the patient's lifetime.
- Gluten-free products are available, e.g. flour, bread, biscuits, and pasta.
- Alternatives can be used, e.g. rice cakes, potato flour.
- Advise patient to check ready-meals, sauces, and soups for gluten content.
- Most restaurants will meet requests.
- Special advice and recipes can be obtained from a dietitian or from the Coeliac Society.
- Other foods are not restricted in achieving a balanced diet.

Calorie-controlled diets

Obesity, p.246.

Principles of feeding dependent patients

This may be necessary for patients who are unable to use upper limbs, who are visually impaired, who have coordination problems, or who are disorientated or confused.

- Assess the patient and encourage them to help themselves or participate in the process as much as possible.
- Place the patient in a comfortable position and protect clothing. This should be appropriate and ensure the patient's dignity.
- Ensure dentures are in place and the mouth is clean and fresh.
- Where possible, all ward activities should cease (e.g. ward rounds, visiting) to ensure time can be spent with patients who need help.
- Ensure that all equipment is clean, perform hand hygiene, and wear an apron to prevent cross infection.
- Use appropriately sized cutlery.
- Test the temperature of the food.
- Communicate with the patient and involve them in deciding what they eat. Explain to the patient what each food is.
- Give small portions of food and, if possible, allow the patient to participate in putting food in their mouth in order to control the rate at which food is taken.
- Relatives may sometimes wish to feed the patient.
- Observe for signs of swallowing difficulties and seek advice from the speech therapist and dietitian on the most suitable diet.
- Provide sips of water to keep the mouth from becoming too dry.
- Ensure used trays are removed immediately and the area is left clean and tidy.
- Ensure that the patient's mouth is cleaned after the meal, there is no collection in gums or cheeks, and the patient is comfortable.
- Note and record what food has been eaten.

Artificial feeding

Enteral feeding

This is the administration of complete nutrition preparations into the GI tract either orally or through tubes. It should be used when the patient has a functioning GI tract. It is indicated for postoperative patients and for patients with GI disease, altered consciousness levels, and anorexia.

Tube feeding
- Nasogastric, nasoenteric (duodenal or jejunal) tube
- Useful for short-term feeding
- May also be used longer term

Gastrostomy
- Used in upper GI obstruction and when long-term feeding is anticipated.
- Reduces discomfort and embarrassment arising from nasogastric tube.
- Percutaneous endoscopically guided gastrostomy (PEG) tubes are commonly used and held in place by an inflatable balloon.
  - Should not be used where there is either a treatable obstruction or malignancy.
  - Carry significant morbidity and mortality risks.
- Liquid food can be administered by the following depending on the facilities available.
  - A bolus with a syringe
  - Gravity infusion: liquid flows through over given period of time
  - Pump-controlled infusion: can be set at different rates
  - Special liquid preparations

Complications
- GI problems (diarrhoea, constipation, nausea and vomiting)
- Tube-related problems (blockage, dislodgement, nasal trauma)
- Respiratory problems (pulmonary aspiration)
- Metabolic problems (hyperglycaemia, electrolyte imbalance, dehydration)

Parenteral nutrition

This is the administration of all nutritional requirements (amino acids, glucose, fat, electrolytes, vitamins, and minerals) via the IV route. It is used for patients who have critical illnesses, e.g. multiple trauma, sepsis and burns, inflammatory bowel disease, GI obstruction, acute pancreatitis. It can be administered via:

- *A central line inserted* in the subclavian or internal jugular vein – this should preferably be a tunneled line.
- *A peripherally inserted central catheter (PICC)* tip in the superior vena cava.

The nutritional solutions may be hospital prepared or commercially produced and should be formulated according to the patient's needs for energy and nutrition.

Complications
- Infection via catheter or line, dressings, or feeding solution
- Septicaemia
- Dislodging
- Blockage of the tube or rupture
- Pneumothorax and air embolism
- Fluid overload and electrolyte imbalance
- Abnormal liver function tests (LFTs)
- Hypo- or hyperglycaemia

Nurse's role in reducing the risks of artificial feeding

General principles

- Have evidence-based protocols in place for the management of enteral and parenteral feeding that follow national guidance and a system to monitor trends and complications.
- Ensure all staff are trained and up-to-date in enteral and parenteral feeding and in the management of central lines.
- Ensure patients are given sufficient information to provide informed consent to the process. Explain the purpose, benefits, and risks of the procedures and treatment.
- Observe for any side effects or complications (e.g. diarrhoea, nausea, and vomiting) and discuss with members of the multidisciplinary team.
- Monitor body weight and fluid balance.
- Test urine for sugar and ketones and blood for electrolytes and glucose.

Enteral feeding

- Use appropriate tubing and syringes that are not compatible with IV or other parenteral devices and have distinct coloured connector ports and male Luer connections that meet national guidance. Three-way taps must not be used.
- Follow local procedures for inserting tubes (📖 Artificial feeding, p.250) and for checking the tube is in the correct position before administering each feed or medication following vomiting, coughing, or retching, after chest physiotherapy, or if there is any doubt about the tube position.
- Follow agreed checking procedures—check if patient is on medication that may increase the pH of the gastric contents. Check length of tube for signs of displacement, and obtain aspirate. If pH is <5.5 administer feed, if aspirate is >5.5 do not administer the feed. Recheck in 1 hour and seek advice if still >5.5.
- Flush the tube with water after each nutritional formula and administration of medication. Check for gastric residue if the patient feels nauseated.

Parenteral feeding

- Screen patients for infection prior to insertion of catheter or line and periodically thereafter (urine, wound swabs, sputum, and any fluid drainage).
- Use strict aseptic techniques for insertion, dressing change, contact with dressing, and connecting feeding solutions. A dedicated line and lumen must be used only for parenteral feeding.
- Ensure type of line and length is clearly documented.
- Ensure the catheter is properly secured.
- Inspect dressing three times a day. Transparent dressings allow the site to be observed for inflammation and infection, and therefore can be left for changing weekly unless loose or wet.

- Change giving set according to local protocols, e.g. every 24 hours unless there are problems such as blockage. Catheters/lines should be changed weekly unless long-term type.
- Use local guidelines for flushing the catheter, e.g. 3 mL of saline using a 10 mL syringe to avoid high pressure; heparin may also be used. Stop if there is resistance; avoid using excessive force as this causes catheter to rupture.
- Observe for signs of tube being dislodged, e.g. patient hearing gurgling sound in ear, chest pain during flushing, and swelling or pain in neck and arm.
- Observe for signs of infection, e.g. fever, raised pulse, feeling unwell, or deterioration in condition.
- Send the tip of the catheter for culture when the tube is removed.

Fluid and electrolyte balance

Fluid balance is closely associated with a disturbance in electrolyte imbalance.

Patients at risk include those with confusion, inability to communicate, dysphagia, artificial nutrition and fluids, specific medical problems (e.g. renal failure), very young and very old, dependent, immobile, or unconscious, and those on drugs such as diuretics.

Dehydration

Too little water alters blood biochemistry (sodium, potassium, calcium) and causes headaches, dizziness, confusion, hypovolaemia, dry skin and mouth, oliguria, and hypotension, and eventually coma, collapse, and death. It may occur as a result of insufficient fluid intake, diuretics, poly-uria, sweating and diarrhoea, hyperglycaemia, or burns.

Overhydration

This occurs when the amount of water ingested exceeds the body's ability to excrete it, e.g. in renal failure and heart failure. Overhydration pro-duces oedema, ascites, hypertension, weight gain, and reduced serum sodium levels.

Electrolyte imbalance

📖 Fluid and electrolyte imbalance, p.257.

Assessment

- Identify patients at risk (📖 Patients at risk, above) and factors contributing to imbalance.
- Take an accurate nursing history to identify symptoms (e.g. thirst, diarrhoea, excess sweating), specific diseases (e.g. GI disorders, renal failure, terminal illness pathology), drugs (e.g. diuretics), and ability to self-care. Ask family about mental confusion, hallucinations, and general mental health status.
- Identify usual diet and specifically foods high or low in sodium and potassium, e.g. orange, tomato or prune juice, stock cubes, added salt. Ask about any restrictions, fasting, or problems with swallowing or eating. Identify normal fluid intake and fluid preferences and recent changes.
- Measure weight daily—identify rapid weight loss or gain.
- Observe skin for elasticity, dry tongue (dehydration), red swollen tongue (sodium excess), sunken eyes, mucous membranes, and oedema.
- Observe urine for amount and colour (concentration and specific gravity—raised in dehydration), and observe for constipation.
- Keep accurate food and fluid intake and output, and chart and compare total fluid intake with output (See Table 8.3).
- Observe for marked increase or decrease in blood pressure and pulse rate.
- Check bowel movements.
- Observe for specific signs of dehydration or overhydration (📖 Dehydration, p.254 and 📖 Overhydration, p.254).
- Check electrolyte levels (📖 Fluid and electrolyte imbalance, p.257).

Table 8.3 Average fluid intake and output

Average fluid intake (mL)		Average output (mL)	
Oral fluids	1500	Urine	1500
Fluids in food	800	Faeces	200
Oxidation of food	300	Lungs	300
		Skin	600
Total	2600	**Total**	2600

Nursing management of fluid balance

Nursing management

- Assess the patient. 📖 Nursing assessment of patients with GI disorders, p.204.
- Explain to the patient the reason for the fluid imbalance and the interventions being given.
- In conjunction with the multidisciplinary team, identify the amount of fluid intake required during the day and the most appropriate route according to patient's condition and prescription (oral, artificial, or IV). Involve patient in choice where possible.
- For oral fluids:
  - Assess patient's ability to be independent.
  - Provide encouragement and assistance if necessary to restrict or increase intake.
  - Determine patient's preferences and give options and choices of fluid.
  - Consider whether specific diet is required, e.g. for a low-calorie diet choose low-calorie fluids.
  - Provide feeding aids, feeders/straws to promote independence or thickened fluids for patient with difficulty with managing free-flowing fluids.
  - Assess intake regularly (e.g. hourly) and involve family, if appropriate.
- Measure fluid intake and output accurately and show patient/carer how to do this.
  - Use calibrated containers of appropriate size and chart.
  - Do not guess amounts.
  - Ensure patient is provided with a commode frequently to prevent incontinence which cannot be measured.
- Consider use of nasogastric or percutaneous endoscopic rehydration for patients who are too weak to ingest fluids or for patients who have permanent dysphagia (📖 Dysphagia, p.206). In some settings subcutaneous rehydration may be given but the nurse should be skilled in the technique.
- Give replacement fluids via infusion for rapid rehydration with acute dehydration or via central venous access in the longer term. Accurate control and management of the infusion is essential.
- Ensure patients are kept comfortable, with frequent mouth care.
- Reassess frequently; evaluate effectiveness of interventions and monitor progress.
- Discuss with patient and family and provide information and advice on fluid intake and output to prevent problems from recurring. Also provide information on food and drink high and low in sodium and potassium.

Fluid and electrolyte imbalance

📖 Chapter 39, Common laboratory tests and their interpretation, p.1167.

Sodium

Sodium is normally lost through the skin, GI tract, and kidneys. The normal range is 135–145 mmol/l. It is closely linked to water loss and retention.

- *Isotonic dehydration*: a balanced loss of water and sodium
- *Hypertonic dehydration*: a greater loss of water than sodium
- *Hypotonic dehydration*: a greater loss of sodium than water

Hyponatraemia (<130 mmol/l)

Is common in hospitalized patients because of salt loss or fluid overload, e.g. in diuretic therapy, vomiting and diarrhoea, heart, liver, or renal failure, inappropriate IV therapy.

Hypernatraemia (>145 mmol/l)

May be caused by inappropriate IV saline therapy, diabetes insipidus, or dehydration.

Potassium

The kidney controls the potassium balance in the blood. The normal range is 3.8–5.2 mmol/l.

- *Hypokalaemia*: occurs due to potassium loss in diarrhoea, laxative abuse, use of diuretics, diabetes, overhydration, or Cushing's syndrome. It may cause muscle weakness, thirst, polyuria, cardiac dysrhythmias, or paralytic ileus.
- *Hyperkalaemia*: occurs in renal failure, Addison's disease, or the use of potassium-sparing diuretics. Concentrations >6.5 mmol/l may lead to cardiac arrest and ventricular fibrillation.

Calcium

Most calcium is found in the bones but approximately 1% is in the blood. Serum levels are 2.10–2.60 mmol/l.

- *Hypocalcaemia*: may be due to inadequate dietary intake, chronic renal failure, pancreatitis, or hypoparathyroidism. It may cause neuromuscular irritability, cramps, confusion, and convulsions.
- *Hypercalcaemia*: may occur as a result of malignancy, dehydration, diuretics, vitamin D intoxication, primary hyperparathyroidism, and sarcoidosis. It may result in muscle cramps and spasms, paraesthesia, abdominal pain, bone pain, peptic ulcers, malaise, renal stones, polyuria, and thirst.

Phosphate

Normal range is 0.8–1.4 mmol/l.

- *Hypophosphataemia*: occurs in alcohol withdrawal, starvation or malnutrition, dextrose infusions, hyperparathyroidism, or overuse of antacids.
- *Hyperphosphataemia*: may occur in renal failure and metastatic bone tumours. Phosphate, magnesium, and calcium levels should be monitored daily in patients who have been malnourished and are commencing feeding. This is to look for re-feeding syndrome.

Health education for the prevention of GI disorders

- Explain to the patient the function of the GI tract and the various structures in simple terms.
- Provide information on factors that increase the risk of GI disorders.
  - Smoking, stress, excess alcohol and coffee intake which may lead to gastric erosion and peptic ulceration
  - Tobacco and alcohol consumption which increase the risk of oral cancer
  - Obesity and impact on morbidity and mortality
  - Ignoring the stimulus to defecate
  - Family history of some bowel disorders
  - Drugs, e.g. NSAIDs, analgesics, iron supplements, antidepressants
  - Lack of dietary fibre, high consumption of red meat
  - Lack of exercise
- Provide information on healthy lifestyles and behaviours that will reduce the risk of GI disorders.
  - Healthy balanced diet with fibre, vitamins, minerals, fresh fruits and vegetables, as well as protein, carbohydrate, and fats
  - Adequate fluid intake, e.g. 2 l/day
  - Stopping smoking and reducing alcohol consumption
  - Using dental services regularly
  - Benefits of exercise on gut motility
  - Importance of hand hygiene before preparing and eating food and after using the toilet
- Provide information on recurring symptoms that patients should seek medical advice for.
  - Anaemia, weight loss or gain, anorexia, epigastric discomfort, indigestion, swallowing problems, persistent vomiting, melaena, diarrhoea, constipation, any altered bowel habit, bloating, abnormal lumps, bumps, and swellings, abnormal bleeding from the GI tract
- Ensure patient has access to specialist support and advice including:
  - Smoking cessation workers
  - Advice on drinking habits and what are safe levels
  - Dietitian for nutritional advice
  - Dental practitioner and hygienist
  - Speech and language therapist for swallowing disorders
- Provide opportunities to ask questions and discuss how patients can realistically implement this information into their lifestyle.

Discharge and continuing care

- Ensure patients and their families have information about their condition, treatment, prognosis, and future care plan, and that they are aware of any side effects.
- Ensure effective communication with the multidisciplinary team to ensure continuity of care, e.g. GP, community nurse, colorectal or stoma nurse specialist, palliative care nurse, nutrition nurse specialist.
- Ensure patients are able to cope with aspects of self-care or ensure arrangements are made with carers, e.g. changing stoma appliances; giving rectal enemas; and managing stool charts, weight charts, artificial feeding regimens.
- Ensure patients/carers understand the diet and fluids required and can adapt this to daily living on discharge. Also make sure they have any aids to assist feeding, e.g. special cutlery.
- Ensure patients and their families understand the importance of hand hygiene and infection control when carrying out care.
- Ensure patients have appropriate supplies of drugs or equipment (e.g. stoma appliances) and know how to use or dispose of these and/or how to get additional supplies.
- Ensure patients understand what to expect during the convalescent period and the activities they can and cannot do. This will vary depending on their age and medical condition.
- Provide information and contact details of professionals responsible for continuity of care and make sure patients know who to contact if problems arise.
- Provide information on support and self-help groups. 📖 Patient information and support, p.261.
- If appropriate, put patients in touch with other patients who are coping well with the same disorder.
- Ensure patients have scheduled follow-up appointments and arranged transport, e.g. sutures removal, home visits, or outpatient appointments.
- Ensure patients have written information on all aspects of the care and treatment of the condition.
- Provide an opportunity for patients to raise concerns and ask questions.

Patient information and support

- Beating Bowel Cancer   www.beatingbowelcancer.org
- British Dental   www.mouthcancerawarenessweek.org.uk
  Associaion
- British Pharmaceutical   www.bpng.co.uk
  Nutrition Group
- Coeliac Society   www.coeliac.co.uk
- Colostomy support   www.webhealth.co.uk
- Crohn's disease and   www nacc.org.uk.
  ulcerative colitis
- Digestive Disorders   www.corecharity.org.uk
  Foundation
- IBD club   www.ibdclub.org.uk
- Ileostomy and Internal   http://the-ia.org.uk/welfare.htm
  Pouch Support Group
- Mouth Cancer   http://rdoc.org.uk
  Awareness, UK
  Mouth Cancer Patient
  Information Forum
- Health professions'   http://nmap.ac.uk/browse/mesh/D010437.html
  gateway to evaluated
  internet resources
  for nurses, midwives,
  and allied health
  professions

Further information

Norton C (2008). *Oxford handbook of gastrointestinal nursing*. Oxford University Press, Oxford.

Common drugs used for gastrointestinal disorders

Common drugs used for gastrointestinal disorders are listed in Table 8.4. **All drug doses listed in this table are adult doses and not children's doses.** This table is only to be used as a guide and the current BNF should be consulted for further advice. Nurses should involve themselves only in the administration of medications which fall within their sphere of competence.

Table 8.4 Common drugs used for gastrointestinal disorders

Drugs used in treatment of obesity	Dose	Common side effects
Orlistat	120 mg immediately before, during, or up to 1 hour after each main meal up to a maximum of 360 mg daily; treatment continued only if weight loss 12 weeks from start of treatment exceeds 5%; omit dose if meal is missed or contains no fat	Oily leakage from rectum, flatulence, faecal urgency/incontinence, liquid or oily stools, abdominal distension and pain (gastrointestinal effects minimized by reduced fat intake), tooth and gingival disorders, respiratory infections, fatigue, anxiety, headache, menstrual disturbances, urinary tract infection
Anti-emetic drugs	**Dose**	**Common side effects**
Metoclopramide	10 mg (5 mg in young adults 15–19 years under 60 kg) 3 times a day	Extrapyramidal effects especially in children and young adults, hyperprolactinaemia, occasionally tardive dyskinesia on prolonged administration
Prochlorperazine	For acute attack: initially 20 mg followed by 10 mg after 2 hours Prevention: 5–10 mg 2–3 times daily	Extrapyramidal effects – particularly in children, elderly, and debilitated; drowsiness, agitation, and electrocardiograph changes; respiratory depression may occur in susceptible patients; many other side effects (See BNF)
Domperidone	10–20 mg 3–4 times daily up to a maximum of 80 mg	Rarely gastrointestinal disturbances (including cramps), raised prolactin concentration, extrapyramidal effects, and rashes

Table 8.4 Common drugs used for gastrointestinal disorders (continued)

Dyspepsia and gastro-oesophageal reflux drugs	Dose	Common side effects
Compound alginate preparations	1–2 tablets chewed (or 5–10 mL of Gaviscon® Advance Liquid) after meals and at bedtime	Few reported; note some alginate preparations contain significant amounts of sodium

Antispasmodics	Dose	Common side effects
Hyoscine butylbromide	20 mg 4 times a day	Constipation, dry mouth, transient bradycardia (followed by tachycardia, palpitations, and arrhythmias), reduced bronchial secretions, urinary urgency and retention, dilatation of the pupils with loss of accommodation, photophobia, flushing, and dryness of skin
Mebeverine	135 mg 3 times daily 20 minutes before meals	Rarely allergic reactions (including rash, urticaria, and angioedema)

Ulcer healing drugs	Dose	Common side effects
Ranitidine	Dose and duration varies depending on aetiology being treated; standard doses are 150 mg twice daily or 300 mg at night for 4–8 weeks	Diarrhoea and other gastrointestinal disturbances, altered liver function tests, headache, dizziness, rash, and tiredness
Omeprazole	Dose and duration varies depending on aetiology being treated; standard dose is 20 mg once daily for 4 weeks in duodenal ulcer and for 8 weeks in gastric ulcer; maintenance dose for acid related dyspepsia is 10–20 mg once daily	Gastrointestinal disturbances (including nausea, vomiting, abdominal pain, flatulence, diarrhoea, constipation), headache, dizziness, and increased risk of bacterial gastroenteritis
Lansoprazole	Dose and duration varies depending on aetiology being treated; standard dose is 30 mg once daily for 4 weeks in duodenal ulcer and for 8 weeks in gastric ulcer; maintenance dose for acid related dyspepsia is 15 mg once daily	As above

Table 8.4 Common drugs used for gastrointestinal disorders *(continued)*

Helicobactor pylori eradication

A range of combination therapies are recommended in the BNF. These normally consist of a proton pump inhibitor, e.g. lansoprazole, plus two antibiotics, e.g. amoxicillin (or clarithromycin if penicillin allergy exists) and metronidazole.

Antidiarrhoeal drugs	Dose	Common side effects
Loperamide	4 mg initially, then 2 mg after each loose stool for up to 5 days (usual dose 6–8 mg daily up to a maximum of 16 mg)	Abdominal cramps, dizziness, drowsiness, skin reactions (including urticaria), paralytic ileus, and abdominal bloating

Laxatives	Dose	Common side effects
Ispaghula husk (bulk forming agent)	Dose varies with preparation	Flatulence, abdominal distension, gastrointestinal obstruction or impaction
Senna (stimulant agent)	15–30 mg at night (initial dose should be low, then increase)	Abdominal cramps, diarrhoea
Lactulose (osmotic agent)	Initially 15 mL twice daily, then adjust according to patient needs	Flatulence, cramps, abdominal discomfort

Drugs for chronic bowel disorders	Dose	Common side effects
Mesalazine	Dose varies according to brand and formulation of preparation used	Diarrhoea, abdominal pain, exacerbation of symptoms of colitis, headache, hypersensitivity reactions (rash and urticaria), nausea, vomiting
Sulfasalazine	Acute attack: 1–2 g 4 times a day until remission occurs, then 500 mg 4 times a day	As above plus loss of appetite, fever, blood disorders, photosensitivity, ocular complications, urine may be coloured orange, some soft contact lenses may be stained, vertigo, tinnitus, insomnia, depression, hallucinations, kidney reactions

Table 8.4 Common drugs used for gastrointestinal disorders *(continued)*

Parasitic infections	Dose	Common side effects
Metronidazole (📖 Table 20.1 Common drugs used for infectious diseases: Other antibacterials, p.729)	Amoebic dysentery: 800 mg 3 times daily for 5 days Amoebic liver abscess: 400 mg 3 times daily for 5–10 days	Nausea and vomiting, unpleasant taste, furred tongue, gastrointestinal disturbances, oral mucositis, anorexia, rashes, darkening of urine, hepatitis; prolonged or intensive therapy may cause peripheral neuropathy, transient epileptiform seizures, and leucopenia
Mebendazole	Threadworm: 100 mg as a single dose (if re-infection occurs, a second dose may be needed after 2 weeks) Roundworm: 100 mg twice daily for 3 days	Rarely abdominal pain, diarrhoea; hypersensitivity reactions also reported

Stoma care

Enteric coated and modified-release drugs are unsuitable for patients with stomas (particularly ileostomies) as there may not be sufficient release of the active ingredient. Laxatives, enemas, and washouts should not be prescribed for stoma patients and antibacterials should not be given for an episode of acute diarrhoea. See the BNF for further information.

Preparations for anal and rectal disorders	Dose	Common side effects
Glyceryl trinitrate rectal ointment	Apply 2.5 cm of ointment to the anal canal every 12 hours; maximum duration of use 8 weeks	Burning, itching, and rectal bleeding. 📖 Table 7.1 Common drugs used for cardiovascular disorders: Nitrates, p.197

A variety of creams and ointments are available for treatment of haemorrhoids. Many contain soothing agents and others are compound preparations including a steroid or local anaesthetic. Steroid containing creams/ointments can cause atrophy of the anal skin and steroid containing products can be absorbed through the rectal mucosa. Excessive application of such compound preparations should be avoided and duration of use limited to a few days only.

Nursing patients with liver and gall bladder problems

Nursing assessment of patients with liver and gall bladder problems

In addition to a general nursing assessment (📖 Chapter 3, Individualizing nursing care practice, pp.32–33) perform the following procedures.

Observe the patient

Are there signs and symptoms of liver disease?
- Nausea and vomiting
- Oedema—check eyes, face, ankles, feet, genitals; check for signs of ascites
- Lethargy, drowsiness, and poor concentration
- Encephalopathy—note grade (I–IV) as follows:
  - Grade I   Altered mood or behaviour
  - Grade II   Increasing drowsiness, confusion, slurred speech
  - Grade III Stupor, incoherence, restlessness, significant confusion
  - Grade IV   Coma
- Pruritus (itching) due to bile salt deposits; check for bruising and signs of bleeding, spider naevi, scratching
- Colour of skin (yellow tinge)
- Liver flap, clubbing, Dupuytren's, xanthelasma, cyanosis, gynaecomastia
- Breathlessness from fluid overload, pulmonary/peripheral oedema, pleural effusion
- Colour of urine and faeces—dark-coloured urine and pale faeces may indicate biliary obstruction
- Muscle wasting (cachexia) from poor nutritional intake
- Weight loss
- Fetor hepaticus (often characterized as a smell like pear drops)

Ask the patient about

Nursing history
- Ability to manage self-care and activities of daily living
- Support or dependants at home
- Past nursing problems
- Psychological, emotional, and spiritual concerns
- History of substance abuse (alcohol or drug related)
- Fears and anxieties about the condition, diagnosis, prognosis, treatment, and care

Medical history
- Recent history of haemorrhage
- Diarrhoea
- Diuretics (causing hypovolaemia—acute renal failure)
- Decreased cardiac output and hypotension (due to MI and heart failure)
- Diabetes
- Hypertension
- Trauma
- Drugs (nephrotoxicity, anticoagulants)
- Blood transfusion
- Neurological disorders

Specific liver history
- Known liver diseases
- Diet and appetite
- Nausea and vomiting
- Assess fluid and alcohol intake
- Drugs (e.g. diuretics, steroids)
- Encephalopathy—note grade (I–IV)
- Pain (location and type)
- Itching
- Jaundice
- Variceal bleeding

Present symptoms
- Abdominal pain
- Nausea, vomiting, or anorexia
- Jaundice
- Lethargy
- Pruritus
- Oedema and/or ascites
- Breathlessness
- Encephalopathy—note grade (I–IV)
- Dark urine and pale faeces
- Weight loss

Assess nutritional status
- Review diet and nutritional intake.
- Use a formal screening tool and refer to dietitian.
- Assess intake of protein (may need to avoid excess protein) and salt (low salt diet indicated with ascites).
- Assess intake of alcohol (patients should be discouraged from drinking alcohol).

Tests and measures
- Blood pressure—low blood pressure (<60 diastolic)
- Temperature—hyperthermia or hypothermia may indicate infection
- Pulse—tachycardia may indicate infection
- Raised blood glucose may indicate diabetes, low blood glucose may indicate liver failure
- Weight—as a baseline to gauge fluid retention
- Urinalysis—presence of blood and protein may indicate infection or renal pathology (this is an important distinction as proteinuria does not occur in hepatorenal syndrome or hypovolaemic renal failure for example)

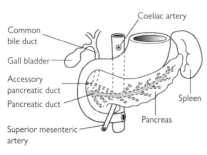

(a)

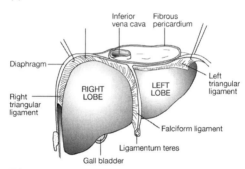

(b)

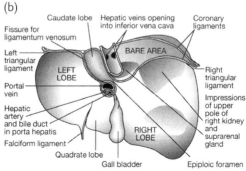

Fig. 9.1 (a) Adult arrangement of the liver and biliary tract. (b) Anterior view of the liver and its peritoneal reflections. Taken from Mackinnon P and Morris J (2005), *Oxford Textbook of Functional Anatomy*, vol 2, Fig 6.6.1b and 6.6.2a. Oxford University Press, Oxford. Reproduced with permission from Oxford University Press.

Special liver tests and investigations

The arrangement of the liver and biliary tract and an anterior view of the liver and its peritoneal reflections are shown in Fig. 9.1.

Laboratory tests
- Liver function tests (LFTs)
- Coagulation screen
- Hepatitis screen
- Anti-mitochondrial antibodies
- Tumour markers, e.g. alphafetoprotein (AFP) if indicated
  (📖 Chapter 39, Tumour markers, p.1183)

📖 Chapter 39, Liver profile, p.1172.

Abdominal ultrasound

Used to detect or investigate:
- Abdominal pain
- Hepatomegaly
- Splenomegaly
- Focal liver lesion
- Hepatic vein thrombosis
- Ascites
- Gallstones

Ascitic tap

This is used to detect spontaneous bacterial peritonitis. It is also used to detect malignancy, nephritic syndrome, CCF, cirrhosis, and portal hypertension.

Imaging
- Abdominal x-ray
- CT – identifies tumours
- MRI – provides detailed structural imaging
- Hepatic angiogram/venogram
- Doppler flow studies of the portal and hepatic vein

Neurophysiological studies

EEG may detect encephalopathy.

Liver biopsy

Percutaneous liver biopsy (may be under ultrasound guidance).

Nursing care of patient undergoing percutaneous liver biopsy
- Ensure patient understands the procedure, the purpose, risks, and benefits of the biopsy and has had time to consider written information.
- Ensure the patient is aware of potential complications (haemorrhage, pneumothorax, pain, and death).
- Encourage the patient to ask questions and express feelings or concern about the biopsy.
- Ensure the patient has given written consent.
- Ensure FBC and clotting profile is taken pre-biopsy and results reviewed.
- Take baseline temperature and blood pressure.

- Ask the patient to lie flat on the bed with their right hand under their head.
- Ensure the patient is given an explanation of what is to take place (insertion of local anaesthetic, location of the biopsy needle).
- Reassure the patient during the procedure.

Post-procedure
- Restrict the patient to bed for 6 hours.
- The patient should lie on their right side for at least 2 hours and then remain on the bed for another 4 hours, sitting up if it is more comfortable.
- Pulse, blood pressure, and observations of biopsy site are taken every 15 minutes for the first 2 hours, every 30 minutes for the next 2 hours, and hourly for the final 2 hours.
- Ensure samples are sent to the laboratory properly labelled with the correct form.

Position
There is controversy over how the patient should lie following this procedure. Some centres nurse patients flat, others on their left side. There have been no studies to prove which is correct, but the argument for the right side is that it may help to compress the puncture site and patients are in the recovery position.

Transjugular liver biopsy
Undertaken if INR >1.4 or more than 4 seconds prolonged, or if the platelet count is <60 000.

Nursing care of patient undergoing transjugular liver biopsy
- Ensure patient is nil by mouth for 6 hours prior to procedure.
- Ensure there is venous access.
- Administer prophylactic antibiotics 1 hour prior to procedure, according to your hospital policy.
- Ensure the patient is aware of potential complications (haemorrhage, infection, and death).
- Ensure that an explanation is given by the specialist radiographer as to what will take place (i.e. insertion of local anaesthetic, location).
- Post-procedure observations and care are the same as for percutaneous biopsy. 📖 Nursing care of the patient undergoing percutaneous liver biopsy, p.272.

Endoscopic retrograde cholangiopancreatography (ERCP)
ERCP gives information about the bile ducts and the pancreatic ducts. It can be undertaken for diagnostic or therapeutic indications. For example, a diagnostic ERCP may show narrowing, obstruction, or gallstones. A therapeutic ERCP enables sphincterectomy, removal of stones, stent insertion or removal, and obtaining biliary cytology.

Nursing care of patient undergoing ERCP
- Ensure patient understands the procedure, the purpose, risks, and benefits of the procedure, and has had time to consider written information.

- Ensure patient is aware of potential complications (cholangitis, pancreatitis, pain, and death).
- Encourage the patient to ask questions and express feelings or concern about the procedure.
- Ensure the patient has given written consent.
- Ensure FBC and clotting profile is taken pre-procedure and results reviewed.
- Take baseline temperature and blood pressure.
- Ensure the patient is given an explanation of what is to take place (i.e. sedation, insertion of endoscope).
- Reassure the patient during the procedure.
- Ensure the patient is nil by mouth for 6 hours prior to procedure.
- Administer prophylactic antibiotics 1 hour before procedure.

Post-procedure
- Administer oxygen therapy until patient is fully awake.
- Monitor blood pressure and pulse every 30 minutes until patient is fully awake and observations are stable. Monitor blood pressure and pulse 4-hourly until discharge.
- Follow eating and drinking protocol unless otherwise directed by medical staff: sips of water only for 4 hours post-procedure; clear fluids for the next 4 hours; patient may eat and drink normally after 8 hours.
- If patient experiences severe pain in abdomen, neck, or chest, contact the medical staff immediately and place patient nil by mouth.

Percutaneous transhepatic cholangiography (PTC)

Nursing care of a patient undergoing PTC
- Ensure patient understands the procedure, the purpose, risks, and benefits of the procedure, and has had time to consider written information.
- Ensure the patient is aware of potential complications (haemorrhage, pain, peritonitis, and cholangitis).
- Encourage patient to ask questions and express feelings or concern about the procedure.
- Ensure the patient has given written consent.
- Ensure FBC and clotting profile is taken pre-procedure and results reviewed.
- Take baseline temperature and blood pressure.
- Ensure the patient is nil by mouth for 6 hours prior to the procedure.
- Ensure there is venous access.
- Administer prophylactic antibiotics 1 hour prior to the procedure.
- Ensure that an explanation is given by the specialist radiographer as to what will take place (i.e. insertion of local anaesthetic, site of insertion of drainage catheter).

Post-procedure
- Restrict the patient to bed for 6 hours.
- Monitor pulse, blood pressure, and puncture site every 15 minutes for the first 2 hours, every 30 minutes for the next 2 hours, and hourly for the last 2 hours.
- Monitor fluid balance and drainage output while external drain is *in situ*.

Nursing problems for patients with liver disorders

Encephalopathy

Due to toxins crossing cerebral membranes and causing cerebral dysfunction. It is graded as follows:
- Grade I   Altered mood or behaviour
- Grade II   Increasing drowsiness, confusion, slurred speech
- Grade III   Stupor, incoherence, restlessness, significant confusion
- Grade IV   Coma

Ascites and/or oedema

Due to portal hypertension together with salt and water retention.
- Breathlessness: fluid retention may lead to development of a pleural effusion
- Increased risk of pressure damage due to lethargy and reduced mobility
- Altered body image due to oedema of eyes, face, and genitalia
- Distended abdomen due to ascites

Abdominal pain

- Varies depending on cause and location, e.g. tumour, spontaneous bacterial peritonitis
- Fever
- Raised temperature or hypothermia may indicate infection of bacterial, viral, or fungal nature

Skin condition

- Jaundice: yellow colouring due to a raised plasma bilirubin level
- Pruritus: itching varies from moderate to severe due to presence of bile salts in skin
- Spider naevi

Impaired nutritional state

Due to nausea, vomiting, anorexia, restricted salt diet and fluid intake, impaired protein, fat, and carbohydrate metabolism.

Anxiety, fear, and depression

Due to long-term prognosis; effects and restrictions on personal, work, and family life; effects of treatment and inability to cope; stigma of diagnosis (e.g. alcoholic liver disease, hepatitis); and fear of receiving donated organs.

Medical interventions

Encephalopathy, ascites, oedema, and abdominal pain are referred for medical treatment.

Pruritis

Administer anti-pruritic agents. Monitor their effectiveness in reducing itching.
- *Colestyramine:* Binds bile salts, which are then eliminated in the faeces. May also bind calcium, fat-soluble vitamins, and other drugs.

Therefore it must be taken 1 hour after tablets and 4 hours before the next tablets. Also causes nausea and flatulence.
- *Ursodeoxycholic acid:* Used in primary biliary cirrhosis to protect the bile ducts in the liver. Unproven as an anti-pruritic agent in other conditions.
- *Antihistamines:* These have some value as a sedative.
- *Naloxone:* Opioid antagonist that is given as an intravenous infusion. Not tolerated by some patients.
- *Rifampicin:* Safety of long-term use not established.

Biliary drainage

Itching can be relieved in 24–48 hours for patients with biliary obstruction by the insertion of a stent (hollow tube), which will allow bile to flow freely. Stenting can be internal, external, or both. If external biliary drainage is required, a percutaneous transhepatic cholangiography (PTC) may be performed. Percutaneous transhepatic cholangiography, p.274.

Non-medical interventions

- Offer regular cool baths.
- Suggest patient wears loose clothing and mittens.
- Keep fingernails short.

Psychological support

- Encourage patients to express their anxieties.
- Give counselling as required.
- May need anti-depressant treatment.

Variceal bleed (melaena or haematemesis)

Portal hypertension

As portal pressure rises above 10–12 mmHg, collateral vessels develop within the systemic venous system. Portal hypertension can be classified according to the site of obstruction. Pre-hepatic obstructions are due to portal vein thrombosis. Intra-hepatic obstructions are commonly caused by cirrhosis. Post-hepatic obstructions can be caused by severe heart failure, pericarditis, and the Budd–Chiari syndrome.

Varices

Varices, which are caused by portal hypertension, are dilated collateral veins (i.e. varices) that occur at sites of porto-systemic anastomosis. They occur in the lower oesophagus, in the stomach, around the umbilicus, and in the rectum. Varices develop in patients with cirrhosis once portal pressure increases. If the portal pressure gradient is >12 mmHg, variceal bleeding may occur. The mortality associated with variceal bleeding is 30–50% per episode. Expert help is needed to manage the event. The patient will need to be resuscitated until they are haemodynamically stable (don't give 0.9% saline). Correct clotting abnormalities, start IV infusion of specialist vasoactive drugs. May require endoscopic sclerotherapy or, if bleeding is uncontrolled, insertion of a Minnesota or Sengstaken-Blakemore tube.

Nursing management

- Monitor vital signs—pulse, blood pressure, and oxygen saturation levels.
- Monitor urine output.
- Maintain airway.
- Insert intravenous line—peripheral or central.
- Obtain blood for group and cross-matching.
- Restore blood volume with plasma expanders or blood transfusion (baroreceptor reflexes are diminished in cirrhosis).
- Administer vasoconstrictor therapy, e.g. terlipressin or octreotide. (Note: Octreotide is rarely used now and is a controversial treatment.)
- Perform urgent endoscopy to establish cause of bleeding, i.e. varices or gastric ulcers. Sclerotherapy or variceal banding is effective in the treatment of variceal bleeding.
- Balloon tamponade (Sengstaken tube) should only be utilized if close supervision of patient can be guaranteed, e.g. in HDU or critical care setting.

Psychological and emotional support is vital. Offer constant reassurance and updates regarding treatment to patients and their families as a variceal bleed will be a frightening and a traumatic experience.

Hepatic encephalopathy

Refers to neuropsychiatric manifestation of liver disease which may be acute or chronic in nature. It is thought to be caused by substances toxic to the brain bypassing the liver and not being neutralized or synthetic dysfunction impairing metabolism, e.g. ammonia not being converted into urea. The exact mechanism is unknown, but several substances have been identified as causative factors by altering the blood–brain barrier to allow toxins to enter and interfere with the normal cerebral metabolism.

Nursing management

- Ensure bowels are kept clear. Aim for two soft stools per day. Administer lactulose and phosphate enemas as needed. Lactulose lowers pH in colon and limits nitrogen utilization.
- Monitor nutritional status. Use food chart to monitor calorie intake. Encephalopathic patients are at risk of malnutrition. Low-protein diets are not recommended now because of their detrimental effects on the patient's nutritional state.
- Monitor fluid balance. Encephalopathic patients are at risk of dehydration.
- Monitor consciousness levels using Glasgow Coma Scale if consciousness levels drop. 📖 Chapter 13, Glasgow Coma Scale, p.475.
- Use the Encephalopathy Grading scale. 📖 Encephalopathy, p.276.
- Maintain a safe environment. One-to-one nursing may be required once a grade III encephalopathic state has been reached. Different patients manifest different signs and symptoms. The patient may be drowsy or agitated and confused. In the latter situation, the patient may be a danger to themselves and other patients.
- Avoid the use of sedatives, if possible, as this will exacerbate the encephalopathy. This is sometimes difficult to achieve and drugs such as haloperidol may have to be used.
- Liaise with the critical care unit once a grade III encephalopathic state has been reached in order to see whether a critical care bed is available. However, most grade III patients are nursed on the ward. A patient may move from a grade III state to a grade IV state (coma) rapidly.
- If moved to ITU, the patient's head is tilted. Also, restrict protein intake and empty bowels. Haemofiltration is indicated if renal failure ensues. Maintain a clear airway (📖 Chapter 33, p.1033.)

Liver failure

Liver failure may occur suddenly in the previously healthy liver (acute liver failure, ALF). More commonly it occurs as a result of decompensation of chronic liver disease (acute-on-chronic liver failure). ALF is classed as liver failure with an onset within the previous 6–8 weeks where encephalopathy is also present.

Causes

- Paracetamol overdose (commonest cause of ALF in the UK)
- Hepatitis A
- Hepatitis B
- Hepatitis C (extremely rare)
- Hepatitis E (20% of women infected in pregnancy in S Asia)
- Drug reactions, e.g. NSAIDs, isoniazid, rifampicin, herbal remedies, 'ecstasy'
- Toxins (e.g. *Amanita phalloides* mushrooms)
- Acute fatty liver of pregnancy
- Rarer causes: infections such as yellow fever, cytomegalovirus, and herpes simplex
- Biliary cirrhosis, haemochromatosis, auto-immune hepatitis, alpha 1 antitrypsin deficiency, Wilson's disease, and liver cancer

Signs and symptoms of acute liver failure

- Encephalopathy/cerebral oedema
- Jaundice
- Fetor hepaticus
- Asterixis (hand-flapping tremor)
- Constructional apraxia (ask the patient to draw a 5-pointed star)
- Signs of chronic liver disease (ascites, variceal bleeding, pruritus)
- Fatigue and lethargy
- Acute renal failure
- Metabolic derangement such as hypoglycaemia
- Drowsiness, stupor
- Signs of infection and fever

Nursing care—management

Patients are typically cared for in an ITU or HDU setting. Specialist liver units may also be consulted with regard to advice and the management or transfer of the patient.

Below are some of the key factors which will be involved in management of the patient with liver failure.

- Insert a urinary catheter and monitor hourly urine output.
- Monitor intravenous fluids.
- Monitor and administer appropriate nutritional regimen.
- Monitor vital signs including central venous pressure (CVP) 1–2 hourly depending on condition.
- Nurse patient with 20–30° head-up tilt.
- Monitor patient's responses.
- Maintain airway.

- Administer nutritional intake via NG tube with restricted protein intake.
- Administer total nursing care and help with activities of daily living.
- Collect daily bloods for FBC, U&E, bicarbonate, glucose, clotting, and LFTs.
- Culture blood, urine, and sputum.
- Assist with x-rays as appropriate.
- Treat the cause of the failure according to medical instructions.
- Avoid all potentially hepatotoxic drugs and those that may worsen complications of liver failure.
- Avoid sedatives (benzodiazepines, opioids).
- Use a low threshold for intubation/mechanical ventilation.
- Consider early referral to renal team.
- Avoid sedatives.

Prognosis

Spontaneous recovery is more likely with hyperacute than subacute presentation. Survival ranges from 10–40%.

Liver cirrhosis

Cirrhosis results from the necrosis of liver cells followed by fibrosis and nodule formation. There is an irreversible loss of normal liver architecture which interferes with liver blood flow and cell function. Liver biopsy confirms clinical diagnosis.

Causes

The most common causes of chronic liver disease in the UK are related to alcoholic liver disease and hepatitis C.

Other rarer causes

- Chronic hepatitis B
- Primary sclerosing cholangitis
- Primary biliary cirrhosis
- Drugs, e.g. methotrexate
- Metabolic liver disease
- Secondary biliary cirrhosis
- Non-alcoholic fatty liver disease
- Haemochromatosis
- Autoimmune hepatitis
- Wilson's disease
- Budd-Chiari syndrome
- Cryptogenic

Compensated cirrhosis

In this type of cirrhosis, the patient has good liver synthetic function (e.g. bilirubin, albumin, and prothrombin time may be normal) without ascites or hepatic encephalopathy. The focus of management is to prevent progression of liver disease (decompensation) and avoid complications. Treating the underlying cause is the best approach, e.g. haemochromatosis, hepatitis B and C, and alcohol dependency.

Decompensated cirrhosis

This type of cirrhosis is indicated by the development of jaundice, hepatic encephalopathy, or ascites. The severity of cirrhosis and risk of variceal bleeding can be graded using the Child-Pugh assessment score.

The Child-Pugh assessment score

Grade A = 5–6

Grade B = 7–9

Grade C > 10

The risk of variceal bleeding is greater if scores are > 8.
Death is common with a 1- and 5-year survival in patients with a Child-Pugh score C of 42% and 21%, respectively, compared with 84% and 44 % in patients with a Child-Pugh score A.

Complications

- Portal hypertension
- Variceal haemorrhage
- Ascites
- Spontaneous bacterial peritonitis
- Encephalopathy
- Hepatorenal syndrome
- Hepatocellular carcinoma

Five-point checklist for assessing patients with chronic liver disease

1. Does the patient have cirrhosis, or non-cirrhotic chronic liver disease?
2. What's the aetiology?
3. In the patient with cirrhosis, is it well compensated or decompensated?
4. What interventions may prevent progression to cirrhosis, or to decompensation in the patient with established cirrhosis?
5. What investigations/interventions are needed to avoid/treat the complications of cirrhosis?

Nursing management of complications

Ascites
- Monitor fluid balance.
- Chart daily weight.
- Administer diuretics.
- Monitor fluid restriction.
- Give no added salt diet (5.4 g or 90 mmol/day).
- Provide post-paracentesis care. 🕮 Paracentesis, p.294.

Nutrition
- Refer to dietitian.
- Give nutritional supplements and high-protein diet.

Encephalopathy
- Monitor consciousness levels.
- Undertake neurological observations if consciousness levels drop.
- Administer lactulose and phosphate enemas. Aim for two soft stools per day. 🕮 Hepatic encephalopathy, p.279.

Pruritus
🕮 Anti-pruritic agents, p.276.

Variceal bleeding
- Administer platelets, fresh frozen plasma, and blood as needed.
- Maintain airway at all times.
- Monitor pulse and blood pressure every 15 minutes until stable. 🕮 Variceal bleed (malaena or haematemesis), p.278.
- Watch for spontaneous bacterial peritonitis.

Liver transplantation

The treatment of choice for patients with end-stage liver failure.

Transplant assessment

- *Phase 1* involves assessment of patient's age, disease, prognosis, and alternatives to liver transplantation. Basic investigations include ultrasound, ECG, CXR, LFTs, U&Es, FBC, arterial pH, clotting, blood group, and virology.
- *Phase 2* involves surgeon and anaesthetist assessing suitability for transplantation.
- *Phase 3* involves patient and relatives receiving education on liver transplantation from the multidisciplinary team. The team includes the liver recipient transplant coordinators, dietitian, pharmacists, chaplain, social workers, and, if relevant, an alcohol or substance abuse counsellor.
- The patient is now ready to be placed on the transplant waiting list.

Donors

- *Cadaveric donor:* from a brainstem-dead donor; usually from patients with acute head or neurological injuries, subarachnoid haemorrhage, CVA, suicide, and brain tumour. Some transplant centres have set up a non-heart-beating donation programme.
- *Living donor:* the donor should be free from infection and cancer, and HIV negative.
- The donor liver is matched in size and blood group to the liver recipient.

Organ allocation and waiting list

All patients waiting for transplants are registered on the UK Transplant National Transplant Database.

- Patients who are in need of transplant as soon as possible due to acute liver failure are given priority over everyone else on the list in the UK.
- The UK is gradually adopting the MELD scoring system and may, in the future, start to prioritize based on the severity of the MELD score.
- Patients can be suspended from the list if they are in an acute ill health situation at present.

Post-liver transplant care

- Monitor and stabilize major organ systems, e.g. cardiovascular, pulmonary, renal.
- Evaluate graft function (primary non-function graft will require re-transplantation).
- Achieve adequate immunosuppression.
- Detect, monitor, and treat complications, e.g. hypothermia, electrolyte imbalance, cardiovascular instability, renal impairment, pulmonary complications, vascular complications, GI complications, biliary complications, neurological complications, infection, diabetes, rejection of the grafted liver.

Discharge home for a patient following liver transplant

The patient should possess:
- The ability to self-medicate safely
- An appointment with a liver clinic
- A supply of medication to take home and an agreement of GP to supply ongoing medication requirements
- A district nurse appointment for removal of surgical clips/sutures and wound care
- Knowledge to recuperate safely, e.g. when to start work, drive a car, travel abroad (information provided by the liver recipient transplant coordinators)

Patients with gall bladder problems

Acute cholecystitis
Usually caused by a gallstone that cannot pass through the cystic duct.

Signs and symptoms
- Pain in right upper quadrant
- Vomiting
- Fever
- Local peritonitis
- Flatulence

Treatment
- Ensure patient is nil by mouth.
- Administer intravenous fluids.
- Monitor fluid balance.
- Administer pain relief and monitor effectiveness (may need opioids).
- Administer antibiotics.
- Cholecystectomy, preferably laparoscopic, if there is no question of gall bladder perforation.

Laparoscopic cholecystectomy is the operation of choice for 90% of patients with gallstones. Patients go home within 24 hours of the operation in most cases and can return to full activity within approximately 7 days. In 10% of cases an open cholecystectomy is performed where full patient activity can take from 6–8 weeks to achieve.

Chronic cholecystitis
Is the more common type and often has an insidious onset.

Signs and symptoms
- Vague abdominal pain
- Distension
- Nausea
- Flatulence
- Intolerance of fats

Complications
- Biliary stones
- Pancreatitis
- Cancer of the gall bladder

Treatment
- Surgery

Acute cholangitis
This is infection of the bile duct.

Signs and symptoms
- Pain in the right upper quadrant
- Jaundice
- Rigors

Treatment
- Antibiotics, e.g. cefuroxime 1.5 g/8 h and metronidazole 500 mg/8 h

Primary gall bladder cancer

This is an adenocarcinoma and represents <1% of all cancers.

Signs and symptoms
- Jaundice
- Right hypochondrium pain

Diagnosis
Often only made at time of operation.

Treatment
Cholecystectomy

Prognosis
Few people survive 1 year.

Acute pancreatitis

Causes
- Gallstones
- Alcohol
- Trauma
- Steroids
- Mumps
- Autoimmunity
- Hyperlipidaemia
- Endoscopic retrograde cholangiopancreatography (ERCP)
- Drugs, e.g. azathioprine, pentamidine, didanosine
- Cardiac surgery
- Idiopathic

Signs and symptoms
- Epigastric or central abdominal pain (radiating to back)
- Vomiting
- Tachycardia
- Fever
- Jaundice
- Shock
- Ileus
- Rigid abdomen

Diagnosis
Serum amylase levels at least 3 times above the laboratory reference range are generally considered diagnostic of acute pancreatitis but must be evaluated along with the history and physical signs. A CT scan or ultrasound may assist with assessing the severity of the condition and may reveal a swollen pancreas, peripancreatic fluid collection, or gallstones.

Complications
- Renal failure
- Shock
- Hypocalcaemia
- Hyperglycaemia
- Pancreatic necrosis
- Pseudocyst
- Abscess
- Paralytic ileus
- Gastrointestinal haemorrhage
- Ascites
- Malnutrition

Nursing management of patients with acute pancreatitis

- Ensure patient is nil by mouth.
- Pass NG tube if abdomen is distended and patient is vomiting. Aspirate tube regularly to remove gastric secretions.
- Administer parenteral feeding if patient remains nil by mouth for a prolonged period of time.
- Administer IV to maintain hydration, cardiovascular stability, and renal function.
- Catheterize patient and monitor urine output hourly. Aim for 30 mL/hour urine output.
- Monitor blood pressure and pulse hourly and observe patient for signs of shock.
- Administer analgesia and monitor effectiveness. Give pethidine rather than morphine (may cause contraction of the sphincter of Oddi).
- Monitor FBC, U&E, calcium, amylase, and blood gases daily. Patient may need a critical care bed if respiratory failure develops.
- Monitor blood glucose levels 4-hourly.

Chronic pancreatitis

Causes
- Alcohol (85% of cases)
- Idiopathic
- Hereditary
- Trauma
- Gallstones
- Pancreatic cancer
- Cystic fibrosis
- Hyperparathyroidism

Signs and symptoms
- Epigastric pain radiating to back. Pain may be chronic or of brief duration. Pain may be mild or acute.
- Steatorrhea, nausea, and vomiting occur due to diminished output of pancreatic enzymes.
- Development of diabetes is common.
- Biliary obstruction leading to jaundice and cholangitis is less common.

Treatment
- Alcohol abstinence
- Surgery (partial or total pancreatectomy)
- Low fat diet
- Diabetic education and treatment
- Pain control

Cancer of the pancreas

Sites of cancer include head of pancreas (60%), tail of pancreas (15%), and body of pancreas (25%). Some patients have cancer affecting more than one part of the pancreas. This type of cancer accounts for <2% of all malignancies with approximately 7000 deaths/year in the UK and rising.

Causes

No definite causes have been identified, but risk factors are thought to include smoking, alcohol, and excessive coffee and fat intake.

Signs and symptoms

Tumours in the head of the pancreas present with painless obstructive jaundice. Tumours in the body and tail present with epigastric pain which typically radiates to the back and may be relieved by sitting forward. Either may cause anorexia, weight loss, diabetes, or acute pancreatitis. Other symptoms include jaundice and abdominal pain.

Management

- Surgery: partial or total pancreatectomy. Gastric bypass to relieve symptoms.
- Chemotherapy and radiotherapy have not been shown to significantly reduce mortality.
- Palliation of jaundice through endoscopic or percutaneous stent insertion.
- Strong analgesic support. Long-acting morphine should be used freely, as addiction will not be an issue for most patients.
- Early referral to palliative care teams.
- Diabetic education and treatment.

Prognosis

Very poor. Most patients survive <6 months. The 5-year survival rate after surgery is <15%. Less than 10% of patients are considered fit for major surgery.

Pancreatic surgery

Prior to pancreatic surgery the patient should be assessed very carefully with particular attention given to their nutritional state. The patient should receive preoperative teaching with regard to the type of operation and their role in recovery.

Whipple's operation

This is the most common operation for cancer of the head of the pancreas (pancreatoduodenoectomy). The surgery involves removing part of the pancreas, the duodenum, part of the stomach, the gall bladder, and part of the bile duct (See Fig. 9.2).

Pylorus-preserving Whipple's operation

This is similar to Whipple's operation, but does not involve removing a part of the stomach.

Total pancreatectomy

This involves removing the entire pancreas, the duodenum, part of the stomach, the gall bladder, part of the bile duct, the spleen, and many of the surrounding lymph nodes.

Distal pancreatectomy

This involves leaving the head of the pancreas and is used to treat cancers of the tail and body of the pancreas.

Postoperative nursing care

Pancreatic surgery is major surgery and patients will require a bed in an HDU on return from theatre.

- Monitor blood pressure and pulse hourly for 24 hours and while analgesic/epidural infusions are in progress.
- Monitor urine output hourly.
- Administer IV fluids while nil by mouth and not drinking freely.
- Ensure abdominal drains are draining effectively.
- Maintain nil by mouth status until the bowel is working normally post-surgery.
- Administer epidural/analgesic infusions and monitor effectiveness of pain relief.
- Aspirate NG tube and ensure effective drainage of gastric secretions.
- Clean and dress wound as required. Sutures or abdominal clips will be removed by the district nurse 2 weeks after surgery.
- Refer to and work with physiotherapists when attempting to sit patients out of bed or when the patient is ready to mobilize.
- Ensure deep breathing exercises are taught to the patient and are practised.
- Refer to dietitians in respect of diabetic and high calorie diets.
- Refer to diabetic nurse specialists, if appropriate.

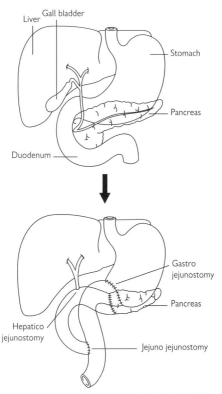

Fig. 9.2 Whipple's procedure. Taken from Bloom S and Webster G (2006). *Oxford Handbook of Gastroenterology and Hepatology*, Fig 2.31. Oxford University Press, Oxford. Reproduced with permission from Oxford University Press.

Nursing interventions

Ascites

Presence of fluid within the peritoneal cavity.

Clinical features

- Abdominal swelling
- Mild abdominal pain or severe pain (may indicate spontaneous bacterial peritonitis)
- Oedema (sometimes present)
- Pleural effusion (sometimes present)

Management

- Fluid balance: daily weights. Fluid balance charts (aim to lose maximum 0.5 kg/day in weight to avoid risk of renal impairment).
- Dietary: sodium restriction and high-protein diet as indicated by dietitian.
- Fluid restriction: often not utilized if serum sodium is <120 mmol/l.
- Diuretics: administer diuretics as prescribed. Spironolactone is the first drug of choice because of its potassium-sparing properties.
- Pain: administer analgesia and monitor its effectiveness. Severe pain may indicate spontaneous bacterial peritonitis (SBP). Prophylactic antibiotics may be indicated if previous episode of SBP has occurred.
- Oxygen therapy may be required if pleural effusion is present or if patient is unable to sit upright.

Paracentesis

If ascites is diuretic resistant, the excess abdominal fluid may need to be drained using a hollow trocar, cannula, or catheter.

Nursing responsibilities

- Establish with medical staff amount of fluid to be drained, i.e. drain until dry or limit to volume drained. (National guidelines instruct to drain until dry, i.e. total paracentesis.)
- Give albumin after the completion of paracentesis, NOT before according to the latest national guidelines.
- Monitor blood pressure and pulse every 30 minutes. Report any drop in blood pressure to medical staff.
- Remove drainage device aseptically after 6 hours to avoid pain and reduce risk of infection.
- Place collection bag over paracentesis site.
- Continue to monitor fluid balance.

Transjugular intrahepatic portosystemic shunt (TIPS)

A TIPS is a small tube about 1 cm in diameter that is placed by a radiologist in the liver to enable blood flowing through the portal circulation to effectively bypass the liver and drain straight into the vena cava. The resulting reduction in portal pressure should lead to a reduced level of ascites.

Nursing care of patient undergoing TIPS

- Ensure patient understands the procedure, purpose, risks, and benefits of the TIPS and has had time to consider written information.
- Ensure the patient is aware of potential complications (haemorrhage, infection, encephalopathy, and death).
- Encourage patient to ask questions and express feelings or concerns about the TIPS.
- Ensure FBC and clotting profile is taken pre-TIPS and results reviewed.
- Take baseline TPR and BP.
- Ensure patient takes no food for 4 hours before procedure. Clear fluids may be taken up to 2 hours before procedure.
- Ensure adequate venous access.
- Ensure prophylactic antibiotics are given 1 hour prior to procedure.
- Post-procedure observation and care—same as percutaneous liver biopsy.

Psychosocial issues for liver patients

Alcohol abusers
Alcohol misuse may result in family disputes, loss of job, financial problems, and loss of self-esteem. Patients who are currently drinking alcohol to excess will also be highly unlikely to be considered for transplantation. Refer patients to a social worker and alcohol experts such Alcoholics Anonymous.

Drug abusers
Patients with hepatitis B and C may well have been involved in the past with illegal drug use. Refer to drug addiction expert for further counselling and advice. Active drug users will not be considered for transplant.

Patients who have taken a paracetamol overdose
Prompt referral to psychiatric services is needed. A social worker referral may be indicated. The family may also need support both during the period of hospitalization and on discharge home.

Patients with an altered body image
Counselling and psychiatric support may be required to address issues of depression and low self-esteem associated with an altered body image, e.g. ascites, jaundice.

Patients with liver cancer
Refer to Macmillan nurses as soon as a definite diagnosis is obtained in order to ensure prompt support for the patient and family is obtained.

Patients with liver transplantation
This major life-changing event is associated with a range of psychosocial and physical issues, e.g. organ donation, care for the patient at home after discharge, and financial implications of a long recuperation.

Stigma of liver disease
Conditions such as hepatitis, drug addiction, and alcoholic liver disease carry a social stigma that can result in low self-esteem. Patients may require counselling and psychiatric support.

Patient education for liver patients

It is the responsibility of the multidisciplinary team to ensure that patients and their families understand the illness and its complexities, or the surgery and its complexities. A multidisciplinary liver team includes medical staff, nursing staff, clinical nurse specialists, Macmillan nurses, social worker, dietitian, pharmacist, chaplain, alcohol or substance abuse expert, and transplant coordination.

- *Diet*: It is vital that the patient and family are given the rationale behind the recommended diet and not just a list of foods. The consequences of non-concordance should also be stressed.
- *Ascites*: Explain the need to monitor the patient's weight at home, adhere to recommended fluid restriction, and adhere to reduced salt diet. Adherence to a fluid restriction and diet is more likely if the consequences of non-concordance are stressed.
- *Encephalopathy*: This can be frightening and traumatic for patients and their family. Explain the need for supervision of the patient when encephalopathic and the importance of ensuring that regular bowel movements are maintained. Reassure the family that behavioural changes are disease related.
- *Support groups*: Inform patients and their families of support groups that are available. Provide telephone numbers and addresses, e.g. alcohol support groups, Macmillan nurses, transplant support groups.
- *Alcohol*: Explain the need for abstinence. Utilize a specialist alcohol expert to educate patient on coping strategies.
- *Liver transplantation*: All members of the multidisciplinary team have a role in preparing the patient and family for the surgery and life after transplantation. This will involve all aspects of organ donations.
- *Liver cancers*: Provide education on the disease process and information on community support services.
- *Surgery*: For postoperative patients, explain the outcome of the surgery and the plan for recovery.
- *Provide information* to the patient and family on treatment options, benefits, and limitations in a way they can understand and make choices.
- *Ensure access* to all members of the liver team for specialist information. Check understanding and provide opportunities to ask questions and have clarification.

Discharge and continuing care

Arrangements vary considerably depending on the patient's disease progression and treatment.

- Check the patient and/or carer:
  - understands their disease and/or surgery and treatment plan and has written information
  - understands their diet and nutritional requirements and can adapt these for home use, e.g. low or reduced salt, high protein, diabetic
  - is confident in managing fluid restriction at home
  - understands the probable course of convalescence, returning to activities and work as appropriate.
- Ensure community support arrangements are in place and contact details have been given, e.g. district nurse, social services, alcohol support, Macmillan nurse.
- Ensure arrangements for wound care and suture removal etc. have been made where appropriate.
- Ensure arrangements for follow-up appointments have been made at clinic or GP.
- Ensure patients have contact details of patient and carer support groups, e.g. alcohol and drug rehabilitation groups, transplant support groups.
- Ensure discharge summaries are communicated to relevant colleagues in primary care and other care sections.
- Explain that patients with medical conditions such as encephalopathy should inform the DVLA Drivers' Medical Unit to advise them of their circumstances.
- Ensure patient and/or carers have been given all medications and education to self-administer safely at home.

Common drugs used for liver and gall bladder disorders

Common drugs used for liver and gall bladder disorders are listed in Table 9.1. **All drug doses listed in this table are adult doses and not children's doses**. This table is only to be used as a guide and the current BNF should be consulted for further advice. Nurses should involve themselves only in the administration of medications which fall within their sphere of competence.

Table 9.1 Common drugs used for liver and gall bladder disorders

Drugs affecting biliary composition and flow	Dose	Common side effects
Ursodeoxycholic acid	Dissolution of gallstones 8–12 mg/kg daily as a single dose at bedtime (or 2 divided doses) for up to 2 years; treatment continued for 3–4 months after stones dissolve	Nausea, vomiting, diarrhoea, gallstone calcification, pruritus
Bile acid sequestrants	**Dose**	**Common side effects**
Colestyramine	Pruritus: 4–8 g daily in water (or other suitable liquid)	Constipation is common but diarrhoea can occur; nausea, vomiting, and gastrointestinal discomfort
Pancreatin	**Dose**	**Common side effects**
Supplements of pancreatin are given by mouth to compensate for reduced or absent exocrine secretion. They are best taken with or immediately before/after food since they are activated by gastric acid. They assist the digestion of fat, starch, and protein. Dosage is according to size, number, and consistency of stools. The most frequent side effects are abdominal discomfort, irritation of the perioral skin, buccal mucosa, and perineal irritation.		
Liver failure/ cirrhosis	**Dose**	**Common side effects**
Lactulose (discourages proliferation of ammonia producing organisms)	30–50 mL 3 times a day (dose adjusted to produce 2–3 soft stools a day)	Flatulence, cramps, abdominal discomfort
Thiamine	Mild chronic deficiency: 10–25 mg daily Severe deficiency: 200–300 mg daily	Few recorded

Table 9.1 Common drugs used for liver and gall bladder disorders *(continued)*

Drugs affecting biliary composition and flow	Dose	Common side effects
Vitamin B+C injection	Coma or delirium from alcohol: 2–3 high potency pairs of ampoules IV every 8 hours	Anaphylaxis may follow injection

Hepatitis B	Dose	Common side effects
Pegylated interferon alfa	Dose depends on product used	Influenza-like symptoms, lethargy, anorexia, nausea, ocular effects, depression
Lamivudine	100 mg daily	Gastrointestinal disturbances, myalgia, arthralgia, fever, rash, urticaria, anorexia, nausea, vomiting, diarrhoea, pancreatitis, liver damage, blood disorders, dyspnoea, cough, headache, insomnia, fatigue, peripheral neuropathy, muscle disorders including rhabdomyolysis, nasal symptoms, alopecia

Transplantation	Dose	Common side effects
Prednisolone	Dose varies	Dyspepsia, oesophageal and peptic ulceration and candidiasis, osteoporosis, adrenal suppression, weight gain, fluid/electrolyte disturbances, hirsutism, increased susceptibility to infection, ophthalmic disorders, impaired healing, bruising (See BNF for more complete list)
Azathioprine	Initially up to 5 mg/kg, then 1–4 mg/kg daily according to response	Hypersensitivity reactions (malaise, dizziness, vomiting, diarrhoea, fever, rigors, myalgia, arthralgia, rash, hypotension, interstitial nephritis – calling for immediate withdrawal), dose-related bone marrow suppression, increased susceptibility to infections and many more (See BNF)

Table 9.1 Common drugs used for liver and gall bladder disorders *(continued)*

Transplantation	Dose	Common side effects
Tacrolimus	Dose varies according to transplant taken place, patient weight, and whether oral or IV (See BNF for details)	Gastrointestinal disturbances, inflammatory and ulcerative disorders, cardiomyopathy, hypertension and many more (See BNF)

📖 Table 25.6 Common drugs used for cancer care, p.854.

Nursing patients with endocrine problems

Hormones

Hormones are chemical substances secreted by cells directly into the blood stream (rather than through ducts). The endocrine glands secrete many of the hormones (See Fig. 10.1). Hormones regulate the metabolic function of other cells in the body. They are classified chemically into one of two large groups of biochemical molecules: amino-acid-based molecules and steroids.

Pituitary gland (anterior lobe)
- Corticotropin or adrenocorticotrophic hormone (ACTH)
- Gonadotropins: luteinizing hormone (LH) and follicle-stimulating hormone (FSH)
- Mammotropin or prolactin (PRL)

Pituitary gland (posterior lobe)
- Oxytocin
- Vasopressin—antidiuretic hormone (ADH)

Thyroid gland
- Thyroxine (T_4), tri-iodothyronine (T_3), and thyrocalcitonin

Parathyroid gland (four parathyroid glands)
- Parathyroid hormone (PTH)

Adrenal glands (two adrenal glands, suprarenal glands)
- Catecholamines, epinephrine and norepinephrine, aldosterone, glucocorticoids, cortisol (hydrocortisone), cortisone, and corticosterone

Pancreas (Islets of Langerhans)
- Glucagon from alpha cells
- Insulin from beta cells
- Somatostatin from delta cells

Gonads

Testes
- Male sex hormones, i.e. testosterone

Ovaries
- Oestrogens: oestrone, oestradiol
- Progesterone
- Testosterone

Thymus gland
- Thymosin
- Thymopoietin

Pineal gland
- Melatonin

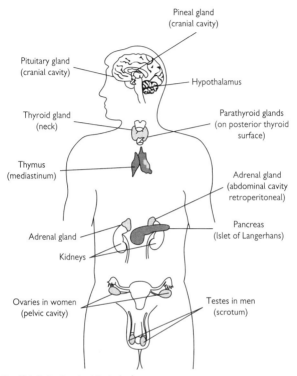

Fig. 10.1 Endocrine glands in the body.

Nursing assessment of patients with endocrine problems

In addition to a general nursing assessment, 📖 Chapter 3, Individualizing nursing care practice, pp.32–33.

Alterations in endocrine function usually lead to problems within the body relating to:

- Energy production
- Energy storage
- Abnormal growth and development
- Abnormal reproductive and sexual function

The anatomical location of the endocrine glands (See Fig. 10.1) limits the ability to perform a direct physical assessment (except for the thyroid gland). Therefore, special attention should be paid to the patient's history regarding the following:

Fluid and nutritional state

- Has the patient's fluid and food intake increased or decreased?
- Has there been any weight loss or weight gain?
- Encourage patient to keep a detailed food diary.

Excretion pattern

- Has the patient experienced urinary frequency, nocturia, or dysuria?
- Has the patient had an increase or decrease in thirst?
- Ask about the colour of stools and frequency of bowel movements. Encourage the patient to keep a stool chart.

Energy level

- What is the patient's normal routine and energy level? Has it changed?
- Has the patient experienced tiredness and lethargy?

Changes in body image

Ask the patient and their family about any recent changes in the physical appearance of the patient:

- Hair distribution
- Skin
- Facial appearance or voice
- Bodily proportions

Reproductive and sexual function

Obtain a reproduction and sexual history relating to menstrual cycle, erectile dysfunction, fertility, and sexual relationships.

Coping with stress

- How is the patient adapting to and coping with problems and changes in their life?
- What are some of the most recent stresses they are experiencing?
- Has the patient had more common colds, infections, bouts of depression, euphoria, anger, crying, or have they been generally feeling under threat or panic?

Physical observations
- Examine muscle mass, fat distribution, skin colour, hair distribution, and fluid retention.
- Note the patient's alertness and response.

Diagnostic tests

These tests are usually carried out because of an oversecretion or undersecretion of the hormone caused by abnormal functioning of the endocrine glands due to disease or injury. Diagnostic tests are used to evaluate:

- Level of hormone in the blood
- Adequacy of endocrine tissue in secreting hormone
- Interrelationships among the various hormonal glands controlled by the anterior pituitary hormones
- Various factors controlled by the endocrine system

Several tests are needed. The routine physical preparation for any test may vary from one organization to the next but the patient should always be informed of the purpose of the test as well as what to expect before, during, and after the test.

Laboratory tests

- Blood tests are used to measure the concentration of hormones (e.g. thyroid hormones, reproductive hormones).
- Urine (24-hour collection) tests may be more appropriate to measure hormones in some conditions (e.g. cortisol in Cushing's syndrome, catecholamines in pheochromocytoma).
- Indirect tests are used to measure the effect of the hormone and not the hormone itself (e.g. serum calcium in primary hyperparathyroidism or blood glucose in diabetes).
- Dynamic function tests may be used to indirectly assess the function of a hormone (e.g. water deprivation test to assess ADH in suspected diabetes insipidus).
- Stimulation tests are used to assess suspected undersecretion of hormones (e.g. ACTH stimulation test in suspected Addison's disease).
- Suppression tests are used to assess suspected oversecretion of hormones (e.g. dexamethasone suppression test in suspected Cushing's syndrome).
- Thyroid function tests are used to diagnose thyroid disorders (hypothyroidism or hyperthyroidism) and include serum free thyroxine (FT4), free tri-iodothyronine (FT3), and thyroid-stimulating hormone (TSH).

📖 Chapter 39, Common laboratory tests and their interpretation, p.1167.

Radiological tests

- Thyroid ultrasound and thyroid scans help diagnose thyroid dysfunction.
- Routine x-rays show how an endocrine dysfunction is affecting body tissues.
- CT scans assess an endocrine gland's structure.
- Nuclear imaging studies help diagnose thyroid dysfunction.

Radioactive iodine uptake test

A tracer dose of radioactive iodine is given orally. At 2, 6, and 24 hours after administration, a special detector is placed over the thyroid gland and the amount of accumulated iodine is measured. Urine is collected for 24 hours. Decreased amounts in urine indicate a hyperthyroid state.

Some key findings in endocrine disorders

General observation
- Personality changes, e.g. disorientation, confusion, drowsiness, depression
- Change in voice
- Overweight, coarse features, muscle wasting, and 'buffalo hump'

Head
- Changes in shape
- Changes in hair growth, e.g. thinning
- Eye and visual changes, e.g. blurred vision, puffy eyes, exophthalmos and lid lag
- Facial flushing and moon-faced dull blank expression
- Acetone on breath

Neck
- Enlargement, i.e. goitre

Chest
- Breast enlargement in men (gynaecomastia)
- Dyspnoea
- Angina, palpitations

Abdomen
- Weight loss or weight gain
- Increased appetite
- Polyphagia, excessive hunger
- Constipation or diarrhoea

Genitals
- Polyuria, polydipsia
- Decreased urine
- Renal calculi
- Cliteromegaly

Upper and lower limbs
- Tremor, weakness, fatigue, muscle cramps, muscle wasting
- Fractures, osteoporosis
- Foot problems
- Decreased tone and reflexes
- Finger clubbing
- Pain in arms and legs

Skin condition
- Profuse sweating or decreased perspiration
- Erythema
- Hyperpigmentation or hypopigmentation
- Poor skin turgor, dryness, pallor, flushing, warmth

Endocrine gland disorders

Hyperthyroidism (thyrotoxicosis)

Hyperthyroidism is excessive production of thyroid hormone caused by disease to the thyroid gland, TSH-secreting pituitary tumour (rare), or over-replacement with thyroid hormone therapy. A common cause of hyperthyroidism is Graves' disease, which affects the eyes, skin, bone, and thyroid gland (gland becomes larger, i.e. goitre). It is more common in women aged 20–30 years. Hyperthyroidism is hereditary and may be linked to severe dietary problems. Cardiovascular involvement such as heart failure, atrial fibrillation, and angina occurs in older patients. Symptoms include heat intolerance, change in menstrual pattern, diarrhoea, skin problems, and exophthalmos. It is diagnosed by low serum T_4, and high TSH.

Treatment
- Reducing hormone levels
- Drugs that inhibit T_3 production
- Radio-iodine (^{131}I) therapy
- Surgery (total or subtotal thyroidectomy)

Hypothyroidism (myxoedema)

Hypothyroidism is a deficiency of thyroid hormone caused by thyroid tissue loss or atrophy (primary) or due to a pituitary defect (secondary). Goitre formation may occur as the pituitary gland secretes more TSH in response to low thyroxine. Goitres may occur naturally in some people or in response to iodine deficiency. Hypothyroidism can be caused by certain drugs. The patient complains of lethargy, weight gain, cold intolerance, constipation, muscle aches and weakness, and anorexia. Other symptoms include puffy face, expressionless face, ivory yellow thick rough scaly skin, dry scalp, coarse brittle hair, thin eyebrows, large tongue, and deep voice. It is diagnosed by low serum F4 and high TSH.

Treatment
- Thyroxine replacement therapy
- Review in 12 weeks
- May need to treat heart disease

Parathyroid disorders

The two types of parathyroid disorders are primary hyperparathyroidism (hyperfunction of glands and high calcium) and hypoparathyroidism (low function and low calcium). The chief complaints of patients with hypoparathyroidism are muscle weakness and tremors. Patients with hyperparathyroidism may be asymptomatic, but complain of abdominal pain and depression. These disorders are diagnosed by measuring serum calcium, phosphate, magnesium, and PTH.

Treatment
Primary hyperparathyroidism
- Surgery
- Monitoring calcium levels and avoiding stone formation
- Fluids

Hypoparathyroidism
- Calcium and vitamin D

Pituitary gland disorders

The pituitary gland plays a crucial role in stimulating other endocrine glands. Problems may occur in the anterior or posterior pituitary lobe or in both. Anterior lobe disorders include developmental abnormalities, congenital defects, circulatory disturbances, and tumours. Posterior lobe disorders include diabetes insipidus and tumours (teratomas and gliomas).

Treatment

- Hormone replacement, if needed
- Surgery for tumours
- Radiotherapy if incomplete removal of tumour

Adrenal gland disorders

Dysfunction of the adrenal gland causes adrenal hormone excess or deficit (e.g. Cushing's syndrome; chronic glucocorticoid excess, in particular a cortisol excess). These disorders can be:

1. Primary—stemming from an intrinsic disorder such as a neoplasm.
2. Secondary (Cushing's disease)—resulting from a pituitary or hypothalamic dysfunction or tumour. Common in women 30–50 years old.
3. Iatrogenic—stemming from excessive or chronic administration of synthetic steroids (e.g. cortisone or prednisone).

Signs and symptoms include an increase in weight, menstrual irregularity, amenorrhoea, facial hair in women, impotence in men, depression, muscle weakness, fractures, thin skin, bruising, water retention, hypertension, and hyperglycaemia. These disorders are diagnosed by laboratory tests (overnight dexamethasone suppression test, serum cortisol levels), imaging, and pituitary MRI. Treatment includes removing the source, i.e. surgery and radiotherapy, plus drugs.

Adrenal crisis (adrenal insufficiency)

This is the most serious complication of adrenocortical insufficiency and can occur gradually or with catastrophic suddenness. It occurs in patients who do not respond to hormone replacement therapy or in those with severe stress and without adequate glucocorticoid replacement. It can occur because of abrupt corticosteroid withdrawal, and therefore, steroid therapy must be withdrawn gradually. Assess for headache, confusion, dizziness, restlessness, apathy, pallor, increased respiratory rate, fatigue, muscle weakness, hypoglycaemia, nausea, vomiting, diarrhoea, abdominal cramps, weight loss, appetite loss, dehydration, reduced urinary output, increased pulse rate, and hypertension. Treatment includes airway maintenance, oxygen, and IV fluids. Replace glucocorticoids by giving IV hydrocortisone 6-hourly until stable.

Addison's disease

This is a rare disorder caused by adrenocortical insufficiency.

Pheochromocytoma

This is a rare tumour which can be benign or malignant and can be of the medulla or both adrenal glands. Middle-aged women are at risk. Patients have hypertension and postural hypotension, and a paroxysm or attack in which they experience strange chest sensations, deep breathing, and pounding heart rate. It is diagnosed by collecting urine for 24 hours for catecholamines and their metabolites. It is treated by surgical removal.

Hyperaldosteronism

This develops from excessive secretion of mineralocorticoids, primarily aldosterone. There are two types: *primary* (Conn's syndrome) which is caused by a benign adenoma; and *secondary* which is caused by a pathological condition outside the adrenal cortex.

Thyroid surgery

Preoperative considerations

- Continue to administer antithyroid drugs (ATDs).
- Achieve euthyroid state; other drugs may be added such as propranolol.
- Occasionally, potassium iodide, 60 mg three times daily may be used to prevent unwanted liberation of thyroid hormones during surgery.
- Inform patient of what to expect following surgery and prepare in the usual way. 📖 Chapter 22, Patients requiring perioperative care, pp.762–770.

Postoperative care

- Assess and monitor the patient's vital signs. Monitor and report any signs of:
  - Laryngeal nerve damage (hoarseness, weak voice)
  - Haemorrhage or tissue swelling (excess bleeding may not appear at the front of the dressing; check back of neck)
  - Respiratory distress
  - Choking sensation
  - Difficulty in coughing or swallowing
- Check for early signs of calcium deficiency (tetany). Patient may complain of tingling sensation around mouth, fingers, and toes.
- Be prepared for an emergency by having the following available:
  - Tracheostomy set
  - Suture removal set in case of obstruction
  - Oxygen and suction equipment
  - IV calcium gluconate or calcium chloride for tetany
- Know what actions to take if the patient becomes distressed and an acute respiratory problem arises.
  - Call for help.
  - Maintain airway.
  - Raise head of bed.
  - Loosen dressing over incision.
  - Give IV calcium if release of dressing does not stop complaint of tingling.
- Involve the patient in their postoperative care by teaching them about their operation preoperatively and re-emphasizing things as they recover from the anaesthetic.
- Support their head and neck when turning 2-hourly postoperatively (i.e. place hands behind the neck and to the sides).
- Ensure the patient has adequate pain control.
- Encourage fluids and a high-carbohydrate high-protein diet.
- Liaise with speech and language therapy team to assess swallowing prior to eating and drinking.
- Later, encourage the patient to exercise their neck.
- Prior to discharge home, ensure patient knows about their lifelong thyroid hormone replacement therapy if they have had a total thyroidectomy.

Nursing care after parathyroidectomy
- Assess and monitor patient's vital signs.
- Observe for any signs of breathing and speaking difficulties.
- Monitor for any signs of calcium loss, e.g. tetany and paraesthesia.
- Monitor for any signs of haemorrhage.
- Encourage patient to express any feelings of pain and discomfort.
- Have a tracheostomy set and IV calcium preparations readily available.
- Monitor intake and output.
- Describe reason for observations and involve the patient in their postoperative care.

Diabetes mellitus

Diabetes mellitus is an irreversible metabolic disorder of multiple aetiolog (WHO 1999). It is a long-term progressive condition characterized by raised blood glucose level. Although a genetic link has been established, universal trigger factor has yet to be determined. There are two types o diabetes mellitus (Table 10.1).

Classification
Type 1 diabetes: insulin insufficiency is caused by autoimmune destruction of insulin-secreting pancreatic beta-cells.
Type 2 diabetes: caused either by defects in insulin secretion or in the way the body utilizes insulin. (This is known as insulin resistance.)

Table 10.1 Characteristics of type 1 and type 2 diabetes mellitus

Characteristic	Type 1	Type 2
Insulin status	Insulin secretion depleted	Deviations in insulin secretion
Age	Under 30 usually	40+ or any age
Presentation	Rapid onset	Slow onset
Body	Underweight or normal	80–90% diagnosed cases overweight
Family history	Weak	Strong
Islet cell antibodies	Present	Absent
Symptoms	Polyuria, polydipsia, weight loss	Asymptomatic or as type 1
Ketones/ketosis	Present or prone (increased risk of)	Rare
Frequency	15% of diagnosed cases	85% of diagnosed cases
Complications	Common related to duration and contributing risk factors	Sometimes present at diagnosis. Common related to duration and contributing risk factors
Treatment	Insulin, diet, exercise	Diet, oral agents, insulin, exercise

In patients with diabetes mellitus, the pancreatic beta-cells fail to secrete insulin and/or the amount secreted is ineffective (insulin resistance). This results in a build-up of glucose in the blood because it cannot be utilized by the cells. A high level of glucose (normal levels 3.5–7.5 mmol/l) in the blood is known as *hyperglycaemia*. People with diabetes are at increased risk of long-term damage to various organs and systems such as kidneys, nerves, vascular system, and eyes.

The incidence is increasing in all age groups worldwide. Type 2 diabetes is one of the most common chronic conditions affecting older people. It is more common in certain ethnic groups (South Asian, African, Afro-Caribbean, and Middle Eastern). Diabetes cannot be cured, but with treatment, support, and education it can be managed.

Causes

Factors that may contribute to the development of diabetes include environmental or genetic factors (for type 1), and obesity and an inactive lifestyle (for type 2).

Diagnosis

- A 2-hour plasma glucose ≥11.1 mmol/l
- A fasting plasma glucose ≥7 mmol/l if patient symptomatic, two results are required ≥7 mmol/l in the asymptomatic patient

Impaired glucose tolerance
- Fasting plasma glucose <7.0 mmol/l and 2-hour post glucose load plasma glucose between ≥7.8 and <11.1 mmol/l

Impaired fasting glycaemia
- Fasting plasma glucose between ≥6.1 and <7.0 mmol/l

Further information

WHO: www.who.org

Presentation and treatment of diabetes

Type 1 diabetes

Signs and symptoms
- Polyuria (excessive urination different to frequency)
- Polydipsia (persistent excessive thirst)
- Weight loss
- Lethargy
- Occasional itching and skin infections
- Elevated blood glucose, urinary glucose, and ketosis (classic presentation)
- Diabetic ketoacidosis (rarely)

Treatment
- Type 1 diabetes requires urgent treatment with insulin.
- There are many different types of insulin which vary in duration of action.
- At present insulin is best administered subcutaneously.
  - Insulin pens are normally used.
  - Pens can be pre-loaded or reusable devices.

Admission to hospital is only required if the patient is acutely unwell (diabetic ketoacidosis, DKA)
- DKA is a life-threatening complication of diabetes characterized by hyperglycaemia, osmotic diuresis, metabolic acidosis, glycosuria, ketonuria, and dehydration (blood glucose >17 mmol/l, ketones >3 mmol/l, acidosis pH <7.3, and bicarbonate <15 mmol/l).
- Treatment includes correcting dehydration, electrolyte imbalance, and ketoacidosis; and lowering blood glucose levels as per local guidelines.
- Explore contributing factors to DKA. Educate the patient and their relatives to prevent reoccurrence where possible.

Type 2 diabetes
Patients may be unaware of their condition because they have only one or two symptoms. Patients are often overweight and may complain of fatigue or reoccurring infections that are slow to heal.
- Refer to dietitian for appropriate dietary advice.
- Assess for hypertension and hyperlipidaemia and treat accordingly.
- Assess lifestyle factors such as smoking, alcohol, and exercise. If lifestyle management (e.g. diet and increased exercise) is not adequate to improve blood glucose levels, consider oral hypoglycaemic agents (See Table 10.2, p.325).
- As Type 2 diabetes is a progressive condition many patients, despite their best efforts, will eventually require insulin by injection.

Specific nursing assessment points

- Determine type of diabetes.
- Note duration of condition.
- Note current treatment.
- Assess nutrition and diet.
- Assess knowledge and self-management skills, i.e. blood glucose monitoring, urine testing, and injection technique if appropriate and any difficulties relating to these.
- Evaluate lifestyle issues, e.g. work, hobbies and activities, exercise, alcohol, and smoking status.
- Identify psychological factors that may affect self management of diabetes, e.g. depression.

Blood glucose monitoring

It is normal for blood glucose levels to fluctuate throughout the day. A simple capillary blood test, performed several times a day, reveals patterns in the body's response to medications, certain foods, and exercise. Based on this information, decisions regarding changes to oral agents and insulin can be made. Optimal blood glucose levels range between 4 and 8 mmol/l. Blood glucose monitoring frequency is determined based on individual needs and local policies should be followed. Poor eyesight, arthritis, or cognitive impairment may indicate difficulty in independent blood glucose monitoring. Long-term blood glucose control can be measured by a glycosylated haemoglobin (HbA1c) test, which requires venous blood. Target range is <7.0% for most patients (See NICE guidelines).

Hypoglycaemia

This refers to a low blood glucose level <2.8 mmol/l. Symptoms include lethargy, severe tiredness, dizziness, weakness, sweating, tachycardia, palpitations, tremor, headache, visual disturbances, and confusion. Treatment includes testing the blood glucose level, giving 15 g quick-acting carbohydrate (e.g. 5 glucose tablets, 5 fruit pastilles, or 100 mL lucozade), followed by 15 g long-acting carbohydrate (e.g. a slice of bread or 2 digestive biscuits). Patients who have an impaired level of consciousness and who are unable to swallow should be placed in recovery position with their airway maintained. IM glucagon may be considered (See Table 10.2) or IV dextrose may be given.

Hyperglycaemia

This refers to a blood glucose level >8.0 mmol/l, whether the result is consistently elevated or a single measurement. Possible causes of hyperglycaemia include undertreatment of diabetes (i.e. insufficient insulin or oral agents), excessive carbohydrate intake, infection or illness, medication that induces hyperglycaemia (e.g. steroids), or inactivity. Treatment includes establishing an underlying cause and treating the cause as necessary.

Nursing management of the patient with diabetes who is admitted to hospital

In addition to natural fears and anxieties caused by admission to hospital individuals may also have fears specific to their diabetes.

Care in outpatient departments

- Avoid delays in appointment times as a delay may interfere with the patient's medication and meal schedule.
- Be aware that patients may have an episode of hypoglycaemia. Know how to recognize symptoms and treat hypoglycaemia, if it occurs.
- Have biscuits, sandwiches, and drinks available.
- Monitor blood glucose level, if appropriate.
- Inquire about the time and dose of the last diabetes medication the patient has taken.
- Ensure the patient knows when to take their next dose of diabetes medication.

Patients undergoing elective surgery

- Blood glucose levels are usually managed with an IV insulin regimen as per local protocol.
- Patients need to be nil by mouth for 6 hours.
- Optimal glycaemic control is preferable preoperatively, i.e. HbA1c in target range (<7.0%) and stable blood glucose levels where possible.
- Surgery should be performed in the early morning to minimize variations from normal control measures.
- Patients should be kept on their usual food, fluid, and medication routine until the night before surgery and re-assessed for possible IV fluids.
- Blood glucose levels should be monitored regularly throughout surgery and postoperatively so that hyperglycaemia and hypoglycaemia are avoided where possible.
- The patient's usual regimen of insulin should be commenced before IV insulin is discontinued so that adequate insulin levels are established. This is done when the patient's condition is stable.
- Blood glucose levels should be optimized to enhance wound healing and recovery.

Nursing interventions for patients with diabetes

Effective management of diabetes requires a multidisciplinary team approach that includes the patient and their family. Education should focus on empowering the patient to achieve day-to-day control of their diabetes.

- Ensure the patient understands their diabetes and how it will impact their lifestyle.
- Ensure the patient knows about the likelihood of complications.
- Assess the level of appreciation the patient's partner, family, and close friends have for the patient's condition.
- Evaluate how the patient monitors and controls their blood glucose levels, according to individual needs.
- Confirm that the patient's blood glucose meter is functioning correctly so that results are accurate.
- Ensure that individual dietary advice is available.
- Emphasize the importance of regular exercise.
- Encourage a reduction, if not cessation, in smoking.
- Emphasize the importance of concordance with treatment.
- Teach the patient what to do in cases of hypoglycaemia and hyperglycaemia.
- Inform the patient of the effects of taking other medications on diabetes control.
- Instruct the patient on what to do if they are admitted to hospital and what information to carry in cases of emergency.
- Inform the patient of the effects of other illnesses and infection on diabetes control.
- Encourage regular checks of blood pressure.
- Emphasize the importance of good eye care and regular eye checks for retinopathy.
- Emphasize the importance of foot and leg care with attendance at a chiropodist if needed.
- Provide travel advice and advise where to obtain information.
- Inform the patient of potential support agencies and where to access evidence based information.

The aim of the National Service Framework for Diabetes in the UK is to maximize the quality of life of all people with diabetes and to reduce their risk of developing long-term complications.

National Service Framework for Diabetes

- Prevention of type 2 diabetes.
- Identification of people with diabetes.
- Empowering people with diabetes.
- Clinical care of adults with diabetes.
- Management of diabetic emergencies.
- Care of people with diabetes during admission to hospital.
- Detection and management of long-term complications.

Common drugs used for diabetes

Common drugs used in patients with diabetes are listed in Table 10.2. **All drug doses listed in this table are adult doses and not children's doses**. This table is only to be used as a guide and the current BNF should be consulted for further advice. Nurses should involve themselves only in the administration of medications which fall within their sphere of competence.

Table 10.2 Common drugs used for diabetes

Insulin—The aim of treatment is to achieve the best possible control of blood glucose concentration while avoiding troublesome hypoglycaemic reactions. The duration of action of a particular type of insulin varies from one patient to another and needs to be assessed individually. Insulin regimens usually consist of one or a combination of the insulin groups below.

	Dose – always expressed in units	Common side effects
Short-acting insulin, e.g. soluble insulin, insulin lispro, insulin aspart, insulin glulisine	Usually injected SC 15–30 minutes before meals – onset of action 30–60 minutes with a peak at 2–4 hours and duration up to 8 hours; if given IV (and can be given IM) the peak is very quick (within minutes) and effectively disappears within 30 minutes	All types of insulin have the potential to cause hypoglycaemia and can also cause transient oedema, local reactions, and fat hypertrophy at the injection site; rarely hypersensitivity reactions (e.g. urticaria) and rash though insulin containing protamine may cause allergic reactions
Insulin of intermediate duration of action, e.g. isophane insulin, insulin zinc suspension	When given by SC injection insulin has an onset of action of 1–2 hours with maximal effect at 4–12 hours and duration of 16–35 hours	
Insulin whose onset of action is slower and lasts for long periods, e.g. crystalline insulin zinc suspension, insulin glargine, insulin detemir		

Oral antidiabetic drugs are used for patients not adequately controlled by diet and exercise. They should be used to augment the effects of diet and exercise, not replace them. These agents generally fall into one of three types – sulphonylureas, biguanides, and a group of miscellaneous agents such as the thiazolidinediones.

Table 10.2 Common drugs used for diabetes *(continued)*

	Dose	Common side effects
Sulphonylureas, e.g. glibenclamide, gliclazide, tolbutamide, glipizide, glimepiride	See individual agent in BNF Used in patients who are not overweight or where metformin is contraindicated; glibenclamide and chlorpropamide are best avoided in the elderly because they may cause hypoglycaemia even at normal doses	Nausea, vomiting, diarrhoea, and constipation; excessive dosage causes prolonged hypoglycaemia
Biguanides, e.g. metformin	Used in patients who are overweight unless contraindicated 500 mg with breakfast for at least 1 week, then 500 mg with breakfast and evening meal for at least 1 week, then 500 mg with breakfast, lunch and evening meal; maximum dose 2 g daily in divided doses	Anorexia, nausea, vomiting, diarrhoea (usually transient), abdominal pain, metallic taste; rarely lactic acidosis but can occur in patients with renal impairment and is an indication for withdrawal of biguanide
Prandial glucose regulators (stimulate beta cell production of insulin), e.g. repaglinide, nateglinide	See individual agent in BNF Used in patients who are not overweight or where metformin is contraindicated	Hypoglycaemia, gastrointestinal disturbances, hypersensitivity reactions, e.g. urticaria, pruritus
Thiazolidinediones	Pioglitazone—initially 15–30 mg daily increased to 45 mg daily according to response	Gastrointestinal disturbances, weight gain, oedema, anaemia, headache, visual disturbances, dizziness, arthralgia, hypoaesthesia, haematuria, impotence

Hypoglycaemic emergency	**Dose**	**Common side effects**
Glucose injection	50 mL glucose 20% injected via a large vein (or 25 mL glucose 50% though this is more viscous and irritant to veins)	
Glucagon injection	1 mg if body weight over 25 kg 500 mcg if body weight under 25 kg NB If no response within 10 minutes IV glucose must be given	Nausea, vomiting, abdominal pain, hypokalaemia, hypotension

For foot and skin care: 📖 Table 12.1, Common drugs used for dermatologic conditions, pp.432–4; Table 20.1 Common drugs used for infectious diseases, pp.728–31. See local dressings/tissue viability policy and BNF for dressings.

Common drugs used for endocrine disorders

Common drugs used for endocrine disorders are listed in Table 10.3. **All drug doses listed in this table are adult doses and not children's doses**. This table is only to be used as a guide and the current BNF should be consulted for further advice. Nurses should involve themselves only in the administration of medications which fall within their sphere of competence.

Table 10.3 Common drugs used for endocrine disorders

Thyroid disease	Dose	Common side effects
Carbimazole	15–40 mg daily in divided doses and reduced when patient is euthyroid (usually after 4–8 weeks) to 5–15 mg daily	Nausea, mild gastrointestinal disturbances, headache, arthralgia, rashes and pruritus are relatively common; agranulocytosis may occur so sore throat, mouth ulcers, malaise, fever, bruising **must be reported immediately**; other side effects include arthralgia and headache
Levothyroxine	Initially 50–100 mcg daily (50 mcg for those over 50 years) before breakfast increased in 25–50 mcg steps every 3–4 weeks until metabolism normalized	Usually at excessive dosage – angina, arrhythmias, palpitation, tachycardia, skeletal muscle cramps, diarrhoea, vomiting, tremors, restlessness, weight loss, flushing, fever, sweating, heat intolerance, excitability, insomnia, headache, muscular weakness
Pituitary	**Dose**	**Common side effects**
Tetracosactide	250 mcg IM or IV as a single dose test for adrenocortical function	As for corticosteroids, e.g. prednisolone
Desmopressin	Dose varies according to illness being treated and route of administration	Fluid retention, hyponatraemia (with convulsions in more serious cases) on administration without restricting fluid intake, stomach pain, headache, nausea/vomiting, allergic reaction, emotional disturbance in children; nasal spray may cause epistaxis, nasal congestion or rhinitis

Nursing patients with renal and urological problems

Nursing assessment of patients with renal problems

In addition to a general nursing assessment (📖 Chapter 3, Individualizing nursing care practice, pp.32–33) perform the following procedures.

Observe the patient
- Nausea, vomiting, anorexia, poor nutrition
- Oedema: check ankles, sacrum, and periorbital areas
- Lethargy, poor concentration, confusion, drowsiness, seizures
- Restless legs
- Pale (anaemia), yellow tinge to skin, dry skin and scratching (pruritis) that may be due to high serum urea
- Easy bruising
- Breathlessness from fluid overload (pulmonary oedema) or acidosis

Ask the patient about

Nursing history
- Ability to manage self care and activities of daily living
- Social circumstances and home support (dependants at home, carer availability)
- Past and present nursing problems or issues
- Psychological, emotional, and spiritual assessment
- Fears and anxieties about the condition, prognosis, treatment, care, and past experiences

Medical history
- Medications, e.g. diuretics, antihypertensives (especially ACE inhibitors), erythropoietin injections (EPO), steroids, NSAIDs, antibiotics
- Previous surgery
- Medical conditions, e.g. diabetes, hypertension (and hypotension), cardiac disease, stroke, infections, connective tissue disorders (e.g. SLE), trauma

Specific renal history
- Hypertension
- Urinary tract symptoms (e.g. UTIs, haematuria)
- Known underlying renal diseases
- Dialysis (haemodialysis or peritoneal dialysis)
- Renal transplant
- Dietary and fluid restrictions

Present symptoms
- Reduced appetite, nausea, and vomiting
- Changes to urine output
- Pain (location and type)
- Lethargy
- Pruritus
- Oedema
- Breathlessness

Test and measure

Blood pressure

- High blood pressure is both a cause and consequence of kidney disease. It may indicate fluid overload (e.g. insufficient fluid removal on dialysis).
- Low blood pressure may be caused by poor cardiac function, antihypertensive medications or excessive fluid removal during dialysis; also occurs with renal trauma (retroperitoneal bleeding).
- Never measure blood pressure in the same limb as an AV fistula.

Urine

- Rapid changes in urine volume occur in acute renal diseases, e.g. glycosuria, leucocytes, haematuria.

Weight

- Used to monitor fluid balance and nutrition.

Nursing problems for patients with renal conditions

Changes in urine output

Anuria: <100 mL in 24 hours. Anuria must be differentiated from retention of urine or a blocked catheter.

Oliguria: <400 mL in 24 hours. Causes are analogous to acute renal failure.

Polyuria: excessive volume of urine (>3 litres in 24 hours); often causes nocturia. It should be distinguished from frequency due to infection or inflammation.

Fluid balance

Monitoring fluid balance is a central skill in renal nursing. 📖 Chapter 8, Fluid and electrolyte balance, p.254.

Concomitant medical conditions

Renal patients often have many co-existing conditions that must always be taken into consideration, e.g. diabetes, cardiac disease, systemic lupus erythematosis (SLE).

Uraemic symptoms

Uraemic symptoms occur when excessive amounts of the metabolic waste products normally excreted by the kidneys accumulate in the blood stream.

- Nausea, vomiting, taste changes, loss of appetite, and malnutrition
- Lethargy, poor concentration, drowsiness, confusion, and seizures
- Headache—may be due to a raised blood pressure
- Breathlessness
- Skin irritation, itching
- Bleeding due to platelet dysfunction

Pain

Renal pain: varies depending on cause; localized loin pain/tenderness may be due to trauma or infection, e.g. in pyelonephritis or kidney stones. Many serious renal disorders are painless.

Chest pain: due to concomitant angina or pericarditis.

Infection

Dialysis and transplant patients are particularly prone to infection. Raised temperature and rigors may also occur with pyelonephritis. Transplant patients are on lifelong prophylactic antibiotics.

Malnutrition

This may result from nausea, vomiting, anorexia, taste changes, dietary restrictions (e.g. protein, phosphate, and salt), restricted fluid intake, or infections. Thorough nutritional assessment is extremely important in renal disease.

Anxiety, fear, and depression

Many renal diseases are chronic. Patients may have concerns regarding long-term prognosis; the effects on personal, work, and family life (especially the impact of dialysis treatment); and their ability to cope.

Special renal tests and investigations

Urinalysis (dipstick testing)
- Protein (albumin) may indicate renal damage (e.g. diabetes, hypertension, glomerulonephritis, SLE).
- Microscopic haematuria has many causes, including trauma, renal and bladder tumours, infections, renal tract stones, and glomerulonephritis.
- Glycosuria usually suggests diabetes mellitus, but also occurs in some forms of renal tubular damage.
- Positive tests for leucocyte esterase and nitrites suggest infection, but require laboratory confirmation by microscopy and culture (MSU).

Common laboratory tests
- Serum U&E
- Estimated GFR (eGFR) (This is now routinely reported with creatinine in all hospital laboratories. No extra blood tests are required. It is calculated from serum creatinine using the 'MDRD' formula adjusting renal function for age, sex, and race [the result must be multiplied by 1.21 in black patients]. It is not validated for use in acute renal failure, in pregnancy, or in patients aged <18, but is used to classify chronic kidney disease into five stages.) 📖 Chronic kidney disease, p.340
- FBC (anaemia)
- Serum bicarbonate (helps assess degree of acidosis)
- LFTs (↓ albumin in nephrotic syndrome and poor nutrition)
- Bone profile and parathyroid hormone (PTH) (disturbances common in renal disease)
- C-reactive protein (CRP) (↑ indicates infection or inflammation)
- Urine protein-to-creatinine ratio
- Urine microscopy for presence of red cells; culture and sensitivity to detect infection and guide antibiotic selection if present

Diagnostic imaging
- *Renal ultrasound* is used to detect kidney(s) and abnormalities, document their size (small kidneys suggest chronic kidney disease), exclude obstruction (causes hydronephrosis: dilatation of renal pelvis or ureter), identify renal calculi (may miss small or ureteric stones), evaluate masses (cysts/tumours) or blood/fluid collections around kidney following trauma (or biopsy). Also commonly used after transplantation. See Fig. 11.1 for diagram of kidney.
- *Abdominal x-ray* may identify renal calculi.
- *Intravenous urography/pyelography (IVU/IVP)* identifies presence and position of kidneys and ureters and detects abnormalities such as calculi, cysts, tumours, and obstruction.
- *CT scan* is increasingly used to characterize renal and peri-renal masses (simple cysts vs. tumours), collections and abscesses, calculi, extent of trauma, and obstruction. Caution: CT contrast is nephrotoxic.
- *MRI* provides detailed structural information. MRI contrast (gadolinium) should be avoided if eGFR <50 mL/min.
- *Renal arteriography* is an invasive procedure that is used to identify a renal arterial stenosis.

Renal biopsy

Used if histological diagnosis is required, especially in unexplained acute or chronic renal failure or nephrotic syndrome. Can also give prognostic information and guide treatment.

Nursing care of the patient undergoing renal biopsy

Pre-procedure

- Ensure that patients understand the biopsy and its potential benefits, that they have had time to consider the procedure, and that they have received written information and have given written informed consent.
- Ensure patient is aware of complications (pain, haematuria, blood clot, infection and, very rarely, loss of a kidney or death) and has been given the opportunity to discuss them. Encourage the patient to ask questions and express feelings about this.
- Undertake the pre-biopsy tests and ensure the patient understands why these are being done (FBC, U&E, LFT, clotting profile, group and save serum). Make sure the results are available and have been reviewed.
- Ensure there is venous access.
- If the patient has significant renal impairment, some units will have a protocol to reduce bleeding risk (e.g. to give IV desmopressin acetate). Check local guidelines.
- Take baseline observations of temperature and blood pressure.
- Ask the patient to empty their bladder pre-biopsy.
- Arrange the patient in a prone position with a pillow or sandbag under the abdomen.
- Explain what the nephrologist will do (infiltration of local anaesthetic, then insertion of biopsy needle) under ultrasound guidance.
- Reassure the patient during the procedure.

Post-procedure

- Ensure the patient remains in the same position for 30 minutes with pressure to the biopsy site for at least 10 minutes.
- Ensure the patient remains on bed rest for 4–6 hours.
- Monitor temperature and blood pressure every 15 minutes for 2 hours, every 30 minutes for the next 2 hours, and then 4 hourly. If any of these parameters change, call for assistance immediately.
- Monitor urine output and observe for presence of haematuria.
- Give analgesia and monitor its effects.
- Repeat FBC may be required to ensure the haemoglobin has not dropped.
- Ensure biopsy samples are sent to the laboratory properly labelled with correct form.
- Advise the patient not to undertake strenuous activity for 2 weeks.
- Ensure the patient knows who to contact if problems arise after discharge.
- Main complication is bleeding.

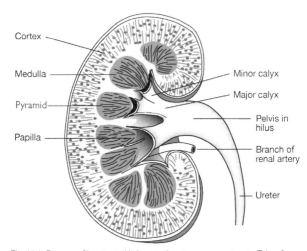

Fig. 11.1 Diagram of hemisected kidney to show its component parts. Taken from MacKinnon P and Morris J (2005). *Oxford Textbook of Functional Anatomy*, vol 2, Fig 6.7.3. Oxford University Press, Oxford. Reproduced with permission from Oxford University Press.

Common disorders and procedures encountered on the renal ward

Renal syndromes

Patients with renal conditions are categorized into one of four clinical syndromes based on their signs, symptoms, and investigation results.

Nephrotic syndrome

This is characterized by heavy proteinuria, hypoalbuminaemia, and peripheral oedema.

- Reduce discomfort from oedema.
- Ensure proper fluid balance and salt restriction (<5 g/day).
- Recognize increased risk of thrombosis (e.g. DVT and PE).
- Prepare the patient for kidney biopsy. 📖 Renal biopsy, p.333.
- Manage multiple medications (e.g. diuretics, corticosteroids).
- Assess pressure areas at risk.

Nephritic syndrome

This is characterized by hypertension, microscopic haematuria, proteinuria, oliguria, and deteriorating renal function.

- Manage multiple medications (e.g. antihypertensives, immunosuppressants).
- Prepare the patient for kidney biopsy.
- Ensure adherence to salt restriction (<5 g/day).
- Prevent fluid overload and pulmonary oedema.

Acute renal failure (acute kidney injury)

This is characterized by a rapid fall in GFR (📖 Acute renal failure, p.338). It is often reversible.

- Ensure strict fluid balance.
- Observe for signs of infection.
- Possibly prepare the patient for acute dialysis.

Chronic kidney disease

This is characterized by irreversible, usually progressive decline in GFR.

- Prevent its occurrence (e.g. good control of blood sugar in patients with diabetes) or delay its progression (e.g. control of blood pressure, smoking cessation).
- Reduce cardiovascular risk (e.g. exercise).
- Monitor for and treat complications (e.g. anaemia).
- Provide symptom relief (e.g. breathlessness).
- Modify patient's diet (e.g. low in potassium and phosphate).
- Prepare patient for dialysis or transplantation.

Surgical procedures

Creation of dialysis access is performed by insertion of a haemodialysis catheter, formation of an AV fistula, or insertion of a Tenckhoff peritoneal dialysis catheter.

Renal transplant may be a planned admission for a live donor transplant or an emergency admission for a deceased transplant.

Nephrectomy is usually undertaken for a renal tumour. It may also be desirable in other situations, especially if the kidney is non-functioning (e.g. recurrent infections, large staghorn calculi). It can be done laparoscopically. Donor nephrectomy is also performed in living donor for transplantation.

Pyelolithotomy is the removal of a stone through the renal pelvis, usually for large staghorn calculi.

Nephrolithotomy is percutaneous removal of a stone from the renal substance.

Pyeloplasty is refashioning of the pelvic-ureteric junction of a kidney when it does not function properly or causes obstruction to urine outflow.

Preoperative care

- Ensure patient understands risks and benefits of surgery, the nature of pre- and postoperative care, and the surgical procedure itself.
- Ensure written information is given.
- Ensure necessary investigations have been undertaken including checks of kidney function (serum creatinine, eGFR), FBC, group and cross-match, urinalysis, urine for microscopy, culture and sensitivity, and imaging (e.g. intravenous urography [IVU], renogram, ultrasound).
- Prepare for general anaesthetic, if appropriate.
- Undertake baseline blood pressure and temperature.
- Ensure consent is signed (📖 Consent to treatment, p.770).
- For renal surgery, ensure the correct side is marked to make certain the correct kidney is operated on; check that consent form and theatre list correspond.
- Explain importance of deep breathing and lung expansion postoperatively even though it may be painful.
- Reassure the patient that adequate analgesia will be given.
- Explain urinary catheter, IV drip, nephrostomy tube, or drainage tubes if they will be present and their purpose.
- Listen to patient's anxieties about operation, prognosis, and impact on daily life.

Postoperative care

- Ensure adequate analgesia is given and monitor effect.
- Observe temperature and blood pressure to identify haemorrhage and infection.
- Observe urine output, colour, and odour.
- Record fluid intake and output.
- Observe drainage from tubes and record output. Check tubes are secure and dressings clean and dry. Discuss how long drains are to remain *in situ* with the surgical team.
- Encourage sitting and deep breathing as soon as the patient is alert.
- Commence sips of water, fluid, and light diet as patient can tolerate.
- Provide regular information, support, and advice to patient and family.

Acute renal conditions

Acute renal failure

Pre-renal causes

Decreased circulating volume resulting from:

- hypovolaemia due to haemorrhage, burns, or diarrhoea
- sepsis causing systemic vasodilatation
- cardiogenic shock (e.g. post-myocardial infarction).

Renal causes

- Acute tubular necrosis (ATN) caused by ischaemia due to decreased renal perfusion (e.g. hypotension, shock) or nephrotoxins (especially drugs, e.g. NSAIDs, IV contrast, gentamicin)
- Malignant hypertension
- Renal artery occlusion due to thrombosis
- Acute glomerulonephritis (nephritic syndrome)
- Systemic diseases such as multiple myeloma and SLE

Post-renal cause

Obstruction resulting from conditions such as:

- stones
- prostatic hypertrophy
- tumours
- retroperitoneal fibrosis.

Nursing care

- Manage fluid balance.
  - Fluid intake restriction may be necessary to prevent fluid overload. To prevent dehydration or hypovolaemia, ensure oral, IV, or NG fluid replacement. The precise parameters of 'overload' and 'dehydration' will vary from patient to patient depending on the degree of renal failure.
  - Monitor and record all fluid intake and output; weigh patient daily.
- Monitor temperature and blood pressure on patient chart.
- If CVP line *in situ*:
  - Measure regularly using consistent reference point.
  - Ensure post-insertion chest x-ray has been reviewed.
  - Observe carefully for signs of line infection.
  - Remove as soon as possible.
- Administer drugs, e.g. diuretics, nitrates, antibiotics.
- Observe for indications for emergency dialysis, e.g. breathlessness due to pulmonary oedema, cardiac arrhythmias from hyperkalaemia or worsening metabolic acidosis.
- Administer oxygen therapy to maintain oxygen saturation >95%.
- If serum potassium >6.0 mmol/l or rapidly rising, place patient on continuous cardiac monitoring. Administer emergency treatments (e.g. insulin and dextrose infusion) as prescribed and without delay.
- Monitor closely for signs of infection, e.g. fever, infected cannulae or dialysis catheters, purulent sputum, cloudy or offensive urine.
- Provide clear explanation of acute dialysis, if necessary.
- Keep patient clean and comfortable, ensure clear explanations are given, and provide support to patient and family.

Acute pyelonephritis

This is acute inflammation of the kidney caused by ascending UTI, often *E. coli*. Symptoms include rigors, tachycardia, hypotension, urinary frequency, dysuria, cloudy and offensive urine, tenderness over kidney, and nausea and vomiting. Renal abscess is an uncommon complication.

- Perform urinalysis and send MSU.
- Administer antibiotics, anti-emetics, and analgesia as prescribed.
- Monitor and record temperature and blood pressure.
- Encourage oral fluids and administer IV fluid, if required.
- Monitor and record all fluid intake and output and weigh patient daily.
- Keep patient clean and comfortable, ensure explanations are given, and provide support to patient and family.

Renal trauma

This may be due to blunt or penetrating injuries and is associated with back and abdominal injuries. Symptoms usually include localized loin pain and tenderness, haematuria, and low blood pressure if there is ongoing bleeding. Colic may result from the passage of blood clots. Resuscitation with IV fluids and transfusion may be necessary; ultrasound or CT scan may be performed to assist diagnosis, and surgery may be required.

Chronic kidney disease

Chronic kidney disease (CKD) is a disease that develops as a result of irreversible renal damage. Progressive deterioration of renal function occurs over months or years and may eventually lead to end-stage renal failure (ESRF). As CKD advances (eGFR <30 mL/min) patients may start to develop a variety of symptoms. However, there is considerable inter-patient variability and symptoms may not appear in some patients until GFR is reduced to 10–15 mL/min (📖 Nursing problems for patients with renal conditions, p.330 for common symptoms). End-stage renal failure is the point at which an individual's kidney function is no longer sufficient to meet their physiological needs and maintain their health (around an eGFR of <15 mL/min) and renal replacement therapy is required. CKD prevalence increases with age and is more common in many ethnic minorities.

CKD is divided into five stages according to eGFR:

Stage of CKD	GFR (mL/min/1.73 m² surface area)	Description
1	>90*	Kidney damage* with normal GFR
2	60–89*	Kidney damage* with mild reduction in GFR
3	30–59	Moderately reduced GFR
4	15–29	Severely reduced GFR
5	<15	Kidney failure

*Must also be evidence of chronic kidney damage, e.g. abnormal urinalysis (blood, protein) or abnormal renal imaging.

Table: NKF K/DOQI classification of CKD (redrawn with permission from National Kidney Foundation). See National Kidney Foundation (2002). 'Part 4. Definition and classification of stages of chronic kidney disease'. *Am J Kid Dis*, **39**(2, Suppl 1), S46–S75.

- Normal GFR is ~100 mL/min/1.73 m² so estimated GFR (eGFR) roughly equates to a percentage of kidney function.
- GFR >60 mL/min alone is not considered as CKD unless coupled with further evidence of kidney damage such as structural abnormalities on imaging or an abnormal urinalysis.
- The early stages of CKD are often asymptomatic and complications such as anaemia usually begin to arise when patients reach stage 3 (GFR 30–60 mL/min).
- Most patients in stages 1–3 will not progress to end-stage renal failure and the clinical priority in these patients is to reduce cardiovascular risk as many will develop serious cardiovascular disease (e.g. MI, stroke).

Common causes

- Diabetes mellitus, which accounts for 20% of all cases, causes thickening (sclerosis) of the glomeruli.
- Glomerulonephritis (i.e. inflammation of the glomeruli) may be triggered by infection (e.g. streptococcal) or auto-immune disease (e.g. SLE).
- Hypertension causes damage to the renal microcirculation.
- Chronic pyelonephritis (or reflux nephropathy), i.e. repeated infections of either or both kidneys in childhood.
- Atherosclerotic renovascular disease is a build-up of plaque in the renal arteries; it is a similar process to coronary artery disease.
- Polycystic kidney is an inherited disease causing enlarged cystic kidneys with disturbed function.

Management

- Identify and treat cause where possible.
- Aim to prevent further damage.
  - If diabetic, maintain good control with regular blood sugar monitoring, effective insulin/oral hypoglycaemic regimen, and diet.
  - Control hypertension with antihypertensives (e.g. ACE-inhibitors), including diuretics if fluid overloaded.
  - Treat dyslipidaemias (usually with a statin).
  - Encourage exercise, weight loss, healthy diet, and smoking cessation.
- Implement appropriate diet (depends on severity of CKD): low salt (<5 g/day), high carbohydrate (30–35 kilocalories/kg/day), and potassium and phosphate restriction. A reduced protein diet may slow progression of CKD, but its use is controversial as it requires extremely careful supervision and may lead to malnutrition.
- Prevent and treat bone disease, e.g. phosphate binders and vitamin D supplements.
- Regularly monitor blood pressure and blood glucose, and test blood for creatinine and eGFR.
- Identify and treat complications, e.g. hyperkalaemia, anaemia, metabolic acidosis.
- Prepare patient for renal replacement therapy, e.g. haemodialysis, peritoneal dialysis, renal transplantation.

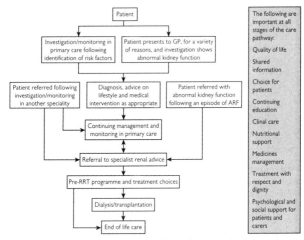

Fig. 11.2 Care pathway for chronic kidney disease. Reproduced with permission from the National Service Framework for Renal Services. See: DH Renal NSF Team (2005). *Part two: chronic kidney disease, acute renal failure and end of life care.* Department of Health, London.

Nursing care of patients with chronic kidney disease

Fig. 11.2 presents a care pathway for chronic kidney disease.

Treatment of symptoms

Anaemia

- Caused by reduced levels of the hormone erythropoietin.
- Requires careful monitoring of haemoglobin.
- May require recombinant EPO injections (SC 1–3 times a week). Note that EPO may increase blood pressure.

Iron deficiency

- Results from a reduced ability to absorb iron from gut, poor nutrition, frequent blood tests, and haemodialysis itself.
- Oral iron (e.g. ferrous sulphate) may not be adequate and IV iron is often required.
- Adequate iron stores are essential to maintain haemoglobin especially for patients on EPO (usually aiming for ferritin >150 mcg/L).

Oedema

- Results from fluid retention.
- Restrict fluid intake to 1000–1500 mL per day.
- Administer diuretics as prescribed.

Calcium and phosphate imbalance (usually ↓ calcium and ↑ phosphate)

- Restrict dietary intake of phosphate.
- Administer phosphate binders with meals and vitamin D analogues (e.g. alfacalcidol) as prescribed.

Hyperkalaemia

- Reduce dietary intake of potassium.

Metabolic acidosis

- Results from inability of kidney to reabsorb bicarbonate.
- Administer sodium bicarbonate tablets as prescribed.
- Administer prescribed treatment to reduce hypertension.

Helping patients cope with treatment and symptoms

Oedema

- Advise on position changes and use of pressure-relieving mattresses and cushions to prevent pressure ulcers.
- Ensure loose-fitting clothing is available for patient to wear.

Fluid restriction

- Help patient divide amounts to last all day.
- Provide measuring jugs so that amounts can be controlled.
- Provide mouthwashes to keep mouth fresh.

Diet and nutrition

- Recognize that a 'renal diet' can be unappetizing.
- Ensure dietitians are in regular contact to determine patient's likes and dislikes.
- Provide a varied and appetizing diet.
- Check food is being eaten.

Anorexia

- Ensure small amounts of food are available that meet strict requirements of diet.
- Encourage use of mouthwashes before and after food.

Nausea and vomiting

- Ensure clean vomit bowl, tissues, and mouthwashes are available.

Weakness, fatigue, and lassitude

- Encourage patient to rest.
- Suggest that patient follows a routine.
- Support patient in self care.
- Explain reason for anaemia and prescribed treatment.

Pruritus

- Keep skin clean and dry, nails short.
- Discourage patient from scratching.
- Suggest using emollient cream or aromatherapy.

Monitoring

- Ensure strict monitoring of fluid balance and dietary intake by ensuring patients:
  - take responsibility for their diet and fluid balance
  - understand the implications of their dietary restrictions
  - know how to achieve dietary restrictions
  - have proper equipment for measuring fluids
  - keep accurate records that are reviewed daily.
- Monitor temperature and blood pressure (↑ blood pressure, ↑ pulse, and ↑ respiratory rate may indicate fluid retention).
- Obtain daily weight.
  - Perform at same time each day.
  - ↑ weight indicates fluid retention.
  - ↓ weight may indicate over-diuresis or poor nutrition.
- Observe feet, ankles, hands, and face for signs of peripheral oedema.

Helping patients cope with the long-term challenge of chronic kidney disease

Patients with CKD have many challenges to face, which include:
- accepting the long-term nature of their condition and adapting to chronic illness
- managing the impact on family, social, and professional life
- increased dependency on others; e.g. health care professionals, family members, and friends
- dependency on dialysis to sustain health (including its considerable time demands)
- possible side effects from treatment.

Nurses can help and support patients and their families.
- Be sensitive and supportive when discussing prognosis and progression of CKD.
- Spend time listening to patients' and their families' concerns.
- Encourage patients to express their feelings.
- Involve patients in care planning, any interventions, and evaluation of their treatment.
- Provide information that is tailored to the individual's circumstances and needs (e.g. age, culture, lifestyle, family circumstances).
- Refer patients to multidisciplinary team as necessary (e.g. dietetic advice, counselling, psychological care, and social support)
- Ensure access to information about options for renal replacement therapy and that they understand the risks, benefits, and implications of the treatment as it relates to them and their family.
- Ensure patients have the opportunity to make informed choices at every stage.
- Share reviews of progress, keep patients up to date with their prognosis, and ensure they have opportunities to revise care plans.
- Encourage patients to take control of their disease.

Renal replacement therapies

Types of treatment available for people with CKD include:
- Haemodialysis
- Peritoneal dialysis
- Renal transplantation – live or deceased donor

Dialysis acts as a partial surrogate for a normal functioning kidney by:
- removing waste products (e.g. urea)
- removing excess salt and water
- correcting acidosis
- removing or regulating electrolytes (e.g. potassium, calcium, and phosphate).

Transplantation completely replaces normal kidney function and is the optimum treatment for ESRF.

Haemodialysis

The dialysis machine is set up with sterile PVC tubing and a dialyser, which contains a semi-permeable membrane through which the patient's blood is pumped. Inside the dialyser, blood flows on one side of the membrane while dialysate fluid (solution containing physiological levels of electrolytes) flows in the opposite direction on the other. Small pores in the membrane allow waste products and electrolytes to pass through. Molecules that are too large to move across the membrane (i.e. protein and blood cells) remain in the blood. A difference in the concentration gradient between the dialysate and the blood allow for waste products to be removed and essential electrolytes to be replaced by diffusion. By varying the pressure across the membrane, water can be removed through a process called ultrafiltration. The standard dialysis prescription is 3 times a week for 4 hours per session.

Venous access

Haemodialysis requires repeated access to large blood vessels in order to provide an adequate flow of blood to the dialysis machine. Types of dialysis access include:

Arteriovenous fistula (AVF)
- An artery is surgically joined to a vein usually at the wrist (radiocephalic AVF) or antecubital fossa (brachiocephalic AVF).
- The vein is left to 'mature' over a 6–8 week period.
- This enlarges the vein and enables two wide-bore needles to be inserted through the skin, one to carry blood to the machine and one to return it to the patient.

Synthetic (PTFE) graft
- A synthetic graft is inserted between an artery and vein, and may be placed in the forearm, upper arm, or thigh.
- Performed when veins are too fragile to form an AVF.
- Can be used within a few days of placement.
- Does not last as long as a native AVF and is more prone to infection.

Blood pressure and blood tests should not be taken on limbs with an AVF or PTFE graft.

Central venous catheter
- Inserted into the internal jugular, subclavian, or femoral vein.
- Can be used immediately, but usually a temporary measure only.
- May be tunneled under the skin to reduce infection risk.
- The catheter is locked with heparin solution (local policies may differ) and capped off between dialysis sessions.
- Often used for emergency dialysis or while waiting for an AVF to mature.
- May be required long term if other vascular access sites have failed.
- Complications include infection, thrombosis, and air embolism.

Where patients dialyse

Renal unit
- Patients who are unable to self care or who have unstable condition.
- Undertaken by specially trained staff.

Satellite unit
- Self-contained units outside the hospital setting for patients who are more stable.
- Often contain minimal or self-care areas where patients can undertake most, if not all, of their own dialysis.
- An important advantage is that these units are often closer to the patient's home.

At home
- Patients undergo special training and a room in their home is adapted to accommodate the dialysis equipment.
- A carer/helper may be necessary.
- Should be offered to all patients (NICE guidelines).
- Allows individual dialysis prescription (e.g. increased hours, daily, or nocturnal dialysis) to better suit a patient's needs.

Complications of dialysis

- Atherosclerotic vascular disease is more common (e.g. ischaemic heart disease, cerebrovascular disease).
- Hypotension during dialysis.
- Disequilibrium syndrome, if urea and electrolytes are corrected too quickly.
- Other complications of advanced CKD may persist and progress (e.g. hypertension, renal bone disease, anaemia).
- Infection at access site.

Haemodialysis patients admitted to general wards

Upon hospital admission, collect the following information:

- Where does their dialysis usually take place? (Inform the patient's parent unit that they have been admitted without delay.)
- How many times a week do they dialyse? (When is the next due?)
- What is the patient's current access for dialysis? (Ensure all staff know to avoid using the same arm as an AVF for phlebotomy or blood pressure measurement. Do not use the patient's dialysis catheter for fluid or drug infusions.)
- What is the patient's post dialysis 'target' weight and how far over it are they at the moment?
- What is the patient's usual post dialysis blood pressure?
- How much residual urine do they pass?
- What is the patient's daily fluid allowance?
- What dietary restrictions do they normally observe?
- Do they take regular EPO injections? If so, do they have the EPO with them? This needs to be stored in the refrigerator.
- How is the patient coping with dialysis?

Nursing care of patients on haemodialysis

Patients experience physical, psychological, and emotional problems that may be interlinked.

Physical problems

The symptom burden in haemodialysis patients is high. They may experience nausea, anorexia, weight loss, fatigue, weakness, bone pain, restless legs, poor sleep quality, and loss of libido. They may develop difficulties with self caring and activities of daily living leading to feelings of frustration and poor self esteem. Haemodialysis patients must comply with rigorous dietary and fluid restrictions to reduce electrolyte abnormalities (e.g. hyperkalaemia) and fluid overload between dialysis sessions. Poor concordance with such restrictions results in increased morbidity and mortality. As well as dialysis treatment itself, most dialysis patients will also have to take many medications.

Nursing care
- Provide supportive care, assist with self-care activities, and encourage the patient to undertake as much activity as possible.
- Fluid intake is often restricted to <1 l/day. Help patients divide this fluid allowance throughout the day.
- Monitor intake and output and weigh daily.
- Medications will include antihypertensives, EPO injections, phosphate binders, and vitamin D analogues. Make sure the patient understands the reason for each medication, when to take them (e.g. phosphate binders are taken shortly before, or with, each meal), and the consequences of not taking them.
- Above all, provide encouragement, particularly if the patient has recently started treatment.

Psychological and emotional problems

Low self esteem, low mood, and anxiety may be present in haemodialysis patients for a number of reasons.
- Changes to body image, e.g. due to venous access and weight changes.
- Disruption to marital, family, and social life.
  - Family members may have to adopt the role of carers.
  - Patients (and carers) may no longer be able to work, with financial implications.
  - Feelings of social isolation may occur.
  - Patients may have stress and anxiety about the future.
  - Relationships (both emotional and sexual) may be affected.
  - Growing dependence on carers, the dialysis treatment, and health care professionals can cause anger and frustration.

Nursing care
- Promote self care and encourage independence.
- Help increase the patient's acceptance of the treatment.
- Spend time listening to the patient's and their family's concerns.

- Involve appropriate members of the multidisciplinary team (dietitians, social workers, psychologists, and occupational therapists). Have discussions about individual patients at team meetings.
- Provide suitable information, which will allow the patient to make informed choices and will help foster a sense of personal autonomy.

Continuous venovenous haemofiltration (CVVHF)

- This is a slower, 'gentler' form of treatment, providing greater haemodynamic stability than haemodialysis. It is used for patients with acute renal failure in a critical care setting.
- Solutes are removed predominantly by convection (ultrafiltration) rather than diffusion (dialysis).
- Large volumes must be ultrafiltered in order to achieve adequate solute clearance. To prevent hypovolaemia, replacement fluid must be administered.
- If fluid removal is desirable (e.g. the patient is in pulmonary oedema), ultrafiltration (UF) rate is set to exceed replacement fluid infusion per hour.
- Venous access is obtained by a central venous (double or triple lumen) catheter.
- Treatment is administered continuously (over 24 hours), rather than in short (e.g. 4 hour) bursts.
- Patients must be closely monitored for transient hypotension, hypothermia, infection, and overall fluid balance.

Peritoneal dialysis

Peritoneal dialysis (PD) is performed by the patient or carer at home. It involves the infusion of hypertonic dialysate solution into the peritoneal cavity via an indwelling PD catheter. The peritoneal cavity is surrounded by the peritoneal membrane which is semi-permeable, allowing fluid and small solutes to move through. The dialysate is left to dwell inside the peritoneal cavity for 4–10 hours. Waste products and solutes pass into the dialysis solution by diffusion from the blood stream, across the peritoneal membrane, and into the dialysate solution (until the concentration on either side of the membrane is equal). Fluid removal (ultrafiltration) occurs as a result of osmosis caused by a high concentration of glucose within the dialysate. There are different types of dialysate fluid containing varying glucose concentrations to enhance the osmotic pull and ability to remove excess fluid. At the end of the dwell time the dialysate fluid is drained out and exchanged for fresh fluid.

Types of peritoneal dialysis

Continuous ambulatory peritoneal dialysis (CAPD)
- The standard prescription is three to five 2 litre exchanges per day (i.e. at 4–6 hour intervals), though there is much interpatient variability.
- Fluid exchanges are relatively simple and only require a clean surface and a nearby sink to wash hands in.
- Exchanges can be undertaken at home or work.

Automated peritoneal dialysis (APD)
- Uses an automated machine to perform the exchanges overnight while the patient is asleep.
- The machine is usually programmed to perform four to six exchanges over an 8-hour period depending on individual need and tolerance.
- Fluid is usually left in the peritoneal cavity for the duration of the day until the patient goes on the machine the following night.
- Some patients also perform an additional exchange during the day.

PD is the treatment of choice for many patients as it offers more flexibility and independence than haemodialysis. It also makes it easier for patients to travel (including abroad). Relative contraindications to PD include the presence of a colostomy, ileostomy or ileal conduit, a rectal or vaginal prolapse, inflammatory bowel disease, and abdominal hernias.

PD catheter insertion
- Must be done by an experienced operator.
- The exit site (point where PD catheter exits onto surface of abdomen) is chosen to enable the patient to clearly see it to change dressings and so as not to be constricted by clothing (especially at the waist).
- Patient should give informed consent.
- Aseptic technique is essential.
- Can be inserted under local or general anaesthetic.
- Local policies will differ but generally the initial dressing is left for 5–10 days unless there are signs of bleeding or infection.
- The PD catheter is usually rested for 2 weeks prior to use to ensure healing, but can occasionally be used sooner.

Patient training

- Adapt training to an individual's needs, ability, and learning style. Training should cover:
  - the procedure for exchange of fluid
  - the importance of aseptic technique
  - how to prevent complications, particularly infections (peritonitis and exit site)
  - how to recognize complications (peritonitis: cloudy dialysate fluid, abdominal tenderness, and/or raised temperature; exit site: localized redness, swelling, tenderness, and purulent discharge).
- Instruct patients on the first line of action and who to contact if they have any concerns.
- Visit the patient's home to observe dialysis exchanges and verify that the patient's technique is satisfactory.
- Provide positive feedback and encouragement at all stages.
- Ensure continuing support is provided by a community PD nurse.
- Ensure proper delivery and storage of dialysate fluid and ancillaries in the patient's home.

Patient and family support

Providing effective communication and support are essential to help the patient adapt to changes in lifestyle, cope with feelings about altered body image, and accept the need for continuous therapy. Explaining that PD can be used more flexibly so that independence and mobility is achieved will give confidence. Stress the importance of continuing diet and medication regimes.

Nursing care for peritoneal dialysis patients on general wards

- Find out from the patient and/or carer what their PD regimen is, their diet, fluid allowance, and medication requirements.
- Contact the local renal/PD unit and seek help from the PD nurse.
- Contact the patient's own PD centre if different from above to inform them of the patient's admission and to seek any special instructions.
- Nurses unfamiliar with PD must be supervised by an experienced PD nurse and should pay particular attention to:
  - washing hands with bactericidal soap before procedure and using non-touch technique throughout
  - warming the dialysate fluid to 36°C before use for patient comfort (do not use a microwave to do this as it will chemically alter the PD fluid)
  - adding drugs to the PD fluid as prescribed (e.g. heparin to prevent fibrin formation or antibiotics to treat peritonitis)
  - ensuring correct strength dialysate fluid is used and stays in the peritoneal cavity for the prescribed time
  - recording time of commencement and completion of exchange, the amount of fluid drained in and out, and the clarity (a cloudy bag indicates peritonitis until proven otherwise)
  - checking fluid balance after each exchange
  - if peritonitis: checking temperature, blood pressure, and temperature every 4 hours
  - sending specimen of peritoneal fluid for microscopy and culture as instructed by PD nurse or physician.
- Weigh patients daily after their first exchange to help determine PD regimen for the day.
- Monitor fluid intake and output.
- Continue with any dietary restrictions and requirements.
- Take care to prevent peritonitis, and exit site and tunnel infections (this is vital) – use local polices for care of catheter site as these vary.
- Encourage patient to shower as baths are not advised due to risk of infection.

Transplantation

If the patient is fit to be a recipient, then transplantation is the treatment of choice for patients with ESRF. A pre-emptive transplant (prior to dialysis) has the best outcome of all.

Transplanted kidneys can now be expected to last many years (average for deceased transplant ~10–12 years and ~15 years for a living donor). The average wait for deceased kidney is 2 years (depending on factors such as recipient blood group), but due to a shortage of deceased organs only 15–20% of patients on the waiting list receive them.

Donors
Living donor
- Can be relative (live related), partner, or friend (live unrelated).
- Must be an adult (age >18) who is in good physical and psychological health and consents to the process willingly.
- Both donor and recipient must undergo 'work up' tests to ensure that they are fit and healthy enough to undergo surgery and to evaluate long-term immunosuppression in the case of the recipient. The donor is screened to identify any potential conditions that could lead to renal problems in their future.

Deceased donor
- Organs retrieved from a donor certified as brainstem dead (usually patients with acute neurological injuries such as trauma or subarachnoid haemorrhage).
- Consent is given either as an advance directive from the donor or by their next of kin. This is a very difficult time for the donor's family, and nurses must provide support and information for family members.
- The donor will normally be on ITU and is maintained with circulatory and respiratory support (e.g. inotropes and ventilation) until the organs are harvested.
- The local transplant coordination team is contacted.
- Organs are perfused with a special solution and cold stored for transport.
- Requires an organ distribution network to select the most suitable recipients from a national database (UK transplants).

Expanding the donor pool
Because of a shortfall in the number of organs available, there is much interest in developing strategies to increase the available transplants.
- Non-heart-beating donors: organs retrieved after circulatory arrest as opposed brain stem death. Outcomes may be less good.
- Transplanting across blood groups: until relatively recently transplants were only carried out in blood-group matched pairs according to 'transfusion rules'. Incompatible transplants are now possible.
- Transplanting across a positive cross-match: removing donor antibodies (e.g. with plasma exchange) that would previously have precluded a particular transplant.
- Live donor exchange schemes: if a patient has a live donor but the transplant cannot go ahead for immunological reasons, donors and recipients agree to swap kidneys with another pair in a similar situation.

Transplant operation

- Graft implantation is usually into right iliac fossa.
- Native kidneys are not removed unless there is a specific reason to do so.
- The donor ureter is joined to the recipient bladder. A double J-stent is usually inserted (and subsequently removed cystoscopically at 12 weeks).
- A drain is usually left in the peri-renal space.

Postoperative period

- Obtain a full handover from theatre team.
- Implement nil by mouth until advised by surgical team.
- Perform chest physiotherapy as required.
- Provide DVT prophylaxis (thromboembolic deterrent [TED] stockings, SC heparin – unit protocols may differ).
- Administer all medications as prescribed.

Fluid balance

- Urinary catheter – to be left *in situ* for 5 days – monitor hourly urine output.
- Central venous pressure (CVP) line; aim CVP 10–12.
- Administer IV normal saline or other physiological solution.
- Monitor blood pressure and temperature closely.
- Maintain accurate fluid balance chart.
- Document drain volumes.
- Obtain daily weight.

Analgesia

- Provide analgesia as prescribed – NSAIDs should be avoided.
- Patient controlled analgesia (PCA) is preferred.

Graft assessment

- Monitor urine output.
- Monitor U&E and FBC daily.
- Maintain therapeutic levels of the anti-rejection drugs (ciclosporin, tacrolimus, rapamycin; blood sample taken pre-dose).
- Ensure that blood supply to both feet is satisfactory.
- Monitor daily blood glucose (steroids may cause hyperglycaemia).
- A duplex ultrasound or nuclear medicine scan to ensure adequate perfusion is usually performed within first 24 hours.

Early complications

- Haemorrhage (rising pulse, falling blood pressure, falling CVP, increase in drain volumes)
- Infection (pyrexia, rising pulse, falling blood pressure, rising white cell count or CRP)
- Vascular thrombosis (pain over graft, falling urine output)
- Acute rejection (falling urine output, rising serum creatinine)

Palliative care

Deciding not to have dialysis

Some patients with significant co-morbidity or dependence on carers may find their quality of life on dialysis unacceptable. Complications and side effects from treatment may outweigh benefits. Survival may be short with unpleasant symptoms and regular hospital admissions. For these patients continuing supportive treatment and choosing not to have dialysis may allow a better quality of life with little or no reduction in actual life expectancy.

The decision whether or not to have dialysis is ultimately made by the patient (if competent), usually with family involvement. It is up to the nursing and medical staff to make sure that the decision is a fully informed one, with complete understanding of the implications of commencing dialysis and the pros and cons of opting not to have it.

Treatment of symptoms

Physical and social support is needed for both patient and family. Ensure all necessary referrals are made, e.g. social worker, district nurses, physiotherapists, home care teams, hospice. Psychological support is extremely important at this time. Symptoms will increase as renal function deteriorates.

- Anorexia
  - This is a common symptom.
  - Dietary restrictions can often be relaxed.
- Nausea and vomiting
  - Administer anti-emetics as prescribed.
  - Constipation may also be a cause, start laxatives early.
- Confusion
  - This is usually a late development.
  - Check for reversible causes (constipation, electrolyte disturbances, drug toxicity).
- Dry skin, pruritus, and excoriation
  - These are common.
  - Hyperphosphataemia is often the cause.
  - Use emollient creams (aqueous cream, Diprobase®, E45®) in bath water.
  - Give antihistamines as prescribed.
- Acidosis
  - Can cause breathlessness and fatigue.
  - Give sodium bicarbonate as prescribed.
- Dyspnoea
  - If pulmonary oedema, give diuretics as prescribed; bronchodilators may also be helpful.
  - Advise to sleep in a more upright position.
- Anaemia
  - Give IV iron and EPO as prescribed.
  - May require blood transfusion.

- Restless legs
  - Treat anaemia.
  - Give other therapy as prescribed; e.g. clonazepam.
- Anxiety and depression
  - These are common.
  - Talk to the patient.
  - Involve counsellor, if available.
  - Give medication as prescribed.

Patient education for renal patients

The aim is to develop patients' and their families' understanding of their illness and treatment, including invasive procedures and surgery.

- Recognize that education for the family and carers is extremely important as many chronic renal conditions will have a significant impact on them.
- Ensure patients have an understanding of the condition, common symptoms, planned treatment, and/or surgery. Encourage them to ask questions and express feelings.
- Ensure that education is culturally sensitive and takes account of the individual's needs and circumstances, e.g. a higher proportion of people from black and minority ethnic groups have diabetes and hypertension leading to renal disease.
- Educate patients in short sessions and focus on the essentials first because patients with advanced CKD often feel unwell and may have difficulty concentrating and retaining information.
- Dietary modification plays a central role in many renal disorders. Tailor dietary advice to the individual, acknowledging their personal likes and dislikes, ethnic variation, who prepares the food, and who eats with the patient. Give recipe ideas and advice on eating out.
- Provide information on benefits and side effects of medications, including which over-the-counter medications should be avoided (NSAIDs!!). Re-iterate the importance of concordance whenever necessary.
- Provide information on treatment options, benefits, and limitations using terminology that patients understand and that facilitates informed choices. Help patients understand why certain options may or may not be best suited to their individual situation.
- Ensure access to all members of the renal team for specialist information. Check understanding and ensure adequate opportunity to ask questions is provided.
- For postoperative patients, explain the outcome of surgery and plan for recovery.
  - Make arrangements for ongoing wound care and suture removal.
  - The convalescent period and timing of return to full activity and work will be dependent on type of operation, patient's condition, and type of work.
  - Advise on complications to watch out for, who to contact if concerned, and what follow-up is necessary.
  - Ensure patients have medications and any special instructions.

Preventative education

Advise patients about the following:

- Prevention of heart disease by diet, exercise, smoking cessation, medication, and lifestyle.
- Importance of keeping blood pressure and, if applicable, diabetes well controlled.

- Early identification of CKD in high risk groups (e.g. diabetics and hypertensives) through urine testing (to identify haematuria and proteinuria), blood pressure measurement, and blood test for eGFR.
- The importance of renal function being monitored if nephrotoxic drugs are being taken.
- The importance of screening and follow up for those with family history and genetic risk of CKD (e.g. adult polycystic kidney disease).

Discharge and continuing care for renal patients

Arrangements vary considerably depending on the individual patient, their renal disorder, and its treatment.

- Check the patient and/or carer:
  - understands the renal disorder and treatment plan (provide written information where possible)
  - understands dietary and nutritional requirements and can adapt these for home use
  - is confident in managing a fluid restriction at home as required
  - has prescribed medications, understands their use, possible side effects, and consequences of non-concordance
  - understands a staged convalescence, with graded return to activities and work.
- Check that all arrangements for patients on home dialysis have been made (e.g. home adaptations, equipment, supplies) and that training has been completed successfully.
- For those on hospital or satellite dialysis, ensure arrangements for dialysis have been made with the appropriate unit and discussed with the patient.
- Ensure support arrangements are in place and that contact details are given, e.g. outreach or community renal nurse, social services support, and other members of the multidisciplinary team.
- Ensure arrangements for wound care, suture removal, etc. have been made, if appropriate.
- Arrange for peer support, e.g. to meet with a patient coping with treatment and dialysis as relevant.
- Ensure patients have contact details of patient and carer support groups and associations.
- Explain that patients on dialysis must inform the DVLA Driver's Medical Unit of their change in circumstances.
- Ensure arrangements for follow-up appointments are made at relevant outpatient clinics, renal unit, or GP.
- Ensure prompt discharge information is communicated to relevant colleagues in primary care and other involved parties.

Nursing assessment of patients with urological conditions

Observe the patient
- Abdomen: distension or masses (a palpable bladder or distended abdomen may be due to retention of urine or constipation and may contribute to incontinence)
- Signs of confusion
- Meatus: discharge, which may indicate infection
- Penis: lesions that could be suspicious
- Scrotum: bruising or swelling which may indicate trauma or infection
- Testes: palpable painful lumps which may be infective in origin, or painless lumps which could represent tumour
- Dry skin for signs of dehydration
- Urine test for glucose, haematuria, proteinuria (observe for haematuria, foul smell, or cloudy appearance)
- Digital rectal examination for tenderness (which may indicate prostatitis) and size, texture, median sulcus and nodules (which may reveal enlargement, abnormality)—this examination should be performed with consent and counselling and should be carried out by properly trained personnel only
- Urinary residual: measure with bladder scanner

Fig. 11.3 shows the base of the bladder and prostatic urethra.

Ask the patient/family

Medical history
Identify predisposing factors for urological disorders.
- Medical conditions, e.g. spinal lesions, spina bifida, cerebral vascular accident, childhood urinary problems, gynaecological/obstetric problems, diabetes, Parkinson's disease, tumours, multiple sclerosis, and heart disease
- Trauma such as road traffic accident
- Previous surgery

Current problems
These descriptions will indicate what investigations to order to diagnose disorder:
- Haematuria
- Back pain or loin pain
- Recurrent urinary tract infection
- Lower urinary tract symptoms (LUTS)
- Genital pain
- Difficulty sitting down
- Erectile dysfunction and onset and duration

Urinary symptom history
- Description of LUTS
- Frequency or urgency
- Nocturia or dysuria

- Urge incontinence, hesitancy, straining, stress incontinence
- Intermittency, poor flow, incomplete emptying
- Any episodes of haematuria

Drug history

- Certain drugs may predispose to certain urological conditions such as bladder cancer.
- Certain drugs may colour urine.
- Diuretics cause frequency.
- Phenothiazides reduce bladder sensation.
- Analgesia can cause constipation.

Social, family, and lifestyle history

- May reveal genetic or environmental predisposition to certain urological malignancies such as bladder, renal, or prostate cancer (e.g. smoking, exposure to rubber, dyes).
- Poor fluid intake may be responsible for urine infection, irritative symptoms, and constipation.
- Certain fluids and foods may colour urine.
- Travel to African countries where parasites that can cause bladder cancer could be contracted.
- Close relative with prostate cancer or being of black descent, which increases risk of developing prostate cancer.
- Use of vulval irritants.
- Sexual history may indicate previous STIs and erectile dysfunction.

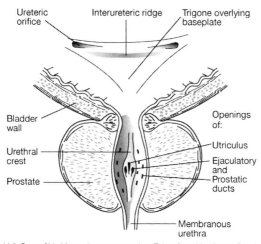

Fig. 11.3 Base of bladder and prostatic urethra. Taken from MacKinnon P and Morris J (2005). *Oxford Textbook of Functional Anatomy*, vol 2, Fig 6.8.5. Oxford University Press, Oxford. Reproduced with permission from Oxford University Press.

Problems for patients with urological conditions

Retention of urine
Acute retention of urine: sudden painful inability to pass urine (differentiate from anuria—no urine produced).
Chronic retention of urine: slower onset (generally painless) and may lead to overflow incontinence.

Incontinence of urine
Nocturnal enuresis: involuntary passing of urine during sleep—usually in children >5 years but could also result from chronic retention.
Stress incontinence: involuntary passing (leaking) of urine during laughing, sneezing, coughing, or strenuous exercise.
Urge incontinence: strong uncontrolled urge to pass urine quickly followed by urinary leakage of moderate-to-large amounts.

Hesitancy
This is prolonged time to initiating flow.

Post void dribbling
This refers to dribbling once finished passing urine.

Urgency
This is a strong urge to pass urine which can be painful and restrict activities.

Feeling of incomplete emptying
Patient may feel that urine has been left behind in bladder leading to increased urge to pass urine and frequency.

Frequency
This is voiding too frequently (normal 4–6 times per day).

Nocturia
This is waking at night to pass urine leading to disturbed sleep patterns.

Dysuria
This is painful passing of urine.

Social isolation
This may occur due to anxiety about leaking or smelling of urine or increased frequency. It may lead to restriction in activities and working.

Emotional problems
Patients may have anxiety, embarrassment, and low self-esteem; may feel unattractive; and may have an inability to share feelings about problems.

Pain and discomfort
Location and type of pain varies, e.g. loin, pelvic, abdominal, or back pain. The pain may be dull ache, colicky, or bone pain.

Weight loss
This may occur in cancer.

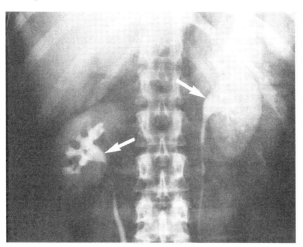

Fig. 11.4 Intravenous urogram. Showing the renal pelvis leading to the ureter. Taken from MacKinnon P and Morris J (2005). *Oxford Textbook of Functional Anatomy*, vol 2, Fig 3.8. Oxford University Press, Oxford. Reproduced with permission from Oxford University Press.

Special urological tests, investigations, and examinations

Urine dipstick test

This is useful for suggesting investigations for certain disorders.

- Protein may indicate renal disease and UTI.
- Glucose and ketones may indicate diabetes.
- Blood may indicate bladder or renal cancer, bladder outflow obstruction, or UTI.
- Nitrites and leucocytes may indicate UTI.
- Bilirubin may indicate hepatobiliary disease.
- pH and urobilinogen are of little value.

Midstream specimen of urine (MSU)

This is a specimen taken for microscopy, culture, and sensitivity if UTI is suspected or to confirm the presence of red blood cells.

Urine cytology

This is of limited use if negative but useful for choosing further investigation if positive for malignant cells or to confirm haematuria.

Blood tests

These include FBC, U&E, blood culture, and blood glucose. Raised levels of prostate specific antigen (PSA) are indication for further investigation to rule out prostate cancer or suggest benign cause.

Flexible cystoscopy

A flexible cystoscope is introduced via the urethra into the bladder to identify lesions, stones, urethral stricture, occlusive or friable prostate, or tumours. This is usually done while the patient is awake using local anaesthetic lubrication and may be done at outpatient clinic appointment.

Rigid cystoscopy with or without biopsy

This is use of a rigid cystoscope while patient is under general anaesthetic. Small pieces of bladder urothelium may or may not be taken for histological analysis. A bladder biopsy may diagnose bladder cancer.

Intravenous urogram (IVU)

This is an x-ray following injection of a contrast medium to view the anatomy of the renal and urinary tract and reveal obstructive pathology (See Fig. 11.4).

Digital rectal examination (DRE)

May be performed for female patients. For male patients this may indicate prostate cancer if grossly abnormal. The prostate may feel hard and knobbly compared with healthy prostate, which feels smooth and slightly soft. Normal DRE does not rule out prostate cancer and slightly abnormal DRE does not necessarily indicate prostate cancer.

Trans-rectal biopsy

Small pieces of prostate are taken and sent for analysis to confirm prostate cancer. This is usually done with ultrasound guidance to visualize internal anatomy and measure the size of the prostate. Complications include rectal bleeding, urinary infection, and blood in the ejaculate and urine.

Urinary tract ultrasound

This is a useful first-line investigation for a number of urological conditions. It may reveal hydronephrosis, bladder or renal stones, renal cysts or tumour, or bladder diverticulae. It is noninvasive without exposing to x-rays.

X-rays (e.g. kidney ureter bladder and chest x-ray)

Kidney ureter bladder (KUB) may be used to evaluate renal colic, often in conjunction with urinary tract ultrasound or IVU. Chest x-ray may be done to check for bone or chest metastases in prostate or bladder cancers. CT also can be used for these investigations and has a higher pick-up rate.

CT and MRI scans

These investigations allow cross-sectional imaging of the body. They are very useful for staging various urological cancers. CT is increasingly used to assess renal colic.

Promoting urinary continence

Incontinence is widespread with estimates that 3–25% of the general population is affected, including 30–50% of older people. In the UK, 5 million people have some form of urinary incontinence; women are at greater risk than men.

There are three main types of incontinence: stress, urge, and mixed (combination of stress and urge). Treatment depends on the type of incontinence present and an assessment to determine the type of incontinence will need to be made with input from a specialist incontinence advisor.

Causes and contributory factors

- Damage or deterioration of the pelvic floor muscles or nerves (these can occur for various reasons):
  - Childbirth
  - Menopause (due to hormonal changes)
  - Abdominal or pelvic surgery (e.g. prostatectomy)
  - Disorders that affect nerve conduction (e.g. diabetes, CVA, Parkinson's disease, spinal disorders)
  - Chronic cough, constipation, heavy lifting, or obesity
  - Uterine prolapse
- Overactive or unstable bladder
  - Hypersensitivity causes the bladder to contract and empty.
  - Occurs in stroke, Parkinson's disease, atrophic vaginitis, or as a primary disorder.
- Urinary obstruction
  - Prevents normal voiding.
  - May result in increased urinary residual and lead to many lower urinary tract symptoms including dribbling, incontinence of urine night and day, and increased frequency, e.g. prostatic hyperplasia.
- Functional causes
  - Immobility
  - Inability to access facilities
  - Cognitive or behavioural problems or confusion

Treatment options

Conservative treatment

- Exercise prescription to improve function of the pelvic floor muscles. Electrical stimulation can be used if patient cannot contract these muscles.
- Use of aids such as pads and sheaths (although many patients find this method difficult to manage). There are many different types available; they must be well-fitting and meet the patient's needs and lifestyle. Expert advice from a specialist is helpful.
- Bladder retraining: these are programmes of education and a scheduled voiding regimen to improve bladder capacity and may enable patient to hold on to urine for longer periods of time.
  - Double voiding—urinating twice to ensure complete emptying of bladder

- Medication, e.g. anticholinergic drugs help prevent muscle contraction; vasopressin may help nocturnal eneuresis
- Transcutaneous electrical nerve stimulation (TENS) to reduce symptoms of overactive bladder
- Use of alarms
- Indwelling catheterization is sometimes used as a last resort when intractable incontinence cannot be managed in any other way. It is not recommended as it can exacerbate symptoms. However, if it is needed to allow healing of excoriated skin, it should be removed as soon as possible.

Surgical treatment

- In women, tension-free vaginal tape (TVT), which is a first-line treatment for stress incontinence, elevates the bladder neck (may be done laproscopically); colposuspension and other sling procedures may also be used.
- Injection of bulking agents to bulk tissues around the bladder neck.
- In men, transurethral resection of the prostate (TURP) may be used for chronic retention and overflow incontinence.
- Artificial urinary sphincters may also be used.
- Newer treatments under trial at present include botulinium toxin type A injection into the bladder tissue. (Botulinium toxin type A injections into the bladder are increasingly used for incontinence secondary to neurological disease and also due to overactive bladder.)

The role of the nurse in promoting continence

- Ensure there is an in-depth assessment for all patients with continence problems.
- Perform thorough assessment.
  - Record symptoms and effect on quality of life. Include quality of life scale and bladder diary to record frequency, volume, times urine is voided, and fluid intake; note episodes of urine leakage with causes (e.g. laughing).
  - Identify any underlying causes, e.g. diabetes, constipation, etc.
  - Examine the patient's abdomen for palpable bladder or mass and perineum to identify prolapse and problems with pelvic floor muscles, and rectal examination for sphincter damage.
  - Perform urodynamic studies to observe pressure changes in bladder.
  - Record patient fluid intake with frequency and volume chart, if possible.
  - Perform urinalysis to exclude infection (and diabetes).
  - Evaluate patient's manual dexterity and environment to identify accessibility and privacy of toilets.
  - Evaluate patient's motivation, willingness, and commitment to treatment alternatives.
- Know when to refer to others with more expertise including multidisciplinary team such as continence nurse specialists or advisers, urology nurse specialists, physiotherapists and occupational therapists, specialist pharmacists, and social workers. Ensure they provide information on aids, treatment options, and support.
- Ensure that women with 3rd and 4th degree perineal tears after childbirth are referred for continence advice.
- Encourage self-help. Advise on:
  - decreasing caffeine intake
  - achieving or maintaining healthy drinking habits
  - losing weight, if obese
  - preventing constipation
  - stopping smoking
  - importance of maintaining prescribed exercises to improve pelvic floor muscles.
- Provide encouragement and support, allow patients to discuss feelings, and suggest coping strategies.
- Involve family members and ensure they are aware of local support, e.g. laundry facilities, supplies, etc.
- Ensure patients are aware of support groups and further advice.

Patients with urinary tract trauma or infections

Bladder and urethral injuries

- This kind of trauma should only be managed by an experienced urological team.
- These injuries may occur due to lower abdominal trauma, pelvic fractures, or perineal trauma.
- Patients with this type of injury may also exhibit blood at the meatus, open injury to penis or perineum, and haematoma or extravasation into the perineum, scrotum, or penis.
- Patients may also have injury to other major organs and treatment of them takes priority. Treat shock (monitor blood pressure pulse, administer IV fluids, or transfusion) as advised; only once patient is stable can urological injury be established.
- A urethral injury may be difficult to distinguish from a bladder injury.
- It needs to be established whether urethral injury is anterior or posterior (by performing ascending urethrogram).
- If anterior urethral trauma is identified, intervention is withheld to determine whether patient can void normally.
- If patient voids normally, no further intervention is needed.
- If patient is unable to void, a single attempt at catheterization may occur; if difficult then the bladder is allowed to fill at which time a supra-pubic catheter is inserted.
- If posterior urethral trauma is diagnosed and trauma is minor, wait for the patient to void. If unable, then supra-pubic catheterization is advised.
- If trauma is severe, it is important to assess whether the bladder, urethra, or both are injured with an ascending urethrogram.
- It is important that everything is explained to patients so that they know what to expect. They need support and reassurance.
- Administer analgesics and antibiotics as prescribed.
- Reassure the patient and family.
- For suspected renal trauma, a CT scan is the first-line investigation. Initial treatment is usually conservative with resuscitation, cardiovascular monitoring, analgesia antibiotics, and blood transfusion supplied as necessary.

Lower urinary tract infections

- Infection may enter the urinary tract via the urethra or may be blood-borne. It may result in cystitis, prostatitis, and urethritis.
- Women are more susceptible than men because of their shorter urethra and its close proximity to the vagina and rectum.
- Risk factors include increasing age, diabetes, pregnancy, sexual intercourse, urinary obstruction and stasis, dehydration, and hospitalization (infection following catheterization, urinary tract procedures).
- Commonly caused by *E. coli*.

Assessment

📖 Nursing assessment of patients with urological conditions, p.366.

Advice and treatment

- Administer prescribed medication.
  - Antibiotic therapy may be single dose, short course (3–4 days or 7–10 days), or longer course for patients with known malformations and men with prostatitis (2–4 weeks).
  - Analgesia, NSAIDs, alpha blockers (for bladder outflow obstruction patients), and antispasmodics may be used to relieve pain and symptoms.
- Ensure patient understands the action and side effects and the importance of completing the whole course of antibiotics.
- Increase fluid intake to prevent future UTI. Cranberry juice is thought to be beneficial but this is not proven.
- Warm baths may help relieve pain but should be soap free.

Prevention

- Maintain proper hygiene.
- Wipe from front to back after urinating.
- Void after intercourse.
- Take showers rather than baths.
- Keep perineum clean and dry.
- Avoid use of irritants (perfumed products).

For upper UTI 📖 Acute pyelonephritis, p.339.

Nursing care of patients undergoing prostatectomy

Benign pathology (benign prostatic hyperplasia)

- Common in men >50 years.
- Prostatectomy, either transurethral (TURP) or open (Millins), is undertaken when medical and noninvasive approaches have been ineffective.
- TURP can also be performed to alleviate urinary symptoms for advanced prostate cancer.
- Transurethral resection removes prostate tissue but leaves the prostate capsule intact.

Malignant pathology (radical prostatectomy)

- Performed for prostate cancer when the tumour is considered to be clinically isolated and life expectancy is >10 years.
- Does not use a urethral approach; it is either open (radical retropubic or perineal) or laparoscopic/robotic (keyhole surgery).
- Removes the whole prostate including the prostate capsule, resulting in the physical removal of part of the urethra requiring reconnection of the bladder to the urethra.

Assessment

Detailed urinary symptom history is important (📖 Urinary symptom history, p.366) to provide the appropriate advice.

Initial treatment and nursing care

- Explain reason for symptoms.
- Advise on fluid intake, bladder retraining programme, and prevention of constipation.
- Administer prescribed drugs and explain function and side effects, e.g. alpha-blockers to relax smooth muscle of the prostate and bladder neck to improve obstructive symptoms (nocturia, hesitancy, post-void dribbling, intermittency), frequently producing retrograde ejaculation.
- Five alpha-reductase reduces size of prostate and improves flow rate for 39% of men (rises to 60% when combined with alpha-blocker), frequently reduces libido, and increases breast size.
- Explain surgical treatment options.

Surgical treatment

The nurse should describe the different treatment options, help the patient understand these and their risks and benefits, and answer any subsequent questions.

Transurethral resection of the prostate (TURP)

This is performed to remove hyperplastic tissues in the prostatic urethra. A resectoscope with a wire loop electrode is inserted into the urethra and cuts away the tissue to remove the obstruction. Haemorrhage and clot retention are risks.

Laser TURP

This is performed as above but with laser technology. Haemorrhage, clot retention, and complications are reduced but it has a shorter treatment history.

Retropubic prostatectomy

A retropubic incision is made into the prostatic capsule, the obstructing lobes are shelled out, and the capsule is re-sutured.

Radical prostatectomy (for cancer treatment)

This involves removal of the prostate, seminal vesicles, and adjacent tissue via the retropubic perineal. This is done for prostatic cancer. Risks include urinary incontinence and erectile dysfunction.

Transurethral microwave thermotherapy (TUMT)

Heat generated by microwave antennae in the urethra is used to coagulate prostatic tissue. It can be done in outpatients. Long-term effects are not fully evaluated; however, complication rate is higher than TURP.

Transurethral needle ablation (TUNA)

Radiofrequency energy is used to generate heat and coagulate prostate tissue. This can be done in outpatients. Long-term effects are not fully evaluated.

Pre- and postoperative care for prostatectomy patients

Preoperative nursing care for transurethral and radical prostatectomy
- Ensure patient understands the type of prostatectomy, the pre- and postoperative care to expect, including catheters and tubes, and the risks and benefits. Ensure written information is provided to supplement explanations.
- Ensure the patient has given written consent.
- Give the patient time to discuss feelings, particularly about sexual activity, potency, and ability to naturally father children. Inform that ejaculation will cease for radical prostatectomy (discuss sperm storage as appropriate to patient need) and that retrograde ejaculation will occur for transurethral prostatectomy.
- Prepare patient for possibility of incontinence with advice about fluid intake, pelvic floor exercises, and bladder retraining.
- Undertake a nursing assessment and obtain baseline measurements of temperature and blood pressure, weight, serum U&E, FBC, and PSA.
- Administer medication to prepare bowel as prescribed. Give advice to prevent constipation and postoperative straining.
- Encourage early postoperative mobility to prevent respiratory and reduced mobility complications.

Postoperative nursing care for radical prostatectomy
- Explain need for discharge with urethral catheter.
- Teach patient how to care for and manage catheter. Check patient's understanding before discharge.
  - Advise on appropriate hygiene, e.g. clean the meatus at least twice a day with plain soap, water, and disposable cloth.
  - Explain that some leakage of blood around the catheter may occur.
  - Describe possible side effects and how to deal with them, e.g. bladder spasm, haematuria, and UTI.
- Assess patient's pain, give prescribed analgesia as appropriate, and monitor effect.
- Encourage patient to sit up as soon as they are stable to assist breathing and urinary flow.
- Monitor urine output and colour to determine extent of bleeding, reporting to clinicians appropriately.
- If a wound drain is *in situ*, monitor drainage and record the amount and colour. Remove drain prior to discharge as instructed by clinician.
- Encourage fluid intake, at least 2 litres per day, and record intake. IV infusion can be removed when intake is sufficient as instructed by clinician.
- Advise patient on high-fibre diet to prevent constipation.
- If available, arrange for patient to be seen by prostate nurse specialist for advice, support, trial of voiding, advice and explanation of possible outcomes, future care plan, and contact details.

- Arrange for district nurse for support, supplies, advice, and care regarding catheter and possible use of pads once catheter is removed.
- Schedule appointment to return for trial without catheter and review prior to discharge if possible but posted at earliest convenience if not.
- Encourage patient to carry out pelvic floor exercises daily to encourage early continence as soon as catheter is removed.
- Give PSA blood testing form to the patient prior to discharge if possible but posted at earliest convenience if not.

Postoperative nursing care for transurethral prostatectomy
- Explain that a saline solution is used for irrigation via a three-way catheter to prevent clot formation and obstruction to urine flow.
- Assess patient's pain, give prescribed analgesia as appropriate, and monitor effect. Ensure the patient is in a comfortable position.
- Encourage patient to sit up as soon as they are stable to assist breathing and urinary flow.
- Monitor the urine output and colour to determine the degree of blood loss. Irrigation will be administered via catheter postoperatively and regulated dependent on the amount of bleeding and clots present.
- Encourage fluid intake, at least 2 litres per day, and record intake. IV infusion can be removed when intake is sufficient.
- Advise high-fibre diet to prevent constipation.
- If patient fails trial of voiding and must be discharged with a catheter, advise patient on self care of catheter (or teach designated other as appropriate), checking understanding.
  - Clean the meatus at least twice a day with plain soap, water, and disposable cloth.
  - Some leakage of blood around the catheter may occur.
  - The catheter can be removed as instructed by the clinician.
- Explain that initially voiding may be uncomfortable or may occur without warning. Advise patients to keep a urine bottle close at hand. Bladder retraining may be required. A small pad may be helpful initially to stop soiling of pyjamas.
- Encourage the patient to do the exercises taught preoperatively, if needed.
- Monitor patient for signs of complications including infection, perforation of the bladder, transurethral syndrome (absorption of large amounts of irrigation fluid into venous system—may lead to hypertension, nausea, vomiting, visual disturbance, bradycardia and confusion).

Urological cancers

Prostate cancer

This is a common cancer for men; risk factors include age, geography, (highest risk in North America and northern Europe), ethnicity (risk greater in black populations than white), diet (high fat intake), and hormones. Cancer is most commonly adenocarcinoma with ductal, mucinous, squamous, transitional cell, and sarcomatoid occurring more rarely. Metastases usually occur in bones initially. It may be slow onset and asymptomatic, followed by urinary symptoms, or there may be symptoms due to metastases (bone pain).

Diagnostic tests
- Digital rectal examination
- Blood for prostate specific antigen (PSA)
- Prostatic biopsy (📖 Special urological test investigation and examination, p.371)
- Transrectal ultrasound

Treatment
- Active surveillance (for patients with clinically insignificant disease or multiple comorbidities)
- Surgical intervention (for curative intent)
  - Radical prostatectomy is performed if tumour is localized and transurethral resection is performed to reduce symptoms in advanced disease (📖 Nursing care of patients undergoing prostatectomy, p.378).
  - Orchidectomy may be done in advanced prostate cancer to rapidly lower testosterone levels and retard the growth of the cancer, which is testosterone dependent.
- Radiotherapy (for curative or palliative purposes)
  - External beam radiation therapy (EBRT) or intensity-modulated radiation therapy (IMRT) or seed insertion (brachytherapy).
  - EBRT side effects include urinary frequency, urgency (rarely incontinence), dysuria, rectal irritation, diarrhoea, and tiredness.
  - Brachytherapy side effects include urinary frequency, urgency, and possibly rectal irritation.
  - May be necessary to perform TURP prior to radiotherapy for bladder outflow obstruction to prevent post-treatment urinary retention.
- Hormonal therapy (for palliative intent)
  - Inhibits the production of testosterone.
  - Given in conjunction with radiotherapy to shrink prostate (hormones given usually for 3 months prior to treatment).

Bladder cancer

Transitional cell carcinoma and carcinoma *in situ* are most common. Squamous, adenocarcinoma, and urachal occur less commonly. Risk factors include smoking, working in textile and rubber industries (aromatic amine exposure), certain analgesic abuse, chronic cystitis in the presence of long-term indwelling catheter, previous pelvic irradiation, and use of cyclophosphamide and schistosomiasis. Painless haematuria, recurrent UTIs, and even irritative urinary symptoms are often the first symptoms.

Diagnostic tests
- Urine for microscopy
- Urine cytology (to be interpreted with caution)
- Cystoscopy and biopsy
- CT scan to stage (📖 Special urological tests, investigations, and examinations, p.370)

Treatment
Depends on staging of the tumour.
- Ta: tumour confined to mucosa. Transurethral resection of bladder tumour (TURBT) may be followed by intravesical chemotherapy or immunotherapy (which may also be used to prevent or prolong time to recurrence) if there are multiple tumours or if tumours recur frequently (for Ta tumours).
- T1: tumour extends to lamina propria. Treatment as for Ta.
- T2 and T3: involvement of muscle. Cystectomy and ileal conduit or neo bladder or TURBT plus radiotherapy.
- T4: spread beyond the bladder. Palliative radiotherapy or TURBT to relieve symptoms.
Regular cystoscopic surveillance is required as tumours can recur.

Testicular cancer
Ninety-five percent of testicular tumours are germ cell tumours. These are subdivided into seminoma, non-seminoma, or mixed. They most often present in men aged 15–35 years. Lifetime risk is 1 in 500. Patients usually present with scrotal mass (painless) or discomfort that can be caused by infective process masking painless lump. In metastatic disease patients may present with back pain, respiratory compromise, or neurological deficit.

Diagnostic tests
- Tumour markers
  - Alpha fetoprotein (AFP) is elevated in some tumours but not in others.
  - Levels of the tumour markers are prognostic, however, the return to normal of markers does not indicate absence of residual disease.
- CT scan to stage and for follow-up of all testis cancer patients.

Treatment
- Radical orchidectomy is initially performed to remove affected testis via an inguinal incision.
- Subsequent treatment depends on the type and stage of tumour.
  - Retroperitoneal lymph node dissection
  - Chemotherapy
  - Radiotherapy
  - Marker surveillance
  - Follow up imaging.

Renal cancer

This is most commonly renal cell carcinoma (RCC), less commonly sarcoma, lymphoma, or leukaemia. There are variants of RCC including Von Hippel Lindau disease, a clear cell variant of RCC. Non-clear cell types of RCC include papillary RCC and chromophobic, collecting duct (Bellinis' duct), and renal medullary (associated with sickle cell trait). All of these subtypes can have sarcomatoid variants. Initially renal tumours are asymptomatic and non-palpable and can remain so until they are advanced. Fifty percent of all renal cancers are discovered incidentally through imaging carried for a range of non-specific symptoms. Flank pain may be experienced once there is local tumour growth, haemorrhage, paraneoplastic syndromes, or metastases.

Treatment

For localized tumours surgical removal (radical nephrectomy) including adrenal gland is the gold standard for curative intent.

• The surgical approach is dictated by the size, location, and habitus of the patient; they are open or laparoscopic.
• Surgery can be nephron sparing (removal of the tumour alone leaving as much of normal functioning kidney as possible) or non-nephron sparing.
• If renal carcinoma is bilateral or if patient has only one kidney, nephron-sparing surgery is encouraged as much as possible.
• Surveillance for recurrence is informed by the initial pathologic tumour stage.

Penile cancer

This is the least common of the urological cancers, usually occurring in older men and peaking at age 80. Neonatal circumcision is the most effective way to prevent penile cancer as it usually develops under the prepuce. Circumcision in adulthood does not prevent penile cancer. It is most prevalent where good hygiene is absent and is of most concern in African, Asian, and South American countries.

Squamous cell carcinoma is the most common cancer found on the penis and must be differentiated from lesions with malignant potential such as cutaneous horn, pseudoepitheliomatous micaceous and keratotic balanitis, balanitis xerotica obliterans, and leukoplakia. Other malignant lesions include bowenoid papulosis, Karposi's sarcoma, verrucous carcinoma, and giant condyloma acuminatum. Basal cell carcinoma, sarcoma, Paget's disease, surface adenosquamous, lymphoreticular, and melanoma of the penis are extremely rare.

Possible predisposing factors include the human papilloma virus (HPV) and exposure to tobacco products. Penile cancer presents as a lesion on the penis. Diagnosis is through biopsy and treatment is not instituted until this is carried out. Presence and extent of inguinal nodes involvement are the most prognostic factors for survival.

Treatment

• Usually partial or total penectomy followed by lymphadenectomy, if lymph nodes are palpable.
• Radiotherapy is used for carefully selected patients and for those who are very comorbid.

- Chemotherapy is of limited use.
- Reconstruction should be considered for patients who are able to have a partial penectomy. Total penectomy is a much more complicated process and candidates for this procedure must meet certain requirements.
- Lymph node dissection for patients without palpable lymph nodes is not evidence guided. It is guided by retrospective and historic data along with the use of recent histopathologic insights.

Psychological and emotional care for patient with urological cancers

Common reactions to urological cancers
- Feelings of anxiety and depression
- Denial
- Fear of death
- Fear of the unknown
- Anxiety at change in body image or altered self-concept
- Feelings of physical mutilation
- Loss of control and despair
- Anxiety about effects on sexuality

Assessment
- Patient's and family's understanding of condition and effects of treatment
- Impact on quality of life
- Anxieties and feelings
- Information needs and desire to know more
- Willingness to talk about themselves—whether embarrassed or have difficulty in expressing feelings

Meeting needs
- Use the assessment to identify priorities.
- Spend time listening to patients and talking through anxieties.
- Provide information as appropriate in a language they can understand and identify where to find additional sources of information (☐ Useful contacts for people with urological problems, p.391).
- Ensure care is coordinated and there is effective communication among members of the multidisciplinary team.
- Refer patients for sperm storage as appropriate (radical prostatectomy, cystectomy, and orchidectomy).
- Discuss future prosthesis as appropriate (testicular cancer).
- Discuss erectile dysfunction treatment as appropriate (usually with nurse specialist).
- Ensure patients are involved in decisions about care. Involve family members when possible if the patient wishes.
- Refer patient to relevant support services according to their needs, e.g. urology specialist nurse, clinical psychologist, palliative care team, social services, etc.

Urinary catheterization

This is insertion of a catheter into the bladder to empty the contents, e.g to relieve retention, to measure output or residual urine accurately, to instill substances (e.g. drugs) for irrigation or to enable bladder function tests to be done, or to relieve incontinence.

Types of catheters
- Foley balloon catheters
  - Two channels, one for drainage, one for balloon inflation—used for bladder drainage
  - Three channels, as above plus channel for continuous fluid irrigation, e.g. after prostatectomy
  - Balloon sizes vary: 2.5 mL for children, 5–30 mL for adults
- Non-balloon catheters
  - Used for intermittent emptying of bladder or installation of solutions
- Catheter materials
  - PVC usually used for intermittent catheterization
  - Latex, Teflon or silicone elastic coating—for short-term use
  - Silicone—suitable for long-term use and patients with latex allergy
  - Hydrogel coatings—for long-term use

Types and principles of catheterization
Urethral catheterization
- Choose smallest size necessary, e.g. 12–14 ch. Check local policy.
- Insert catheter via the urethra.
- Use sterile anaesthetic lubricating gel for males and females: insert into meatus in males and massage upwards; apply to catheter tip in females.
- Main risks are infection, urethral trauma, bladder spasm, encrustation, and lifestyle changes.

Suprapubic catheterization
- Insertion of the catheter (usually 16 ch) into bladder via the abdominal wall under GA or LA for urinary retention when urethral entry not possible due to urethral stricture, trauma, or surgery to the pelvis; also to allow urethral recovery postoperatively.
- Benefits over urethral catheterization are reduced infection, easier assessment of natural voiding, reduced risk of urethral trauma, easier sexual intercourse, and easier management.
- Main risks are encrustation, bladder spasm, infection, and altered body image.

Intermittent self catheterization (CISC)
- Used for incomplete bladder emptying and urethral dilatation maintenance and prevention.
- Benefits include freedom from indwelling catheter and incontinence aids, and promotes better quality of life, independence, and sexuality.
- Must be done according to purpose (dilatation or retention).
- For retention, CISC carried out anywhere from 1–6 times per day depending on volume of urinary residual.
- Appropriate for patients with good manual dexterity and understanding of cause.

Principles of catheterization and catheter care

- Use aseptic technique.
- Select appropriate catheter.
- Explain procedure and obtain consent.
- Ensure privacy and dignity.
- Use lubricating gel to encourage ease of passing and reduce urethral trauma. This is compulsory (usually anaesthetic gel).
- Keep closed system of drainage.
- Avoid unnecessary emptying or changing of bags.
- Decontaminate hands.
- Use sterile gloves to take samples and only from sampling ports using aseptic technique.
- Position urine bag below bladder level, and hang on stand.
- Use clean containers for emptying bags and good hygiene measures for cleaning meatus.

Education/discharge information for patients with urological disorders

- Assess the patient's understanding of the condition, treatment, and/or surgery, prognosis, and future. Determine what patients want to know. Include family as needed or at patient request.
- Use models, diagrams, and written information to help patients learn.
- As appropriate and where available, arrange visits with expert patients or provide patients the opportunity to meet others who are successfully coping with similar conditions, e.g. people with long-term indwelling catheters, intermittent catheterization, prostatectomy, recurrent cystitis.
- Encourage patients to achieve self care where possible.
  - Demonstrate techniques the patient may have to undertake, e.g. catheter care, self-catheterization. Supervise to ensure safe practice and encourage confidence.
  - Ensure the patient understands the reason for and is able to carry out effective hygiene measures, e.g. meatal care and handwashing.
- Advise patient on how to avoid constipation and why it is important to do so. Explain the importance of consuming a high-fibre diet (e.g. fresh fruit, wholemeal bread, cereals, bran) and taking sufficient fluids (2 litres per day minimum) or adjusting fluid intake to manage continence and lifestyle (e.g. car and air travel). Advise patient to take more fluids if urine becomes concentrated.
- Advise on complications that may arise (e.g. signs of wound infection, urine infection, catheter blockage) and how to manage them.
- Ensure patient is aware of where to get more supplies of pads, catheter bags, dressings, etc. and where to dispose of these.
- Ensure patient understands the use of medications, side effects, and consequences of non-concordance.
- Give advice on travelling.
  - How to cope with long distances—managing continence problems.
  - Taking supplies (if going abroad a letter from GP explaining what and who catheters are for may be helpful).
  - Finding accessible toilets.
- Advise on suitable clothing to assist with continence problems, e.g. wrap-around skirts, Velcro fastenings.
- Listen to the patient's concerns about body image and sexuality and advise that incontinence or catheterization does not necessarily rule out sexual intercourse.
- Listen to the patient's concerns about hygiene and odours and advise on taking supplies of wipes and clean underwear when out.
- Be sensitive; patients often find it embarrassing to talk about bodily functions.
- Ensure there is continued care as appropriate when the patient goes home including psychological and emotional support as well as physical care or, for some patients, palliative care.
- Ensure detailed discharge information is communicated to the GP, community nurse, and nursing home as relevant.

- Ensure the patient has contact details of the ward, specialist nurse, palliative care team, or primary and community staff as appropriate.
- Ensure follow-up appointments have been made.
- Ensure referrals are made as appropriate in clinics for patients with erectile dysfunction after prostatic surgery or cancer treatment.

Patient information

Information for patients going home with catheters

- Ensure patients have catheter equipment (bags, etc.) and know where to get further supplies.
- Ensure the patient understands:
  - the importance of handwashing before and after dealing with the catheter
  - to empty the catheter bag before it gets too full to prevent leakage and anatomical trauma (show how to empty into a container or the toilet and observe patient doing this correctly)
  - that the tubing should not be kinked, that the bag should not be obstructed by straps, and that the bag is kept lower than the bladder level.
- Demonstrate how to change the catheter bag and emphasize washing hands first and not touching the connector. Advise to use for 7 days before changing it.
- Advise on using unscented soap and water to wash around the meatus twice a day using downward strokes. Clean from front to back to reduce the risk of spread of bacteria from the anal area.
- Advise not to try to remove the catheter, which should be done by a physician or nurse.
- Explain how sexual intercourse can be achieved. In women the catheter is taped to the stomach and her partner should wear a condom to prevent the risk of infection. Men should fold the catheter along the erect penis and wear a condom over the top. A water-soluble lubricant may be helpful. Additional hygiene measures should be taken afterwards.
- Advise patient to drink 2 litres per day and take a high-fibre diet to reduce risk of urinary tract infection.
- Patients should be told of the risks leading to urinary tract infection, and to seek advice if any of the following occur:
  - offensive smell
  - cloudy urine
  - pain or discomfort
  - no drainage for 6–8 hours
  - soreness or redness
  - haematuria for more than 12–24 hours.

Useful contacts for people with urological problems

- Is There an Accessible Loo?   www.cae.org.uk/itaal.html/
- Association of Continence   www.aca.uk.com
  Advice
- Continence Foundation   www.continence-foundation.org.uk
- Cancer Help UK   www.cancerhelp.org.uk
- Enuresis Resource and   www.eric.org.uk
  Information Centre (ERIC) UK
- Chartered Physiotherapists   www.csp.org.uk
  Promoting Continence
- Incontact   www.incontact.org.uk
- Patient UK   www.patient.co.uk
  Genital/Urinary/Prostate
  Patient Support
- Prostate Cancer Charity UK   www.prostate-cancer.org.uk
- Prostate Help Association   www.prostatecancer.org.uk
- PromoCon   www.disabledliving.co.uk
- Radar (Royal Association for   www.radar.org.uk
  Disability and Rehabilitation)
- RCN Continence Care Forum   www.rcn.org.uk
- The UK Parauresis Association   www.shybladder.org.uk
  (Shy Bladder)
- UK Interstitial Cystitis   www.interstitialcystitis.co.uk
  Support Group

Common drugs used for renal and urinary disorders

Common drugs used for renal and urinary disorders are listed in Table 11.1. **All drug doses listed in this table are adult doses and not children's doses.** This table is only to be used as a guide and the current BNF should be consulted for further advice. Nurses should involve themselves only in the administration of medications which fall within their sphere of competence.

Table 11.1 Common drugs used for renal and urinary disorders

📖 Table 7.1 Common drugs used for cardiovascular disorders: diuretics (not potassium-sparing diuretics), p.192; beta-blockers, p.194; alpha-blockers, p.195; vasodilators, p.195; angiotensin-converting enzyme inhibitors, p.196; angiotensin-II receptor antagonists, p.197; calcium channel blockers, p.198.

Drug	Dose	Common side effects
Renal disease		
Erythropoetin	Aimed at increasing haemoglobin concentration to stable level of 10–12 g/100 mL	Dose-dependent increase in blood pressure and platelet count; influenza-like symptoms, thromboembolic events
Calcium salts	Used as a phosphate binder; dose dependent on product used	Gastrointestinal disturbances, bradycardia, arrhythmias
Vitamin D, e.g. alfacalcidol	1 mcg daily (500 ng in elderly) adjusted to avoid hypercalcaemia; maintenance normally 0.25–1 mcg	Anorexia, lassitude, nausea and vomiting, diarrhoea, weight loss, polyuria, sweating, headache, thirst, and raised concentrations of calcium and phosphate

📖 Table 9.1 Common drugs used for liver and gall bladder disorders: Transplantation, p.300.

Drug	Dose	Common side effects
Malignant prostatic disease		
Goserelin	3.6 mg SC into anterior abdominal wall every 28 days or 10.8 mg every 12 weeks	Hot flushes, sweating, sexual dysfunction, gynaecomastia
Bicalutamide	50 mg daily (in gonadorelin therapy start 3 days beforehand) or 150 mg as monotherapy	Gynaecomastia, hot flushes, impotence, weight gain
Leuprorelin	3.75 mg IM every month or 11.25 mg IM every 3 months	Hot flushes, sweating, sexual dysfunction, gynaecomastia

Table 11.1 Common drugs used for renal and urinary disorders
(continued)

Drug	Dose	Common side effects
Urinary frequency, enuresis, incontinence		
Anticholinergics	e.g. oxybutinin – initially 2.5–5 mg, 2–3 times daily to a maximum of 5 mg, 4 times daily	Dry mouth, gastrointestinal disturbances, blurred vision, difficulty in micturition, palpitation, skin reactions; CNS stimulation and facial flushing (both more common in children); many more (See BNF)
Urinary retention		
Alfuzosin	2.5 mg 3 times daily maximum up to a maximum of 10 mg daily NB First dose to be taken on retiring to bed as it may cause collapse due to hypotensive effect. Patients should be warned to lie down if symptoms such as dizziness, fatigue, or sweating develop and remain lying down until symptoms abate	Postural hypotension, syncope, depression, erectile disorders (See BNF for more side effects)
Benign prostate disease (separately or in combination)		
5 α reductase inhibitor: finasteride (5 mg), dutasteride (500 mcg)	Once daily (may require several months' treatment before benefit is obtained)	Erectile dysfunction, decreased libido, ejaculation disorder, breast tenderness and enlargement
Alpha blocker: tamsulosin (400 mcg), alfuzosin (10 mg), doxazosin (8 mg)	Dose depends on preparation used. NB First dose to be taken on retiring to bed as it may cause collapse due to hypotensive effect. Patients should be warned to lie down if symptoms such as dizziness, fatigue, or sweating develop and remain lying down until symptoms abate	Postural hypotension, syncope, depression, erectile disorders (See BNF for more side effects)
Sodium bicarbonate	3 g in water every 2 hours until urinary pH exceeds 7; maintenance of alkaline urine 5–10 g daily	Belching, alkalosis on prolonged use

Drugs used in nephritis: 🕮 Table 20.1 Common drugs used for infectious dieases: penicillins, cephalosporins, tetracyclines, aminoglycosides, macrolides, pp.728–9.

Chapter 12

Nursing patients with dermatology and skin problems

Nursing assessment of patients with dermatology and skin needs

Skin disorders can affect all parts of the body; thorough observation and examination of the total body skin surface, nails, and hair is necessary. In addition to a general nursing assessment (📖 Chapter 3, Individualizing nursing care practice, pp.32–33) perform the following procedures.

Observe the patient

- General skin characteristics (fair complexion, blond hair, freckles, blue, green, grey eyes are more at risk of melanoma)
- Changes in the skin—variation in colour, bruising, pallor, inflammation and new lumps, bumps, raised patches, moles, or naevi with changes in pigmentation, shape, or bleeding
- Breaks in the skin, sores, lesions, or ulcers. (Describe and take measurements and photographs, if relevant.)
- Texture of the skin—turgor, dryness, flakiness, or oiliness
- Temperature of the skin
- Signs of infestation, e.g. lice and nits on the head, lice on body, scabies burrows on skin
- Rashes and skin eruptions (📖 Rashes and skin eruptions, p.398)
- Scratching and signs of infection
- Nail features (📖 Nail changes, p.399)

Ask the patient about

Nursing history

- Ability to manage self care and activities of daily living
- Home circumstances (dependants or carers)
- Current coping and self-care strategies that are effective
- Lifestyle, particularly sun exposure (recent and from childhood) and sun protection
- Leisure and social activities (may affect how the patient accepts and manages their care)
- Use of artificial tanning equipment
- Involvement in sporting activities including skiing (sun exposure)
- Anxieties about communal showers
- Occupation, e.g. exposure to irritants, chemicals, and allergens
- Family history of skin conditions
- Diet
- Aggravating factors, e.g. light

Medical history

- History of disorder
- Age of onset
- Chronic or acute
- Allergies and their triggers and effects (e.g. rashes, itching, wheezing, sneezing, and watery eyes)
- Episodes of anaphylaxis treatment and management

- Family history, particularly hay fever, asthma or eczema
- Other skin problems
- Drug therapy
- Results of prior tests, e.g. skin (patch) testing

Current and potential nursing problems
- Rash (duration, previous episodes, known causes)
- Pruritis
- Pain, wounds, pus
- Patient's level of knowledge about the disorder, treatment, and future
- Infection, oedema, wounds, pressure damage
- Concordance with skin care products and hygiene

Anxieties and feelings
- Perceptions of skin disorder
- Concerns about body image, peer acceptance or recognition
- Feelings about the treatment and its impact on lifestyle
- Level of embarrassment about the condition
- Difficulties discussing condition

Assessing skin characteristics

- Colour: Observe for any bruising, discoloration, erythema, pallor, jaundice, cyanosis.
- Texture: Note mobility, thickness, roughness, smoothness, tendency to break down, scales.
- Turgor: Pinch skin gently—note whether it returns to normal shape.
- Moisture: Observe for excessive dryness, moisture, warmth, or coolness.
- Lesions: Observe vascular changes, petechiae, purpura, and skin lesions.
- Symmetry: Observe location and for grouping

Rashes and skin eruptions

- *Eczema:* vesicles (tiny blisters) develop in the epidermis and fluid accumulates between the epidermal cells (spongiosis); dry flaky skin (xeroderma), skin thickened, cracked with an opaque scale, lichenification (increased thickness resembling bark of tree as a result of oedema and inflammation). Infected eczema appears as small cracks or fissures that lead to yellow crusted patches of raw oozing areas. 📖 Eczema: causes, p.404.
- *Atopic dermatitis:* lesions at elbow and knee flexures, and for children on extensor surfaces and face.
- *Contact dermatitis:* erythematous (red), sore, dry, and itchy skin.
- *Scabies:* mites produce a burrow on the surface of the skin that appears as a greyish scaly lesion that is about 0.5 cm in length. The burrow looks like a brownish twisted line with a vesicle at one end. Excoriation, papules, and nodules are present. Occurs at wrist, between fingers, around umbilicus and waist, axilla, palms of hands, and soles of feet. Crusted scabies may occur and resemble psoriasis or eczema.
- *Acne vulgaris:* comedones (blackheads and white heads); superficial papules and pustules; deep pustules and nodules; sinuses form between nodules.
- *Rosacea:* redness over cheeks, nose, and chin; papules, pustules, and telangiectasia develop. 📖 Acne and rosacea, p.414.
- *Psoriasis:* erythema (redness), induration (raised from skin surface), desquamation (scaling), plaque (raised flat topped lesions); lesions vary in size and coalesce (merge); affects all body areas but particularly elbows, knees, and nails. 📖 Psoriasis, p.408.
- *Fungal infections:* single or multiple plaques with scaling.
- *Drug eruptions:* commonest type is erythema with itchy pink wheals or measles-like rash.

• Nail changes – Observe colour and shape

Features	Possible causes
Longitudinal pigmentation (normal in dark skin)	Malignancy (melanoma, Kaposi's sarcoma)
Smaller bands of pigmentation, splinter haemorrhages	Trauma or infection
Pitting	Psoriasis
Hyperkeratosis (thickening)	Tinea (athlete's foot)
Paronychia (thickening of skin folds around nail)	*Candida*
Terry's nails (difference in colour between proximal and distal nail bed)	Congestive cardiac failure, renal failure
Beau's lines (transverse depressions)	Acute, severe illness
Periungual telangectasia (capillary loops become tortuous and dilated)	Repeated injury, infection, dermomyosotis, lupus erythematosus
Mee's lines (transverse white lines)	Acute, severe illness, arsenic poisoning

Nursing problems

Skin rash and eruptions
Skin may have pustules, papules, bumps, pimples, and scales that may be uncomfortable or lead to psychological problems. ☐ Psychological problems, below.

Itching and irritation
Itching and irritation may result from rash, infestation, bites, or allergic reaction.

Risk of infection
Cross-infection from person to person may occur (e.g. scabies, impetigo, and fungal and bacterial conditions) and secondary infection may occur due to excoriation of the skin from scratching.

Pressure damage or risk of pressure damage
Pressure damage (also referred to as bedsores, pressure ulcers, and decubitus ulcers) are areas of localized damage to the skin and/or underlying tissues caused by pressure, shear force, friction, and moisture. ☐ Pressure ulcers: assessment and prevention, p.424.

Wounds
A wound is a break in the skin. Wounds may be acute (e.g. due to incision or trauma) or may be chronic (i.e. a wound fails to progress past the initial stage of healing and becomes a complex condition). ☐ Care of surgical wounds, p.784 and ☐ Pressure ulcers: management, p.426.

Psychological problems
Psychological problems may result from discomfort associated with the skin condition itself, from the appearance of the skin disorder, or from the reaction of others. These problems may lead to:
• Low self-esteem
• Distorted self-perception
• Depression
• Anxiety
• Relationship problems (e.g. family, friends and social contacts may believe the skin condition is contagious or unsightly, which may lead to isolation and loneliness for the patient)

Lack of knowledge about the skin condition
Patients' lack of knowledge about their condition may lead to non-concordance with treatment, may limit their involvement in decisions about care and treatment, or may keep them from taking responsibility for self care.

Specific skin and allergy tests

Skin patch tests

Skin patch tests are used to identify substances that cause contact allergy. Allergens are placed on skin (usually the back), covered by discs, and left for 48 hours. Patch tests are read at the time the allergen is removed (i.e. 48 hours after the allergen was applied) and again 48 hours following removal of the allergen (i.e. 96 hours after the allergen was applied). Test substances vary depending on the clinical problem. These tests are only performed in allergy or dermatology clinics.

Skin prick testing

Skin prick tests are used to detect immediate hypersensitivity reactions and may cause an anaphylactic reaction (i.e. an antigen–antibody reaction that produces a release of histamine causing reduced cardiac output, low arterial pressure, wheeze, laryngeal oedema, and cyanosis).

Skin and wound swabs

Skin and wound swabs are used for culture and sensitivity to identify bacterial infections, e.g. *Staphylococcus* which may be a trigger for atopic eczema or *Streptococcus* in psoriasis. They can also be used to identify a viral infection that occurs on top of a bacterial infection, e.g. herpes simplex virus spreads much more easily in skin affected by eczema.

Skin biopsy

Punch biopsy is used to assess full thickness of the skin. Excisional biopsy is used if the lesion is too large for a punch biopsy or curettage. Skin samples are sent for histology and culture for bacterial infections or immunofluorescence to detect presence of substances, e.g. antigens.

Mycology for fungus or yeast

Skin scrapings, nail clippings, and hair debris are taken to identify fungus or yeast. Microscopic investigation takes 2 weeks. If microscopic investigation suggests a possible positive, mycology culture is performed, which takes 4–5 weeks.

Laboratory tests

- U&E, LFTs, FBC and ESR
- Serum IgE and LFTs
- Serum TSH and FT4
- Fasting lipids

📖 Chapter 39, Common laboratory tests and their interpretation, p.1167.

Wood's light examination

A Wood's light examination can be used to detect bacterial, fungal, and yeast infections and to measure the depth of melanin in the skin. An ultraviolet light handset is used in a darkened room to fluoresce the skin.

Ascarus hunt

An Ascarus hunt test is used to identify scabies. A few drops of 5% potassium hydroxide are applied to the skin over a burrow site. Cells are scraped onto a microscope slide and examined under a microscope to detect mites or larvae.

Eczema: causes

Eczema, also known as dermatitis, is a group of skin conditions that can affect both males and females of all ages. The term eczema is derived from the Greek meaning 'to boil over'. The National Eczema Society estimates that up to 1 in 5 children and 1 in 12 adults suffer from eczema.

Eczema produces dry, itchy, and hot skin that can cause great discomfort and distress to both the sufferer and their carers. In its most severe form eczema can cause patients to scratch excessively, leading to broken skin. Localized and sometimes systemic infection may result.

The cause of eczema can be exogenous (i.e. due to an external source) or endogenous (i.e. due to an internal source).

Endogenous eczema

Atopic eczema is the most common eczema and is thought to be due to a genetic predisposition. A family history often reveals eczema, asthma, or hay fever. The scratch-itch cycle can result in secondary infection.

Varicose eczema affects the lower legs of patients who suffer from varicose veins and associated venous hypertension. Poor venous return results in stasis of venous blood, oedema, and subsequent irritation and inflammation of the skin.

Discoid eczema affects adults and presents as itching circular patches. Its cause is unknown.

Seborrhoeic eczema affects the face, scalp and flexures of adults. The ill-defined greasy, erythematous, scaly patches are not particularly itchy. It is believed to be exacerbated by an overgrowth of yeast on the skin.

Pompholyx (a bubble) affects the hands and feet. Tiny blisters on the soles, palms, toes and fingers cause intense irritation.

Exogenous eczema

Allergic contact dermatitis is caused by an external allergen such as nickel or fragrance.

Irritant contact dermatitis is commonly associated with specific occupations, e.g. hairdressing, nursing, cleaning, and mechanics. It is caused by repeated contact with chemicals on the skin. The most common irritants are detergents and soaps.

Photosensitive eczema can occur due to a systemic or topical photosensitizer. Typically, an area exposed to UV rays will become inflamed and eczematous.

Unclassified eczema

Asteototic eczema, also known as eczema craquelée, presents as dry 'crazy paving' eczema with scale and often deep fissures (cracks).

Lichen simplex presents as an area of lichenified (thickened) eczema. Constant scratching or rubbing causes thickening, and often crusting, of the skin.

Eczema: treatments and care

Treatments

Treatments for eczema are multifactorial and the basic principles can be applied to all types of eczema.

- Maintenance of basic hygiene without using soap (soaps and detergents can be very drying).
- Regular use of emollient/moisturizer to the whole body. Guidelines suggest 500 g per week for an adult. Patient concordance is improved by allowing patients to use the moisturizer of their preference.
- Application of topical steroid to the affected areas. Topical steroids reduce inflammation, relieve itching, and promote comfort. The appropriate potency of steroid should be selected based on the patient's age as well as the site and severity of eczema. Patients should be instructed to use a sufficient amount of steroid preparation. Under use is far more common than over use due to the misconception of the term 'use sparingly'. Fingertip units are used as a measurement of application of topical steroid.

The fingertip unit method: 1 adult fingertip = ½ g of cream or ointment

FACE & NECK	ONE ARM	ONE HAND	ONE LEG	ONE FOOT	TRUNK (front)	TRUNK (back)
2 ½	3	1	6	2	7	7

- Topical immunosuppressive creams such as tacrolimus and pimecrolimus may be effective in sufferers who have failed to improve with topical steroids. Long-term side effects are unknown.
- As eczema is often a chronic condition, intermittent, long-term use of topical steroid is necessary. However, patients should be educated on the risks of over use.
- Applying an occlusive dressing over topical treatment can be helpful in reducing the itch-scratch cycle. Wet wraps may be helpful in the young and paste bandages may be helpful in older children and adults.
- Antihistamines can often help reduce the itch and irritation.
- Removal of any known irritant is essential.
- Patients should keep cool, wear cotton clothing, and avoid wool and synthetic materials.
- Severe eczema may require administration of oral steroids and dermatologists may also prescribe courses of UVA and UVB light therapy to relieve symptoms. In very severe cases systemic drugs such as azothioprine and ciclosporin may be prescribed.
- Suspected contact dermatitis will often require patch testing to identify allergens. Skin prick testing and radioallergosorbent testing (RAST) may also be performed on some patients. Allergies, p.416.

Nursing care

- The main role of the nurse is to support and educate patients with eczema.
- The nurse should teach patients about their medications and how to use them correctly.
- Listening to patients and providing support is essential as the psychological effect of living with eczema can often be very debilitating and cause misery to both patients and their families.
- The nurse should advise patients on reducing the impact of house dust mites. 📖 Allergies, p.416.
- Providing dietary advice, such as the use of exclusion diets, can be helpful in some children with widespread atopic eczema. A dietitian should always be consulted if changes in diet are to be advised.

Psoriasis

Psoriasis is a chronic inflammatory non-infectious condition that affects 2–3% of the population. It can occur at any age but most commonly occurs in individuals who are in their mid-teens to early 20s or who are between 55 and 60 years. Psoriasis is a genetically linked condition, and may be triggered by streptococcal infections, physical trauma, stress, certain drugs (e.g. beta-blockers, anti-malarials, NSAIDs, lithium), high alcohol consumption, burns, sunburn, or injury.

Physical effects

Psoriasis produces redness of the skin (erythema), scaling (desquamation), thickening (induration), fissures, raised flat-topped lesions (silvery plaques), excoriation, merged lesions (coalescence), and onycholysis (nails separate from the nail bed).

Psychological and social effects

Visibility of psoriatic lesions is associated with feelings of poor physical health. Patients may have low self-esteem, a distorted self-perception, and may be depressed or anxious. Patients may be angry at the reactions of others who misunderstand the nature of the condition. Relationships with family and friends and new contacts may be difficult, and patients may experience problems with sexual relationships due to fears of rejection. Psoriasis may lead to social isolation as patients avoid sports, swimming, using communal showers, and hairdressers. Patients may also experience work-related issues due to employer or co-worker prejudice.

Treatment

- Emollients can be used as a soap substitute to help moisturize dry skin and ease itching.
- Coal tar has anti-inflammatory and anti-proliferative actions but may cause staining, burning, or smell.
- Dithranol, which is applied to the plaques only, is used under the supervision of a dermatologist. It is applied for 24 hours, and then removed with oil. Dithranol also causes staining, burning, and smells.
- Vitamin D derivatives (e.g. calcipotriol) are also applied to plaques only; they may cause increased irritation.
- Topical corticosteroids have anti-inflammatory and anti-proliferative effects and can be used on all sites of psoriasis.
- Topical retinoids (e.g. tazarotene) have been found to improve chronic plaque psoriasis in the short term. Retinoids are teratogenic and should not be used in pregnant women or pre-conceptually.
- Phototherapy (UVA and UVB) will produce remission. UVA may be linked with psoralen (PUVA) for effective clearance and long-term maintenance.
- Systemic drugs (e.g. ciclosporin, methotrexate, acitretin, and hydroxycarbamide) are used to clear the psoriasis but should be prescribed by a dermatologist and carefully monitored for side effects.

Role of the nurse in supporting psoriasis patients

- Listen to patients' feelings, fears and anxieties, and identify emotional barriers.
- Ensure patients and their families have information necessary to understand the condition, its chronic relapsing nature, as well as treatments and their side effects.
- Ensure patients and their families have realistic expectations of the future.
- Demonstrate the application of treatments to the patient and/or carer and ensure their ability to properly apply the treatments. Ensure patients and carers are aware of any side effects and how to prevent or minimize them.
- Where possible, align the treatment regimen with the patient's lifestyle to promote concordance.
- Provide information and discuss how to manage lifestyle, including how to overcome psychological problems.
- Refer to specialist services, e.g. chiropody or specialist nurse.
- Ensure patients have written materials on the condition, including information on support networks, e.g. Psoriasis Association.

Skin infections and infestations

The human skin is host to a wide range of bacteria, both harmless and potentially harmful, but normally provides a barrier against infection. Skin infections can vary from small localized lesions such as pustules and abscesses to life-threatening conditions such as bacteraemia.

Folliculitis is a pustular inflammatory condition caused by bacteria in the hair follicles that can affect any part of the body. The condition can be triggered by shaving or by using some topical preparations, e.g. tar. Typically there are small pustules which discharge and can be uncomfortable and embarrassing. Simple strategies such as a more delicate approach to shaving or applying treatments in the direction of hair growth can help. Oral antibiotics may be required.

Impetigo is a superficial bacterial skin infection caused by *Staphylococcus* aureus or a mixture of *Staphylococcus* and haemolytic *Streptococcus*. Lesions of impetigo produce yellow exudate which dries to a crust on the skin surface. Lesions most commonly affect the face but can spread quickly to other parts of the body if untreated. Impetigo is contagious and care must be taken to use separate personal items, particularly towels. First line treatment is usually application of a topical antibiotic such as mupiricin or sodium fusidate. Because resistance to these antibiotics can be rapidly acquired, it is recommended that only a 2-week course be prescribed. Systemic antibiotics may be required in severe cases.

Cellulitis is an infection of the subcutaneous tissues that can spread rapidly if untreated. It is potentially life threatening. Bacteria commonly gain entry via breaks in the skin surface due to insect bites, wounds, and fissures. Bacterial enzymes cause rapid spread of the infection which presents as localized heat, swelling, pain, and erythema (redness). The patient will often feel systemically unwell with pyrexia and sometimes rigors. The cellulitic area may produce blisters or necrosis. Skin swabs and blood cultures are taken to identify the pathogen and sensitivity. Management includes either oral or parenteral antibiotics depending on the severity and spread of cellulitis. Nursing care should focus on vigilant monitoring of the patient's condition (observations of temperature and blood pressure as well as observing spread of cellulitis) and on patient comfort (e.g. pain management and relief of pyrexia). Dressings may need changing frequently due to leakage of serous fluid. Patient's position must also be changed often to prevent venous pooling in legs.

Fungal infections are very common and are usually caused by dermophytes (*Tinea*) or yeasts (*Candida*).

Tinea is often referred to as ringworm and commonly affects the web spaces of feet and may spread to other areas. Skin scrapings and/or nail clippings are taken to confirm the diagnosis. Once confirmed treatment with topical antifungals such as miconazole or clotrimazole is usually sufficient. Systemic therapy with terbinafine may be required in resistant cases, particularly for nails and scalp.

Candida (thrush) commonly infects the gastrointestinal tract and can cause problems in all mucosa. It can also affect skin, especially in skin folds and nails. *Candida* presents particular problems in severely unwell and immunosuppressed patients. It can also occur during and after antibiotic treatment. Lesions cause discomfort and soreness and, when present in skinfolds (groin, under breasts, natal cleft and under stomach folds), causes skin to become red and shiny (intertrigo). In persistent cases diabetes should be excluded. Mycology cultures are taken to confirm diagnosis. Treatment includes application of topical agents (clotrimazole, nystatin) or use of systemic antifungals (fluconazole).

Infestations

Scabies (Sarcoptes scabie) is a common parasitic infection. Mites burrow 1 cm along the epidermis, usually via web spaces, and lay 2–3 eggs a day over a 4–6 week lifespan. Patients experience intense itch and irritation of the skin which is worse at night. The skin shows signs of excoriation from itching combined with a rash, and burrows may be visible. Secondary infection can occur and antibiotics may be required. Scabies is highly contagious and is acquired from physical contact with infected persons, even those who have not yet developed symptoms. It is important that patients understand the mode of spread. Poor hygiene is NOT a cause of scabies. Diagnosis is normally made by clinical presentation and history of symptoms, but sometimes an ascarus hunt is performed. Treatment of scabies is with topical malathion lotion which must be applied to the whole body. Others who have close contact with the patient must also be treated, whether or not they show symptoms. Patients' bedding, towels and clothing should be changed following treatment and washed at a high heat. Itch and irritation can continue for some time after treatment.

Body lice are flattened wingless insects that can be spread through bedding and clothing. Infestations tend to be associated with poor social hygiene and poverty. Treatment is with topical malathion or permethrin. Topical steroids and antibiotics may be required if itching and irritation from the lice has caused secondary eczema or impetigo. Washing bedding and clothing is required to eradicate lice.

Head lice are transmitted by close contact and are more common in children. The adult female louse lays eggs (nits) that adhere to the hair about 0.5 cm from the scalp. The nits hatch producing more lice which cause itching, particularly at the nape of the neck and behind the ears. Treatment is mainly with permethrin and malathion lotions. However, lice have been reported to be resistant to these treatments. Other strategies such as using conditioner and combing every 3 days have proved to be successful. Treatment of the family and close contacts is essential, but concordance is not always achievable. In very severe cases of long-term infestation, excoriation of the neck and secondary infection can occur resulting in secondary infection and discharge. Sufferers may become systemically unwell and may require antibiotics.

Nursing management of scabies

Early recognition is critical to prevent outbreaks, but scabies is difficult to diagnose.

- Topical anti-scabies treatment can have a drying effect on the skin, but moisturizers and oral antihistamines may help.
- Seek the expert advice of the infection control team who will provide guidance on treatment and monitoring of patients and outbreaks, and will provide up-to-date training for staff.
- Infested people and close physical contacts should be treated whether or not they are symptomatic.
- Treatment consists of the application of a scabicide over the entire body surface (e.g. malathion lotion or permethrin) with special attention to the area between the fingers and undersides of nails. The scabicide should be left to dry for 8–12 hours, and should be reapplied after handwashing. Although mites should be killed in a few hours, itchy rash may remain for 3–4 weeks. A repeat application is required after 1 week. Ensure patients understand how to use lotions and can apply them correctly.
- Universal infection control measures and protective clothing should be worn when dealing with a patient, including when the creams and lotions are being applied to the skin.
- Oral antihistamines (e.g. chlorphenamine) may be prescribed for symptomatic relief or calamine lotion may be used. Patients need to understand the purpose for the drugs and any side effects.
- Discourage patients from scratching as this may lead to secondary infection. If secondary infection occurs, antibiotics may be required.
- If the patient is hospitalized, sheets, bedding, and clothing should be changed daily.
- If the patient is home, sheets should be changed on the day of treatment. Patients at home should be advised that sheets, bedding, and clothing should be washed in hot water and dried at a high heat. Hot ironing will also help kill the mites.
- Ensure patients and contacts understand the mode of spread of scabies and refrain from prolonged physical contact. Children should be kept away from school until treatment is completed. It may help to reassure patients and their carers that a lack of cleanliness does not cause scabies.
- Patients with Norwegian scabies are highly contagious. This form of scabies is found in patients who are immunocompromised or severely incapacitated. These patients need to be isolated and their laundry must be treated as infectious.

Acne and rosacea

Acne vulgaris

Acne vulgaris is a common inflammatory condition that affects 80% of adolescents but also occurs in those over 30 as mature acne. Increased sebum excretion causes a blockage of the pilosebaceous ducts, and colonization with *Proprionobacterium acnes* bacteria results in inflammation.

Patients develop spots, blackheads, whiteheads, red papules and pustules, nodules, and cysts on the face, back, and shoulders. Sinuses may be formed between the nodules, and the skin appears oily. Scarring from old lesions may be present.

The effect acne has on the sufferer's body image and self-esteem is an important consideration when treating patients. Adolescence is already a time of insecurity and having a visible skin disease can increase anxiety and depression.

Treatment

The treatment of acne depends on the severity of the acne, the psychological impact of the acne to the patient, and the patient's preference.

- Benzoyl peroxide, applied twice daily, has a strong antimicrobial effect and some anti-inflammatory effect. It may cause dry skin, bleaching, and sometimes contact dermatitis.
- Topical antibiotics (e.g. erythromycin, tetracycline) are available in liquid, gel, ointment, or lotion formulations and may be suitable for inflammatory acne.
- Systematic antibiotics (e.g. tetracycline, doxycycline, or erythromycin for 6 months) may be used when topical treatment is not effective or may be used in conjunction with topical treatment, especially when the risk of scarring is high.
- Anti-androgen therapy co-cyprindiol (cyproterone acetate 2 mg and ethiyloestradiol 35 mg) is commonly used for females with moderate acne. This oral contraceptive helps to reduce sebum production.
- Topical retinoids (e.g. isotretinoin) act by removing non-inflamed lesions and reducing development of inflammation. It is important that the patient avoids the sun and is advised that scaling and erythema may occur but that this will settle.

When the above strategies have failed, *oral retinoid therapy* may be considered. Oral retinoid treatment is prescribed by a consultant dermatologist. This treatment has serious adverse effects including dry lips and skin, muscle aches, depression, and liver changes. The treatment is potentially teratogenic (i.e. may cause benign or malignant tumours) and carries a high risk of birth deformities. Females must use contraception and monthly pregnancy tests must be performed.

Nursing management of patients on oral retinoid therapy

- Observe for signs of depression.
- Provide psychological support.
- Ensure contraception is being taken by females.
- Advise on the use of moisturizers.

Rosacea

Rosacea is a chronic disorder of unknown cause that mainly affects middle-aged people. Initially, redness of the cheeks, nose, chin, and forehead occurs sporadically, but then gradually becomes more severe and permanent with the development of telangectasia, papules, and pustules. Swelling of the nose may occur. Treatment includes topical and systematic antibiotics, and laser therapy may be used to reduce flushing and redness. Patients should be advised to use moisturizing cream and to identify and avoid triggers (e.g. spicy foods, sun exposure, hot weather, or alcohol).

Nursing advice and support for patients with acne

- Assess the effect on the patient's self-confidence, relationships with peers, school work, and leisure activities. Identify signs of anxiety or social isolation, and encourage patients to talk about their feelings.
- Ensure the patient understands the causes of acne, what the condition is, and that it is common in their age group.
- Ensure the patient understands that treatment may take weeks or months to have an effect and that continued concordance with the treatment plan is essential or acne will recur.
- Advise the patient on the importance of local hygiene (i.e. washing with soap and water twice daily to remove surface sebum); of applying moisturizer; and avoiding unnecessary touching of the lesions.
- Advise the patient against wearing tight, restrictive clothing.
- Avoid conditions of high humidity and heavy sweating.
- Ensure the patient knows how to apply topical treatments and understands their side effects.

Allergies

An allergy is an over-reaction or hypersensitivity to an allergen (antigen) that is harmless in most people but causes an abnormal reaction in a susceptible person. Common allergies include pollen, mould, house dust mites, food (e.g. eggs, shellfish, peanuts), pets, bee stings, drugs (e.g. antibiotics), and materials (e.g. latex, plasters). A predisposition to allergy includes genetics, exposure to allergen, and exposure to pollutants.

Allergic response

On first exposure to an allergen no perceptible response occurs, but a process of sensitization occurs. Upon a subsequent exposure to the allergen, an allergic and inflammatory response occurs. Allergic responses result in a range of symptoms from rash, itching, sneezing, runny nose and eyes, local or generalized oedema, constriction of bronchi, and difficulty in breathing to anaphylaxis—a severe allergic response causing laryngeal oedema, bronchospasm, profound respiratory distress, vasodilation, low blood pressure, and shock. Anaphylaxis may progress to respiratory and cardiac arrest.

Nursing advice and support

- Characterize the allergy: obtain a detailed clinical history of signs and symptoms and relationship to allergens, e.g. symptoms occurring with the seasons, with food or with contact with animals.
- Perform a skin patch test to assess a person's sensitivity to a range of allergens.
- Advise patients on avoiding triggers.
  - Reduce exposure to pollen—keep house and car windows closed; stay indoors if possible; avoid activities that increase exposure (e.g. mowing the lawn or gardening when pollen count is high), wear mask, and use air conditioning.
  - Reduce exposure to mould—clean showers and baths regularly with bleach solution, use dehumidifiers, avoid cleaning gutters.
  - Reduce exposure to house dust—vacuum rather than dust; use dust proof covers on pillows and mattresses. Wash bedding at 55°C or higher, and leave floors bare of rugs and carpets or have washable ones. Use washable curtains and blinds.
  - Avoid pets or bath them weekly.

Treatment

- *Desensitization* occurs by injecting minute amounts of allergen and increasing the dose as tolerance builds up. Government restrictions apply and the process must only be done in specialist clinics.
- *Antihistamines* are given orally or topically to inhibit the allergic reaction, e.g. acrivastine, chlorphenamine. IV chlorphenamine can be used in anaphylaxis.

Bullous diseases (blistering)

Common causes of blistering include burns, friction, and insect bites.

Bullous pemphigoid

Bullous pemphigoid is the most common autoimmune blistering disease. It normally occurs in the elderly, affects both males and females, and may have a possible association with certain drugs, e.g. diuretics, and some antibiotics. Patients present with large intact blisters (bullae) over the limbs and trunk that have often been preceded by red inflamed itchy patches over the body. The mouth is sometimes affected. The blisters are sub-epidermal, and have a thick roof. Diagnosis is confirmed by biopsy and immunofluorescent tests on blister fluid and blood samples.

Treatment
- Very potent topical steroids
- Systemic steroids
- Oral minocycline and other immunosuppressive drugs
- Potassium permanganate baths to dry out blisters

Pemphigus

Pemphigus is a chronic blistering disease that affects males and females, usually during middle age. It has a high mortality rate if left untreated. The two main types of pemphigus are pemphigus foliaceus and pemphigus vulgaris, both of which present with blisters in the mouth, on the genitals, larynx, pharynx, oesophagus, and anus. Blisters can rupture leaving large erosive and painful areas.

Treatment
- High doses of systemic steroids
- Immunosuppression (azothiaprine, ciclosporin, and methotrexate)
- Topical corticosteroids
- Potassium permanganate baths to dry out blisters

Dermatitis herpetiformis

Dermatitis herpetiformis (DH) is a rare blistering condition that causes intense irritation and itch. It affects the young and middle aged. DH presents as clusters of erythematous urticarial papules or small vesicles. The blisters cause intense itching and are easily ruptured by scratching, leaving areas of sore eroded skin. Affected areas include knees, elbows, buttocks, shoulders, scalp, and axillae, with occasional lesions in the mouth. DH is linked to gluten sensitivity and coeliac disease.

Treatment
- Gluten-free diet is advised.
- Dapsone is used but close monitoring is required due to potential severe side effects (rash, anaemia, motor neuropathy, hepatitis).
- Antihistamines may help decrease irritation.
- Iodine dressings should be avoided as they may exacerbate disease.

Nursing care
- Attend to hygiene.
- Apply topical treatments.
- Monitor diet and fluid intake.
- Lance large tense blisters with a sterile scalpel at the underside of the blister. Apply non-adherent dressings to open blisters to promote comfort and to reduce risk of secondary infection.
- If oral blisters are present, attend to mouth care and offer a soft diet.
- Provide psychological and emotional support for patients and family.

Skin cancer

Skin cancer is currently the main condition treated in dermatology units. its incidence and prevalence has soared throughout the world. Excessive exposure to ultraviolet radiation is linked to malignant melanoma and to other forms of skin cancer.

Basal cell carcinoma

Basal cell carcinoma (BCC), the most common type of skin cancer, is most commonly seen in older people who have a history of long-term sun exposure. BCC presents as lesions that crust over, heal, and then reappear. It commonly occurs at sun-exposed sites such as the face, bald scalps in men, and shins in women. If untreated the lesions will ulcerate and are referred to as rodent ulcers. Diagnosis is confirmed by biopsy.

Tumours are classified as high risk or low risk. High risk tumours should be managed by a dermatologist and include:
- Tumours on eyes, nose, naso-labial folds, ears
- Tumours >2 cm diameter, ill defined
- Recurrent
- Infiltrative
- Immunosuppressed

Treatment
Treatment varies depending on whether the tumour is high or low risk.

High risk
- Excision
- Mohs (micrographic surgery which enables the surgeon to excise layer by layer, analysing each section under a microscope until full clearance is achieved)
- Radiotherapy in frail/elderly or for palliation
- Curettage and cautery for small nodular lesions or for palliation
- Cryotherapy (for small nodular types)

Low risk
- Excision
- Curettage and cautery
- Radiotherapy
- Cryotherapy
- Topical therapy (5-flurouracil, imiquimod)

Squamous cell carcinoma

Squamous cell carcinoma is an invasive tumour that can spread (metastasize) if untreated. It is often related to sun damage but can also occur in patients with chronic diseases that affect the skin (e.g. lupus erythematosus) or at sites of previous or ongoing damage (e.g. burns, leg ulcers). Immunosuppressed patients are more susceptible. *Diagnosis* is confirmed by biopsy. *Treatment*, which should be prompt, normally includes excision of tumour, and may be followed by radiotherapy.

Malignant melanoma

Malignant melanoma is the most common cause of cancer related death in the 25–35 male age group. It affects the pigment producing cells (melanocytes) and is the most dangerous form of skin cancer as it can spread rapidly through the lymphatic and circulatory system. Melanoma is related to short bursts of intense sunshine, is most common in fair skinned blue eyed people, and often has a family history. Other risk factors include large numbers of pigmented naevi and previous history. The most common site for women is the legs.

Diagnosis and treatment

Diagnosis typically begins by identification of a suspicious mole which changes in shape and colour including inflammation, crusting, bleeding, irregular borders, asymmetric lesions, irregular colour, and sensation (pain, tenderness, itch). ◻ ABCDE guide to melanoma diagnosis, below. Treatment includes complete wide excision of the lesion with a good margin of unaffected skin around the lesion. Histology will reveal whether the melanoma has been completely removed. The patient's general health should be checked and lymph nodes palpated. A chest x-ray may also be ordered. Regular review is imperative, initially with a specialist who will carry out a full body check for mole changes and a lymph node check.

The diagnosis of malignant melanoma can be daunting and requires a sensitive approach. It will inevitably be life changing for the patient as sun avoidance, mole watching, and potential socioeconomic issues with insurance and mortgage companies are often unavoidable. Patients may require specialist counselling in order to come to terms with their diagnosis. Support groups exist for those who need them.

ABCDE guide to melanoma diagnosis

Asymmetry
Border (irregularity)
Colour (1 colour OK, 4 colours suspicious)
Diameter (>5 mm is suspicious)
Evolution (growing mole)

Nursing advice and support for patients with skin cancer

Support the patient following diagnosis

- Support the patient through periods of adjustment, understanding, and acceptance of diagnosis and prognosis. Provide information and explanations.
- Ensure the patient understands the specific type of cancer, e.g. with basal cell carcinoma the cancer does not metastasize; with squamous cell carcinoma and malignant melanoma it is not possible to give reassurances that treatment will prevent metastases.
- Reassure patients that frequent follow up is not necessary for patients with basal cell carcinoma.
- Discuss concerns about scarring and resulting impact on confidence, depression, and anxieties.
- Discuss impact on lifestyle, e.g. concerns about future support to family (e.g. mortgage), and refer to specialist help if necessary.
- Ensure opportunity to see skin cancer nurse specialist.
- Skin cancer specialist nurse should teach how to examine lymph nodes.

Educate about sun care habits

- Advise to limit further exposure to sun and cover up, using hats, long-sleeved shirts, and trousers. Avoid sunburn at all costs.
- Use sunscreen factor 15+ minimum on all exposed skin including face, tips of ears, scalp, backs of hands, and legs. Apply every 2–3 hours in summer and winter even if it appears cloudy. Use when exposed at high altitude, e.g. when skiing.
- Give advice to family and carer.
- Avoid sun beds and tanning tables.
- Teach patient how to examine the skin.

Other advice

- Check drugs in case they cause photosensitivity, e.g. antihypertensives, diuretics.
- Watch for further lesions, especially rough lumpy areas, changes to lesions, and any lesions that fail to heal.
- Be aware of the significance of any enlarged lymph nodes and advise patient to seek advice.
- Contact support groups.

Pressure ulcers: assessment and prevention

Risk assessment

Pressure ulcers (also referred to as bedsores, pressure sores, decubitus ulcers and pressure damage) are areas of localized damage to the skin and/or underlying tissues (muscle and bone).

Factors contributing to pressure ulcers

- *Extrinsic factors:* pressure, shear (layers of skin or tissue slide over one another, e.g. when patient slides down the bed or chair), friction, moisture, or a combination of these.
- *Intrinsic factors:* disease (e.g. diabetes, peripheral vascular disease), age, reduced mobility, poor nutrition, and poor mental alertness.

Assessing a patient's risk

- Risk assessment should be done on first contact with the patient, e.g. on admission.
- Follow local policy and assessment tools used.
  - Weight and height—obese and extremely thin patients are most at risk.
  - Level of mobility—the more restricted the greater the risk.
  - Continence—the degree of urinary or faecal incontinence raises the risk.
  - Skin condition—look for discoloration (blue/purple areas), erythema, non-blanching hyperaemia, blisters, broken areas, oedema, dryness, friability.
  - Age—elderly patients (≥80 years) are more at risk.
  - Nutrition—poor nutritional state, dehydration, or restricted food and fluid intake increase risk.
  - Mental state—confusion, apathy, poor cognition and unconsciousness increase risk.
  - Coexisting diseases (e.g. diabetes, peripheral vascular disease, spinal injuries, anaemia, cardiac failure, cancer) increase risk.
  - Neurological deficits and sensory impairment (e.g. paraplegia, multiple sclerosis, stroke) increase risk.
  - Surgery, particularly orthopaedic surgery or critical care surgery, increases risk.
  - Certain drugs increase risk, e.g. steroids and anti-inflammatory drugs.
- Assessment should be repeated as necessary depending on the patient's condition and level of risk.
- All areas should be visibly inspected.
- For patients who are at risk and who are being discharged, relatives and carers should be taught how to assess risk.
- Document findings of assessment and act on them.

Prevention

Prevention is aimed at reducing risk. The risk assessment is an essential guide to making decisions about which interventions should be used. Frequent reassessment is essential to evaluate the effectiveness of interventions.

Patient involvement

- Gain patients' cooperation by explaining the factors involved in pressure ulcer development and the preventive measures being taken.
- Explain how they can help themselves, e.g. changing position, redistributing weight, eating, and drinking.

Mobility

- Encourage mobility as much as possible, e.g. walking around bed area, changing position from bed to chair frequently, or being repositioned in bed or chair.
- Changing position should be determined by risk level but normally at least 2-hourly.
- Avoid positioning on bony prominences or on areas of existing pressure damage or wounds.
- Seek specialist advice from a physiotherapist or tissue viability specialist.
- Make a record of positions used and changes.

Skin care

- Keep patient's skin clean, dry, and moisturized.
- Check for incontinence frequently and attend to patient's hygiene immediately.
- If incontinent, plan measures to reduce effects and seek help from continence specialist, if necessary.

Nutrition

- Use nutrition assessment tool to determine the level of risk.
- Find out patient's food preferences and provide these where possible.
- Ensure patient has appropriate assistance with eating and drinking.
- Seek advice from a dietitian as necessary.

Pressure-relieving devices

- The use of pressure-relieving devices is determined by the level of risk, causative factors, susceptible sites (e.g. heels), and acceptability and comfort to the patient.
- Select the appropriate devices according to the risk and local availability. At a minimum, all vulnerable patients should be placed on a high-specification foam mattress/cushion with pressure-reducing properties and a high-specification foam mattress with alternating pressure overlay. A sophisticated continuous low-pressure system, e.g. low air loss, air flotation, or viscous fluid, is used for patients at a greater risk.

Pressure ulcer classification scales, examples	
European Pressure Ulcer Advisory Panel (EPUAP)	The management of pressure ulcers in primary and secondary care. NICE Clinical Guidelines, September 2005
Pressure ulcers	*Best Practice Statement for Treatment/Management of Pressure Ulcers.* NHS Quality Improvement Scotland, March 2005
Stirling Pressure Sore Severity Scale (SPSSS)	Reid J, Morrison M (1994) Towards a consensus classification of pressure sores. *J Wound Care* **3**(3): 157–60
Pressure Ulcer Scale for Healing (PUSH)	Stotts NA, Rodeheaver GT, Thomas DR, Frantz RA et al. (2001) An instrument to measure healing in pressure ulcers: development and validation of the pressure ulcer scale for healing (PUSH). *Journals of Gerontology Series: A Biological Sciences and Medical Sciences* **56**(12): 795

Pressure ulcers: management

- Ongoing risk assessment and preventative measure are important aspects of the management of pressure ulcers.
- The management of pressure ulcers should be the responsibility of a first level registered nurse.
- Seek advice from a tissue viability specialist, if necessary.
- Assess the pressure ulcer.
  - The NICE clinical guideline indicates that the European Pressure Ulcer Advisory Panel classification system of pressure ulcer grades should be used (📖 European Pressure Ulcer Advisory Panel classification system of pressure ulcer grades, p.427).
  - Assessment of the ulcer should also include a description of the wound, its size (maximum length, depth, and width—use calibrated ruler), location/site, grade, exudate (amount, consistency, colour, and odour), signs of infection (pus, cellulitis, and malodour), undermining, presence of tracking sinus or fistula, pain (type and duration), and condition of surrounding skin (healthy, macerated, oedematous, and eczema).
  - Supplement description with photography and/or tracings.
  - Document all findings.
  - Reassess as frequently as necessary.
- The reaction of the patient and any concerns and anxieties should be noted and considered when deciding on treatment.
- Choose the most appropriate method of treatment, e.g. dressing or topical agent, debridement, or adjunct therapy based on the assessment. Check whether there is a local wound formulary to follow.
- Dressings may include:
  - Contact layers—prevent adherence to the wound bed, used on superficial wound with exudates, e.g. paraffin gauze.
  - Passive dressings—used to control exudates, prevent contamination, and control odour, e.g. films, foams, and hydrogels.
  - Interactive dressings—produce a gel-like covering on the wound surface to promote healing, e.g. hydrocolloids and alginates.
  - Active dressings—promote cell growth (e.g. collagen and hyaluronic acid), used with skin grafts, human or animal skin replacements.
  - Antimicrobial dressings, e.g. iodine.
- Topical preparations may be applied to compensate for a deficiency in an element important for wound healing, e.g. zinc oxide.
- Debridement is the removal of dead or necrotic tissue (slough). This may be done in several ways—using specific agents (e.g. enzymes) to digest the slough, hydrogels, maggots (larval therapy), wound irrigation, ultrasound, or laser therapy.
- Referral for surgery may be required if conservative management fails.
- Antimicrobial therapy may need to be prescribed if there is an infection.

European Pressure Ulcer Advisory Panel classification system of pressure ulcer grades[1]

Grade 1

Non-blanchable erythema of intact skin. Discoloration of the skin, warmth, oedema, induration, or hardness may also be used as an indicator, particularly on individuals with darker skin.

Grade 2

Partial thickness skin loss involving epidermis, dermis, or both. The ulcer is superficial and presents clinically as an abrasion or blister.

Grade 3

Full-thickness skin loss involving damage to, or necrosis of, subcutaneous tissue that may extend down to but not through underlying fascia.

Grade 4

Extensive destruction, tissue necrosis, or damage to muscle, or bone, or supporting structures, with or without full-thickness skin loss.

1 Royal College of Nursing and National Institute for Health and Clinical Excellence (2005). *The prevention and treatment of pressure ulcers.* London. Reproduced with permission from the European Pressure Ulcer Advisory Panel.

Formal risk assessment scales, examples

Braden Scale	Bergstrom N, Braden BJ, Laguzza A, Holman V (1987) The Braden scale for predicting pressure sore risk. *Nurs Res* **36**(4): 205–10
Knoll Scale	Towey AP, Erland SM (1988) Validity and reliability of an assessment tool for pressure ulcer risk *Decubitus* **1**(2): 40–8
Norton Scale	Norton D, Mclaren R, Exton-Smith AN (1962) *An investigation of geriatric nursing problems in hospital.* The National Corportion for the Care of Old People, London
Pressure Sore Prediction Score	Lowthian P (1989) Identifying and protecting patients who may get pressure sores. *Nurs Standard* **4**(4): 26–9
Waterlow Risk Assessment Score	Waterlow J (1988) The Waterlow card for the prevention and management of pressure sores: towards a pocket policy. *Care Science and Practice* **6**(1): 8–12
Pressure Ulcer Risk Assessment Tool (PURAT)	Wicks G (2006) PURAT: is clinical judgement an effective alternative? *Wounds UK* **2**(2): 14–24
Pressure ulcer risks assessment scales for children: Bedi, Cockett, Garvin, Braden Q, Pickersgill, the Pattoid pressure scoring system, the paediatric pressure sore/skin damage risk assessment (Waterlow)	Wilcock J (2006) Pressure ulcer risk assessment in children. In: White R, Denyer J, eds. *Paediatric Skin and Wound Care.* Wounds UK, Aberdeen: 79–86

Leg ulcers

A leg ulcer is usually described as loss of skin on the leg (below knee) or foot that has not healed within 6 weeks. Approximately 70% of leg ulcers are due to venous problems, 20% are due to arterial disease, and the remainder are due to other aetiologies, e.g. neuropathy, trauma, obesity, malignancy, self-inflicted, or osteomyelitis. 🕮 Venous ulcers, p.185.

Assessment

Proper assessment is essential for correct diagnosis and treatment.

Holistic assessment includes social circumstances, age, sex, mobility, nutrition, underlying diseases (e.g. diabetes, rheumatoid arthritis, circulatory problems), medication, smoking, family history, pregnancy, previous ulcers, and coping and adjustment strategies.

Limb assessment includes observing the condition of the skin (shiny, tight skin, brown discoloration due to venous staining, varicosities, colour changes when limb is dependent and when elevated); check for signs of previous ulceration, trauma, surgery, oedema, and cellulitis; note size and shape of limb and range of movement in leg and ankle. Note any local lymphadenopathy.

Ulcer assessment includes identifying the site, size, shape and duration; observe for signs of infection, exudates, colour consistency, odour, appearance of surrounding skin, pain, and stages of wound healing.

Doppler assessment (i.e. use of Doppler ultrasound via a hand-held mini-Doppler) is used to measure the arterial flow to the limb by calculating the ankle brachial pressure index (ABPI) and should only be done by specially trained practitioners.

Assessment of quality of life includes recognizing that the condition may cause significant disruption to lifestyle leading to lack of mobility, social exclusion, loneliness, lack of self-esteem and confidence, and preoccupation with ulcer and treatment regimen.

Management

Compression has been found to heal venous ulcers more effectively than no compression. The correct treatment type must be decided by a specialist as incorrect compression may result in loss of limb. It can be applied through multi-layer compression bandages; examples are short-stretch bandaging, four-layer system, and long-stretch bandaging. Compression hosiery may also be used. These must be applied appropriately by trained practitioners. Concordance may be poor as some patients cannot tolerate certain bandages, or if bandages are too thick to wear with fashionable shoes, or if dressing change is painful. Hosiery may be difficult to put on, uncomfortable to wear, especially in hot weather, or result in allergic reactions, e.g. to nylon or Lycra®. Wearing compression hosiery helps to prevent recurrence of ulcers.

Other treatments include drug treatment. Oral pentoxifylline may have a positive effect on ulcer healing. Treat the cause, optimize nutrition, and encourage smoking cessation.

Nursing advice and support for patients with leg ulcers

- Ensure the patient understands the nature of the leg ulcer and has sufficient information about treatment options to make informed choices and participate in their own care.
- Identify the patient's circumstances and preferences for treatment. Previous experiences, lifestyle, social circumstances, and age will influence this. Tailoring treatment to these is essential for concordance.
- Ensure patient has specific instructions relating to the treatment, e.g. not to remove or loosen compression bandaging or to interfere with dressings.
- Advise on infection prevention.
- Give advice on nutritious diet that will aid healing and, if necessary, discuss ways of controlling or reducing weight.
- Teach specific exercise that will aid venous return, e.g. ankle flexing and foot rotation.
- Emphasize the need for elevating the leg and avoiding prolonged periods of standing to promote venous return.
- Advise on maintaining personal hygiene.
- Ensure patient is measured accurately for compression hosiery to promote comfort, concordance, and reduce the risk of trauma. Nurses should be specially trained to do this and use local guidelines.
- Demonstrate how to apply compression hosiery (turning the stocking almost inside out, easing over the foot so that the heel is in place, and then easing up the leg to finish just below the knee). Observe the patient carrying out the procedure. Advise that applicators can be obtained if patient has limited mobility or dexterity. Advise on care and washing of the stockings.
- Ensure the patient has written information.
- Discuss ways of coping and adjustment and listen to concerns and anxieties.
- Ensure patient is referred to a tissue viability nurse specialist, if necessary.
- Make arrangement for follow-up and give contact details in case of concerns.

Patient education for dermatological problems

The aim is to promote healthy skin.

- Encourage patients to stop smoking.
- Ensure the patient understands their condition, prognosis, and what the treatment is designed to achieve. Provide information materials to support explanations.
- Take time to listen to the patient to identify particular concerns and focus education on these.
- Avoid dehydration as it causes dryness of skin.
- Advise on washing and drying skin thoroughly, particularly at flexures and between toes (warm damp conditions promote fungal infections).
- Use unperfumed soap with moisturizer, or for patients with dry skin use emollients instead of soap. Water should be warm and not hot. Use moisturizer after washing. Dry the skin by patting rather than rubbing.
- Advise that cotton clothing is often more comfortable than synthetic fibres and to avoid restrictive clothing.
- Demonstrate how to apply treatments and observe self-application.
- Identify any triggers to the condition and avoid them.
- Keep nails clean and short to reduce skin damage.
- Keep towels, flannels, etc. separate.
- Protect the skin from the sun, using hats, high-factor sun cream, tee-shirts, and long sleeves and avoid over-exposure.
- Avoid using tanning machines.
- All patients, especially those at high risk of melanoma, should do a skin self-examination from head to toe every month after a shower or bath and watch for changes in moles. Seek medical advice if changes noted. Check **A**ppearance, **B**leeding, **C**olour, **D**iameter.
- Advise about risks of pressure damage and use of pressure-relieving aids and where to obtain these.
- Use good wound care practices using up-to-date research and evidence-based practices to achieve effective healing.
- Refer to chiropody for foot problems, e.g. long deformed nails.
- Refer to tissue viability nurse or dermatology nurse specialists for specific advice and for complex problems.
- Raise awareness of risk factors of skin disorders, e.g. increased risk of fungal infections in swimming pool users; medicines may precipitate conditions; head lice and scabies common in children working in close proximity or where there is overcrowding.

Discharge and continuing care

- Use locally developed care pathways to ensure continuity of care on discharge, e.g. handover made to community nurses, appointments with tissue viability and skin care specialists, chiropodist, and attendance at outpatients or nurse-led clinics.
- Ensure patient understands the nature of the condition and the purpose of the treatment.
- Ensure patient knows how to maintain a healthy skin by carrying out prescribed treatment.
- Encourage patients to manage their own skin care and checks to detect recurrence and to limit flare-up.
- Check that patient has the correct medication and knows where to get further supplies.
- Provide an opportunity to discuss coping strategies.
- Provide contact numbers for advice and help.
- Ensure access to local support and self-help groups and patients with similar conditions.
- Provide information to share with employers and occupational health service if condition is related to working conditions or environment.
- Refer to specialists who may be able to help with self-confidence, e.g. camouflage, and make-up specialists or counselling service.
- Ensure patient's family has information that will help them understand the patient's condition and emotional reactions and responses.

Common drugs used for dermatologic conditions

Common drugs used for dermatologic conditions are listed in Table 12.1. **All drug doses listed in this table are adult doses and not children's doses.** This table is only to be used as a guide and the current BNF should be consulted for further advice. Nurses should involve themselves only in the administration of medications which fall within their sphere of competence.

Table 12.1 Common drugs used for dermatologic conditions

Topical antibacterial preparations	Dose	Common side effects
Mupirocin	Apply up to 3 times daily for up to 10 days	Local reactions including urticaria, pruritus, burning sensation, rash
Fusidic acid	Apply 3–4 times daily	Rarely hypersensitivity reactions

Pruritus – the underlying cause should be treated. Where there is dry skin an emollient (e.g. aqueous cream) may be effective.

Acne – 📖 Table 20.1 Common drugs used for infectious diseases: Tetracyclines, pp.728–31.

Parasiticidal preparations	Dose	Common side effects
Carbaryl	Head lice: rub into dry hair and scalp, allow to dry naturally, shampoo after 12 hours and comb wet hair; repeat after 7 days Crab lice (NB unlicensed indication): as above but apply *aqueous solution* over whole body	Skin irritation
Permethrin	Scabies: apply 5% preparation over whole body and wash off after 8–12 hours	Pruritus, erythema, stinging

Common treatment for Psoriasis	Dose	Common side effects
Coal tar preparations	Apply 1–3 times daily starting with low strength preparations	Skin irritation, acne-like eruptions, photosensitivity (NB stains skin, hair, and fabric)

Table 12.1 Common drugs used for dermatologic conditions
(continued)

Common treatment for psoriasis	Dose	Common side effects
Dithranol	As above; preparations are usually washed off after 5–60 minutes depending on formulation	Local burning sensation and irritation (NB stains skin, hair, and fabric)
Salicylic acid	As above	Sensitivity, excessive drying, irritation, systemic effects after widespread use

Common topical steroid preparations (See BNF for product examples under each potency grouping)	Dose	Common side effects
Mild steroid	Apply thinly once or twice a day	Very few
Moderately potent steroid	As above	Few
Potent steroid	As above	Absorption through the skin can rarely cause adrenal suppression and Cushing's syndrome (absorption is greatest where skin is thin, raw or occluded); local side effects include spread of untreated infections, thinning of skin, striae atrophicae, telangiectasia, dermatitis, acne, depigmentation, hypertrichosis
Very potent steroid	Apply thinly once or twice daily for up to 4 weeks	

Drugs used in skin cancer: 📖 Table 25.6 Common drugs used for cancer care, p.854–859.

Nursing patients with neurological problems

Nursing assessment of patients with neurological problems

When assessing the patient, remember that the nervous system is like an electrical conduction system that coordinates and controls all human functions. Components of the neurological system include the brain, spinal cord, and peripheral nervous system. There are pathways for voluntary, autonomic, and reflex activity. The 'neuron' is the basic cell that facilitates movement and sensation. It also processes and retains information. Absent or abnormal responses provide information that helps in determining which neurological structure or pathway may be impaired. Table 13.1 lists the cranial nerves and their function.

Observation of the patient is key to recognizing and interpreting subtle deviations from normal. In addition to a general nursing assessment (Chapter 3, Individualizing nursing care practice, pp.32–33) perform the following procedures.

History
- Observe the patient's general behaviour and personality.
- Consider speaking with the family/close partner for additional information.
- Ask about any recent significant changes in mood or any signs of memory loss.
- Encourage the patient to talk about the illness, including the onset, progression, and nature of symptoms.
- Investigate key symptoms such as complaints of pain, headache, seizures, vertigo, numbness, visual changes, weakness, and changes in conscious level.
- Ask about recent fits, falls, faints, or 'funny turns'. Check with partner, family, and friends.
- Discuss the nursing implications of the condition including functional problems the patient is experiencing.
- Ask how the patient's condition has affected their partner, family, and lifestyle.
- Note any family history relating to such conditions as epilepsy, migraine, multiple sclerosis, and vascular disease.
- Note previous medical history.
- Note social history, e.g. smoking.
- Note prescribed and over-the-counter medications.
- Record other therapies used, i.e. herbal or complementary.
- Note allergies.

Table 13.1 Cranial nerves

Nerve	Function
I Olfactory	Smell
II Optic	Vision
III Oculomotor	Eye movement—all eye muscles except superior oblique and external rectus. Also controls iris, sphincter, and ciliary muscles
IV Trochlear	Superior oblique eye muscle movement
V Trigeminal	Sensory and motor function—face, sinuses, tooth area
VI Abducens	External rectus eye muscle movement
VII Facial	Facial movement
VIII Acoustic	Hearing
IX Glossopharyngeal	Sensory—posterior area of tongue, tonsil, and pharynx. Motor—pharyngeal musculature
X Vagus	Motor—palate and vocal cords
XI Accessory	Shoulder, neck movement
XII Hypoglossal	Tongue movement

Physical examination

Observe the patient carefully.

- If ambulant, note their gait. (Abnormalities such as hemiparesis and Parkinsonism cause specific types of walking difficulties.)
- Note the patient's position sitting and lying down. Identify warning postures (See Fig. 13.1).
- Compare the patient's right and left sides.
- Check the two key functional components of consciousness.
  - Arousal (alertness)—eyes should open spontaneously when spoken to.
  - Awareness of self and environment—ask patient who they are, what time it is, day, month, and year.
- Assess the output of spontaneous speech, fluency, and use of inappropriate words.
- Head: Check movement and any signs of pain (neck movements may be restricted due to meningeal irritation). Note any loss of sensation in forehead and face.
- Eyes: Check pupillary responses to light, any signs of visual disturbance such as blurred or double vision, redness, discharge, sensitivity to light, use of spectacles and contact lenses.
- Nose: Note any bleeding, discharge, injury, blockages, changes in sense of smell.
- Mouth: Note changes in taste, difficulty swallowing, changes in speech, condition of inside of mouth, dentures and tongue.
- Ears: Note any hearing impairment, discharge of blood or fluids, ringing or unusual sounds.
- Chest: Assess breathing and respirations, movement of chest, any abnormalities.
- Abdomen and groin: Assess bowel and bladder function.
- General musculoskeletal: Inspect muscles for tone and strength, any strange sensations, numbness or tingling, weaknesses, muscle stiffness, aching, cramps, wasting, joint movement, deformities.
- Evaluate deep tendon reflexes (See Fig. 13.2) (role of doctor or specialist nurse).
- Note plantar (sole of foot) response (Babinski's reflex): upward movement of great toe and fanning of the little toes is abnormal.
- Perform special neurological tests for numbness, sensations, Romberg's test for position sense, paralysis or weakness, tics, tremors, myoclonus, fasciculation, coordination, cerebellar function, joint position sense, and vibration sense.
- Examine skin for colour, tone, and breakdown/injury.
- Review the patient's functional capabilities to perform their activities of daily living, grooming, and hygiene.
- Take and record vital signs. A slow heart rate may suggest pressure on brain and rising systolic blood pressure may suggest increasing intracranial pressure. Neurological dysfunction alters respiration.

a) Decorticate (abnormal flexion)

In the decorticate posture, the patient's arms are adducted and flexed, with the wrists and fingers flexed on the chest. The legs may be stiffly extended and internally rotated, with plantar flexion of the feet.

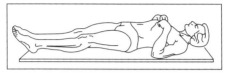

The decorticate posture may indicate a lesion of the cerebral hemisphere or diencephalon.

b) Decerebrate (extension)

In the decerebrate posture, the patient's arms are adducted and extended with the wrists pronated and the fingers flexed. One or both legs may be stiffly extended, with plantar flexion of the feet.

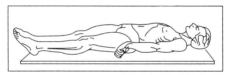

The decerebrate posture may indicate a lesion of the upper brain stem.

Fig. 13.1 Identifying warning postures.

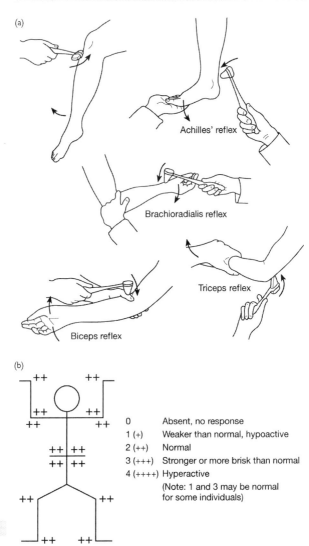

Fig. 13.2 (a) Procedures for testing deep tendon reflexes. (b) Grading of deep tendon reflexes.

Diagnostic tests

Clinical neurophysiology is an area of medicine that is concerned with testing the electrical functions of the brain, spinal cord, and the nerves in the limbs and muscles.

Lumbar puncture A needle is passed into the lumbar spine, below the level of the spinal cord at L4–L5 or L5–S1 interspaces. After removal of the inner needle, cerebrospinal fluid (CSF) is collected and pressure is measured. After explaining and gaining consent for the procedure, no special pre-test preparation is needed. Assist the patient either to lie in the fetal position near the edge of the bed or to sit upright on the side of the bed, with chest and head extended toward the knees. After the procedure, keep the patient flat for several hours, monitor vital signs, needle insertion site, and any complications such as neck stiffness and change of consciousness. Treat any headache with analgesics. A lumbar puncture is not performed if increased intracranial pressure is suspected (See Table 13.2).

Electroencephalogram (EEG) is a recording of the electrical activity of the brain. Electrodes are placed on the patient's scalp and a tracing is made in the form of wavy lines. It takes 45–60 minutes with the patient lying or sitting. The patient is encouraged to relax during the procedure and may sleep if they want to. However, the patient will be encouraged to open their eyes for part of the test and over-breathe. No special preparation or aftercare is needed.

Evoked potentials are recordings of the electrical responses of the brain and spinal cord to stimulation of the senses (sight, hearing, and touch). Patients should be sent for the tests with any glasses they own.

Nerve conduction studies are recordings of the passage of electrical signals along nerves in the limbs.

Electromyography (EMG) is a recording of the electrical activity of the muscles. Make sure the neurophysiologist is informed if the patient is anticoagulated.

Radiological tests are plain radiographs of the skull and spine that can detect developmental, traumatic, or degenerative bone abnormalities. The radiologist must be informed in advance if the patient might be pregnant as some of these tests involve exposure to radiation. The radiology department should also be informed in advance if patient suffers from claustrophobia or would be unable to keep still. Internal metal is a contraindication, including surgically implanted devices, for MRI scanning.

Computed tomography (CT) is a sophisticated x-ray detector that takes a series of images of the various layers of the brain and spinal cord. No special preparation is needed. The patient removes glasses, jewellery, dental braces, and any other metal objects. The patient lies on scanner couch and keeps still, but is allowed to talk. The procedure takes minutes. Injection of contrast media may be needed for certain areas. Patients with allergies may need 48-hour steroid cover. No special aftercare is needed.

Magnetic resonance imaging (MRI) can be useful for certain conditions. The patient lies in a very strong magnetic field and echoes from radio-waves are converted to an image. Contrast media may be needed, but no special preparation is needed. The patient must be able to lie still in supine position. The MRI is a rather noisy machine.

Cerebral angiography (angiogram) is an x-ray test that involves injecting a contrast medium into the cerebral arterial circulation. A catheter is inserted into the femoral artery and advanced upwards to the neck. Patient consent is needed. The patient is nil by mouth 4–6 hours prior to test. Premedication is given as a sedative. The procedure lasts approximately 1 hour. Surgery may then follow or, in some cases, immediate treatment may follow after x-rays are taken. When the test is finished, pressure is applied and the femoral or other puncture site is observed for bleeding. The patient remains recumbent for 6 hours, then is allowed up with usual diet and fluids.

Positron emission tomography (PET) scans are a new nuclear medicine scan performed after the injection of a radioactive isotope.

Isotope brain scans are similar to PET scans. The patient is given an IV radionuclide which is scanned by the camera. Patients who have been given radioactive substances should be nursed in a side room for the first 24 hours, during which time they should not have contact with pregnant staff or visitors.

Myelography is the introduction of a radio-opaque liquid into the spinal subarachnoid space, following a lumbar or cisternal puncture. Fluoroscopy monitors the flow of the dye. Food and fluids are restricted for 4–8 hours prior to the procedure. Any allergies must be noted, especially to iodine or dyes. The patient remains supine for several hours post-test. Vital signs and fluid balance are monitored.

Doppler ultrasound is a noninvasive test that can be used to evaluate blood flow. It may identify narrowing (stenosis) or blockage (occlusion) of vessels. No particular preparation or nursing care is required for the patient.

Table 13.2 Signs of increasing intracranial pressure (ICP)

	Early signs	Late signs
Level of consciousness	Not easily rousable Some orientation loss Restlessness and anxiety	Unrousable
Pupil reactions	One pupil constricts then dilates Sluggish to light Unequal	Pupils fixed and dilated
Motor response	Sudden weakness Motor changes Profound weakness	Abnormal posturing
Vital signs	Rise in blood pressure Fall in pulse Change in breathing pattern	High systolic blood pressure Profound bradycardia Abnormal respirations

Neurological nursing problems

Assessing level of consciousness

The Glasgow Coma Scale is the standard method used to assess a patient's level of consciousness. ☐ Glasgow Coma Scale, p.475.

- Ask patient their name and orientation to place, time, and person. Disorientation affects sense of time first.
- Begin by measuring the patient's response to verbal commands, light tactile touch, or painful nail bed pressure stimuli.
- Response to painful stimuli may be purposeful or non-purposeful movement, or patients may be unresponsive.
- Eye movement—inspect each pupil for size and shape, and compare for equality (See Fig. 13.3).
- Test response to light. Pupil should constrict when a light from a pen torch is shone into eye.

Pain ☐ Chapter 23, Pain assessment, pp.794–8

- Pain is a key symptom in neurological nursing care. Assess by considering the patient's description. Also observe the patient's physical and behavioural responses to their pain.
- Use a pain assessment tool or scale and ask key questions.
- Record behavioural responses such as crying/calling out, restlessness, moaning, sighing, grimacing, muscle twitching, and rocking. Pay particular attention to the part of the body involved.
- Sympathetic responses associated with mild or moderate pain include pallor, elevated blood pressure, dilated pupils, muscle tension, dyspnoea, and tachycardia.
- Parasympathetic responses associated with severe deep pain include pallor, decreased blood pressure, slow pulse, nausea, vomiting, dizziness, weakness, and loss of consciousness.
- Assess pain 2-hourly in neurological patients and monitor its course throughout the day and night.

Headache

Headache is a common symptom of many neurological conditions.

- Primary headaches are not associated with any known pathology, e.g. migraine, tension, and cluster headaches.
- Secondary headaches are caused by an underlying pathology, e.g. meningitis, tumours, or subarachnoid haemorrhage.

Equipment needed to perform a neurological examination

- Cotton wool
- Pen torch
- Ophthalmoscope (check batteries and bulb are working)
- Otoscope
- Pins with sharp and blunt ends, e.g. Neurotips
- Reflex hammer
- Tongue depressors
- Tuning forks 128 Hz and 256 Hz
- Snellen chart

May be useful

- Tape measure
- Taste and smell kits (to be used only by a specialist) with stoppered vials (check dates of expiry)
  - Peppermint, oil of cloves, coffee, soap (smell)
  - Sugar, salt, vinegar, quinine (taste)

Note: It is the nurse's responsibility to ensure that the patient has reading glasses and hearing aids, if used.

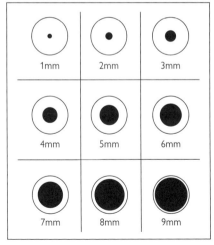

Fig. 13.3 The pupils are typically equal in size, with an average diameter of 3.5 mm. To ensure accurate evaluation of pupil size, compare your patient's pupils with the scale above. Keep in mind that maximum constriction may be <1 mm and maximum dilation >9 mm.

Epilepsy/seizure

Seizures are paroxysmal events associated with abnormal electrical discharges of neurons in the brain.

Partial seizures (focal, local)

Partial seizures are contained in one part of the cerebral hemisphere and are classified as simple or complex.

- Simple—consciousness remains intact.
- Complex—some loss of consciousness may occur.

Absence (petit mal) seizures

Absence seizures begin with a brief change in the level of consciousness, indicated by blinking or rolling of the eyes, or a blank stare, and slight movements. These seizures are very brief, lasting 1–10 seconds, and may not be noticed by the patient or onlookers.

Generalized tonic–clonic (grand mal) seizures

This type of seizure may start with a loud cry—the patient falls to the ground and loses consciousness. The body may stiffen (tonic phase) and then alternates between episodes of muscle spasm and relaxation (clonic phase). Tongue biting, urinary incontinence, laboured breathing, apnoea, and cyanosis may occur. These seizures last 2–5 minutes. When the patient recovers they may be confused, drowsy, and suffer from headaches.

Nursing care

Aim is to protect the patient from injury and prevent serious complications.

- If you are with a patient who knows a seizure is imminent (i.e. aura is present), help them to lie down and use pillows or blankets to protect them.
- Turn the patient on their side, if possible.
- If time allows it may be possible to insert an airway, but DO NOT force anything into the patient's mouth once the seizure has started.
- Provide privacy if possible.
- Stay with the patient and observe and protect them.
- Time the seizure.
- Move any surrounding objects dangerous to the patient's safety.
- Do not try to restrain the patient.
- After the seizure, put the patient in the recovery position; apply suction and oxygen if needed.
- Check for injuries.
- Care for incontinence.
- Maintain IV access if necessary.
- Re-orient and reassure the patient.
- Document carefully what happened.
- Refer for medical assessment and treatment if needed.

Care of the unconscious patient

- Remember ABC (airway, breathing, circulation). (📖 Chapter 33, Nursing care of patient emergencies, pp.1029 and 1098.)
- Assess the airway for signs of obstruction and protect if necessary. You may need to seek additional expertise.
- Apply suction if needed.
- Monitor oxygen saturation.
- Monitor and document vital signs according to the condition of the patient.
- Monitor and record the level of consciousness using the Glasgow Coma Scale. 📖 Glasgow Coma Scale, p.475.
- Keep strict fluid balance chart. Maintain fluid and nutrition via the most suitable access.
- Always speak to patient before touching (hearing is possible though the patient may seem unresponsive).
- Perform passive and active range of motion exercises.
- Reposition side-to-side 2-hourly.
- Apply elastic stockings to prevent deep vein thrombosis.
- Provide mouth and eye care 2-hourly.
- Monitor bowel and bladder movements.
- Maintain hygiene and daily bathing.
- Monitor and care for skin.
- Support family and friends when they visit.

Paralysis

Paralysis is the complete or partial loss of the power to move part of the body due to injury or disease of the nerves supplying the relevant muscles.

Paralysis involving one half of the body is known as *hemiplegia* and paralysis involving all four limbs and the trunk is known as *quadriplegia*.

- *Plegia* signifies loss of power, i.e. true paralysis.
- *Paraplegia* is paralysis of both legs, sometimes part of the trunk.
- *Paresis* refers to a significant weakening of the affected muscle(s).
- *Upper motor neuron damage* causes an increased tightening up of the muscles (spasticity).
- *Lower motor neuron damage* causes a reduction or loss of normal tone in the muscles (flaccidity).

Paralysis is caused by stroke; brain tumour; brain abscess; brain haemorrhage; damage to parts of the nervous system or the spinal cord; diseases such as multiple sclerosis and poliomyelitis; muscle disorders such as muscular dystrophy; and nerve disorders or neuropathies.

- The impact of paralysis is influenced by whether it affects the patient's dominant (preferred) side.
- Paralysis affects the patient's functioning and their ability to carry out their daily living activities.
- Paralysis is at its most severe in the early stages after injury or disease, and recovery of movement may occur over time.
- There is no known cure for paralysis.

Treatment

Treatment of the cause is the key to recovery.

- Treat spasticity by having the patient avoid factors that make it worse, e.g. anger, anxiety, stress. Complementary therapies may help.
- Adopt best positions for limbs and support carefully.
- Avoid very cold weather and encourage the patient to wear warm clothing.
- Keep the paralysed muscles from wasting from lack of use by exercises and physiotherapy techniques. Temporary splints may be used to provide support around a joint.
- Treat flaccid paralysis similarly to the above.

Most people come to terms with their paralysis and body image disturbance (📖 Chapter 24, Nursing patients with body image problems, p.822).

Further information

Various voluntary agencies help people with their paralysis:
Disabled Drivers Association   Tel: 01508 489449
Spinal Injuries Association   Tel: 0208 444 2121

Meningitis

- Inflammation of the coverings of the brain (the meninges) caused by viruses, bacteria, or fungi.
- Symptoms and signs are fever, headache, neck stiffness, photophobia, nausea and vomiting, +/− disorientation, seizures, Kernig's sign (See Fig. 13.4), and rash (in meningococcal meningitis).

Bacterial meningitis

Most common are:
- *Neisseria meningitides* (meningococcal)
- *Streptococcus pneumoniae* (pneumococcal)
- *Haemophilius influenzae* (haemophilus)
- *Escherichia coli* meningitis

During epidemics many people may carry the bacteria in their throats and noses, but do not get meningitis. It affects people of any age.

Meningococcal meningitis

- Rash may be present, which appears as small red/purple spots 1–2 mm in diameter which do not disappear (blanche) when pressed, or large purple/black bruises found in or around the armpits, groin, and ankles.
- Close contacts may need specialist advice on prophylaxis.
- Possible complications are deafness, epilepsy, hydrocephalus, and brain damage.

Viral meningitis

- Most common viruses are enteroviruses (e.g. Coxsackie), glandular fever (Epstein-Barr virus), herpes simplex, human immunodeficiency virus, and cytomegalovirus.

Fungal meningitis

- Is rare and usually only occurs in people whose immune systems have become weakened.
- Diagnosis involves examining and antigen testing the CSF which is obtained by lumbar puncture.
- Presents over weeks rather than days.

Nursing care

- Nurse in quiet darkened calm environment.
- Provide analgesics for pain.
- Use tepid sponging and electric fans to keep patient cool.
- Encourage fluids.
- Monitor vital signs.
- Maintain general hygiene and mouth care.

(a)

(b)

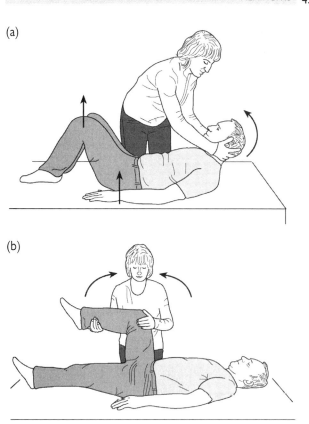

Fig. 13.4 (a) Brudzinski's sign is elicited as the examiner passively flexes the patient's head and neck. A positive sign is indicated by the involuntary flexion of the hips and legs. (b) Kernig's sign (the inability of the patient to tolerate knee extension when the hip is flexed).

Encephalitis

Encephalitis is an inflammation of the brain that is usually caused by a viral infection of the brain (herpes simplex or no specific virus identified). Infection can involve one area of the brain (focal) or many scattered areas (diffuse). Patients typically present with a flu-like illness followed by strange behaviour, altered consciousness, or seizures. Encephalitis is rare.

Nursing care
• Similar to that of patients with meningitis.

Chronic neurological conditions

Migraine

Migraine is a headache, often one sided, that is accompanied by nausea and sometimes vomiting. Sensitivity to light, sound or smell may occur. Patients with classic migraine may experience a warning or aura, which often disturbs vision, e.g. flashing lights and zigzags. Aura only occurs in about 20% of migraine patients.

Migraine differs from person to person. The headache may be unilateral or bilateral, is typically exacerbated by movement, and may or may not throb or be severe. Some patients experience numbness and tingling on the face or arm, or, in rare cases, paralysis of the arm and leg on one side of the body. Migraine headaches typically last hours to days.

Migraine tends to run in the family, and may be associated with menstrual cycle in women. Those women with migraine with aura should not take the combined oral contraceptive pill. Migraine may be brought on by fasting, irregular meals, alcohol, exercise, dehydration, stress, or too much or too little sleep. The cause is not really known.

Further information

British Association for the Study of Headache (BASH) Guidelines www.bash.org.uk
Migraine Trust www.migrainetrust.org

Medication overuse headache

Medication overuse is a common and often under-recognized type of headache. This type of headache is caused by regular use of any analgesic or caffeine and may have features similar to migraine or tension type headaches. Patients diagnosed with medication overuse headache should be supported in completely withdrawing from medications and caffeine. Headaches may become worse for the first few weeks, but severity usually then diminishes.

Cluster headaches

Cluster headaches are much less common than migraine, and are more common in men and smokers. Pain is shorter and much more severe. Episodes may be clustered together in quick succession over several days or weeks, and last minutes to several hours. Patients experience intense unilateral pain usually associated with intense agitation and restlessness. The ipsilateral eye (the eye on affected side) may water and become blood shot. The nose may become stuffy or run.

Tension headaches

Tension headaches are usually mild, featureless, bilateral, and have a variable duration. They are treated with common analgesics, relaxation techniques, and amitriptyline (if chronic).

'Red flag' headaches

The following may indicate an underlying cause in need of urgent medical intervention:

- Thunder clap headache – sudden severe headache
- Any headache associated with loss of consciousness
- Headaches that have changed substantially in character
- Headaches that are caused by coughing
- New headaches with neurological signs
- Headaches that are worse on lying down and improved by standing
- Headaches associated with significant superficial scalp temporal tenderness, e.g. pain on combing hair

Trigeminal neuralgia

Trigeminal neuralgia is irritation of the 5th cranial nerve. It has a varied aetiology and creates brief spasms of very severe pain along a nerve in the face and/or jaw. It can be triggered by chewing, eating, speaking, touching the face, or even by the wind. This type of headache is common in older people and is treated by anticonvulsants, tricyclics, or surgery.

General treatment of headaches and migraines

- Encourage regular hydration, food, and sleep.
- Avoid excessive analgesics.
- Consider abstaining from caffeine.
- For acute infrequent attacks, use analgesics or NSAID with anti-emetics (metoclopramide or domperidone). Consider domperidone suppositories for patients who are vomiting. Consider a triptan if analgesics or NSAIDs are ineffective.
- Patients may be prescribed regular medication for frequent or disruptive headaches, e.g. beta-blockers.
- Suggest use of biofeedback. Person concentrates on certain ways to relax, lower blood pressure, etc., and the therapist gives them feedback as to how they are achieving their aim.
- Consider acupuncture.
- Consider nerve blocks.

Bell's palsy

Bell's palsy affects the 7th cranial nerve and causes paralysis of the facial nerve muscles on one side of the face, often with inability of the eye to close properly. It has an unknown aetiology, affects adults, and is usually reversible within several weeks. There is no real treatment, although prednisone and acyclovir may be useful. Teach the patient how to cope, protect eye from injury and infection (eye drops for dryness, and consider patch), facial exercises, and instruction regarding medications.

Multiple sclerosis

Multiple sclerosis (MS) is the most common physically disabling neurological disease that affects young people. The term 'multiple sclerosis' originates from 'sclerosis', which means 'scarring', and 'multiple', which relates to the sites of the scarring throughout the brain and spinal cord. It is a chronic neurodegenerative disease of the central nervous system, and is of unknown aetiology. It attacks the protective sheath of fatty protein (myelin) which protects the neurons and axons.

Epidemiology

- In the UK, 90,000 individuals are affected
- Female-to-male ratio is 2 to 1
- Rare before puberty and after the age of 60 years
- Peak incidence in 30s and 40s
- Incidence higher with increasing latitude above the equator

Symptoms

MS is a complex and unpredictable condition. Its course varies from person to person and does not follow a set pattern. Common symptoms include fatigue, loss of vision in one eye, blurred or double vision, dragging feet, weakness of limbs, poor coordination, balance problems, numbness, pins and needles, and burning sensations. (These may be continuous or intermittent.) Symptoms may also include bladder symptoms, vertigo, depression, and pain.

Types and pathogenesis

There are three types of MS. Patient's lifespan is generally similar across the different types of MS.

- Relapsing remitting MS (RRMS) – relapses are followed by periods of complete or partial remission.
- Primary progressive MS (PPMS) – gradual deterioration from onset.
- Secondary progressive MS – gradual deterioration that follows on from RRMS.

MS may also be 'benign' with no significant disability despite long duration of illness. An environmental factor may trigger the condition in patients with genetic susceptibility to the disease.

Diagnosis

No single test or procedure can be used to diagnose MS. Diagnosis is usually based on symptoms, signs, and results from a series of tests (e.g. MRI scanning, evoked potentials, and lumbar puncture).

Medical management

- Corticosteroids may be used to treat an acute attack of MS.
- Various treatments may be used for the symptoms of MS, e.g. spasticity, bladder dysfunction, and fatigue.
- Disease modifying therapies such as beta interferon may be used.

Nursing care

Nursing care of patients with MS includes bladder and bowel management, pelvic floor exercises, fatigue management, aerobic training, emotional support, psychological therapy for depression, health promotion, and liaison with a multidisciplinary team and a specialist MS nurse. 📖 Key symptoms and nursing points for MS, below.

Further information

MS Trust   www.mstrust.org.uk
MS Society   www.mssociety.org.uk
MS Society (Scotland)   www.mssocietyscotland.org.uk

Key symptoms and nursing points for MS

- *Fatigue.* Fatigue usually worsens as the day progresses and is markedly affected by temperature, particularly heat. It can be exacerbated by poor sleep, pain, stress, lack of exercise, and medications. Educate and support the patient, encourage exercise, suggest timed rest periods, and recommend avoidance of factors that worsen fatigue.
- *Weakness.* The most feared symptom of MS is weakness, which implies paralysis, loss of walking, and disability. Assess patient's performance at activities of daily living and ask questions about particular difficulties. What aids do they use? Any specific problems like rising from a chair? Refer to physiotherapist for muscle strength assessment and appropriate exercises.
- *Mobility.* Assess spasticity and ataxia—encourage an exercise programme, arrange for ambulation aids if appropriate, and assess mobility in bed.
- *Vertigo, imbalance, and incoordination.* Patients at risk of falling require a careful assessment of their environment in hospital and at home.
- *Cognitive and emotional disorders.* Assess carefully to determine whether memory is affected. Evaluate abstract thinking and problem solving, attention and concentration, and verbal fluency. Emotional problems include depression (especially as the condition progresses), stress, and mood swings (anger, irritability, and euphoria). Encourage the patient to talk and express their problems. Provide support to the family, if necessary.
- *Bladder dysfunction.* Encourage the use of aids and special devices. Assess the extent of the problem; encourage skin care for incontinent patients. Advise on adequate fluid intake, caffeine avoidance, and bladder drill. Drug therapy may be useful, sometimes surgery. Avoid long-term indwelling urethral catheters if possible.
- *Dysphagia.* Assess extent of problem. Encourage patient to eat small amounts slowly. Patient may tire through a long meal and swallowing becomes worse. Refer for speech and language therapy if concerned about aspiration.
- *Spasm.* Review patient exercises and drug therapy.
- *Pain.* Assess and manage patient's pain. 📖 Chapter 23, Nursing patients with pain, pp.794–8.

Parkinson's disease

Parkinson's disease is a chronic progressive degenerative disorder that damages the substantia nigra area of the brain. There is currently no cure; however, many options are available for treating the symptoms which can vary in their degree of severity. Parkinson's disease is one of the most common neurological conditions affecting older people, but it can affect young people as well. Men and women are equally affected.

Signs and symptoms

The main symptoms include slowing of movement, stiffness of muscle, and sometimes tremor. Other symptoms include small writing (micrographia), mask like expression, speech difficulties, loss of balance, bowel and bladder problems, depression, and anxiety. As the disease progresses, patients often develop cognitive problems.

Diagnosis

At present the diagnosis is made clinically; however, PET and dopamine transporter (DAT) scans are available in some centres to confirm the diagnosis (a small amount of radioactive dopamine is injected and scanned in the brain).

Treatment and management

- Drugs that replace dopamine, mimic its action, or stop its breakdown plus drugs that inhibit the action of acetylcholine.
- Medication should not be abruptly discontinued or withdrawn.
- If patient is unable to swallow or is nil by mouth, consider apomorphine subcutaneous therapy.
- Surgery may be performed in specialist centres.
- Patients often remain at home with care centred on maintaining safety and well being.
- Encourage patients to use cues or walking aids if needed.
- Requires a multidisciplinary health team approach, including a social worker and Parkinson's disease specialist nurse.
- As the disease progresses, family/carers may need help and the patient may need to go into a nursing home to allow periods of respite for the family.

Further information

Parkinson's Disease Society   Tel: 0808 800 0303

Key nursing interventions for patients with Parkinson's disease

- Timing of medication is important. Monitor effectiveness and side effects.
- Try to maintain independence and self caring.
- Observe diet and fluid intake.
- Monitor activity and movement.
- Encourage mobility and exercise.
- Help with activities of daily living such as bathing, shaving, mouth and dental care, etc., if necessary.
- Help the patient communicate, if necessary.
- Involve the multidisciplinary team.
- Consider monitoring the patient hourly using an 'on-off' chart or diary. Patient's mobility and ability to self care may vary from hour to hour, often known as 'on-off' phenomena.
- Consider 2-hourly position change if necessary, particularly overnight as patients find it difficult to turn in bed.
- Monitor ability and take precautions to prevent falls. As the patient's illness progresses, balance becomes affected.
- Observe for features of psychosis and memory problems in late stages of the disease.

Degenerative diseases

Creutzfeldt–Jakob disease

Creutzfeldt-Jakob disease (CJD) is a very rare disease with approximately 100 new cases diagnosed every year. It is one example of a human progressive fatal transmissible spongiform encephalopathy (TSE). This term describes the spongiform change seen in the brain in these conditions. Transmission can only occur by consumption of, or injection with, nervous tissue, or, in the case of variant CJD, from other organs and blood. It is not transmissible by ordinary contact with affected individuals. Diagnosis is made by brain biopsy. Variant CJD was identified in 1996 and was originally called 'new variant CJD' or 'nvCJD'. This is the only form to have resulted from bovine spongiform encephalopathy (BSE) in cattle.

Further information

National CJD Surveillance Unit	www.cjd.ed.ac.uk
National Prion Clinic	www.nationalprionclinic.org
CJD Support Society	www.cjdsupport.net

National Prion Clinic in London is the specialist centre of care for patients with CJD.

Motor neuron disease

Motor neuron disease (MND) is an uncommon disease that causes progressive degeneration of the motor system, leading to weakness and wasting of the muscles. It is a slow progressive disease with an unknown cause and no real effective treatment. The extent to which the lower motor neuron system and the upper motor neuron system are affected determines the varying patterns of disability. The patient has stiffness and twitching (fasciculation), speech and swallowing difficulties, respiratory muscle weakness, muscle cramps, and muscle weakness. Some patients experience emotional lability and may laugh or cry inappropriately. There are several types of MND. Race, diet, and lifestyle are not determining factors of the disease. A small minority have familial MND.

Diagnosis and treatment

Diagnosis is made by a neurologist, using blood tests, EMG, and MRI scans. Treatment includes drugs, therapy support, feeding by gastrostomy tube in some cases, and ventilatory support in some cases. Although MND affects lifestyle and occupation, it does not affect intelligence and therefore the patient should be involved whenever possible in their nursing care.

Myasthenia gravis

Myasthenia gravis is a rare chronic disease characterized by excessive fatigability relieved by rest. It is caused by an autoimmune response that blocks the receptors at the neuromuscular junction. Patients experience weakness and fatigue of selected voluntary muscles. The peak onset is 20–40 years with a smaller peak at 50–60 years. The severity of the disease depends on the number of receptors involved. Diagnosis is confirmed by laboratory tests, neurophysiology, and sometimes a test involving an injection of edrophonium under suitable specialist supervision. Treatment is by medicated symptom control, by surgical intervention, by plasmapheresis, or by IV immunoglobulins, depending on type and severity of the condition. Acute ventilatory support may be necessary in the hospital on rare occasions. Self care and patient education are key to nursing in the community.

Guillain–Barré syndrome

Guillain–Barré syndrome is an acute inflammatory polyneuropathy, characterized by varying degrees of motor weakness or paralysis. It is a rare disorder with an unknown cause, but may be an autoimmune response to a viral infection. The disease affects people of all ages. Patients experience weakness and numbness (usually distal); the weakness may progress over hours or days. Patients usually make a full recovery. Careful nursing is crucial and includes monitoring for respiratory muscle weakness and respiratory failure by forced vital capacity (FVC) every few hours. Severe cases also require cardiac monitoring for autonomic abnormalities.

Huntington's disease

Huntington's disease is a chronic progressive dementia that causes movement abnormalities (i.e. chorea and dystonia), cognitive deterioration, and affective disturbances. The disease affects people 35–45 years upwards. Huntington's disease is a genetic condition that has no known cure.

Stroke and transient ischaemic attack (TIA): overview

Stroke

Stroke is a clinical syndrome of presumed vascular origin that is typified by rapidly developing symptoms or signs of focal, and sometimes global, loss of cerebral function lasting more than 24 hours or leading to death (World Health Organization 1978). Stroke is a source of significant morbidity and is the largest cause of adult disability. It affects between 174 and 216 people per 100,000 population in the UK each year, and accounts for 11% of all deaths in England and Wales. There are two types of stroke.

Ischaemic stroke and primary intracerebral haemorrhage

Ischaemic stroke, whether caused by an embolus or thrombosis of a cerebral artery, accounts for 80–85% of strokes, primary intracerebral haemorrhage for 10–15%, and subarachnoid haemorrhage for 5%. For those with a first stroke, up to 20% will have a recurrent event within 3 months and up to 43% will have a recurrent stroke within 5 years.

Subarachnoid haemorrhage

Although this is technically a stroke, it has a different aetiology, requires different interventions, and is addressed later (📖 Cerebral aneurysm, p.478).

Transient ischaemic attack

Transient ischaemic attack (TIA) is a clinical syndrome characterized by an acute loss of focal cerebral or ocular function with symptoms lasting less than 24 hours. It is due to inadequate cerebral or ocular blood supply as a result of low blood flow caused by a thrombosis or embolism. It is associated with diseases of the blood vessels, heart, or blood.

TIA affects 35 people per 100,000 of the population each year. The risk of stroke is very high (up to 30%) in the first month of the event. However, the greatest risk of stroke is within the first 72 hours. Patients who have an ABCD2 score ≥4 are at highest risk.

The distinction between stroke and TIA is becoming redundant, as all patients with suspected stroke or TIA should be treated as a medical emergency and should undergo specialist assessment in the hospital. Those with stroke and those with TIAs at high risk of completed stroke with ABCD2 scores ≥4 will require immediate specialist assessment and rapid access to a comprehensive specialist stroke service. Those with TIA with ABCD2 scores <4 should be given aspirin 300 mg (with proton pump inhibitor, if necessary) and be instructed not to drive. They should be assessed and investigated in a specialist service (e.g. neurovascular clinic) as soon as possible within 7 days of the event. Patients should also be told that if another event occurs, they should immediately return to the hospital.

Whether the patient has had a stroke or TIA, they should receive a rapid diagnosis, a detailed assessment, acute treatment, and later rehabilitation according to an agreed written local protocol based on national guidelines.

ABCD2 score—sum total score as follows:

Age >60 years	1
Systolic blood pressure >140 mmHg	1
Diastolic blood pressure >90 mmHg	1
Unilateral weakness	2
Speech impairment without weakness	1
TIA duration >60 minutes	2
TIA duration 10–59 minutes	1
Diabetes	1

Patients with ABCD2 <4 have about 1% risk of stroke at 7 days post TIA but those with high score >5 have about 12% risk.
(from the Lancet, 366, PM Rothwell, MF Giles, E Flossman, CE Lovelock, JNE Redgrave, CP Warlow and Z Mehta. A simple score (ABCD) to identify individuals at risk of stroke after transient ischaemic attack, 8. Copyright (2005) with permission from Elsevier.)

Signs and symptoms

Stroke and TIA classically present with the *sudden* onset of one or more of the following symptoms:
- Limb weakness
- Difficulty speaking or understanding speech
- Possible loss of vision, clumsiness, or numbness of arms or legs

For suspected stroke or TIA, use the ***FAST*** test:
- ***Facial movements***: Ask the patient to smile or show teeth. Look for NEW lack of symmetry.
- ***Arm movements***: Ask the patient to lift their arms together and hold. Does one arm drift or fall down?
- ***Speech***. If the patient attempts a conversation, look for NEW disturbance of speech.
- ***Test all three.*** If one or more is abnormal, suspect a stroke.

Common symptoms
- Face, arm, leg weakness
- Dysarthria (slurred speech)
- Expressive and/or receptive dysphasia
- Sensory or visual inattention (visuospatial defect)
- Hemianopia (visual field defect)
- Diplopia (double vision)
- Transient monocular visual loss/disturbance (amaurosis fugax)
- Incoordination (past pointing, heel to shin)
- Unsteady gait
- Cognitive problems

Risk factors for stroke and TIA

Patients with any risk factors should be assessed, monitored, and treated.

Common risk factors
- Hypertension
- Atrial fibrillation (AF)
- Diabetes
- Dyslipidaemia
- Ischaemic heart disease
- Age >75 years
- Valvular problems
- Obesity
- Smoking
- Peripheral vascular disease (PVD)
- Alcohol misuse
- Unhealthy diet (high fat and/or salt)
- Previous stroke and/or TIA

Stroke and transient ischaemic attack (TIA): prevention

Lifestyle advice
- Stop smoking.
- Reduce alcohol intake.
- Take regular exercise.
- Ensure diet low in fat and salt.
- For those with diabetes, ensure good blood sugar control (plasma glucose 4–7 mmol) and regular review by diabetes services.
- Preclude patients from driving. Advise patient to inform Driver and Vehicle Licensing Agency (DVLA) and insurance company. A specialist assessment is required before driving may recommence.

Blood pressure
Regardless of initial blood pressure, for every 8 mmHg drop in systolic pressure there is a 42% risk reduction in stroke risk. Therefore, even though a specific target will be set, the message to the patient is 'lower, lower, lower'.
- All patients should be on a blood pressure lowering medication (a thiazide diuretic is the first line treatment with addition of an ACE inhibitor and A2 antagonist).
- Target blood pressure:
  - For most patients the goal is 140/85 mmHg.
  - For patients with established atherosclerotic disease or chronic renal failure the goal is 130/80 mmHg.
  - For patients with diabetes the goal is 130/80 mmHg or below.

Antithrombotics and anticoagulants
All patients with ischaemic stroke/TIA should be prescribed antithrombotics or anticoagulants.
- Current NICE guidelines should be followed. Presently, ideally, a combination of low dose aspirin (50–150 mg daily) and dipyridamole modified release 200 mg should be taken for a period of at least 2 years.
- Patients intolerant of dipyridamole should continue on low dose aspirin.
- Patients unable to take aspirin should take clopidogrel 75 mg daily.
- Patients intolerant of aspirin (e.g. with gastrointestinal problems) should continue aspirin and be considered for a proton pump inhibitor.
- Patients who are in atrial fibrillation should be considered for warfarin within 2 weeks of event.

Antilipid agents
- All patients with ischaemic stroke should be taking a statin (e.g. simvastatin 40 mg daily) unless contraindicated.

Carotid stenosis

- Carotid imaging (doppler and magnetic resonance angiography)
  - should be performed in all patients who have had a carotid artery TIA or who have had a minor stroke and are making a good recovery and who are good surgical candidates
  - should be performed within 24 hours for high risk and within 7 days for lower risk patients regardless of the setting (i.e. inpatient or attending specialist clinic).
- Carotid endarterectomy
  - should be considered in all patients who have a significant carotid stenosis.
  - should be performed within 48 hours of the event for high risk and within 7 days for low risk TIA patients.
- Referral to the appropriate specialist should be made.

Echocardiogram

An echocardiogram is required to exclude a cardiac cause (e.g. thrombus) in patients who:

- are in AF or who have cardiac disease
- do not have identified cause or risk factors for stroke (e.g. young, or without known health problems).

Primary prevention

- Control blood pressure
- Control dyslipidaemia
- Antiplatelet/anticoagulant therapy for AF
- Smoking cessation
- Reduced alcohol consumption
- Low fat/salt intake
- Exercise

Stroke and transient ischaemic attack (TIA): diagnosis and management

Specific diagnosis
- Made from clinical history and examination.
- The location of the artery or arteries affected should be determined.
- A CT scan excludes stroke due to primary intracerebral haemorrhage.
- Time of onset should be determined in order that time dependent treatments (e.g. thrombolysis for ischaemic strokes) can be considered.
- For those with ischaemic stroke, start aspirin 300 mg.

Thrombolysis
Thrombolysis is offered to suitable patients with ischaemic stroke (platelet aggregometry therapy) at certain centres (registered with Safe Implementation of Thrombolysis in Stroke Monitoring Study—SITS-MOST) by staff with specialist training. Specialist nursing care is required for these patients, including protocol guided assessment and treatment of complications.

Acute nursing management
Active management in the initial hours after stroke onset saves the ischaemic brain from infarction and may prevent the worsening of stroke.
- Admit patients to a specialist area for stroke care (acute stroke unit).
- Perform acute physiological and neurological monitoring for the first 72 hours.
- Perform an assessment 2-hourly for the first 24 hours and 4-hourly thereafter.
- For those with ischaemic stroke, begin aspirin 300 mg.

Reduction of the impact of the initial event and preventing stroke progression

Physiological monitoring
- Perform repeated assessments of blood glucose, oxygen saturation level, hydration, and temperature and maintain parameters within normal limits. Actively manage infection unless the patient is receiving palliative care.
  - Blood glucose – monitor 4 hourly. If plasma glucose >8 or <2 mmol/l, get medical assessment.
  - Oxygen saturation – if low (<95%) oxygen therapy should be prescribed. Consider positioning patient to improve lung expansion.
  - Hydration – ensure adequate fluids either by oral, subcutaneous, or intravenous route. Monitor fluid balance.
  - Temperature – treat raised (≥38°C) temperature with paracetamol. Carry out infection screen (blood cultures).
- Perform repeated assessments of heart rate and blood pressure.
  - Monitor pulse and cardiac functioning and manage arrhythmias – treat any significant tachycardia, bradycardia, or atrial fibrillation.
  - Reduce blood pressure only during the acute phase where there are likely to be complications from hypertension, e.g. hypertensive encephalopathy, aortic aneurysm with renal involvement.

Neurological monitoring
- Perform a baseline detailed neurological assessment.
- Perform frequent assessment using a standardized scale (e.g. the Scandinavian Neurological Stroke Scale).
- If neurological deterioration is recognized, increase the frequency of physiological monitoring, identification of abnormalities, and medical review.

Early management

Swallowing assessment
- Keep the patient nil by mouth until a swallow screening assessment has been performed by a competent health professional (at least within 24 hours of admission).
- Assess risk of aspiration with patient sitting upright.
- If a patient fails the swallow screening assessment, keep the patient on nil by mouth and refer to speech and language therapy who will advise on thickened fluids/modified diet.
- Manage persistent swallowing problems with a nasogastric tube in the acute phase within 3 days. It may be necessary to insert a PEG tube later.
- Refer to dietitian.
- If nil by mouth, perform regular mouth care and oral assessment.

Positioning, mobility, and risks from immobility

- Sit out of bed and mobilize as early as possible.
- Assess manual handling – use good manual handling techniques to prevent complications (e.g. shoulder or limb pain). It is better to use a hoist when transferring patients as it may not be safe to transfer with just the aid of two nurses.
- Assess pressure ulcer risk – review patient's position regularly and return back to bed after short periods, no longer than 2 hourly.
- Refer to physiotherapy so that patient is seen within 24 hours (movement and mobility can be assessed and exercises recommended).
- Apply anti-embolus stockings unless contraindicated (leg ulcers, broken skin, peripheral vascular disease), and/or consider pharmacological therapy.
- Refer to occupational therapy (daily living activities can be assessed and managed).
- Refer to speech and language therapy so patient is seen within 7 days for any communication problems.

Bladder and bowel management

- Perform a full assessment of patient's level of continence.
- Implement an active management plan to promote continence.
- Use aids for communication and provide a call bell or buzzer.
- Assist the patient to the toilet, and encourage a 2-hourly toileting regimen – prompt urinary voiding.

- Consider further tests if incontinence persists.
  - Bladder scan checking for residual volume – if residual volume is above 90 mL, exclude constipation and consider intermittent catheterization.
  - Per rectum examination for constipation – consider laxatives, suppositories, or enemas (🔲 Chapter 8, Constipation, p.224).
  - Use indwelling catheter only for retention of urine.
  - Refer to appropriate continence services and specialists.

Psychological assessment and management

- Assess social and psychological needs by observing, listening, and talking to the patient. (Early intervention by a social worker and a clinical psychologist may help.)
- Assess mood weekly using a screening tool.
- Allow patients the opportunity to talk about how they are feeling, make time to sit with them and explore ways to improve their emotional state. Involve relatives and friends.
- For patients with severe emotional problems as a consequence of the stroke (troublesome tearfulness or laughing inappropriately), consider treatment with antidepressants.
- Consider antidepressants for patients who have low mood (should be continued for 6 months for a good response).
- For those with low mood consider further treatment by an appropriately trained professional.

Cognitive problems

- Screen for cognitive problems using standardized assessments and if necessary, ensure that trained personnel perform a detailed assessment.
- Offer cognitive rehabilitation.
- Perform comprehensive re-assessment by the multidisciplinary team prior to discharge. Discuss results and implications with the patient and their future carer, and arrange for rehabilitation and support packages.

Difficulties with spatial awareness (neglect/inattention)

- Ensure that therapy and nursing sessions encourage attention to the affected side.
- Offer assessment by an orthoptist.
- Offer rehabilitation.
- Ensure patient is not socially isolated in the ward and ensure a bed position where they receive input from both sides of the bed.

Information and support for patients and carers

Information for patients and their families following stroke can be offered in a variety of formats. Patient organizations have a variety of leaflets and web-based materials on stroke.

- Consider information and support needs from admission and start preparation for discharge as soon as possible.
- Give information on the likely diagnosis, prognosis, investigations, treatment, and expected care pathways.

- Give information on recommendations for lifestyle and secondary prevention measures.
- Provide information that takes into account each individual's needs.
- Assess carers for carer strain using a standardized tool.
- Discuss with carers the burden they feel and their anxieties and concerns. Give relevant advice.
- Offer tailored carer support, if available (e.g. Stroke Family Support, aids and adaptations, advice on housing and financial support).
- Provide information in a variety of languages and formats specific to patient and carer needs.
- Inform patients and their carers of the local availability of support services and agencies, with contact details.

Head injury

Head injuries can be due to trauma, stroke, or internal cranial bleeding. This may result in decreased level of consciousness which is associated with severe potentially life-threatening complications. Treatment of disordered consciousness is focused on care of the airway, breathing, and circulation.

Nursing care and monitoring of the patient with a head injury should be guided by clinical assessments and protocols based on the Glasgow Coma Scale (GCS) 📖 Glasgow Coma Scale, pp.475 and 1034 (Nursing Care of patient emergencies, Chapter 33). When using the GCS, quantify the patient's response to stimulation in descriptive terms, rather than a numerical value. If the GCS <9, or if falls by 2 points, call for senior help.

The AVPU (Alert, Verbal, Painful, Unresponsive) system can provide a rough guide to whether patients need airway protection, but full assessment is still required.

Frequency of observations

This is dictated by the patient's level of consciousness and should take into account any of the following risk factors:

- Seizure at any time after injury
- Focal neurological signs
- Severe headache or other neurological symptoms
- Continuing amnesia
- Continuing nausea and/or vomiting
- Irritability or abnormal behaviour
- Clinical or radiological evidence of a recent skull fracture or suspected penetrating injury
- Significant medical problems, e.g. anticoagulant use

Initial stages

- Administer oxygen, if prescribed.
- Monitor vital signs, rate, rhythm, and pattern of breathing.
- Elevate head of bed 30°.
- Administer intravenous fluids as prescribed.
- Monitor input, output, and electrolyte balance.
- Assess skin integrity using Waterlow Scale or appropriate tool.
- Perform position changes as indicated by the patient's condition.
- Assess nutrition using an appropriate tool; consider nasogastric feeding.
- Carry out oral care as patient's condition indicates.
- Catheterize if required and assess bowel function as per local policy.

Later stages

Any of the following examples of neurological deterioration should prompt urgent reappraisal by a doctor:

- GCS falls <9 or if falls by 2 points.
- New or evolving neurological symptoms or signs appear, such as pupil inequality or asymmetry. **A widely dilated, unreactive pupil on one side suggests a unilateral space occupying lesion—this is a medical emergency.**
- Seizures.
- Development of severe or increasing headache or persistent vomiting.
- Development of agitation or abnormal behaviour.

Glasgow Coma Scale

Eye opening

4 Spontaneously open
3 Open to verbal request
2 Open with painful stimuli
1 No opening

Best verbal response

5 Oriented to time, place, person; converses appropriately
4 Converses, but confused
3 Words spoken, but conversation not sustained
2 Sounds made, no intelligible words
1 No response

Best motor response

6 Obeys commands
5 Localizes to painful stimulus
4 Withdraws to painful stimulus
3 Abnormal flexion to pain (decorticate posturing)
2 Abnormal extension to pain (decerebrate posturing)
1 No response

Brain tumour

A brain tumour is an abnormal growth of cells. Brain tumours are classified as primary if they originate in the brain or secondary (metastatic) if they originate from cells that have spread to the brain from a cancerous tumour in another part of the body.

- Cancers of the lung, breast, stomach, and melanoma (skin) commonly metastasize to the brain.
- Tumours that arise within the brain are named after the cell from which they are thought to arise.
- The commonest primary tumour is glioma (a tumour arising from the glial – or supporting cells of the brain).
- Gliomas can be slow growing (low grade) or fast growing (high grade).
- Low grade gliomas can grow over many years.
- A more benign type of brain tumour is a meningioma, a tumour that arises from the surrounding coverings (meninges) of the brain.

Symptoms
- Headache
- Drowsiness or altered consciousness
- Blurring of vision
- Memory problems
- Weakness in limbs
- Visual and speech problems
- Epileptic fits
- Seizures
- Odd behaviour

Treatment
- Cerebral metastases can sometimes be treated with radiotherapy and/or surgery.
- High grade gliomas can be treated with surgery, radiotherapy, and chemotherapy.
- Meningiomas can sometimes be removed completely and cured.
- Steroids, anticonvulsants, and analgesics may be used.
- Patients may not be allowed to drive for up to 2 years after a malignant brain tumour has been diagnosed.

Nursing care
📖 Craniotomy, p.479 describes the principles of pre- and postoperative care for surgery for brain tumours.
- Some patients have chemotherapy implanted into the tumour cavity, requiring appropriate cytotoxic wound care.
- Patients and family often need extra counselling and support.
- Support services including Macmillan nurses, district nurses, social workers, and occupational therapy are often needed.
- The patient and their family may benefit from joining an appropriate support group.

Cerebral aneurysm

A cerebral aneurysm is a balloon-like pouch occurring in the wall of one of the blood vessels that supplies the brain. Aneurysms typically develop at points of bifurcation of the blood vessels, and the vessels of the circle of Willis are affected most often. If the aneurysm ruptures, bleeding into the subarachnoid space usually ensues (known as a **subarachnoid haemorrhage**).

Signs and symptoms
- Sudden onset headache, often with rapidly developing meningism
  📖 Pain, p.446; Meningitis p.452.
- Typical signs of meningism include neck stiffness, photophobia, and positive Kernig's sign
- Feeling a 'sudden sensation' of being hit on the back of the head or neck
- Vomiting
- Possibly coma or sudden death

Diagnosis and treatment
- Diagnosis of a bleed is confirmed by CT scan or blood in the CSF detected by lumbar puncture.
- May be treated with neurosurgery or endovascular treatments.

Nursing management
The focus of nursing care is careful patient monitoring and implementation of aneurysm bleeding precautions.
- Nurse patient in a quiet, darkened room.
- Administer nimodipine, usually by mouth and only if necessary; infused intravenously via central catheter.
- Enforce strict bedrest.
- Monitor vital signs hourly.
- Check pupils.
- Monitor mental and conscious level using Glasgow Coma Scale hourly.
- Strictly monitor fluid balance.
- Administer analgesics to reduce pain.
- Provide nursing care with most activities.
- Rehabilitation after surgery is similar to that after stroke.

Craniotomy

A craniotomy is an operation to open the skull in order to expose the brain. It is used to treat any pathology requiring surgical intervention within the cranial cavity (i.e. tumours, strokes, aneurysms, and trauma).

Preoperative care

In addition to the usual routine (📖 Chapter 22, Nursing patients requiring perioperative care, pp.762–70), the following should be performed:
* Full assessment of neurological observations.
* Full assessment of vital signs.
* Removal of any hair will be done in theatre.
* Provide patient and family with information regarding postoperative care.

Postoperative care

* Monitor conscious level using Glasgow Coma Scale.
* Administer oxygen as prescribed.
* Monitor vital signs, rate, rhythm and pattern of breathing.
* Elevate head of bed 30°.
* Administer intravenous fluids as prescribed.
* Monitor input, output, and electrolyte balance.
* Provide analgesics and anti-emetics as required.
* Observe wound and drainage.
* Assess skin integrity using Waterlow Scale or appropriate tool.
* Change position as indicated by patient's condition.
* Assess nutrition using appropriate tool.
* Carry out deep vein thrombosis risk assessment using appropriate tool.
* Carry out oral care as patient's condition indicates.
* Turn 2-hourly from side to side.
* Encourage early mobilization.

Discharge and continuing care

- Assess and compare the patient's functional status and mobility. Use special guidelines according to local policy.
- Note patient's abilities in relation to grooming, toilet use, feeding, transfer from bed to chair and back, sitting and standing balance, mobility about house or ward, use of aids and wheelchairs, dressing ability (e.g. help with buttons), bathing independently or supervised, and bowel and bladder function. Document incapacity and pass on details to the community nursing team.
- Perform a psychosocial needs assessment, including any anxiety, depression, mood swings, and cognitive impairment.
- Consider that patients with some conditions, e.g. memory loss, may be unable to perform an everyday task. Fatigue, weakness, and lassitude may impair prolonged physical or mental function when at home.
- Consider referring patients with sexual problems to a specialist (if patient wishes).
- Consider limitations in activities that may result from neurological conditions.
  - In many cases, especially following craniotomy, the patient's driving licence may be suspended, and this will need to be reviewed following recovery.
  - Air travel may be contraindicated for at least 8 weeks.
  - Contact sports such as boxing and rugby should be avoided. However, swimming is allowed, especially when any wounds have healed.
  - There may be a risk of fitting if alcohol is taken in large amounts.
- Encourage patients to pace themselves, set new objectives, and possibly alter their former lifestyle. Some patients may benefit from keeping a reflective diary of their progress. Others may need to take regular rest breaks.
- Consider level of supervision required by patients. Patients with minor head injuries are usually sent home with strict guidelines to follow if their symptoms worsen. Those with severe injuries may well need longer-term care and supervision at home.

The nurse has a significant role in teaching neurological patients, alongside other members of the multidisciplinary rehabilitation team. Specialist nurses also play a major role in supporting patients in the community and may be involved in instituting changes in patient care and treatment, e.g. MS nurses and specialist epilepsy nurses help monitor patients in the community.

Further information

Brain and Spine Helpline: Tel: 0808 808 1000
                                www.brainandspine.org.uk
DVLA Drivers' Medical Group: Tel: 01792 783686

Nursing interventions and useful equipment for patients

Assess the need for special aids and devices that may improve the patient's life in hospital and at home.

- Bathing and showering aids (e.g. seats and handrails)
- Special beds for ease of moving, rising from, and sitting up in
- Commodes at the correct height for the patient, or a special foot stool if using standard hospital or home toilet and patient's feet do not reach the ground
- Powered armchairs
- Communication aids
- Word processor
- Page turners for reading
- Remote controls for electrical devices in the home, e.g. stereo, DVD, television, kettle
- Special neck collars for support
- Feeding aids
- Stair lift
- Handrails and ramps
- Outdoor and indoor wheelchairs
- Special personal alarms for emergency care
- Mobile telephones
- Specially adapted vehicle for transport

Common drugs used for neurological disorders

Common drugs used for neurological disorders are listed in Table 13.3. **All drug doses listed in this table are adult doses and not children's doses.** This table is only to be used as a guide and the current BNF should be consulted for further advice. Nurses should involve themselves only in the administration of medications which fall within their sphere of competence.

Table 13.3 Common drugs used for neurological disorders

Control of epilepsy	Dose NB Plasma monitoring of blood levels used to adjust dose	Common side effects
Phenytoin	Initially 150–300 mg daily as a single dose (or 2 divided doses) with or after food Usual dose range 200–500 mg (dependent on plasma level)	Nausea, vomiting, constipation, paraesthesia, headache, tremor, transient nervousness, anorexia, and insomnia are common; ataxia, slurred speech, nystagmus, and blurred vision are signs of overdose; gingival hypertrophy can also occur
Sodium valproate	Initially 600 mg daily in 2 divided doses after food, increasing at 3 day intervals by 200 mg to a maximum of 2.5 g daily in divided doses; usual maintenance dose 1–2 g daily	Gastric irritation, nausea, ataxia and tremor, diarrhoea, hyperammonaemia, increased appetite, transient hair loss (regrowth may be curly), oedema, thrombocytopenia and inhibition of platelet aggregation, impaired hepatic function – withdraw immediately; many more side effects (See BNF)
Migraine	**Dose**	**Common side effects**
Prophylaxis – use beta blockers (📖 Table 7.1 Common drugs used for cardiovascular disorders: Beta blocker drugs, p.194)	Propranolol most commonly used at dose of 40 mg 2–3 times daily	📖 Table 7.1 Common drugs used for cardiovascular disorders: Beta blocker drugs, p.192

Table 13.3 Common drugs used for neurological disorders *(continued)*

Migraine	Dose	Common side effects
Treatment – use sumatriptan if simple analgesia is ineffective	50 mg (some patients may require 100 mg) as soon as possible after onset; dose may be repeated in not less than 2 hours if migraine re-occurs but do not give second dose for *same* attack; maximum dose 300 mg in 24 hours	Sensations of tingling, heat, heaviness, pressure or tightness of any part of body (if intense in throat/chest – discontinue), flushing, dizziness, feeling of weakness, fatigue, nausea and vomiting (See also BNF)

Parkinson's disease	Dose	Common side effects
Co-beneldopa and Co-careldopa	Dose varies according to preparation used	Excessive daytime sleepiness and sudden onset of sleep; anorexia, nausea, vomiting, insomnia, agitation, postural hypotension, dizziness, tachycardia, arrhythmias, reddish discoloration of urine; many more side effects (See BNF)
Cabergoline	Initially 1 mg daily, increased by increments of 0.5–1 mg at 7–14 day intervals; usual range 2–6 mg daily	Excessive daytime sleepiness and sudden onset of sleep; nausea, constipation, headache, nasal congestion, dyspepsia, epigastric pain, syncope, depression; many more side effects (See BNF)
Selegiline	10 mg in the morning or 5 mg at breakfast and mid-day (elderly patients should start at 2.5 mg)	Nausea, dry mouth, postural hypotension, dyskinesia, vertigo, sleeping disorders, confusion, hallucinations

Alzheimer's disease	Dose	Common side effects
Donepezil	5 mg once daily at bedtime, increased if necessary after 1 month to 10 mg daily (maximum 10 mg daily)	Nausea, vomiting, anorexia, diarrhoea, fatigue, insomnia, headache, dizziness, syncope, psychiatric disturbances, muscle cramps, urinary incontinence, rash, pruritus

Multiple sclerosis	Dose	Common side effects
Prednisolone (📖 Table 9.1 Common drugs used for liver and gall bladder disorders: Prednisolone, p.301)		
Baclofen	5 mg 3 times daily with or after food, increased gradually to a maximum of 100 mg daily; discontinue if no benefit within 6 weeks	Frequently sedation, drowsiness, muscular hypotonia, nausea, urinary disturbances

Table 13.3 Common drugs used for neurological disorders *(continued)*

Myasthenia gravis	Dose	Common side effects
Pyridostigmine	30–120 mg at suitable intervals throughout the day; total daily dose 300–1200 mg though inadvisable to exceed 450 mg daily	Nausea and vomiting, increased salivation, diarrhoea, abdominal cramps; signs of overdosage include bronchoconstriction, increased bronchial secretions, excessive sweating, involuntary defaecation and micturition, nystagmus, agitation (See BNF for more)

Trigeminal neuralgia	Dose	Common side effects
Carbamazepine NB May also be used for epilepsy (See BNF)	Initially 100 mg 1–2 times daily, increased gradually according to response; usual dose 200 mg 3–4 times daily, up to 1600 mg daily in some patients	Nausea and vomiting, dizziness, drowsiness, headache, ataxia confusion/agitation, visual disturbances; many more side effects (See BNF)

Nursing patients with sensory system problems (eyes, ears, nose, and throat)

Nursing assessment of patients with eye problems

In addition to a general nursing assessment (📖 Chapter 3, Individualizing nursing care practice, pp.32–33) perform the following procedures.

Observe the patient

- Infection of the eye: redness, watering, discharge (note amount and consistency), crusting, swelling, abscess, and styes. Is infection unilateral or bilateral? Does the patient rub their eyes?
- Exophthalmos: protrusion of the eyeballs, most commonly associated with thyroid eye disease. Also consider eyelids, ptosis, ulcers, ectropions, blepharitis.
- Pupils should be round, central, of equal size, and respond equally to light. Observe for abnormal pupil shape and size.
- Squint: eyes are not correctly aligned with each other; in children it is of particular concern because they may not develop normal vision (amblyopia or 'lazy eye').
- Signs of injury: penetrating wounds, bruising around eye, or corneal abrasion.
- See Fig. 14.1 for diagram of the eye.

Ask the patient about

Nursing history

- Ability to manage self-care and activities of daily living
- Coping strategies
- Social situation (any dependants at home or anyone to care for them or is the patient isolated)
- Past and present nursing problems
- Psychological and spiritual assessment
- Fears and anxiety about the eye condition and what they understand about it, and possible care and treatment

Medical history

- Renal disease and hypertension (retinal vein occlusion may occur)
- Diabetes (diabetic retinopathy)
- Rheumatoid arthritis (keratoconjunctivitis—dry eye and scleritis)
- Visual disturbances, diplopia, and optic neuritis in multiple sclerosis
- Use of specific drugs (e.g. anticoagulants, antihypertensive, recreational drugs)

Specific eye history

- Prescription glasses, reading, distance, both, varifocals, bifocals
- Contact lenses, artificial eye, methods of removal, cleaning, and storage
- Whether registered as visually impaired or severe visual impairment
- Whether under the care of an ophthalmologist

Present symptoms
- Visual disturbances including blurred or distorted vision, dark spots in the visual field, flashing light, floaters, rainbow colours or halos around bright lights
- Photophobia
- Headaches, irritation, discharge, pain, inflammation
- Changes in vision

Family history
- Glaucoma
- Visual impairment and causes
- Diabetes
- Coronary heart disease
- Hypertension

Test and measure

- Blood pressure—high blood pressure increases risk of a variety of retinal problems especially in patients with diabetes.
- Urine—protein may indicate renal disease and glucose or ketones may indicate diabetes.
- Pupil reaction—asymmetry of the pupils may indicate serious disease.
  - Causes of an abnormally constricted pupil include drugs, nerve damage (Horner's syndrome), and previous iritis (inflammation of the iris which can lead to it being stuck down onto the lens).
  - Causes of an abnormally dilated pupil include drugs, nerve damage (third nerve palsy which is serious or Adies pupil which isn't), trauma, and glaucoma.

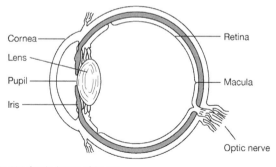

Fig. 14.1 Simple diagram of the eye.

Nursing problems of the eye

Impaired vision
The degree of impaired vision varies—blindness, blurring, patchy or cloudy vision, distortion of vision.

Photophobia
This is painful sensitivity to light.

Eye pain
Pain is often severe if it is due to corneal abrasions, foreign bodies, scleritis, or acute glaucoma. It is less severe in conjunctivitis, keratoconjunctivitis, and optic neuritis. Eye pain may also be due to referred pain, trigeminal neuralgia, shingles, migraine, and tension headaches. It may also occur postoperatively or after laser treatment.

Dry eyes
Dryness causes irritation and redness and is due to reduced secretion of tears, evaporation of tears, or mucin deficiency in tears.

Eye discharge
Discharge may be watering or purulent due to infection. It may result in sticking of eyelids, especially on waking.

Anxiety
This may be due to concerns about possible deterioration in sight leading to blindness or due to fears that treatment and tests may be painful.

Social isolation
This may result from lack of confidence with other people (inability to recognize familiar faces) and difficulty undertaking activities (problems with driving, getting about, hobbies, e.g. writing, sewing). Some eye problems can be visible to others and this can lead to inappropriate attention to the patient causing discomfort and embarrassment.

Lack of appropriate visual aids
These include ill-fitting spectacles, difficulty inserting or removing eye prosthesis, or contact lenses.

Common terms in ophthalmology

- **Conjunctivitis**: inflammation of the conjunctiva (the delicate transparent membrane that lines the eyelids and the eyeball)
- **Diplopia**: double vision
- **Entropion**: inversion of the eyelid—the lashes are in contact with the eyeball
- **Enucleation**: removal of the eye
- **Exophthalmos**: protrusion of the eyeball
- **Nystagmus**: involuntary rhythmic movement of the eyeball
- **Papilloedema**: unilateral or bilateral oedema of the optic disc due to raised intracranial pressure
- **Photophobia**: painful sensitivity to light
- **Scleritis**: inflammation of the sclera (the white of the eye)

Eye tests and investigations

Visual acuity
Visual acuity is tested with most recent glasses on (if worn) using either Snellen's test board or LogMAR visual acuity (with distance glasses, bifocal, varifocal, or contact lens). Near vision can be tested by reading a book or newspaper (with reading glasses). Record the smallest type or object read or named.

Ophthalmoscopy
This is mainly used to look at the retina. It may detect retinal haemorrhages, or exudates (e.g. in diabetic retinopathy), retinal detachment, cupped discs (indication of glaucoma), abnormal vitreous and blood, loose floaters, or red reflex. Additionally it can be useful to spot opacity of lenses (cataract) or abnormal pupils. When viewing the retina, it helps to darken the room and use appropriate prescribed mydriatic drops to dilate the pupil. Before administering these drops patients should be warned that their vision will be blurred and that they should not drive until this wears off (commonly a few hours but occasionally until the next day).

Examination with slit lamp
This provides a slit of light of variable thickness and angulation that is viewed through a binocular microscope that gives a magnified view of the structures of the front of the eye. Additional hand-held lenses are required to view the back of the eye (e.g. retina, optic disc).

Tonometry
This is used to check intraocular pressure (IOP). Use either Goldmann's tomometry or Tono-Pen®. It is essential that the patient keeps eye still and open. The Tono-Pen or the Perkins Tonometer is good to use to check IOP for bed or wheelchair bound patients. All these instruments should only be used after a drop of topical anesthetic has been administered.

Fundus fluorescein angiography
Dye is injected into veins to highlight retinal blood vessels to detect leakage and dilation. Take precautions in case of anaphylactic shock. Observe for 30 minutes post-procedure. Skin and urine turn yellow.

Fundus photography
This is used to record the retinal appearance.

Visual field test ('perimetry')
Visual acuity tests evaluate only a patient's very best central vision. Visual field tests assess the peripheral vision as well. The final result is a map of the quality of the whole of the patient's vision.

CT scan
Computed tomography (CT) of the head is used to identify tumours affecting the occipital lobe and optic nerve.

X-rays
X-rays are used to detect associated problems (e.g. chest x-ray in ocular inflammation to look for sarcoidosis or TB).

Ultrasound scan
These scans are used to measure structures inside the eye (e.g. before cataract surgery) and to examine the eye when you cannot see the back (e.g. haemorrhage or cataract).

Laboratory tests
FBC, blood glucose, U&E and a lipid profile may be indicated. 📖 Chapter 39, Common laboratory tests and their interpretation, p.1167.

Eyelid and corneal disorders and eye infections

Styes (hordeolum)

External styes: due to infection of lash follicle in lid margin. Treatment is with lid hygiene and warm compresses, and commonly topical antibiotics.
Internal styes: less common, due to infected meibomian gland. May produce cysts that point and discharge inwards onto conjunctiva. Treatment is with lid hygiene, warm compresses, and commonly topical antibiotics.

Chalazion (meibomian cyst)

This is a hard and pip-like lump that often follows a staphylococcal infection. It usually resolves on its own. Treatment includes lid hygiene and lid massage using warm flannel. Persistent cases may require incision and curettage of chalazion under local anaesthetic.

Basal cell carcinoma

This is the commonest malignancy of the eyelid. It may start as a pearly nodule that becomes ulcerated with time. Treatment includes excision, curettage, cryotherapy, or radiotherapy.

Blepharitis

This is an extremely common chronic infection of the eyelid margins. It causes red, itchy, crusted, and scaly lids. It is sometimes associated with conjunctivitis. Treatment includes removing crusts and scales by frequent soaking with compresses of sodium bicarbonate. Antibiotics and also steroid drops may be required if the condition persists.

Lacrimal duct problems

Dacryocystitis is inflammation of the lacrimal sac causing redness, swelling, and watering of eye due to a blocked tear duct. Pus may regurgitate from the tear ducts. It may spread to surrounding tissue and lead to systemic infection. A swab of discharge should be taken before antibiotics are prescribed.

Orbital cellulitis

This may follow sinusitis or periorbital injury. Patients present with fever, eyelid swelling, pain, general malaise, and discharge and congestion of the eye. Blood cultures should be taken before IV antibiotics. A CT scan and ENT opinion regarding involvement with paranasal sinuses may be required. Complications include meningitis, retinal vein occlusion, optic nerve compression, blindness, and cavernous sinus thrombosis. Check patient's temperature. More common and less serious is 'preseptal cellulitis'. This is infection of the lid that has not spread back into the orbit. Although the lid may appear very swollen, the other features of orbital cellulitis are present. In adults it is normally treated with oral antibiotics as an outpatient; in children, however, it should be managed as for orbital cellulitis.

Conjunctivitis

This may be due to allergy, bacterial infection (e.g. *Staphylococcus*, pneumococci), viral infections (e.g. adenovirus), or chlamydia. Eyes are often gritty, sticky, itchy, and sore, with discharge and mild photophobia but no change in vision. Conjunctivitis is usually bilateral. Remove discharge with moist cotton wool balls; avoid cosmetics and eye lotions. Scrupulous handwashing is required. Antibiotic eye drops (e.g. chloramphenicol) are usually prescribed for bacterial and viral infections (to prevent secondary bacterial infection). If conjunctivitis is of particular concern or if it persists, an eye swab may be taken. In allergic conjunctivitis a range of anti-allergy drops are available; in severe cases topical steroids or antihistamine drops may be prescribed by an ophthalmologist. Advise patients not to share towels at home to minimize risk of cross infection.

Ectropion

Ectropion is a turning-out of the lower eyelid. This condition can cause eye irritation and watering. Surgery may correct the deformity.

Entropion

Entropion is a turning-in of the lower eyelid. This condition can cause eye irritation and watering. The in-turned eyelashes may irritate the cornea. Taping the lower eyelid to the cheek can give relief temporarily; surgery may be required.

Other common eye problems

Macular degeneration

This is the leading cause of blindness in patients >65 years. It affects both eyes with deterioration in central vision (blurring, distortion, dark spots, problems in bright sunlight, and difficulty adapting between dark to light) and causes problems with reading, writing, and recognizing faces. Risk factors include age, sunlight, family history, smoking, and diet. Prevention is aimed at reducing risks. Advise patients to use magnifying devices, large print, and talking equipment (books, clocks, etc.). Patients should consider registering as 'severely sight impaired' (blind) or 'sight impaired' (partially sighted). Treatment involves laser photocoagulation. Acute macular degeneration (AMD) is treated by photocoagulation. Some centres treat wet AMD with photodynamic therapy and (most recently approved by NICE) by Lucentis injection.

Cataract

Cataract refers to lens opacity. It is usually progressive and patients have reduced ability to focus and perceive colour, blurring or loss of vision, halos around objects, and increased glare. Causes include congenital infection (rubella), familial, senile, traumatic, radiation exposure, and drug induced, e.g. long-term steroids. Diabetes may give similar symptoms and should be excluded. Treatment includes extraction combined with plastic lens implant, normally as day case with local anaesthesia. The patient must be able to lie still for 30 minutes. The affected eye is dilated. Postoperative antibiotics and steroid eye drops are given 4 times per day, commonly for 2–4 weeks. The first eye dressing is worn 24 hours postoperatively, and may be removed by the patient. For the first few weeks the patient should avoid lifting, bending, smoky atmosphere, make-up, hairspray, and swimming. An eye shield should be worn at night for 2 weeks to prevent inadvertent rubbing.

Glaucoma

Raised intraocular pressure causes damage to the optic nerve leading to loss of vision. Glaucoma is usually chronic (primary open angle glaucoma or POAG). The pressure is not so high as to cause pain, but it can cause considerable damage to the optic nerve. However, because it affects the peripheral vision first, the patient may be unaware. It is usually first noticed by an optician at a routine test. Risks include increased age, African origin, family history, diabetes mellitus, thyroid eye disease, and short-sightedness. Medical treatment includes lowering the pressure with topical prostaglandin agonists and/or beta-blockers (e.g. timolol). Surgery (trabeculectomy) may be necessary in some cases. Patients who are >40 or who have a family history of glaucoma should have an annual eye check for glaucoma. For patients being treated for glaucoma, it is very important to stress the importance of drop concordance. Assess and teach drop instillation techniques.

Much less common is acute 'angle closure' glaucoma. This is an ophthalmic emergency in which the intraocular pressure is extremely high causing the patient substantial pain. The eye is red and hard, the cornea is cloudy, and the pupil is unreactive. This requires urgent treatment with drops (including pilocarpine) and intravenous medication (commonly acetazolamide). Once things have settled, the definitive treatment is with laser 'peripheral iridotomy' which usually prevents recurrence.

Retinal detachment

Initially, patients see a shadow across the vision of one eye. They may see bright flashes or floaters beforehand, but there is no pain. Risks include middle age, short-sightedness, and previous detachment. At a very early stage this may be treated by laser or cryotherapy under local anaesthetic. Most cases, however, require surgery by 'vitrectomy' (i.e. repair from the inside) or by 'Cryo-buckle' (i.e. repair from the outside). In vitrectomy the vitreous is removed and either a gas or silicone oil is used to 'inflate' the eye, which pushes the retina back in place. This operation is done mostly under general anaesthesia but can be done under local anaesthesia. The extent to which the patient is able to see afterwards depends partly on whether the retinal detachment extended to affect the central vision. If so, the ability to see fine detail may not return. Preoperative education is important to alleviate anxiety. Patients are given strict instruction following vitrectomies where a gas bubble is injected. The patient is advised to inform the anaesthetist if admitted to hospital for another operation within 6 weeks post-vitrectomy. Patients should not travel by plane while gas is in the eye. The gas bubble takes an average of 6 weeks before it is absorbed. Advice on resuming normal activities should be sought from the surgeon and supporting team.

Diabetic retinopathy

Background diabetic retinopathy—blocked, dilated, or leaky retinal capillaries become fragile and haemorrhage; usually asymptomatic and not sight threatening
Proliferative diabetic retinopathy—damaged blood vessels reduce blood supply to retina, which leads to new fragile blood vessels developing, scarring, and detached retina
Diabetic maculopathy   ischaemia and/or leakage of fluid reduce the function of the macula affecting central vision

Appropriate treatment of the underlying diabetes is required. Photocoagulation by laser can be used to treat both maculopathy and proliferative retinopathy. Patients following retinal surgery are also advised to keep their heads in a certain position postoperatively for 5–10 days to enable the internal tamponade (gas or silicone oil) to work on affected part of the retina to keep the retina flat.

Nursing care of patients with visual impairment

Visually impaired people may lack confidence out of their normal environment. The nurse should aim to minimize stress of an unfamiliar hospital setting. Patients may have fluctuating vision or difficulty adjusting to sudden changes in light. Remember not all people with visual impairment are the same.

Communication

- Use the patient's name as an introduction; introduce yourself by name and role.
- Talk to the person, not their companion or guide.
- Use the patient's name or touch them so they are aware of being addressed.
- Give them time to speak and listen to them.
- Recognize that visually impaired people may be more alert to tone of voice.
- Provide 'talking' information, e.g. ward information, visiting information.
- Let the patient know when you are leaving.

Guiding

- Introduce yourself and ask if assistance is required—verbal guiding or by touch.
- Allow person to hold your arm just above the elbow.
- Be aware of obstacles that are at head height.
- Walk at person's pace and describe what they are approaching (e.g. doors, level change, narrow passage, flooring).
- For stairs, indicate whether going up or down and guide to handrail. Warn patient when top or bottom is approaching and reached.
- For seating, place guiding hand onto chair back or seat—patient can do the rest.
- Never distract a patient's guide dog or feed a working dog.

Ward orientation

- Describe bed area and how items work—radio, headphones, call bell.
- Show location of bed, locker, toilets, and internal layout.
- Offer to guide to facilities.
- Describe meal times—make patient aware of meal times and describe how food is laid out, e.g. use clock (peas at 10 o'clock etc.). Ask whether help is needed, e.g. with choosing menu, feeding.
- Replace objects in the exact place they were found.

Nursing care of patients undergoing eye surgery

Pre- and postoperative education
Preoperative education is important to alleviate anxiety.

Preoperative nursing care
Approximately 80% of eye surgery is performed under local anaesthetic as day cases. An individualized plan should be developed.

- Assess suitability for day case surgery according to local criteria, e.g. type of surgery, living alone, support, access to telephone, mobility, ability to return for postoperative visit, ability to self-care.
- Obtain a nursing history and assessment. 📖 Nursing assessment of patients with eye problems, p.486.
- Orient patient to environment.
- Gain cooperation during surgery. Patient must be able to lie flat and keep still. Carefully explain procedures; what they will see, hear, and feel during the operation; how long it will take. Retain hearing aids for communication.
- Advise patients to wash hair preoperatively as this may be restricted after.
- Teach postoperative techniques, e.g. instilling eye drops.
- Prepare eye area according to local policy. This may or may not include conjunctival swabs for culture and sensitivity, instilling prescribed eye drops (e.g. antibiotics; mydriatic drops to dilate pupils; local anaesthetic drops; and miotic drops to constrict pupils), and marking eye to be operated on.
- Encourage patient to be mobile pre- and postoperatively, unless there are any contraindications, e.g. bed rest in retinal surgery.
- Check that the consent form has been signed and ask if there are further questions about risk and consequences of the surgery.
- Discuss the patient's anxieties (e.g. pain, loss of sight, return home) and plan care appropriately or make referrals for further support, e.g. social worker.
- Follow principles for preoperative preparation, if general anaesthetic is being used.
- Highlight any relevant problems to the medical team.

Perioperative care
- If possible the patient may walk in and walk out of theatre.
- The patient's head must be correctly positioned and supported to prevent unnecessary movement.
- A nurse should sit and hold the patient's hand to provide support and observe patient's condition, e.g. skin colour, sweating, pulse rate, and chest movements.
- For patients with local anaesthetic, agree a sign (e.g. squeeze nurse's hand) to indicate a concern (e.g. impending sneeze, need to speak).
- Provide explanations during surgery to help reduce anxiety, prevent disorientation, and keep patient informed of what is happening.

Postoperative nursing care of eye patients

Day case surgery

Most patients have day case surgery, usually under local anaesthetic, and can begin mobilizing to prepare for discharge home shortly after surgery is finished. Ensure patients have information and medication including eye drops prior to discharge. 📖 Discharge and continuing care for patients with eye problems, p.502.

Inpatients

Most inpatients will have had a general anaesthetic, more complex surgery, or do not have the support systems at home to enable them to have day surgery. Nursing care is determined by the type of surgery but commonly will include:

- Resting in bed for the first day but allowed up for toilet. Should be gradually mobilized to prepare for discharge from complex retinal surgery.
- Preferred position when lying is for the operated eye to be uppermost to relieve pressure; for some operations the patient must lie on their stomach.
- Assessing the patient's pain and administering prescribed analgesia.
- Eating and drinking may be resumed an hour after return if there is no nausea or other contraindications.
- If eyes are covered, guiding patients to bathroom and around ward; and helping to locate belongings and perform aspects of care.
- Normally the dressing and eye shield, if used, is left for 24 hours.
- Providing explanations about surgery and what happened.
- Preparing for discharge and providing information. 📖 Discharge and continuing care for patients with eye problems, p.502.

Eye dressing and eye check

- Inspect dressing pad for blood or discharge.
- Ask about pain.
- Compare the eyes. Observe the operated eye for swelling, discharge, stickiness, bruising, and redness of the eyelid; redness of the conjunctiva for subconjunctival haemorrhage; the cornea for clarity or abrasions; the pupils for abnormality of shape and size, and reaction to light; and observe the suture line. Record findings.
- Bathe the eye according to local policy, e.g. with gauze swabs and sterile normal saline from inner to outer eye margins, to remove discharge, blood, and any stickiness.
- Insert eye drops as prescribed (📖 Instillation of eye drops, p.501). Replace dressing and eye shield if required or dark/shaded glasses.
- Discuss registering as partially blind/fully blind.

Education for patients with eye problems

Patient with existing eye problems

- Use a model of the eye to explain patient's condition and planned effects of treatment and surgery.
- Explain the importance of handwashing and other actions to prevent infection before, during, and after eye care.
- Teach patient and carer how to instill eye drops; supervised practice is preferable. Give large-print instructions.
- Teach eye cleaning when eyes are sticky. Use cooled boiled water; make up enough for the day and keep in refrigerator. Use gauze or cotton wool balls and wipe from inner to outer eye—one swab per wipe.
- Give information about medication.
- Explain 'what to do' and 'what not to do' to protect the eye and prevent complications, e.g. haemorrhage, infection. This will vary depending on the condition. Instruct patients to avoid bending down, lifting heavy weights, constipation, activities that may induce coughing or sneezing, and washing hair, unless backwash is used. Instruct patients to avoid smoky atmosphere, to be cautious with make-up and hair spray, and not to rub eyes.
- Encourage patients to ask questions and express fears about care and treatment and longer-term prognosis.
- Suggest practical help for patient to improve vision—large-print books, prescribed magnifying glasses, better illumination.
- Explain about eye dressing/eye protection: when it will be removed, what the eye will look like, and whether dressing will be replaced.

Preventive education

This is aimed at reducing the risk of eye problems developing and/or deteriorating.

- Educate on early detection of eye disease by regular eye tests which include slit lamp examination/ophthalmoscopy (to examine the optic disc), tonometry (to measure the intraocular pressure), and perimetry (to examine the field of vision) at least every 2 years but more frequently if deterioration is noted.
- Ensure leaflets on a variety of eye diseases and their prevention are available in a range of languages.
- Advise patient to:
  - Wear sun glasses and brimmed hat when in excessive sunlight to prevent cell damage and subsequent macular degeneration.
  - Eat a healthy diet rich in fruit and green vegetables. Limit saturated fats and cholesterol to reduce risk of age-related macular degeneration.
  - Limit alcohol intake to recommended daily level.
  - Stop smoking.
  - Keep blood pressure down.
- Advise diabetics that glycaemia and blood pressure control are important, including managing insulin regimen, adhering to diet, and exercising with modifications, if necessary. Advise patients to participate in retinal screening programmes.

Instillation of eye drops

- Wash and dry hands and ensure this is done between treating each eye if both eyes are involved.
- Collect equipment (correct drug, prescription sheet, sterile swabs).
- Identify patient, explain procedure and effect of eye drops, and gain consent.
- Cross-check drug with prescription sheet, patient, and identify correct eye.
- Wash and dry hands.
- Ask the patient to look up and gently evert the lower lid and put a drop into the lower conjunctival fornix.
- Putting gentle pressure over the lacrimal sac (just below the medial aspect of the eye) improves absorption to the eye and can reduce systemic absorption
- Ask the patient to close their eyes and wipe away any excess.
- Wash and dry hands.
- Record that the drug has been given.
- Wait 5–10 minutes before further drugs are given in the same eye.
- Make sure that the patient is happy doing this for themselves.

Discharge and continuing care for patients with eye problems

- Follow the discharge process. 📖 Chapter 38, Discharge planning, p.1164.
- Check patient and carer understand eye care requirements.
- Check patient knows how to instill eye drops properly.
- Check patient has medication and understands use, effects of non-concordance, possible side effects, and where to obtain further prescriptions.
- Explain when to resume driving. This varies with type of condition or operation. Seek ophthalmologist's guidance—normally patient must be able to read at level 6/9 on the Snellen Chart (📖 Appendices, Eye Chart, p.1210). May be able to drive with only one functioning eye but insurance company should be informed.
- Give phone number for hospital in case of problems.
- Air travel may be restricted for a period in certain conditions, e.g. following complicated retinal surgery.
- Advise patient to rest if tired—the convalescence period will vary depending on individual and condition. Seek advice on resuming normal activities (e.g. driving) from the surgeon and supporting team.
- Arrange for patient to be visited by specialist nurse or return for dressing check and removal, or give patient information on how to remove own dressing.
- Arrange outpatient appointment with ophthalmologist and for sight test 2–4 weeks postoperatively for cataract patients.
- Encourage patients to have eye tests at least every 2 years and explain how this might save sight.
- Provide list of ophthalmic opticians who make domiciliary visits for housebound patients.
- Provide information on who is exempt from eye test charges.
- Ensure patient has details of Royal National Institute for the Blind, social service, and local and national voluntary organizations to assist in maximizing remaining vision.
- Provide information on how to register as partially sighted or blind if sight loss is serious.

Further information

Royal National Institute for the Blind (RNIB):	www.rnib.org.uk
International Glaucoma Association (IGA):	www.iga.org.uk
Macular Disease Society:	www.maculardisease.org
Driver and Vehicle Licensing Agency (DVLA):	www.dvla.gov.uk
Diabetes UK:	www.diabetes.org.uk

Nursing assessment of patients with ear problems

In addition to a general nursing assessment (📖 Chapter 3, Individualizing nursing care practice, pp.32–33) perform the following procedures.

Observe the patient

- Signs of trauma to the ear, e.g. skin or cartilage damage to the pinna. Is there any bleeding or discharge due to injury to the external ear canal or eardrum, or from a skull base fracture?
- Discharge from the ear canal that may indicate bacterial or fungal infection.
- Swelling or deformity around the ear due to subperichondrial haematoma, mastoiditis, or furunculosis (infected hair follicle).
- Nystagmus, imbalance, unsteadiness, nausea, vomiting, and sweating—may indicate problems with the inner ear.
- Facial nerve palsy—may be due to acoustic neuroma, acute or chronic otitis media, herpes zoster, or Bell's palsy.
- Use of hearing aid or problems with communication—may indicate degree of hearing impairment.
- Evidence of recent surgery.
- See Fig. 14.2 for a diagram of the ear.

Ask the patient about

Nursing history

- Ability to manage self-care and activities of daily living
- Coping strategies, such as how they manage communication if there is hearing impairment (e.g. lip reading, sign language)
- Social situation (any dependants at home or anyone to care for them)
- Past and present nursing problems
- Psychological and spiritual assessment
- Fears and anxiety about the ear condition and prognosis, what they understand about it, and the care and treatment planned

Potential nursing problems

- Hearing impairment (gradual or sudden onset)
- Dizziness or loss of balance
- Episodes of nausea, vomiting, pain, or headaches
- Communication problems (inability to follow conversations, saying pardon frequently, turning up the radio and TV, people appear to mumble)
- Sleep problems

Specific ear history

- Use of hearing aids
- Hearing tests
- Previous ear surgery or procedures, e.g. removal of wax
- Frequent swimmer
- Recent ear infections or trauma
- Foreign bodies
- Exposure to loud noises

Past medical history

- Infectious diseases, e.g. herpes zoster, meningitis, measles—may result in hearing impairment
- Drugs—ototoxic drugs may cause deafness
- Family history of ear problems
- Trauma
- Past surgery

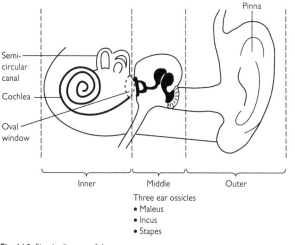

Fig. 14.2 Simple diagram of the ear.

Ear tests and investigations

Examination of the ear

An auroscope is used to examine the external canal and eardrum (See Fig. 14.3). Use the largest speculum that will fit comfortably in the entrance of the canal; ensure batteries are working. Gently pull the pinna upwards and backwards to straighten the canal. It will be possible to see wax, debris, foreign bodies, and the eardrum (unless wax is impacted against it).

Hearing tests

Voice tests

These gauge the patient's ability to hear speech. One ear is occluded with finger; words or numbers are whispered in the other ear and the patient repeats.

Tuning fork tests

These are used to distinguish between conductive and sensorineural deafness. 📖 Types of hearing loss, p.514.

- Rinne's test: This test compares the patient's ability to hear a tone conducted by air and bone. Patients are asked whether a vibrating fork is louder when placed on the mastoid process (bone-conduction) or when placed in line with the external canal (air-conduction). In normal hearing the tuning fork is heard more clearly when held in line with the external canal (i.e. the sound is louder by air conduction and this is called a Rinne positive test). In conductive hearing loss, the tuning fork is heard more clearly when placed on the mastoid process (i.e. the sound is louder by bone conduction and this is called a Rinne negative test).
- Weber's test: This test compares bone conduction in both ears to determine whether a unilateral hearing loss is conductive or sensorineural. A vibrating fork is placed in the centre of the forehead.
  - Patients who perceive the sound in the midline have normal hearing.
  - Patients who perceive the sound better in the poorer ear have conductive loss.
  - Patients who perceive the sound better in the better ear have sensorineural loss.

Audiometry

- Pure tone audiometry: assesses hearing loss by air and bone conduction. Pure tone signals are fed to the patient either by a vibrator attached to the mastoid process (bone conduction) or via ear phones (air conduction). Used for a general assessment of hearing.
- Speech audiometry: assesses the patient's ability to understand speech. A tape of words at varying intensities is played; the percentage of correct words repeated is plotted against a speech audiogram.
- Tympanometry (impedance test): tests for middle ear compliance. The pressure in the external canal is altered; at each setting, sound is passed to the ear and the reflected sound energy is measured.
- Audiometry electric response: surface-recording electrodes are placed on the head and used to study the response of different auditory pathways to sound.

(a)

(b)

(c)

(d)

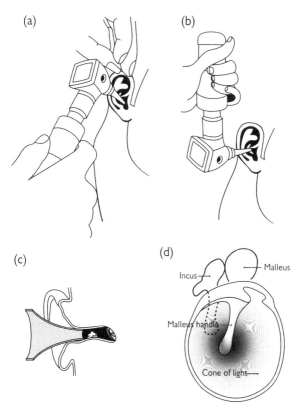

Malleus

Incus

Malleus handle

Cone of light

Fig. 14.3 Examination of the ear with an auroscope. (a) Straighten the ear canal as much as possible and select the largest speculum that fits comfortably in the patient's ear. (b) If the patient is uncooperative or restless hold the handle upwards. (c) Position of the speculum in the ear. (d) Diagram showing the ear drum as seen through the auroscope.

External ear conditions

Trauma

Foreign body causes pain, discomfort, hearing loss, and infection if left. Remove with instruments if the foreign body is superficial and the patient is cooperative. If the patient is uncooperative, there is a danger of eardrum damage and removal under general anaesthesia may be needed.

Blunt trauma to the pinna may cause bleeding and haematoma. It must be aspirated under local anaesthesia and dressed with firm pressure to prevent deformity. Antibiotics are given to prevent infection.

Perforated eardrum can result from sharp object, fracture to base of skull, blast injury, or changes in barometric pressure (e.g. in scuba diving). Patient has pain, conductive deafness, and sometimes bleeding. Do not attempt to clean ear and keep dry. Antibiotics are given to prevent infection. Referral to ENT specialist is usual.

Infections and other non traumatic conditions

Impacted ear wax against the eardrum causes hearing loss. It develops due to difficulty in shedding debris and wax in people who have narrow ear canals, who wear earplugs, or who have hearing aid moulds. Treatment includes irrigation or microsuction. Advise on prevention.

Otitis externa is a bacterial or fungal infection due to scratching (e.g. in eczema) or exposure to water (swimmer's ear). It results in pain, discharge, and swelling of the ear canal and often the surrounding lymph nodes. Treatment includes aural toilet to remove debris, antibiotic and steroid ear drops, or antifungal drops and pain relief. Advise on keeping ears dry. Referral to ENT specialist may be required.

Furunculosis is an infection of a hair follicle in the ear canal. It causes severe pain. Treatment includes pain relief, topical antibiotics and steroid drops, and oral antibiotics if there is surrounding inflammation. Aural toilet is required if there is a discharge of pus. Test urine for sugar to detect diabetes mellitus.

*Herpes zoster (*Ramsay-Hunt syndrome): vesicles appear in the external canal and around the ear. Pain, deafness, vertigo, and 7th nerve palsy may occur. A history of chickenpox or previous shingles is usual. Pain relief is essential. Antivirals (e.g. acyclovir) and steroids may be helpful for palsy.

Nursing care

- Focuses on individual needs and identified problems.
  - Pain relief
  - Support and presence during procedures
  - Explanations of condition, care, procedures, treatment, and next steps
  - Information on further prevention
- Use aseptic techniques for dressings and make arrangements for removal/change of dressings and appointments for follow-up.
- Ensure patient understands medications and can insert drops.

Middle and inner ear conditions

Acute otitis media

This is common in children due to bacterial or viral infections. Patients present with earache, conductive deafness, pyrexia, and general malaise. Spontaneous perforation of the eardrum may occur resulting in pain relief and discharge of pus. Management includes pain relief (e.g. paracetamol); antibiotics if there is no improvement after 2–3 days; and nursing care to monitor and reduce fever, including fluids and keeping the patient comfortable. Mastoiditis is a complication.

Glue ear

Otitis media with effusion may follow acute episode of otitis media due to inadequate drainage via the eustachian tube. It results in deafness and speech and language problems. Long-term antibiotics and mucolytics may help. Surgery includes insertion of grommets with or without adenoidectomy.

Mastoiditis

Infection from the middle ear extends into the mastoid air cells resulting in pyrexia, tenderness and swelling over the mastoid, discharge, and hearing loss. Treatment is usually IV antibiotics. Nursing care depends on symptoms and includes pain relief, reduction of fever, aural toilet, encouraging fluids, and keeping the patient comfortable. Cranial nerve palsy, meningitis, and brain abscesses are complications.

Tinnitus

This refers to any sound heard in the ear not from an external source normally described as ringing, buzzing, and whistling. The cause is often unknown but may be linked to exposure to loud noises, hearing loss, head injuries, Ménière's disease, raised blood pressure, or drugs. In severe cases it interferes with daily life and causes depression. It is always investigated by an ENT surgeon to ensure that there is no sinister cause such as an acoustic neuroma. Reassurance and psychological support is important. Suggest support group and contacting help lines.

Ménières disease

This is a relatively rare inner ear disorder presenting with episodes of vertigo, fluctuating hearing loss and tinnitus, and a sense of fullness in the ear; patients may also have nausea and vomiting. The cause is unknown, but may be due to overproduction of endolymph fluid. Initial management includes diuretics, low-salt diet, avoiding triggers (e.g. stress, fatigue, alcohol, flashing lights). Anti-emetics may help. Psychological problems (e.g. loneliness, isolation, and anxiety) are common. Endolymphatic sac surgery and vestibular nerve section are surgical treatments but the vast majority are treated medically and conservatively and do not require surgery.

Acoustic neuroma

This is a rare benign neoplasm of Schwann cells of the 8th cranial nerve that causes tinnitus, asymmetrical sensorineural deafness, and vertigo later. Treatment may be conservative, gamma knife surgery, or microsurgery. Patients tend to be nursed on a neurological ward.

Patients undergoing ear surgery

Myringotomy and insertion of grommets

A small incision is made in the tympanic membrane and a small tube (grommet) is inserted to ventilate the middle ear and prevent fluid and pressure accumulation. This is undertaken for glue ear mostly in children or malfunction of the eustachian tube in other age groups.

Specific preoperative care includes baseline assessment audiogram, and impedance test, explanation of surgery and pre- and postoperative care for general anaesthetic as day case.

Specific postoperative care includes lying in semi-prone position and resumed eating and drinking when awake. Pain is unusual and immediate improvement in hearing is common. Keep ears dry by using cotton wool and petroleum jelly when hair washing and bathing—remove afterwards. Advise not to clean ears with cotton buds and contact GP if earache occurs.

Myringoplasty

This is an operation under general anaesthesia to repair a perforation in the tympanic membrane (eardrum) using a small graft. Preoperative care is as for myringotomy and postoperative care is as for mastoidectomy. Avoid raising pressure in middle ear by avoiding vigorous nose blowing and keeping mouth open during sneezing.

Mastoidectomy

Surgical removal of affected tissue from the mastoid cavity under general anaesthesia.

Specific preoperative care
- Obtain x-ray of mastoid area and hearing tests to act as baseline.
- Explain surgery and pre- and postoperative care including sutured wound behind the ear and possibility of drain and pain relief.
- Explain risks of surgery, e.g. slight risk of facial nerve damage and infection.

Specific postoperative care
- Instruct patients to avoid lying on the operated side.
- Monitor blood pressure, and pulse, and observe for facial nerve damage.
- Administer pain relief and anti-emetics as required.
- Patients may resume eating and drinking when conscious, if no vomiting.
- Advise patients not to make sudden head movements.
- Mobilize patient as soon as possible.
- Remove pressure dressing using aseptic technique the following day and drain after 1–2 days.
- Remove ear pack 10 days to 6 weeks later.
- Explain about surgery and continuing care including suture removal after 1 week.
- Advise to keep ear dry and inform GP if discharge is more than minimal or is offensive.

Stapedectomy

This is the removal of the stapes ossicle in the middle ear under general anaesthesia and replacement with a plastic prosthesis as a result of otosclerosis (fixation of the stapes at the oval window). Usually results in dramatic improvement in hearing but risk of deafness and balance problems in 2% of patients.

Preoperative care includes audiogram and impedance tests, explanation of operation, risks and benefits, pre- and postoperative care.

Postoperative care as for mastoidectomy.

Patients with hearing impairment

Types of hearing loss
Sensorineural hearing loss: caused by disorders of the inner ear, cochlea, acoustic nerve, or central auditory pathway.

Conductive deafness: caused by disorders of the external or middle ear that prevent sound from reaching the cochlea including congenital deformities (e.g. atresia of external ear), wax, perforation of eardrum, ossicular chain disorders, eustachian tube disorders, otitis media, and cholesteatoma (cystic growth in middle ear).

Presbycusis: age-related hearing loss due to degeneration of the fine hair cells of the cochlea. High-frequency sounds are affected first.

Degree of hearing loss
Deaf: people who are unable to use hearing for communication.

Hearing impaired: people who can use hearing to some degree for communication. May be mild, moderate, severe, or profound, based on softest sound level (decibels) an individual can hear without amplification (mild 16–30 dB; moderate 31–70 dB; severe 71–90 dB; profound over 91 dB). A whisper is about 10 dB.

Aids to interpreting speech
Hearing aids: are electronic battery-operated devices that are worn externally. They amplify and change sound and send it to the ear through a speaker. All sounds, including background noises, are amplified. Types of hearing aids include:
- 'Behind the ear' (most common) and 'body worn' (best for profound hearing loss—the aid is attached to an ear mould)
- 'In the ear' and 'in the canal'—the aid is incorporated into the ear mould itself

Analogue hearing aids are being replaced by digital ones which can be programmed precisely to meet an individual's hearing loss. 📖 Hearing aid care, p.515.

Cochlear implants: are small electronic devices that are surgically implanted underneath the skin behind the ear. They convert sound waves into electrical impulses that the brain recognizes as sound.

Listening equipment
- Loop and infrared systems help the listener hear sounds more clearly by reducing background noise. They may be found in theatres, cinemas, banks, and shopping centres. Smaller systems can be set up in the home.
- Neckloops, earloops, loop amplifiers, or headphones can make listening to videos, TV, radios, and stereos easier by making sounds louder and clearer.
- Subtitles on TV, videos, DVDs.

📖 Communicating with hearing-impaired patients, p.516.

Hearing aid care

Ear moulds
These are made to fit each ear and are not interchangeable. Cleaning should be undertaken regularly.

- Detach the ear mould from the hearing aid.
- Remove any wax that is blocking the tube and wash with soap and water.
- Rinse the mould well and dry it thoroughly. Ensure the tubing is free of moisture. A special 'puffer' can be obtained from audiology departments for this purpose.
- Do not detach the tubing from the ear mould unless it is being changed.
- Replace the tubing about every 6 months as it becomes hardened and affects the performance of the hearing aid.

Batteries

- Ensure that the battery is inserted correctly in the battery drawer. If there is any resistance, check that it is inserted with the proper side facing up. Incorrectly inserted batteries can cause extensive damage and, if privately bought, can be expensive.
- To check the battery is working, turn the hearing aid on and turn the volume to maximum with the hand cupped round the aid. If it whistles, the battery is working. Never do this while the hearing aid is in the ear.

Controls

- Usually consists of on–off switch (O=off), volume control, (M=microphone/on), and battery holder. There may be a 'T' setting which is for a telecoil loop system. The volume generally goes from 1–4 with 1 being the quietest. Adjust for the individual's need at the time.

Communicating with hearing-impaired patients

Problems in communication

- Staff often fail to recognize hearing impairment, which may be due to:
  - poor observation and history taking
  - difficulty in communication because of culture or language barriers
  - failure to communicate with each other.
- Patients may conceal their disability.
- Staff may lack skills or knowledge of how to communicate effectively with hearing-impaired people; may be due to poor training.
- Facilities (e.g. minicoms, hearing loops, etc.) may be inadequate or staff may be unaware of how to use them.

Improving communication

- Ask the patient if they are hearing impaired and what devices or techniques they use. Be aware that they may deny their disability.
- Observe for signs of impaired hearing (e.g. inappropriate response to a question, smile, nod). This may be confirmed by turning away from the patient to ask a question so they cannot lip read.
- Gain the patient's attention by calling their name. Introduce yourself and others if present.
- Create a conducive environment; reduce background noise (e.g. turn off TV, radio), use a quiet room with the door shut, and use a well lit room with adequate lighting for lip reading.
- Speak slowly and clearly and at normal volume to increase clarity. This should not be done to the extent that makes the person feel stupid. Do not shout.
- Face the patient and make sure your mouth is visible at all times and not hidden behind a hand. Do not wear sunglasses.
- It may be helpful to state the topic of conversation to set the context.
- Face the person with the hearing impairment if possible at about 1 m distance and at the same level. Use natural facial expressions, gestures, and body language and make sure these match the message.
- Check that the person can follow you and rephrase if necessary.
- Give time for the patient to interpret what is being said and to make responses. Be patient.
- Follow up important discussions with written information and repeat conversations if necessary.
- It may be helpful to have a sign language interpreter if the patient uses sign language.

Special communication techniques and equipment

British Sign Language and Sign Supported English
British Sign Language (BSL) is the most widely used method of signed communication in the UK. It uses both manual and non-manual components and hand shapes and movements, facial expression, and shoulder movements.

Finger spelling
Often used in conjunction with BSL. Certain words, often names of people and places, are spelled out on fingers.

Equipment
- Alarm clock with flashing lights and vibrating pads.
- Fire alarms with flashing lights.
- Extra loud door bells or combined with flashing lights.
- Telephones with flashing lights, extra amplification, and induction loop to enable people with hearing aids to use the 'T 'setting on the aid with the phone.
- Text phones.
- Video phones to communicate with sign language.
- Subtitles on TV.
- Hearing loops attached to TV, radio, and hi fi equipment.
- Hearing loops set up in theatres, community halls, etc.

Nursing care of patients with ear problems

Ear pain

Pain may be severe if due to trauma, furunculosis (infected hair follicle) in external canal, and otitis media. It may be less severe in otitis externa and perforation of the eardrum. Pain, swelling, and tenderness behind the ear occur with mastoiditis. Give prescribed analgesics and monitor and record effects. Insulated heat pad may help make the patient feel more comfortable.

Ear discharge

Bleeding may occur as a result of trauma, infection, perforation of eardrum, or basal skull fracture. Cerebropsinal fluid (CSF) may leak with basal skull fracture. Offensive discharge occurs in infections of the outer and middle ear, and with foreign bodies (📖 External ear conditions, p.508). If due to infection give prescribed antibiotics, and record and monitor effects. Explain effects and side effects of antibiotics. Perform aural toilet using cotton wick to gently remove debris. Remove foreign body with instruments only if specifically trained and if superficial. 📖 Chapter 13, Head injury, p.474.

Impaired hearing

The degree of hearing loss varies from mild to profound and may be temporary or permanent, gradual, or sudden onset. It may result in long-term speech and language problems. 📖 Patients with hearing impairment, p.514.

Communication problems

Some patients may have to interpret speech without sound and use a combination of lip reading, body language, facial gestures, and the context of the conversation. Others rely on visual communication, e.g. sign language. Some may be helped by hearing aids. Hearing aids may not work because of flat batteries, blocked tubes, and ill-fitting ear moulds. 📖 Communicating with hearing-impaired patients, p.516.

Loss of balance, vertigo

This is caused by inner ear problems. It may be accompanied by dizziness and giddiness; patient may experience falls or 'drop attacks' if vertigo is sudden and intense. Attacks vary in severity and vary in duration from a few minutes to hours. Administer anti-emetic and vestibular suppressant if prescribed in severe cases. Do not move the patient's head unless essential; support the head. Advise the patient to lie on the unaffected side; keep the room dark and free from noise. Speak calmly and quietly. Physiotherapy and specific exercise may help.

Nausea and vomiting

These may occur as a result of disturbances in balance associated with problems of the inner ear; may also occur in infections. Keep vomit bowl close by and change after use. Apply cold face cloth to forehead if the patient is sweating. Give prescribed anti-emetics and give mouthwashes as required.

Anxiety

This may be due to possible deterioration of hearing leading to profound deafness or due to fears that the treatment and tests may be painful or that the condition may have a poor prognosis. Encourage patient to discuss fears and listen to them. Give information to enable patient to make decisions, understand prognosis, treatment, care, and the future.

Social isolation

This may occur because people may be impatient with hearing-impaired people and treat them as less intelligent. Inability to follow conversations may lead to lack of confidence and being ignored by others. Encourage patient to share their disability, and what it means to them, with others. This will enable family, friends, and work colleagues to understand why they are behaving as they do, to be patient, and to take special measures to ensure more effective communication.

Safety risks

Patients with hearing impairment may not hear alarms, e.g. smoke detector fire alarms, car horns, etc. While in hospital special precautions must be made for patients with hearing impairment, e.g. patient needs to be informed in person when fire alarm sounds.

Preoperative care

Follow the principles for preoperative preparation. Teach postoperative techniques, e.g. instilling ear drops. Follow local procedures for preparation of the ear area—a small area behind the ear may be shaved, e.g. in mastoidectomy. Check the consent form has been signed and answer any further questions about risks and consequences of surgery.

Postoperative care

Position the patient in the most comfortable position but avoid lying on operated side; observe temperature and blood presure, and for bleeding and damage to the facial nerve (weakness on side of face). Advise avoiding sudden head movement which may result in dizziness, nausea, and vomiting. Give pain relief. Encourage patient to resume eating and drinking when nausea and vomiting subsides. Time to start to mobilize will vary depending on patient and operation—support patient in case of dizziness.

Removal of ear wax

Impacted ear wax is one of the most common ENT reasons people visit their GP.

- To examine the external canal:
  - Explain to the patient what is planned.
  - Use an auroscope with the largest speculum that will fit comfortably into the canal.
  - Gently pull the pinna upwards and backwards to straighten out the canal.
  - The tympanic membrane should be visible but may be obscured by impacted wax.
  - Observe for any inflammation or infection.
- Take history to determine whether the eardrum has been perforated (📖 Nursing assessment of patients with ear problems, p.504) or whether there have been any injuries or previous surgery or infections.
- In certain circumstances irrigation may be contraindicated, e.g. uncooperative patient, acute otitis externa, previous ear surgery, cleft palate (repaired or not), perforation of eardrum, complications with previous irrigation, or recent or current middle ear infections.
- Use ear drops to soften the wax for 5–7 days and 2–3 times per day. Olive oil, water, and saline drops or commercial drops can be used (none has been found to be more effective than others).
- Insert the drops at night and ask the patient to lie with the treated ear uppermost for a time to allow the drops to penetrate the wax.
- If this fails to clear the wax, irrigation is necessary using an electrical pulsed water irrigator.
  - An internal pump sends pulses of water through a nozzle into the canal.
  - The operators should have training in using this technique and cleaning and care of the equipment.
  - Explanations should be given to the patient and consent obtained.
  - Examination of the external canal immediately before and after syringing is required.
- Auroscopes, speculums, and irrigators should be decontaminated following use.
- Ensure the procedure, result, treatment, and advice given are documented following local policy.
- If contraindicated, failure, or complications arise refer to ENT for microcsuction.

Education for patients with ear problems

Patients with existing ear problems

- Use a model of the ear to explain the patient's condition and what will happen during and as a result of treatment and surgery.
- Explain the importance of handwashing and other actions to prevent infection before, during, and after ear care.
- Teach the patient and carer how to instill ear drops, care for hearing aid and change batteries, and ensure they know how to use any other equipment (📖 Special communication techniques and equipment, p.517). Supervised practice is preferred.
- Explain how to keep the ears dry during bathing, hair washing, and swimming by using petroleum jelly on cotton wool plugs. Advise that these should be removed afterwards.
- Explain 'what to do' and 'what not to do'. These will vary depending on the condition. Avoid strenuous exercise, heavy lifting, and straining following stapedectomy; keep ear dry following myringotomy. Avoid air travel, diving, or other situations causing pressure changes in the ear for a specified period.
- Encourage patients to ask questions and express fears about their condition, care, treatment, and the future and longer-term prognosis.
- Discuss the possible consequences of concealing deafness from others. Advise that family, friends, and work colleagues can give support if they are aware of the disability.
- Suggest ways of improving communication and overcoming problems (📖 Communicating with hearing-impaired patients, p.516).
- Ensure patient is seen by specialists (e.g. speech and language therapists, audiologist for specialist education) and arrange for programmes such as sign language, lip reading.

Preventive education

- Advise patients not to clean ears or attempt to remove wax with cotton buds or any similar equipment because of the danger of impacting wax or damaging the eardrum.
- Advise patients to wear ear protection if working in a noisy environment. This should be provided by the employer and they may be eligible for compensation if protective equipment has not been provided.
- Advise patients to contact their GP if they think they have a hearing loss or another ear problem.

Discharge and continuing care for patients with ear problems

- Follow the discharge process. 📖 Chapter 38, Discharge planning, p.1164.
- Check the patient (and/or carer):
  - Understands their condition and plan for the future.
  - Understands their ear care requirements.
  - Is able to instill ear drops properly.
  - Has the required medication, understands the use, side effects, and consequence of non-compliance and where to get repeat prescriptions.
  - Has their hearing aid, knows how to use and maintain it, and where to get batteries and other help and advice.
  - Has received specific instructions relevant to their condition.
- Arrange for dressing changes or removal; removal of sutures; return to ward; visit to outpatients; or visit by community nurse or specialist nurse.
- Convalescence period will be determined by the individual and their condition.
- Arrange for follow-up at outpatients with the nurse specialist or consultant, or with GP, or with the audiology department.
- Provide information on how to register as hearing impaired or deaf.
- Ensure patient and carer have information about the legal obligations of:
  - Employers who are required to treat deaf people as favourably as hearing people and to make reasonable adjustments to ensure deaf people are not disadvantaged.
  - Education providers to make reasonable adjustments to support deaf students.
- Ensure patient and carer are aware of local and national voluntary and support services and networks (📖 Further information on ear disorders, p.525) and are aware of Disability Employment Advisers at Job Centres who can assist people with hearing impairment to find jobs.
- Ensure the patient is aware of support that social workers can provide for deaf people.
- Ensure the patient and carer know how to access equipment, programmes, and interpreters that will help improve communication and ensure safety, e.g. smoke detectors with flashing lights and vibrating pads.

Further information

Royal National Institute for the Deaf (RNID): www.rnid.org.uk Links to:
    RNID Tinnitus Helpline (information and advice on tinnitus)
    RNID Sound Advantage (range of equipment for deaf and hard of hearing)
    RNID information line (range of information on deafness and hearing loss)

Vestibular Disorders Association:	www.vestibular.org
Ménière's Society:	www.menieres.org.uk
National Institute on Deafness and Other Communication Disorders:	www.nidcd.nih.gov/health/pubs
British Deaf Association:	www.bda.org.uk
Hearing Concern:	www.hearingconcernlink.org
National Deaf Childrens' Society:	www.ndcs.org.uk
ENT Nursing information sheets:	www.entnursing.com
Information regarding ear care:	www.earcarecentre.com

Nursing assessment of patients with nose and throat problems

In addition to a general nursing assessment (□ Chapter 3, Individualizing nursing care practice, pp.32–33) perform the following procedures.

Observe the patient

- Signs of trauma to the nose, e.g. swelling, deformity, dislocation, epistaxis, and soft tissue injury.
- Signs of injury to the throat, e.g. airway injuries causing stridor, cough, obstruction, haemoptysis, pain, internal and external bleeding, tissue damage.
- Epistaxis: note the amount and location of bleeding, whether bleeding is from both nostrils; does the patient spit blood out? Take blood pressure, and pulse.
- Nasal discharge: whether clear, purulent, bloody, foul smelling, from one or both nostrils, any excoriation around nostrils.
- Dysphonia: difficulty with speech and hoarseness, e.g. due to inflammation of the larynx, pharynx, tonsillitis.
- Dysphagia: difficulty swallowing, e.g. in tonsillitis, foreign body, or due to neurological cause.
- Airway obstruction due to infection, swelling (e.g. epiglottitis), foreign body. Check respirations (rate, depth, stridor) and patient's colour as patients may deteriorate rapidly and require immediate medical intervention.
- Signs of fever, e.g. in tonsillitis, peritonsillar abscess, epiglottitis. Take temperature and pulse.

Ask the patient about

Nursing history

- Ability to manage self-care and activities of daily living
- Social situation (dependants at home, anyone to care for them)
- Past and present nursing problems
- Psychological and spiritual assessment
- Lifestyle, e.g. sports (e.g. rugby player, boxer), singer, actor, use of recreational drugs (cocaine)
- Fears and anxieties about the nose and throat condition and prognosis; effects on appearance, lifestyle, and ability to sleep; what they understand about the condition and the care and treatment planned

Potential nursing problems

- Epistaxis—duration of previous episodes, known causes
- Nasal discharge and irritation
- Sore throats—whether recurrent, the duration, known causes
- Dysphagia, dysphonia, hoarseness—duration, extent
- Fever—duration, whether accompanied by nausea, headache, anorexia
- Pain—location, duration, methods of pain relief used
- Breathing problems—obstruction in nasal passages or larynx
- Loss of smell and taste disturbances

Medical history
- Drugs (aspirin, NSAIDs, warfarin, cocaine, and nasal sprays are linked to nose bleeds, antibiotics)
- Hypertension
- Recent upper respiratory infections
- Tonsillitis
- Dental problems, allergies, and rhinitis (associated with polyps)
- Previous nose and throat surgery and tracheostomy.

Nursing patients with nose and throat problems

Epistaxis

This is a nose bleed. With anterior epistaxis, blood drips from the nose (one or both nostrils). With posterior epistaxis, blood drains down the back of the throat. Blood can be profuse and may be swallowed and therefore not visible. 📖 Epistaxis, p.530.

Nasal discharge

This may be clear, CSF (after trauma and fracture; 📖 Trauma, p.530) serosanguinous, offensive, infected, and may be from one or both nostrils. Post-nasal drip is common in sinusitis and polyps and may give rise to a sore throat.

Dysphagia

This is difficulty in swallowing fluids and/or solids.

Dysphonia and hoarseness

These refer to difficulty in speech and changes in the quality, volume, and resonance of the voice.

Pain

This may be sore throat, earache (referred pain from tonsillitis or peri-tonsillar abscess), headache and facial pain (sinusitis) located over site of trauma (e.g. nose, throat), or due to infection (e.g. furunculosis of nose).

Fever

This is raised temperature, often with malaise.

Airway obstruction

The extent of the obstruction is variable depending on the cause. A foreign body in the nose or nasal deformity may cause an obstruction to the airflow through the nasal passages, but conditions such as epiglottitis obstruct the laryngeal opening causing complete obstruction.

Loss of smell and taste

This may result in loss of appetite.

Anxiety

This may be due to recent events (e.g. trauma event); fear of prognosis or that the treatment and tests will be painful; or about arrangements for dependants.

Social isolation

Difficulty with speech and hoarseness may make the individual reluctant to join conversations.

Nose and throat tests and investigations

For all tests and investigations explain the procedure to the patient, obtain consent, and provide support throughout.

Laryngoscopy

Indirect laryngoscopy is used to assess the mobility of the vocal cords or to rapidly assess the hypopharynx to exclude or locate foreign body. A warmed laryngeal mirror is introduced onto the soft palate and the laryngeal structures are viewed by tilting the mirror; the image is reversed.

Fibre-optic laryngoscopy is used to visualize the entire nasopharynx and larynx. A flexible endoscope is introduced through the nose after topical anaesthesia (e.g. cocaine) has been applied. This is valuable in patients who experience severe gagging or who are uncooperative. It is essential for patients who need thorough laryngeal examination, e.g. when cancer is suspected.

Rigid endoscopy is performed under general anaesthesia. Check for loose teeth, caps, crowns, or bridges; warn of small risk of tearing of the oesophagus and the possibility of a sore throat and swallowing difficulty. A biopsy may be taken. The patient may notice spotting/streaking of blood mixed with secretions. Advise to seek advice if voice changes or new symptoms develop, e.g. neck lumps, earache, facial pain.

Laboratory tests

These will vary depending on operation, age, and any underlying condition and may include FBC, group, cross-match and save, prothrombin time (PT), and partial thromboplastin time (PTT). 🕮 Chapter 39, Common laboratory tests and their interpretation, p.1167.

X-rays

Plain x-rays of sinuses are taken to identify fluid levels and mucosal thickening in sinusitis. Lateral pharyngeal (neck) x-rays may be taken to evaluate the size of the adenoids. CT scans are used to evaluate sinus disease and to identify the size and location of tumours.

Culture and sensitivity tests

Throat culture is performed if bacterial infection is suspected, e.g. high temperature, abrupt onset of symptoms, patient appears ill, or elevated WBC. Depress patient's tongue with a spatula, use flashlight to see inflamed area, sweep swab over area without touching lips or tongue. Transport in transport medium that has been correctly labelled.

Nasal and nasopharyngeal cultures are used to identify carrier organisms or to screen for infection. For nasal culture a flexible swab is inserted into the nose and rotated against anterior nares. A longer flexible swab is required to collect specimens from the posterior pharynx. Transport in transport medium that has been correctly labelled.

Sinus washout refers to the introduction of water or saline solution into the maxillary sinus to remove infected material under local anaesthetic or general anaesthetic. Send material for culture. Introduction of the trocar causes cracking noise. This is an unpleasant procedure under local anaesthetic.

Conditions of the nose

Foreign body

Usually occurs in young children—beads, cotton wool, seeds, and sweets are common. It is usually unilateral and may be asymptomatic or produce offensive or blood-stained discharge. If accessible in the anterior part of nose, it can be removed with instruments by a specially trained practitioner. There is a danger of dislodging with subsequent inhalation. Removal under general anaesthesia may be necessary if child is uncooperative.

Trauma

This may result in fracture of nasal bones, nasal septum, or septal haematoma. Fractures may be simple (skin and mucosa intact) or compound (cartilage and bone are exposed). Patients may present with nasal deformity, swelling, obstruction, epistaxis, and soft tissue injury. Reduction of the fracture may be done immediately or after 7–10 days when the swelling subsides.

Nasal polyps

These are pedunculated sacs that are usually bilateral and often allergy related. They cause nasal obstruction, watery discharge, post-nasal drip, and sneezing. They may develop purulent discharge, if infected. They are more common in men. Treatment includes topical steroid drops or systemic steroids or surgical removal. They may recur.

Sinusitis

This is inflammation of mucous membrane of the paranasal sinuses due to obstruction, infection, or allergy. It may present with headache, facial pain, blocked nose, post-nasal drip, and changed voice resonance. Treatment is with antibiotics, analgesia, decongestant, and possible irrigation under general anaesthesia.

Epistaxis

Anterior is commonly seen in children. Blood drips from one or both nostrils. It is usually due to nasal dryness, facial injury, sneezing violently, nose blowing or picking, foreign bodies, or common cold.

Posterior is seen more often in older people. It may be caused by underlying health problems (e.g. hypertension, diabetes, tumours) or may be aggravated by drugs (e.g. warfarin, cocaine, aspirin). Use digital pressure to stop bleeding (📖 Control of epistaxis by digital pressure, p.531). If unsuccessful, invasive measures may be necessary, e.g. nasal packing, topical vasoconstrictor, cauterization with chemical agent such as silver nitrate sticks, or using intranasal balloon pack, balloon tamponade, or arterial ligation under general anaesthesia.

Tumours

Benign tumours include nasal ostoma (rare), nasal papilloma (common wart-like growths), and nasal angioma (causes epistaxis, requires surgical excision).

Malignant lesions are not common. They may cause blood-stained discharge, nasal obstruction, facial swelling, and lymph nodes in neck. Prognosis is poor because of late presentation.

Control of epistaxis by digital pressure

- Pinch the fleshy part of the nose, using the thumb and forefinger to reduce the blood supply for 10 minutes; it may require up to 30 minutes.
- Keep the patient sitting up with their head forward to prevent blood entering the post-nasal space.
- Use an ice compress over the bridge of the nose, back of neck, or both to promote vasoconstriction.
- Do not allow the patient to blow their nose or to sniff. Provide a bowl to expectorate.
- Wear protective clothing—gloves, mask, and eye protection as coughing or sneezing may result in blood particles being aerosolized.
- Note the duration, amount, and location of bleeding.
- Act in a calm manner and reassure the patient who will be anxious and frightened.
- Assess the patient's vital signs for decrease in blood pressure and increased pulse and respirations; observe colour and temperature of skin and nail beds for pallor and cyanosis.

Prevention of further epistaxis

Advise the patient to:

- Not blow their nose for a week.
- Not lift heavy objects for a week.
- Keep the head upright when bending down.
- Not use nasal sprays unless prescribed by doctor.
- Avoid people with influenza or colds.
- Avoid smoky atmosphere.
- Not pick nose.
- Avoid hot fluids immediately after nose bleed (causes vasodilation).

Nursing care of patients undergoing nose surgery

Surgery of the nose

Nasal polypectomy
Polyps are removed under local or general anaesthesia and sent for histology. Unilateral polyps are more often malignant.

Nasal septoplasty
The septum between the nostrils may become damaged after trauma. Surgery involves lifting the mucosa, trimming the cartilage, and replacing the mucous membrane. Silastic nasal splints may be used to prevent adhesions and are removed by the nurse 7 days later.

Functional endoscopic sinus surgery (FESS)
Chronic sinusitis results in abnormal mucus production and drainage. FESS aims to restore normal drainage by correcting anatomical abnormalities, removing mucosa if diseased, removing polyps, and enlarging drainage via an endoscope.

Specific preoperative care
Preoperative assessment may be carried out 1–2 weeks before and the patient is usually admitted on the day of operation.
- Ensure patient understands operation, risks, and benefits and that consent form is signed.
- Perform blood tests (e.g. FBC) and x-rays of nose/sinuses.
- Check on allergies and baseline vital signs.
- Obtain CT scan of sinus to provide an anatomical road map.
- Note medication, particularly use of nasal sprays, anticoagulants, aspirin.
- Advise that packs will be in place postoperatively and that mouth breathing will be necessary and takes time to get used to.
- Ask about loose teeth, caps, crowns, and bridges that may become dislodged.
- Encourage questions and discussion about fears and feelings.
- Instruct patient to fast as necessary.

Specific postoperative care
- Nurse patient in most comfortable position.
- Provide reassurance to help patient cope with feelings of not being able to breathe due to packs.
- Observe for bleeding and signs of infection; take temperature and blood pressure.
- Give mouthwashes to keep mouth fresh.
- Encourage patient to eat and drink when recovered; lack of appetite may occur because of mouth breathing and difficulty in swallowing.
- If blood oozes through nasal packs, prepare 'nose-bag' (pads of gauze).
- Nasal pack is usually removed after 24 hours; warn patient that a long length of gauze may have been used and bleeding may occur.
- Discharge should be after packs have been removed.
- If necessary, give mild pain relief (e.g. paracetamol).
- Convalescence will vary but patient should be at work after 2 weeks and should be fully recovered by 6 weeks.

Complications
- For nasal polypectomy—haemorrhage and infection.
- For nasal septoplasty—infection and haematoma, which presents with severe pain and total nasal blockage, and requires readmission, incision draining, and usually antibiotics.
- For FESS—haemorrhage, haematoma, pain, infection, and rarely CSF leak or loss of vision. Rapid eye swelling due to bleeding into the eye socket is an emergency post FESS and must be recognized and treated promptly to prevent blindness.

Conditions of the throat

Tonsillitis

This is commonly caused by group A beta-haemolytic streptococci. Patient typically presents with sore throat, dysphagia, fever, malaise, headache, cervical lymph glands, and exudate on the tonsils. Throat swabs do not give instant results; antibiotics are not always given as side effects outweigh benefits. Give prescribed analgesia, antipyretics, and antibiotics if prescribed (usually penicillin); encourage fluids and rest. May develop into:

- *Peritonsillar abscess* (quinsy) occurs unilaterally mostly in adults, resulting in worsening of symptoms, earache, dysphagia, and trismus (difficulty opening jaw). Requires antibiotics and drainage of abscess under general or local anaesthesia.
- *Recurrent or chronic tonsillitis* refers to repeat or prolonged episodes of tonsillitis.
- *Tonsillectomy* is considered for patients with recurrent tonsillitis, airway obstruction, sleep apnoea, quinsy, suspected malignancy.
  📖 Tonsillectomy (removal of tonsils), p.536.

Laryngitis

This is inflammation of the larynx. It is usually viral and is exacerbated by overuse of the voice, smoking, and drinking spirits. It causes hoarseness and laryngeal pain; larynx is red and dry. Management includes resting voice, inhaling steam, and avoiding precipitating factors. Antibiotics are rarely needed.

Acute epiglottitis

This is a localized bacterial infection, usually *Haemophilus influenzae*. It is more common in children, but is less common since HIB vaccination. It causes swelling of the epiglottis, increasing dysphagia, stridor, and obstruction of the larynx. High-dose IV steroids are prescribed; humidified oxygen is essential. Emergency intubation or tracheostomy may be required. A calm atmosphere and support is required for parents and child.

Foreign body

Fish and meat bones, sharp objects, and button batteries are common. These may impact in tonsil, pharyngeal wall, obstruct the airway, or be swallowed. It results in sharp local pain, retrosternal pain, worsening dysphagia, increased salivation, and airway obstruction. The foreign body may be identified on x-ray. An ENT specialist is required for removal; an emergency laryngotomy or tracheosotomy is necessary for complete airway obstruction. Observe for raised temperature, and chest or back pain suggesting perforation.

Laryngeal carcinoma

This is the most common head and neck tumour, usually squamous cell carcinoma. Smoking is main risk factor. Patient presents with hoarseness, pain, dysphagia, sore throat, and stridor. Diagnosis is by laryngoscopy and biopsy; treatment is by surgery and radiotherapy. Prognosis is good if detected early.

Advice for patients with voice problems

- Save your voice as much as possible—speak quietly and limit talking.
- Avoid speaking for long periods, shouting, or raising your voice. Stop speaking if voice deteriorates. Do not whisper—this strains the voice more.
- Keep throat and mouth moist with soft drinks but avoid tea, coffee, and alcohol which have a drying effect. Avoid very hot drinks.
- Do not smoke and avoid smokey atmospheres as these damage the throat.
- Keep air humidified by using a humidifier or keeping a bowl of water nearby or wet towel on radiator to produce steam.
- Try to relax; use yoga or relaxation techniques to reduce tension in back, neck, and jaw.

Nursing care of patients undergoing throat surgery

Laryngectomy

This is removal of the larynx, usually because of malignancy. Patients will not be able to speak using their vocal cords and need a new method of communication.

Preoperative care

Preoperative assessment may be carried out 1–2 weeks before and patient is usually admitted a day before operation.

- Obtain FBC, group and cross-match, chest x-ray, and baseline temperature and blood pressure.
- Ensure patient understands surgery, risks, and planned outcomes, particularly about loss of voice and the presence of a permanent stoma with tracheostomy tube.
- Explain how coughing and breathing will occur and that an IV infusion, fine-bore nasogastric tube, and drains will be *in situ*.
- Discuss prognosis and encourage patients to ask questions and express feelings.
- Refer patients to a physiotherapist and a speech and language therapist to learn about care postoperatively.

If appropriate, arrange a visit by a person with a laryngectomy who is leading a full life for the patient and family to talk to.

Postoperative care

- In immediate period, as for tracheostomy. 📖 Nursing care of tracheostomy patients, pp.540–1.
- Drains are removed 2–3 days after operation.
- Hydration and nutrition is through enteral feeds and IV infusion until wound heals; check with barium swallow, then commence soft diet (after 10–14 days).
- Removal of sutures is after 7–10 days.
- Teach patient how to care for stoma and provide alternative methods of communication (📖 Communicating with patients following laryngectomy, p.538).
- Be patient, provide support in helping patient towards self-care, and take time to listen to their feelings and anxieties.
- Any ventilatory support in resuscitation must be given via stoma.

Tonsillectomy (removal of tonsils)

Specific preoperative care

- Ensure patient (and parents) understand the surgery, care, and potential benefits and risks including postoperative haemorrhage, hypernasal speech, airway obstruction, and very rarely death.
- Explain what they might feel like postoperatively, e.g. soreness, reluctance to eat.
- Obtain preoperative blood test for FBC and cross-match.
- Identify recent respiratory problems, e.g. asthma, sleep apnoea.

- Check for medications (e.g. aspirin) and discontinue these, and for allergies.
- Encourage parent(s) to stay with child.
- Check baseline temperature and blood pressure.

Specific postoperative care

- Nurse semi-prone initially.
- Observe for bleeding (check mouth, throat for excessive swallowing, raised, weak pulse, low blood pressure), fever, respiratory distress, pain (analgesia and mild sedatives might help).
- Encourage sips of cold clear fluid when alert, then ice cream and jelly, then introduce normal diet as soon as possible.
- Keep mouth clean, brush teeth as normal.
- Give pain relief.
- Patients are usually discharged home the next day. Provide discharge instructions on complications (e.g. earache, dehydration, secondary bleeding), keeping mouth clean, pain relief, return to activities, school, and work, and action to take if problems arise.

Communicating with patients following laryngectomy

Probably the greatest cause of concern for both tracheostomy patients and laryngectomy patients is the loss of speech and ability to communicate verbally and subsequent isolation. Explanations are important.

- Patients with permanent tracheostomy and laryngectomy need to understand that alternative means of communication should be developed. Staff need to be sensitive to the impact of this news on both the patient and their family and give time for questions and discussion about what it means to them.
- In the immediate postoperative period a writing board and pens, signs, boards, and picture boards will help with communication and the patient may be able to mouth words.
  - Allow additional time for the patient to respond as writing takes longer.
  - Speak in a normal tone. Although the patient cannot speak they may not be deaf.
- Provide a bell or buzzer that will enable the patient to alert staff.
- Remember the general principles of communication: speak in normal voice and at normal rate, face patient, and keep normal levels of eye contact. If you do not understand the message, say so.
- In the longer term patients may use artificial means of communication.
  - Oesophageal speech—pockets of air are retained in the oesophagus and forced into the mouth while words or syllables are mouthed.
  - Electrolarynx—a hand-held battery-operated device produces electronic vibrations that are placed on the throat and the patient forms words which the vibrations turn into sounds.
  - Tracheo-oesophageal puncture—a voice prosthesis is inserted into a surgically created fistula and the patient speaks by forcing air through the prosthesis into the oesophagus and into the mouth where words are formed. The vast majority of patients attain speech using this method.
- Speech and language therapists are essential to advise, support, and teach the patient and family.
- Give information about help and support groups.
- Provide written information as well as giving explanation and having discussions.
- Suggest the patient uses text messaging if possible, instead of phoning.

Nursing care of tracheostomy patients

Tracheostomy

This is an opening in the anterior wall of the trachea; it may be temporary or permanent to facilitate ventilation, e.g. reduce effort of breathing in respiratory failure, bypass upper airway obstruction, support assisted ventilation, and remove bronchial secretions.

Nursing care and overcoming problems

- Patient will be in a high-dependency area or ITU initially; closely monitor blood pressure, pulse, and respirations every 30 minutes to 1 hour.
- Prevent accidental extubation. Ensure tracheostomy ties are secured. Keep emergency equipment at hand—tracheal dilators, spare tracheostomy tubes (one same size and one smaller), suction and suction catheters, syringe, scissors, and stitch cutters if tracheostomy is stitched in. Tracheal opening is held open with dilators until the replacement tube is inserted.
- Suction if cough reflex is ineffective or secretions are thick. Choose correct catheter, Fg10–12 should be sufficient; use 80–120 mmHg pressure. Should be done only by experienced staff trained in technique. 📖 Tracheostomy suctioning, p.541.
- Provide artificial warmth and humidity. Initially humidified oxygen is given, then air can be provided through heat–moisture exchanger. This helps to prevent respiratory distress from inhaling cooled air and drying and thickening of mucus. Keep patient well hydrated and give saline nebulizers frequently.
- Reduce risk of infection. Follow a sterile or non-touch technique and hand decontamination for dealing with the tracheostomy and suctioning. Change humidification equipment daily. Monitor for signs of infection, take temperature, send swabs for culture as appropriate (e.g. secretions, wound). Ensure regular physiotherapy, change of position, and deep breathing to inflate lung bases.
- Perform wound care. Keep clean and dress with tracheostomy dressing to absorb drainage and prevent damage to neck tissue. Clean skin around tube with normal saline to prevent collection of secretion and soreness. Change tapes as necessary when soiled. May require two people to prevent accidental extubation and respiratory arrest. Teach patient self-care if permanent tracheostomy.
- Manage blocked airway, e.g. by mucus plug. Summon help urgently, use suction; if still not removed, deflate tracheostomy cuff with syringe to allow small volume of air to bypass. Give oxygen at 100%. Remove and replace tracheostomy tube by skilled practitioner.
- Provide pain relief. May be IV or through syringe pump for 1–2 days, then IM.
- Patient can mobilize from first postoperative day if fit.
- Diet and fluids to start as soon as patient is able.

Tracheostomy suctioning

Should only be undertaken by specially trained experienced professional.

Indications

- Ineffective cough or no cough (ventilated patient)
- Thick secretions
- Chest sounds wet or 'bubbly'
- Increased coughing and ineffective airway clearing

Catheter size

Should be no more than half the diameter of the inner lumen of the tracheostomy tube.

Suction pressure

- 80–120 mmHg
- If too low, suction is ineffective
- If too high, damage to mucosa, airway collapse, or ulceration may occur

Procedure

- Explain and reassure the patient as this can be a frightening procedure and it may make them cough.
- May need to pre-oxygenate with 100% oxygen to prevent hypoxaemia during the process.
- Use sterile technique with gloves, protective goggles, and mask.
- Use a fresh catheter each time and insert about 13 cm (approximately 6 inches) into the trachea. Do not apply suction during insertion, only on withdrawal.
- Time from insertion to removal of the catheter should be no longer than 10–15 seconds.
- Patient should rest between each suction application.
- Correctly dispose of the catheter.

Education for patients with nose and throat problems

- Use diagrams and models to help explain condition, procedures, and planned effects of treatment, care, and/or surgery.
- Provide written information to supplement verbal explanations.
- Discuss with patients what it is like to have bilateral nasal packs and the need for mouth breathing or loss of voice following tracheostomy and laryngectomy.
- Explain the importance of handwashing and other actions to prevent the spread of infection when administering nasal drops, changing tracheostomy tubes, etc.
- Teach the patient and/or carer how to undertake specific aspects of care, e.g. administer nasal drops, nasal sprays, care of tracheostomy.
- Advise on how to keep nose clean, e.g. use saline in a nasal spray to loosen dried mucus rather than picking and blowing, which may lead to damage or bleeding.
- Explain about pain, how it should diminish, and pain relief to be used.
- Explain 'what to do' and 'what not to do' to prevent complications.
  - Avoid alcohol for one week after polypectomy, nasal surgery, and tonsillectomy (causes vasodilation and risk of bleeding).
  - Use mouthwashes as well as brushing teeth to keep mouth clean and fresh to prevent infection and halitosis.
  - Drink fruit juices and water to ensure adequate hydration.
  - Do not allow water into stoma.
  - Protect scars with scarfs or sunblock.
- Encourage patient to ask questions and express fears and feelings about prognosis, care, and treatment.
- Ensure patient understands the use and effects of medication prescribed and any side effects.
- Ensure parents/carers know what to do in emergency situations, e.g. accidental extubation of tracheostomy tube, secondary bleeding following tonsillectomy.

Preventive education

- Suggest patients with recurrent nose bleeds and tracheostomy consider using humidifiers at home, especially when air is cold and dry, to prevent drying of mucosa.
- Advise patients to use protective equipment for sports to avoid head and nasal trauma.
- Advise patients and parents how to use digital pressure to stop nose bleeds.
- Ensure patients and parents understand why antibiotics are not prescribed in certain circumstances, e.g. in viral causes of sore throat, laryngitis.

Nasal douching

Aims to remove debris following surgery and keep nose and sinuses clean and healthy. Use the following solution:

- 1 teaspoon salt
- 1 teaspoon sugar
- Pinch bicarbonate of soda
- ½ pint tepid water

Procedure

- Put solution in a saucer or shallow bowl.
- Block off one nostril with a finger.
- Sniff up the solution into the other nostril.
- Let the solution run out.
- Sniff hard to clean out old blood clots or mucus.
- Continue until debris is no longer being washed out.
- Repeat on other nostril.
- Douche 3 times a day; then reduce as nose becomes clearer.
- Nose drops, if prescribed, should be taken after douching.

Discharge and continuing care for patients with nose and throat problems

- Follow the discharge process. 📖 Chapter 38, Discharge planning, p.1164.
- Check patient and/or carer:
  - Understands the specific ongoing care required, e.g. tracheostomy care.
  - Knows how to instill nasal drops, use nasal or throat spray.
  - Has medication, knows use and side effects, and where to get additional prescriptions.
  - Has specific written information relevant to their condition and discharge arrangements and support.
  - Knows action to take in the event of complications.
- Ensure patient education has been undertaken. 📖 Patient education for patients with nose and throat problems, p.542.
- Explain typical convalescence and when to resume activities. Varies with type of condition, age, and general condition.
  - Swelling, nasal obstruction, and discomfort subsides and sense of smell returns over 2 week period for nose operations.
  - Sore throat and discomfort following tonsillectomy returns over 2 weeks.
  - Return to work and school should be around 2 weeks; longer for tracheostomy and laryngectomy patients.
  - Advise to rest when tired.
- Arrange follow-up appointment with ENT, GP, specialist nurses, and speech and language therapist.
- Ensure patient and carer have information about local and national support groups, e.g. National Association of Laryngectomy Patients.
- Ensure patient is aware of support social workers can provide for people with communication problems.
- Advise patient on use of MedicAlert bracelet for stoma and need for resuscitation to be via stoma.
- Ensure patients with tracheostomy and/or laryngectomy have information on and/or appointments with agencies to support alternative means of communication.
- Ensure patient has contact number to ring for concerns and queries.

Common drugs used for ear conditions

All drug doses listed in this table are adult doses and not children's doses.

Table 14.1 Common drugs used for ear conditions

	Dose	Common side effects
Betamethasone drops	2–3 drops every 2–3 hours, reduce frequency when relief obtained	Few recorded
Steroid drops combined with antibacterial, e.g. Gentisone HC®, Predsol N®, and Sofradex®	2–4 drops 3–4 times daily (NB Gentisone HC is administered 3–4 times daily and at night)	Local sensitivity reactions
Cerumol® drops	Apply a generous amount (normally 5 drops) while patient lying down with affected ear uppermost for 5–10 minutes	Possible irritation
Betahistine tablets	Initially 16 mg 3 times daily preferably with food, maintenance 24–48 mg daily	Gastrointestinal disturbances, headache, rashes, and pruritus

Common drugs used for eye conditions

All drug doses listed in this table are adult doses and not children's doses.

Table 14.2 Common drugs used for eye conditions

Antibiotics	Dose	Common side effects
Chloramphenicol 0.5% drops	Apply 1 drop every 2 hours; reduce frequency as infection is controlled and continue for further 48 hours after healing	Transient stinging

Anti-inflammatory	Dose	Common side effects
Betamethasone	Apply 1 drop every 1–2 hours until inflammation is controlled, then reduce frequency	Potential 'steroid glaucoma' and/or 'steroid cataract' in susceptible patients; thinning of the cornea and sclera

Mydriatics/ cycloplegics	Dose	Common side effects
Cyclopentolate drops 0.5% and 1% Tropicamide drops 0.5% and 1%	Single or normally short-term use	Transient stinging, raised intra-ocular pressure; on prolonged administration local irritation, hyperaemia, oedema, and conjunctivitis may occur; toxic systemic reaction to cyclopentolate (and atropine eye drops) may occur in the very young and very old

Treatment of glaucoma	Dose	Common side effects
Beta blocker drops, e.g. betaxolol and timolol	Apply twice daily	NB Systemic absorption may occur, therefore see side effect profile (□ Table 7.1 Common drugs used for cardiovascular disorders: Beta blocker drugs, p.194); other side effects include ocular stinging, burning, pain, itching, dry eyes, erythema and allergic reactions
Prostaglandin analogue drops, e.g. latanoprost	Apply once daily in the evening	Brown pigmentation, blepharitis, ocular irritation and pain, darkening/ thickening/lengthening of eyelashes, conjunctival hyperaemia, transient punctate epithelial erosion, skin rash

Table 14.2 Common drugs used for eye conditions *(continued)*

Treatment of glaucoma	Dose	Common side effects
Dipivefrine drops	Apply twice daily	Severe smarting and redness of the eye (NB Use with caution in patients with hypertension and heart disease)
Acetazolamide tablets/capsules	0.25–1 g daily in divided doses	Nausea, vomiting, diarrhoea, loss of appetite, taste disturbance, paraesthesia, flushing, headache, dizziness, fatigue, irritability, depression, thirst, reduced libido, metabolic acidosis and electrolyte disturbances on long-term therapy
Pilocarpine drops	Apply up to 4 times a day depending on preparation used	Ciliary spasm leading to headache and browache which may be more severe in initial 2–4 weeks of therapy; ocular side effects include burning, itching, blurred vision, conjunctival vascular congestion, vitreous haemorrhage, papillary block and lens changes with chronic use
Tear deficiency	**Dose**	**Common side effects**
Hypromellose drops	Use hourly or as required	Few recorded

Common drugs used for nose, throat, and mouth conditions

All drug doses listed in this table are adult doses and not children's doses.

Table 14.3 Common drugs used for nose, throat, and mouth conditions

	Dose	Common side effects
Topical nasal decongestants	Ephedrine: 1–2 drops in each nostril up to 3–4 times daily when required Xylometazoline: 2–3 drops into each nostril 2–3 times daily when required; maximum duration 7 days	Local irritation, nausea, headache; after excessive use – tolerance with diminished effect, rebound congestion, and possibly cardiac effects
Pseudoephedrine	60 mg 4 times daily	Tachycardia, anxiety, restlessness, insomnia
Beclometasone	100 mcg (2 sprays) into each nostril twice a day; when symptoms controlled, 50 mcg (1 spray) 3–4 times daily; maximum 400 mcg (8 sprays) daily; when symptoms controlled, 1 spray into each nostril twice daily	Dryness, irritation of nose and throat, epistaxis; nasal septal perforation can occur usually following nasal surgery
Mupirocin nasal ointment NB Reserve for eradication of nasal carriage of MRSA	Apply 2–3 times daily to inner surface of each nostril for 5 days	Few recorded
Chlorhexidine and neomycin cream	Eradication of nasal staphylococci: apply to nostrils 4 times daily for 10 days Prevention of nasal carriage of staphylococci: apply to nostrils twice a day	Few recorded
Hexetidine, mouthwash/gargle	15 mL undiluted 2–3 times daily	Occasional numbness or stinging
Nystatin suspension	100,000 units held in mouth 4 times daily after food for 7 days (continue for 2 days after lesions resolved)	Oral irritation and sensitization; nausea also reported

Nursing patients with rheumatologic problems and connective tissue disorders

Metabolic bone disease

Osteoporosis

Osteoporosis is a systemic skeletal disease characterized by low bone density and micro-architectural deterioration of bone tissue that causes skeletal fragility and increases the risk of fracture. In the UK, one in three women and one in twelve men are likely to have a fracture due to osteoporosis by the age of 90 years. Osteoporosis can affect the whole skeleton but the wrist, hip, and spine are most frequently affected. It is estimated that it costs the NHS and government in the UK over £1.7 billion each year. Bone density can help to determine the risk of fracture and is measured by dual energy x-ray absorptiometry (DEXA).

Risk factors
- Female
- Early menopause (📖 Chapter 19, Nursing patients with reproductive and gynaecological needs, p.668)
- Smoking
- High alcohol intake
- Lack of exercise
- Thin (📖 Chapter 8, Nursing patients with nutritional and gastrointestinal needs, p.244)
- Family history
- Other factors include: rheumatoid arthritis (RA), thyrotoxicosis, amenorrhoea

Primary osteoporosis
Postmenopausal osteoporosis results from bone loss for 3–5 years after menopause due to a loss of oestrogen. Osteoporosis may also occur due to age related bone loss which can affect both men and women.

Secondary osteoporosis
Secondary osteoporosis accounts for 40% of cases in women and 60% of cases in men. Causes of secondary osteoporosis include:
- Thyrotoxicosis
- Primary hyperparathyroidism
- Cushing's syndrome
- Hypogonadism
- Malabsorption
- Liver disease
- Inflammatory arthritis, e.g. RA and ankylosing spondylitis
- Multiple myeloma
- Drugs, e.g. steroids and heparin

Investigations
- Spinal x-rays
- Bone densitometry (DEXA scan)

Tests to screen for underlying causes:
- Serum calcium, alkaline phosphatase, parathyroid hormone, and creatinine, U&E, and biochemical bone profile

- Serum protein electrophoresis and urinary Bence-Jones protein to exclude myeloma
- Thyroid stimulating hormone to exclude hyperthyroidism
- Serum testosterone to exclude hypogonadism in males

Prevention

Education about the risk factors related to osteoporosis should include:

- Ensure adequate intake of calcium.
- Avoid excessive alcohol.
- Discourage smoking.
- Encourage physical activity.
- Reduce the risk of falls by assessing mobility, eyesight, footwear, and home environment.
- Regularly assess the need for steroids.
- Monitor thyroid therapy to ensure the levothyroxine dose does not require reduction and to avoid over-replacement.

Drug treatments

- Antiresorptive agents are used to reduce fracture risk, e.g. bisphosphonates, calcium and vitamin D, calcitonin, and selective oestrogen receptor modulators.
- Parathyroid hormone injections are used to stimulate bone formation.
- Compound analgesia or low dose tricyclic antidepressants are used to reduce pain.
- Hormone replacement therapy is not now recommended as treatment for osteoporosis due to the affiliated risk of breast cancer and should be used to treat menopausal symptoms only after a full discussion with the patient about risks and benefits.
- Calcium supplementation.

Further information

Osteoporosis helpline: Tel: 01761 472721

Osteomalacia

This is a reversible metabolic disease in which there is a defect in the mineralization of bone. It is the adult equivalent of rickets or vitamin D deficiency in children. It is very rare in Western countries but may occur in older isolated people, in those who do not expose their skin to the sun, in those with liver disease, and as a response to some medications. An increase in vitamin D and calcium in the diet is encouraged, as is careful exposure to the sun and drug supplementation where necessary.

Paget's disease

This is primarily a disease of older age affecting bone turnover in which increased bone formation and reabsorption results in pain, bony enlargement, increased fracture risk, and risk of primary bone malignancy. It commonly occurs in the spine, femur, skull, sternum, and pelvis. The cause is unknown, but it has a tendency to occur in families. It occurs more frequently in Europe and less often in Asia and Scandinavia. Drug therapy includes analgesia or bisphosphonates depending on the severity of symptoms and bone involvement. Typical appearance on x-rays and scans indicates localized enlargement of bone.

Benign bone tumours

These tumours are often asymptomatic and discovered on routine x-ray examination or following a pathological fracture. Their cause is unknown. They are classified according to the type of tissue involved, e.g. osteochondroma from cartilage (most common) or osteoid osteoma, osteoblastoma from bone. Treatment includes drug therapy and surgical excision to the margins of the tumour, if benign.

Malignant bone tumours

A primary tumour originates in the bone; secondary tumours originate in other tissues and metastasize to the bone. The cause is unknown. Types of primary tumours include osteosarcoma, Ewing's sarcoma, and chondrosarcoma. Tumours are diagnosed by bone biopsy, x-ray, and CT scan. Treatment includes reducing the size of the tumour by chemotherapy and radiation. Surgical intervention includes reconstructive surgery and allografts or amputation if unamenable to limb-sparing surgery. Intractable pain is treated surgically with cordotomy (cutting of the spinal nerve roots). Cryosurgery may reduce pain and tumour size.

Osteoarthritis

Osteoarthritis (OA) was once thought of as a degenerative condition resulting from the ageing process. It is now known that OA involves a number of processes in which there is destruction of the joint cartilage with incomplete repair and formation of new bone (referred to as osteophytes or bony spurs). OA is the commonest condition to affect the synovial joints and is a major cause of disability. There are two types; primary and secondary. OA is classified as primary when there is no secondary cause. The latter can be caused by trauma or an inflammatory condition such as rheumatoid arthritis. The commonest age of onset is between 50 and 60 years and it occurs in more women than men. Osteoarthritis can affect any joint but areas commonly affected include the carpometacarpel of the thumb, specific finger joints (the distal phalangeal joints, DIPs), spine, and weight bearing joints (hips and knees). Table 15.1 summarizes the characteristics and treatment for osteoarthritis.

Signs and symptoms

Symptoms occur over time and consist of joint pain and stiffness which can restrict mobility and cause difficulties with everyday functions. Crepitus, bony enlargement, deformity, and a loss of function reflect structural changes. Inflammatory symptoms include warmth, effusion, and thickening of the synovium. If the patient is less able to use a particular joint, then muscle wasting can occur. Changes to the fingers can include Heberden's nodes of the DIPs and Bouchard's node of the proximal interphalangeal joints (PIPs). Fig. 15.1 shows common nodes and Fig. 15.2 shows joint deformities. Squaring of the thumb, known as a Z thumb, can also occur.

Diagnosis

Diagnosis is made by the identification of structural changes clinically or from a plain radiograph. X-ray changes include loss of cartilage, joint space narrowing, the presence of osteophytes, and sclerosis.

Nursing care

- Educate the patient about their condition.
- Ensure adequate pain management, including the use of analgesia such as paracetamol or topical NSAID creams.
- Encourage the patient to perform exercises to improve muscle strength, to reduce muscle wasting, and to maintain joint stability.
- Encourage use of deep and supportive footwear.
- Encourage weight reduction.
- Manage mood symptoms such as anxiety and depression.
- Consider intra-articular hyaluronic or corticosteroid injections.
- Consider joint replacement to reduce pain and improve mobility. Hip and knee replacements are highly effective.
- Surgical techniques include cartilage transplantation.

Key nursing interventions for patients with joint replacement

In addition to routine postoperative care (📖 Chapter 22, Nursing patients requiring perioperative care, pp.762–70), the following interventions are used for patients who have undergone joint replacement:

* Use special abduction pillows or splints to prevent abduction.
* Keep the patient's heels free from pressure.
* Monitor temperature and any signs of infection.
* Beware of postural hypotension when moving and mobilizing patient.
* Encourage early mobilization out of bed.
* Ensure effective pain relief is provided.
* Provide psychosocial support and monitor any signs of emotional upset or confusion.
* Support the physiotherapist in educating the patient regarding leg exercises and weight bearing, depending on operation and surgical instructions.
* Consider thromboprophylaxis if high risk.

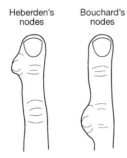

Fig. 15.1 Common nodes.

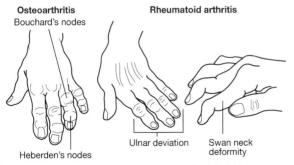

Fig. 15.2 Joint deformities. Reprinted from Hoeman S (2001). *Rehabilitation nursing*, p.143. Elsevier. Copyright (2001) with permission from Elsevier.

Rheumatoid arthritis

Rheumatoid arthritis (RA) is the commonest type of inflammatory arthritis. It occurs in 1–3% of the Western population and affects three times more women than men. It is a chronic, progressive, autoimmune, systemic, inflammatory condition that affects the synovial joints. Symmetrical swelling, pain, and tenderness of the peripheral joints of the hands and feet are the predominant features in the early stages. As the condition progresses other joints can also become affected. Extra-articular features can also occur. The cause of RA is unknown but there is a clear genetic link with infection, stress, trauma, and smoking acting as triggers. The condition commences in the synovial lining of the joint capsule, which becomes inflamed and congested with cells involved in the immune process. These cells (including B and T lymphocytes) attack the joint leading to erosion of the cartilage and bone. Table 15.1 summarizes the characteristics and treatment for RA.

Signs and symptoms

RA is characterized by active and latent periods of disease activity. When the condition is in an active phase the following symptoms are likely to be more intense.

- Pain and stiffness of the affected joints
- Fatigue
- Early morning stiffness
- Joint inflammation (heat and swelling)
- Inactivity stiffness occurring after periods of rest
- Extra-articular features include anaemia, muscle wasting, subcutaneous nodules, dry eyes and mouth, and vasculitis
- Also, systemic symptoms such as raised temperature and nausea.

Patients can experience a range of emotions including anxiety, anger, shock, and depression.

Diagnostic tests

No single test can diagnose RA. Investigations are used to support the clinical diagnosis based on the presence of symptoms already discussed. When considering rheumatoid arthritis, useful diagnostic tests include:

- High erythrocyte sedimentation rate (ESR) and C-reactive protein (CRP) levels usually reflect the degree of inflammation.
- Rheumatoid factor is positive in 70–80% of patients.
- X-rays: erosions are often seen in the metacarpophalyngeal joints. Findings of erosions in hands and feet are significant
- Joint aspiration: a large-gauge needle is inserted into a joint to acquire a sample of synovial fluid for analysis.

Treatment

RA can impact physical, psychological, and social function and management requires involvement of the multidisciplinary team.
- Drug treatment involves use of:
  - Symptom modifying agents including analgesics and NSAIDs
  - Disease-modifying drugs to induce remission, the commonest agents being sulfasalazine and methotrexate. (These drugs can be taken in combination.)
  - Biological agents for patients who do not respond to disease modifying drugs. (See NICE guidelines for specific details.)
  - Intra-articular and intramuscular steroids to provide temporary relief of active symptoms.
- Patient education particularly managing pain, stiffness, and fatigue.
- Joint protection techniques.
- Surgery for pain and reduced function.
- Physiotherapy and occupational therapy (will include regular exercise for joint health).
- Household aids and personal aids.

Nursing care

- Carry out a physical examination, noting which joints are inflamed or which joints the patient says are affected. Feel joints and note temperature.
- Record baseline observations.
- Assess and address any mobility problems.
- Assess and provide effective pain relief.
- Administer prescribed medication and observe for any side effects; educate the patient about possible side effects.
- Reinforce importance of therapeutic joint and muscle exercises; refer to the physiotherapist where appropriate.
- Assist the patient with any activities of daily living as necessary and encourage independence.
- Refer the patient to an occupational therapist for assessment for aids and/or adaptations in the home to maximize independence.
- Show empathy and understanding, and listen to the patient's worries and anxieties.

Table 15.1 Characteristics and treatments of osteoarthritis, rheumatoid arthritis, and juvenile arthritis

Osteoarthritis	RA	Juvenile RA
Onset		
Usually women ≥40 years	Can begin at any age; both sexes, usually between 20–50 years	Both sexes <16 years
Types of disease		
Localized and degenerative	Systemic and inflammatory	Systemic and inflammatory
Typical joints affected		
Weight-bearing joints, e.g. pelvis, spine	Multiple joints, e.g. hands and fingers, shoulders	One or more joints, often large ones
Non-pharmacological treatment		
• Mobilization of affected area by gentle moderate exercise; swimming can be useful • Hot and cold therapy • Sometimes surgery, e.g. arthrodesis, arthroscopy	• Immobilization of affected joints during acute flare-ups • Splints can be worn to give support to joints • Hot and cold therapy • Hydrotherapy • Sometimes surgery, e.g. arthroplasty	• Rest periods and exercise within comfort zone • Physiotherapy

Systemic lupus erythematosus

Systemic lupus erythematosus (SLE) is one of the most common connective tissue disorders. It is a multi-systemic, autoimmune condition of unknown cause with a wide variety of manifestations. The condition is characterized by the development of auto-antibodies, deposition of immune complexes, and raised anti-native DNA antibody binding. The condition is more common in women and black people.

General symptoms

- Fatigue
- Skin rashes: butterfly rash of the face (raised red rash that can be itchy, sore, and sensitive to sunlight) and discoid lesions (red plaques that become thick and scaly)
- Hair loss
- Arthritis
- Joint and muscle pain that is rarely destructive
- Ulcers on the mouth and vagina
- Raynaud's phenomenon
- Weight loss
- Pleurisy
- Vasculitis such as nail fold lesions
- Psychiatric features such as depression, paranoia, and fits

Other systems can become affected including the chest, heart, nervous system, and kidneys. Kidney and central nervous system involvement are associated with a poor prognosis. Certain drugs can cause a type of SLE in individuals with a genetic predisposition to the condition. Diagnosis is complex and is based on the presence of a number of clinical symptoms and immunological events such as raised anti-native DNA antibody binding.

Treatment

Treatment depends on which systems are affected. Patients may require referral to other hospital specialists (e.g. dermatologist or renal physician).

- Topical cortisone creams help reduce inflammation of skin and redness.
- Analgesia and NSAIDs are used to relieve joint pain.
- Anti-malarial medication such as hydroxychloroquine help with joint pain.
- Steroid therapy can be used in low doses to reduce the activity of the condition.
- Immunosuppressive agents such as azathioprine or methotrexate are used as steroid sparing agents. Mycophenolate mofetil reduces disease activity and cyclophosphamide is used in patients who have vasculitis or renal disease. Regular blood tests are needed to monitor potential side effects of these medications.
- Raynaud's phenomenon is treated with calcium channel blockers and local nitrate creams if the symptoms are mild to moderate. If severe, intravenous epoprostenol infusions can be used.
- Skin should be protected from exposure to sunlight. Sun should be avoided or sunscreen should be used.

Nursing care

- Perform a physical examination, noting any skin rashes or blemishes, shininess, and tautness.
- Ask the patient about any joint or muscle pain.
- Ask the patient to describe their symptoms.
- Record baseline observations.
- Perform a urine dipstick and MSU.
- Teach the patient to avoid exposure to solar radiation.
- Teach the patient to assess their skin for changes—any skin ulcers should be treated according to type and location.
- Encourage wearing of gloves and keeping hands warm, where Raynaud's phenomenon is present.
- Give prescribed medication, observing for side effects, and educate patient about possible side effects.
- Refer patient to occupational therapist or physiotherapist if indicated for further assessments.

Further information

Lupus UK, St James House, Eastern Road, Romford, Essex RM1 3NH www.lupusuk.org.uk

Other connective tissue diseases

Polymyositis

This is characterized by weakness of the proximal muscles due to inflammation. If accompanied by a skin rash the condition is classified as dermatomyositis. The peak age of onset is between 30 and 60 years. Symmetrical wasting and weakness of the limb girdle muscles is common which restricts movement. Joints can become painful and swollen. Muscle weakness can result in respiratory failure. Diagnosis is made by a muscle biopsy, electrophysiological studies, and the presence of elevated muscle enzymes (creatine kinase) and serum inflammatory markers. Management involves the use of high dose steroids (up to 60 mg daily). If remission does not occur with steroids alone, then disease modifying drugs are used, e.g. azathioprine or methotrexate. Biologic therapy may also be useful. Exercises help to improve muscle weakness.

Polymyalgia rheumatica

This is a common condition of older people that causes pain and stiffness in the neck, shoulder, and proximal limb muscles. Other symptoms can include fatigue, fever, and weight loss. The female-to-male ratio is 2:1 and diagnosis is by an elevated ESR and CRP (📖 Chapter 39, Common laboratory tests and their interpretation, p.1167). Polymyalgia rheumatica can be associated with giant cell arteritis, which can affect the temporal artery and lead to blindness. Steroids are used to reduce the inflammation. In some rare cases if the symptoms are slow to subside, disease modifying drugs are used, e.g. azathioprine or methotrexate. The condition can resolve after 2 years.

Giant cell (cranial/temporal) arteritis (GCA)

This is associated with polymyalgia in 25% of people. It is common in older people and is rare in people <55 years. Symptoms include headache, scalp and temporal artery tenderness (e.g. on combing hair), and sudden blindness in one eye. Treatment must be prompt and includes prednisolone. Temporal artery biopsy is performed. Patients go into periods of remission approximately every 2 years. Osteoporosis prophylaxis is essential. 📖 Metabolic bone disease, p.550.

Spondyloarthropathies

Ankylosing spondylitis

This causes inflammation of the axial skeleton (sacroiliac joints and vertebral column). The condition affects three times more males than females and is associated with the gene HLA B-27. The inflammation causes bone erosion and bone fusion resulting in pain, stiffness, and reduced mobility in the spine. Sleep is often disturbed. As the stiffness progresses body posture alters as it becomes more difficult to straighten out the spine. Eye symptoms can occur such as iritis and conjunctivitis. Patients with an aggressive condition can also experience pulmonary fibrosis and aortic incompetence. Regular exercise is essential to maintain movement of the spine and hips. Drug therapy involves the use of NSAIDs, disease modifying drugs, and biological agents. (See NICE guidelines for specific details.)

Reactive arthritis

This type of arthritis results from exposure to sexually transmitted disease or a GI infection. It commonly affects the knees, ankles, and feet which become red, painful, and swollen. The triad of arthritis, conjunctivitis, and urethritis is commonly known as Reiter syndrome. Males and females are equally affected. It mainly occurs in patients who are between the ages of 16 and 35 years, and in one third of patients no infectious cause is found. Symptoms generally resolve over 3–6 months but can become chronic. Treatment may include:

- Analgesia and NSAIDs
- Antibiotics to treat infection
- Disease modifying drugs to treat the arthritis
- Steroid injections to affected joints
- Exercises to improve muscle strength
- Rest
- Splinting the affected joint

Psoriatic arthritis

This is a chronic inflammatory arthritis and is associated with the presence of psoriasis in 75% of cases. The usual age of onset is between 20 and 50 years. Clinical features include inflammation of the finger joints (DIPs and PIPs), enthesitis (inflammation of the site of insertion of the tendon or ligament into bone), spinal pain, swollen and red toe (known as sausage toe), and the presence of psoriasis. One third of patients have some eye involvement. Treatment is similar to RA and includes NSAIDs to reduce pain and stiffness and disease modifying drugs or biologic agents to reduce disease activity (methotrexate can work on both the arthritis and the psoriasis). Specific treatment for the psoriasis may involve the dermatologist.

Crystal arthropathy gout

Gout is a disorder characterized by monosodium urate crystal deposits mainly in joints (notably in the foot), which cause inflammation. Hyperuricaemia (high levels of urate in the blood) makes gout more likely to occur.

Presentation

Gout often affects men who are between 40 and 50 years, and affects females later in life. Acute attacks of gout present suddenly with severe pain most commonly in the big toe, though the ankle, knees, wrist, and hands can be affected. Episodes of flares and remission result in chronic gout, particularly when hyperuricaemia is not controlled.

Clinical features

- Swollen joint(s), often with accompanying redness
- Constant and severe pain in the affected joint(s)
- Tophi (nodular swellings) on the fingers, toes, and ears which can produce a chalky exudate

Causes

- Acute illness, e.g. infection
- Trauma
- Excessive alcohol intake
- Obesity
- Hypertension
- Drugs that alter plasma urate concentration (e.g. salicylates, thiazides, furosemide and pyrazinamide)
- Starvation

Management

- Avoid excessive alcohol.
- Drug management includes the use of NSAIDs and colchicine to treat acute attacks. Allopurinol is used to reduce hyperuricaemia, but must not be started until at least 10–14 days after an acute attack.
- The joint can be injected with steroid if the use of NSAIDs or colchicine is contraindicated, although this is rare.

Pseudogout

Pseudogout occurs when calcium pyrophosphate crystals are deposited in the joints. The knee is the most commonly affected joint and other joints including shoulders, wrists, elbows, hips, and ankles can also be involved. The condition can be acute with attacks lasting for months and recurrence can lead to chronic disease. Management involves aspiration and injection of affected joints with steroids. Oral steroids can be used for short periods.

Bone infections

The most common type of bone infections are osteomyelitis, septic arthritis, and tuberculosis (TB) of the bone.

Osteomyelitis

This is a term used to describe any infection of the bone. There are two types of osteomyelitis.

- *Acute*: symptoms include fever (temperature above 38°C), swelling and heat around affected area, reddening of the skin, tenderness, and pain.
- *Chronic*: symptoms include ulceration of the skin, sinus tract formation, pain, and drainage or discharge from affected area.

Osteomyelitis is treated by drug therapy (IV antibiotics), good wound and infection control care, and surgery (drainage of the abcess).

Septic arthritis

This refers to infection in a joint caused by osteomyelitis tracking into a joint, a penetrating wound, or bacteraemia from a distant source of infection or recent surgery. The symptoms are a hot, swollen, red, and painful joint that the patient is reluctant to move. Treatment includes intravenous antibiotics, arthroscopy, or open surgery to drain the joint. Late detection of septic arthritis or poor management leads to destruction of the joint and a reduction in mobility.

Tuberculosis (TB)

TB usually occurs in the lungs but may spread, especially to the vertebral column. It develops slowly and symptoms may not be present at first. Local tenderness may occur. Diagnosis is by blood tests, X-ray, and MRI. Treatment is by drug therapy. Surgery may be necessary as TB can cause vertebral collapse and even paralysis. Spinal fusion may be necessary.

Common drugs used for rheumatologic problems and connective tissue disorders

Common drugs used for rheumatologic and connective tissue disorders are listed in Table 15.2. **All drug doses listed in this table are adult doses and not children's doses.** This table is only to be used as a guide and the current BNF should be consulted for further advice. Nurses should involve themselves only in the administration of medications which fall within their sphere of competence.

Table 15.2 Common drugs used for rheumatologic problems and connective tissue disorders

Gout	Dose	Common side effects
Colchicine	For treatment of gout – initially 1 mg then 500 mcg no more frequently than every 4 hours until pain relieved or vomiting/diarrhoea occur; maximum 6 mg per course; course not to be repeated within 3 days	Nausea, vomiting, abdominal pain; excessive doses may cause profuse diarrhoea, gastrointestinal haemorrhage, rashes, renal and hepatic damage
Allopurinol	Initially 100 mg daily preferably after food, then adjusted according to plasma or urinary uric acid concentration; maintenance dose 100–200 mg daily in mild conditions, 300–600 mg daily in moderate conditions, 700–900 mg daily in severe conditions; doses over 300 mg daily given in divided doses	Rashes (withdraw therapy though if mild re-introduce gradually – discontinue immediately if recurrence); hypersensitivity reactions occur rarely (See BNF for further details and more side effects)

Rheumatoid arthritis	Dose	Common side effects
Methotrexate	7.5 mg once weekly (as a single dose normally of 3 × 2.5 mg tablets) adjusted according to response, maximum total weekly dose 20 mg	Mucositis, myelosuppression, anorexia, abdominal discomfort, intestinal ulceration and bleeding, diarrhoea and many more (See BNF)
Hydroxychloroquine	Administered on expert advice; initially 400 mg daily in divided doses, maintenance 200–400 mg daily; maximum 6.5 mg/kg but not exceeding 400 mg daily	Gastrointestinal disturbances, headache and skin reactions (rashes, pruritus); many more less common side effects (See BNF)
Sulfasalazine	Administered on expert advice and normally as enteric coated tablets; initially 500 mg daily, increased by 500 mg at intervals of a week to a maximum of 2–3 g daily in divided doses	Rashes, gastrointestinal intolerance, and occasional leucopenia, neutropenia, and thrombocytopenia; hypersensitivity reactions ⮡ Table 8.4 Common drugs used for gastrointestinal disorders: Sulfasalazine, p.264

Nursing patients with haematology problems

Nursing assessment of patients with haematology problems

In addition to a general nursing assessment (📖 Chapter 3, Individualizing nursing care practice, pp.32–33) perform the following procedures.

Observe the patient

- Skin and mucous membranes for pallor, slight jaundice, bruising, ulcers, and dryness
- Nails for changes (brittle, spoon-shaped in iron-deficiency anaemia)
- Hair for texture and condition
- Mouth for painful cracks, infections (angular stomatitis, glossitis, *Candida*), bleeding gums, and taste changes
- Temperature, pulse, respiration (infection, cardiac failure, shock), and weight
- Urine volume, colour, and presence of blood

Ask the patient about

Nursing history
- Ability to manage self-care
- Skin and hygiene needs, normal mouth care, and recent problems
- Problems with mobility
- Dietary assessment including type and quality of diet, problems with food intake or appetite, and special diets (e.g. vegetarian)
- Weight changes
- Normal bowel habits and any changes in bowel habits
- Alcohol consumption and smoking
- Menstrual cycle problems
- Bleeding and bruising
- Sweating
- Recent long-distance travel or immobility
- Ability to cope
- Feelings and worries about the condition
- Dependants and carers at home
- Normal lifestyle and priorities for the patient, including hobbies and usual daily activities, to help establish the potential impact of the illness on patient's lifestyle

Medical history
- Malabsorption disorders
- Renal conditions
- Gastric or bowel disorders and surgery
- Pancreatic and blood disorders (e.g. sickle cell disease or coagulation disorders)
- Family history of blood disorders
- Inherited and autoimmune diseases
- Treatments such as radiation, transfusions

Current problems
- Tiredness or lethargy
- Headaches

- Dyspnoea
- GI bleeding
- Haematuria
- Menorrhagia
- Epistaxis
- Pregnancy
- Bone pain or abdominal pain
- Nausea and vomiting
- Infections
- Neurological problems, e.g. numbness, paraesthesia, or recurrent infections
- Usual current daily activities that have been impacted by the current problem

Medications and allergies
- Aspirin or other pain relievers
- Iron and vitamin supplements
- Anticonvulsants and sulfasalazine (folate deficiency)
- Antibiotics, e.g. penicillin and cephalosporins
- Oral contraceptives
- Steroids
- Anticoagulants
- Over-the-counter medications or herbal remedies
- Any known allergies

Understanding of the condition, treatment options (risks, benefits, side effects), and prognosis. Asking the patient about their understanding helps identify their needs.

Tests and investigations

Laboratory tests
- Haemoglobin (Hb)
- White blood cell count (WBC)
- Platelets
- Coagulation screen
- Erythrocyte sedimentation rate (ESR)
- Mean corpuscular volume (MCV)
- Packed cell volume (PCV)
- Other blood tests:
  - Haematinic assays (serum ferritin, vitamin B_{12}, folate)
  - U&E, liver function tests
  - Immunoglobulins
  - Direct antiglobulin test
  - Paraprotein (serum and urine)
  - Specific factor assays to differentiate types of haemophilia
  - DNA tests to detect genes for factor VIII and factor IX
  - Grouping and cross-matching for blood transfusions

  📖 Chapter 39, Common laboratory tests and their interpretation, p.1167.

Bone marrow examination
Bone marrow examination provides a great deal of information about blood-forming tissue and is useful for diagnosing haematologic disorders. Bone marrow examination may be performed by aspiration or biopsy. Aspiration involves inserting a needle into the marrow to obtain a liquid sample of marrow and biopsy involves using a specialized needle to remove a core of the marrow. The most common site for the procedure is the posterior or anterior iliac crest.

Nursing care of patient undergoing bone marrow aspiration or biopsy
- Ensure patient understands the procedure, the purpose, risks, and benefits of the procedure.
- Encourage patient to ask questions and express feelings or concern about the procedure.
- Ensure the patient has given written consent.
- Give analgesic or sedative as instructed before the procedure. (May not be necessary for aspiration.)
- Ask the patient to lay on the abdomen (prone) or on the side with top knee flexed.
- Ensure the patient is given an explanation of what is to take place.
- Reassure the patient during the procedure.
- Following the procedure, apply pressure dressing and watch for bleeding and haematoma formation.

Other investigations
- Barium studies
- Endoscopies
- Faeces for occult blood
- Sigmoidoscopy, if bleeding
- Chest and abdomen x-rays

Nursing problems

Problems associated with anaemia
- Fatigue
- Headache
- Shortness of breath, especially on exertion
- Dizziness
- Palpitations
- Brittle spoon-shaped nails (koilonychia)
- Pica (eating abnormal substances, dirt, coal, ice)
- Peripheral neurological problems, e.g. numbness and tingling in pernicious anaemia
- Loss of appetite
- Inability to perform daily activities
- Inability to work, which may impact financial and social aspects of the patient's life as well as the physical

Risk of infection
Infection risk is directly related to the severity and duration of neutropenia. Several factors can increase the risk:
- Impaired immune response due to underlying bone marrow disease
- Immunosuppression as a result of radiotherapy, chemotherapy, or steroid therapy
- Multiple invasive procedures
- Poor nutrition
- Known previous infection, e.g. varicella zoster virus, fungal infection

Bleeding
Haemorrhagic problems occur as a result of both disease and treatment. They may be chronic and more easily controlled or may be acute and potentially life threatening. Bleeding may be due to low platelet count, platelet dysfunction, erosion of a blood vessel, or coagulation disorders.

Nausea and vomiting
Nausea and vomiting are side effects of chemotherapy and radiotherapy and lead to dehydration, poor nutrition, low morale, and poor concordance with treatment.

Oral problems
These include pain, discomfort, infection (e.g. fungal, bacterial, and viral), bleeding, glossitis, and stomatitis. They are caused by the disease, treatment, and side effects. Patients may experience potential taste changes.

Malnutrition
Anorexia, oral and gastrointestinal complications of treatment, and abnormalities of glucose, fat, and protein metabolism contribute to malnutrition.

Psychological problems

These include grief, fear, loneliness, anger, powerlessness, depression, despair about the prognosis and treatment, and fear of dying. Low self-esteem and poor self-image may occur in relation to hair loss, skin and nail changes, and features of the disorder and treatment. Patients may experience a loss of role and independence.

Lack of knowledge

Lack of understanding about the disorder, treatment, or prognosis may result in anxiety and inability to make decisions about and participate in managing their own care.

Anaemia

Anaemia is a decrease of Hb in the blood below the normal range for the age and sex of the individual.

Anaemia due to blood loss

- Causes include trauma, gynaecological problems (e.g. menorrhagia), GI bleeding, haematuria, and bleeding disorders (e.g. coagulation problems, haemophilia, von Willebrand's disease).
- Acute haemorrhage produces hypovolaemia, shock, and hypoxia.
- Treatment is by replacement of fluid (IV infusion or blood transfusion depending on severity). Anaemia occurs when blood plasma volume returns to normal, often after several hours or days. Red cells are normal size and colour. If bleeding is stopped and iron stores are sufficient, red cell concentration is normal within 3–4 weeks.

Anaemia due to increased destruction of red blood cells

- Premature destruction of red blood cells.
- May be due to disorders of structure or synthesis of Hb, deficiencies in enzymes, and cell membrane.
- Hereditary factors
  - Haemoglobinopathies (e.g. sickle cell, thalassaemia, 🕮 Sickle cell disease, p.580)
  - Cell membrane defects (e.g. spherocytosis)
  - Enzyme defects (e.g. glucose-6-phosphate dehydrogenase deficiency)
- Causes of acquired haemolytic anaemia
  - Immune and autoimmune factors (e.g. drugs, chemicals, toxins, infections, snake venom, prosthetic heart valves)
  - Obstruction in the microcirculation (e.g. thrombocytopenic purpura)

Anaemia due to reduced red cell production

Reduced proliferation

- Iron deficiency anaemia due to inadequate iron for red cell formation is commonest type.
  - Hb <9–10 g/dl blood.
  - Symptoms include tiredness, headaches, breathlessness, dizziness, tachycardia, palpitations, spoon-shaped nails, angular stomatitis, smooth sore tongue, and dysphagia.
  - Treatment includes dietary advice and iron supplements.
- Macrocytic anaemias, e.g. B_{12} (pernicious anaemia) or folate deficiency.
  - May be caused by diet (e.g. vegan), malabsorption, renal loss, and drugs.
  - Treatment is with B_{12} replacement (hydroxocobalamin) or folic acid. The underlying cause should be corrected where possible.
- Bone marrow disease—aplastic anaemia due to exposure to radiation, chemicals, infections and toxins, leukaemia, cancer.
  - Symptoms include weakness, fatigue, pallor, bruising, petechiae, GI bleeding.
  - Treatment includes blood transfusion, bone marrow transplant, and immunosuppressive therapy.
- Blood disorders, e.g. myeloproliferative disorder, myelodysplastic syndrome.

Nursing care of patients with anaemia

A detailed patient assessment may help identify the cause of anemia.

Patient support

This will vary depending on the severity of the anaemia.

- Encourage the patient to rest.
- Assist the patient with self-care deficits (e.g. hygiene, mouth care).
- Monitor the patient for improvement or deterioration.
- Observe for pallor, breathlessness, and bleeding.
- Manage blood product transfusions, use of growth factors, and oral therapy.
- Discuss the patient's concerns and wishes.
- Check for evidence of iron deficiency, e.g. ferritin, folate, and B_{12}.

Education and information

The aim is to relieve anxiety and to encourage the patient to take responsibility for their care and to be able to make decisions about treatment options.

- Give information about the investigations, blood tests, and bone marrow samples, including interpretation of the results.
- Ensure that patients understand their anaemia, i.e. what may have caused it and how it might affect their future lifestyle.
- Provide patients with written information.

Dietary advice

A general healthy balanced diet is necessary to reduce the risk of anaemia. A full nutritional assessment is required and specific dietary advice is necessary depending on the cause of the anaemia. This must be linked to patient's likes and dislikes and examples of menus might be helpful.

- *Iron deficiency:* Advise patients and their carers on foods that are rich in iron, e.g. meat, lentils, hazelnuts, apricots, whole grain rice, spinach, prunes. Explain that vitamin C enhances iron absorption and advise on where it is found, e.g. oranges and tomatoes. Explain that iron absorption is decreased by antacids, tetracyclines, and phytates (found in chapatti flour).
- *B_{12} deficiency:* Advise that vitamin B_{12} is found in fish, meat, eggs, and milk. Vegans are at particular risk and usually need to take supplements.
- *Folate deficiency:* Advise that folate is found in liver, yeast extract, and green vegetables.

Dietary supplements

- *Iron supplements:* usually ferrous fumarate or ferrous sulphate. Injections of iron can also be given. Ensure patient has information on side effects of oral iron (i.e. nausea, vomiting, abdominal discomfort, constipation, diarrhoea, black stools) and of IM and IV injections (i.e. thrombophlebitis, hypotension; should not be given to patients with asthma).
- *B_{12}:* IM hydroxocobalamin. Advise the patient that the injections are needed because the vitamin cannot be absorbed orally. Explain that continuing treatment can help reverse the symptoms and stop deterioration.
- *Folic acid:* orally 5 mg daily.

Sickle cell disease

This is a group of blood disorders where patients inherit sickle Hb, which has a different structure to normal Hb. The Hb becomes rigid and elongated with reduced elasticity. These deformed cells block small blood vessels, causing damage to tissues and organs and resulting in recurrent and unpredictable pain (crisis). It is most prevalent in Caribbean and African people and in some from the Mediterranean and Middle East.

- HbSS (sickle cell anaemia)—haemolytic anaemia with fatigue, breathlessness, mild jaundice, and risk of severe infection, e.g. pneumococcal septicaemia. Crises are common.
- HbSC (HbSC disease)—mild anaemia, retinopathy, and fewer crises.
- SB Thal (sickle beta thalassaemia)—variable degrees of anaemia and possibly splenomegaly.
- HbAHbS (sickle cell trait)—less than half the Hb carries the sickle trait (HbS); therefore carriers are normally not anaemic and have no clinical abnormalities.

Sickle cell crisis

- Takes varying forms and may be triggered by:
  - Respiratory or GI infections
  - Dehydration
  - Alcohol
  - Menstruation
  - Anaesthesia
  - Severe hypoxia due to shock
  - Vigorous exercise at high altitude
- Results in:
  - Severe bone, joint, and abdominal pain
  - Hand and foot syndrome (swelling and pain)
  - Acute chest syndrome (chest pain, pleurisy, and shortness of breath)
  - Priapism
  - Stroke
  - Aplastic crisis (reduction in bone marrow production)
  - Splenic and liver sequestration (enlarged due to pooling of blood)
  - Gallstones
  - Chronic leg ulcers
  - Renal failure
  - Depression and isolation in some cases

Nursing support and advice

- Ensure patient understands the nature of the disorder, treatment, and complications.
- Help the patient identify factors that exacerbate the condition and ways to avoid these.
- Give advice about immunization and prompt treatment of infections.
- Monitor temperature for signs of infection, blood pressure and pulse for signs of shock (indicates sequestration), respiratory rate, and oxygen saturation.

- Provide support for the patient during a crisis by assessing pain and administering:
  - Analgesics (may be done using PCA and checking effectiveness)
  - IV fluids to reduce blood viscosity
  - Oxygen therapy to reduce hypoxia
  - Antibiotics for infections
  - Blood transfusions, if prescribed (may be done if Hb is ≥2 g/dl below normal but depends on symptoms and how well the anaemia is tolerated)
- Give hydroxycarbamide to reduce painful crises and complications.
- Observe for complications, monitor urine output, and dress leg ulcers.
- Discuss concerns with patient and encourage them to express feelings, e.g. effects on development, relationships, working life, and life expectancy.
- Ensure access to specialist nurses, if available, to discuss treatment and care options.
- Discuss the value of premarital and early pregnancy screening.
- Ensure patient is aware of the significance of good oral fluid intake, keeping warm during cold weather and the need for rest in order to reduce the risk of developing a sickle cell crisis.

Coagulation disorders

Acquired coagulation disorders

These include vitamin K deficiency (in GI malabsorption), liver disease and cirrhosis (synthesis of coagulation factors, thrombocytopenia), renal disease (platelet dysfunction), and amyloidosis (acquired factor X deficiency).

Disseminated intravascular coagulation (DIC)

This is caused by shock, sepsis, and malignancy, and results in depletion of clotting factors and platelets leading to thrombocytopenia, increased bleeding tendency, and loss of haemostasis. The patient may become acutely unwell with fever, acidosis, and hypoxia, and end-organ failure may occur from widespread thrombotic damage. Treatment is aimed at managing the underlying disease as well as restoring and maintaining circulation with plasma products and heparin to control thrombotic formation.

Congenital disorders

Haemophilia

Haemophilia A and haemophilia B (Christmas disease) are congenital bleeding disorders caused by deficiencies of factor VIII and factor IX, respectively. They are inherited but rare diseases and may be mild or severe. Family history may or may not be known. Diagnosis is usually before 9 months of age. Patients present with more bruising than would be usual for age. Less common symptoms include bleeding into joints, which become hot, swollen, and painful with reduced range of movement and deformity; haematuria; and petechial haemorrhage. It is always worth checking clotting screen with or without an ultrasound or CT scan.

Treatment

- Factor VIII or factor IX
- Clotting factor concentrates from plasma
- Genetically produced recombinant factors VIII and IX
- Deamino-D-arginine vasopressin desmopressin for mild haemophilia A only
- Tranexamic acid (antifibrinlytic drugs)
- Pain relief
- Prophylaxis is with factor VIII three times and factor IX infusions twice a week
- Resting joints and avoiding weight-bearing until acute bleed recovers
- Pressure and elevation for minor bleeding (avoid NSAIDs and IM injections)

von Willebrand's disorder

This is a common inherited disorder and most cases are mild. It may present with nose bleeds, bleeding following dental treatment, surgery, and, in females, menorrhagia or childbirth. There is profuse bleeding from cuts. Treatment includes desmopressin (IV or SC infusion or intranasal spray), tranexamic acid, or blood products with von Willebrand factor.

Nursing role in patients with coagulation disorders

Ensure patient and/or parents:

- Understand the nature of the disease, treatment, risks, and complications (bloodborne viruses hepatitis A, B, C, HIV).
- Are able to recognize early signs of bleeding.
- Can administer treatment and prophylactic regimen via an implantable central subcutaneous access system, if possible at home, to prevent spontaneous bleeding and minimize long-term disability, disruptions to school, employment, and home life.
- Have access to specialist nurses and centres to provide specialist education, e.g. physiotherapy to prevent articular contractions.
- Receive information on support groups.
- Receive advice on vaccinations (hepatitis A and B) and wearing alert bracelets.
- Are given treatment before invasive or dental treatment is performed, as described above.
- Have emergency contact numbers and know what to do in case of an emergency.

Venous thromboembolism (VTE)

This is the blocking of a blood vessel by a clot that has been dislodged from its site of origin. It includes deep vein thrombosis (DVT), which is a venous thrombosis in the deep veins of the legs and pelvis, and pulmonary embolism (PE), which occurs when a clot breaks off and travels round the circulation to block the pulmonary arteries. VTE has high mortality rate—25,000 deaths in England occur from VTE arising during hospital care, annually.

Risk factors
- Immobility (bed rest, long-haul flights)
- Acute illness
- Malignancy
- Pregnancy and caesarean section
- Thombophilia
- Increasing age and obesity
- Contraception
- Hormone replacement therapy (HRT)
- Previous DVT
- Smoking
- Dehydration (leads to hypercoagulation)
- Surgery, especially orthopaedic surgery

Presenting symptoms

Approximately 50% of patients with DVT are asymptomatic.
- Abnormal calf swelling/oedema and increased warmth of the affected limb
- Lower limb pain
- Dilation of the veins
- Colour changes of the leg (e.g. pallor, redness)
- Pyrexia

Patients with PE may present with:
- Dyspnoea or tachypnoea
- Pleuritic chest pain
- Haemoptysis

Diagnostic tests
- Ultrasound doppler to measure venous flow
- Plethysmography to detect obstruction to venous flow
- Haematology screening to detect the fibrin degradation product (D-dimer assay)
- Chest x-ray and ECG
- Venography to detect a thrombus using radio-opaque IV injection is rarely done

Prevention
- Identify patients at risk—all patients should have risk assessment.
- Stop contraceptive pill prior to planned surgery.

- Administer prophylactic anticoagulation, e.g. aspirin, low-dose unfractioned heparin, synthetic pentasaccharide, oral anticoagulants (warfarin), dextrans.
- Recommend use of anti-embolism stockings.
- Recommend use of intermittent pneumatic devices, e.g. foot pumps.
- Vena cava filters may be inserted by radiologists.
- For patients planning long-haul flights—recommend exercise, avoiding alcohol and dehydration, and using compression hosiery, if appropriate.
- Nursing measures include early mobilization, foot elevation, and hydration.

All the above are subject to review by NICE.

Treatment

- Anticoagulation therapy, e.g. heparin (low-molecular-weight heparin [LMWH] followed by warfarin)
- Physiotherapy
- Use of compression hosiery
- Observation for signs of complications, e.g. bleeding due to anticoagulation (gums, bruising, intracranial, joints, muscle), signs of PE (📖 Chapter 6, Patients with respiratory needs p.118; Chapter 16, Presenting Symptoms, p.584.
- Nursing care (📖 Nursing care of patients with VTE, p.586).

Nursing care of patients with VTE

- Perform a risk assessment using a local risk assessment tool that includes such aspects as information about the patient's gender, age, build, BMI, mobility, past medical history, family history, trauma risk factors, surgical interventions (planned or recent past), specific risk category (e.g. pregnancy), contraceptive, thrombophilia, specific high risk disorders, haemolytic anaemias, myocardial infarction, malignancy, CVA, and varicose veins.
- Observe the patient for signs of DVT. 📖 DVT, p.184.
- Check for signs and symptoms of VTE. 📖 VTE, p.584.
- Ensure anti-embolism stockings are used.
- Follow guidelines to accurately measure and fit anti-embolism stockings to knee or thigh length. Teach the patient how to use the stockings and caution them that they must not be rolled down as this can cause a tourniquet effect on the femoral circulation and cause a DVT. Teach the patient how to fit the stockings, and their care. Nurses should be trained in fitting these for patients.
- Ensure anticoagulation is carried out appropriately and the patient understands the use and benefits of the medication and, if on heparin, understands that they should contact their physician if they:
  - have chest pain or shortness of breath
  - injure themselves, especially eyes, joints, and head
  - cut themselves and bleed heavily
  - have severe nose bleeds
  - develop bruises
  - vomit blood or coffee-ground vomit
  - pass blood in the urine or the stool becomes black (melaena)
  - have a sudden deterioration in health
  - have heavy menstrual periods.
- Ensure early ambulation following operations and encourage mobility as far as is possible. Liaise with physiotherapy to implement a programme of activities.
- Watch for PE. First presentation may be shortage of breath or leg tenderness.
- Provide patients with information including written materials to help reinforce verbal information.
  - *Lifestyle information*: Encourage a balanced healthy diet, low in fat (avoid saturated fat in particular) to help keep cholesterol levels down and reduce the risk of blood clotting. Explain why reduction of dairy products, fried foods, cakes, and biscuits is necessary.
  - Advise on how to lose weight, if obese.
  - Encourage exercise, particularly regular gentle exercise, as part of daily routine.
  - Encourage reduced alcohol consumption and smoking cessation. Provide information and contact details on who can help with this.
  - *Specific information*: Teach about clinical condition, treatment, prognosis, and provide contact numbers for specific health and advice.
- *Listen to patients*: Encourage them to verbalize their fears and concerns and to ask questions.

Leukaemia

This is a neoplastic disorder of the blood-forming tissues. Some genetic disorders including Down syndrome, radiation, chemicals (e.g. cigarette smoke, benzene), drugs (e.g. choramphenicol, phenylbutazone, and chemotherapy), and viruses (HTLV-1) may carry an increased risk.

Acute leukaemia

Acute leukaemia is a clonal (derived from a single cell) malignant disorder resulting in the proliferation of immature blast cells in the bone marrow and other body tissue resulting in bone marrow failure. There are two common types: acute myeloid leukaemia (AML), commonest in adulthood, and acute lymphoblastic leukaemia (ALL), commonest in those aged 2–10 years and over 40 years.

Features: It is always serious and life-threatening. It usually presents with a short history of anaemia (tiredness, pallor, lethargy, dyspnoea), neutropenia (bacterial infections of mouth, throat, skin and chest), thrombocytopenia (bruising and bleeding), bone pain, splenomegaly, hepatomegaly, headache, nausea, vomiting, and blurred vision.

Investigations: These include FBC, coagulation and biochemical screen, chest x-ray, bone marrow aspiration, and cytogenetics. Acute leukaemia may also be detected during a routine blood test as part of a routine health check.

Treatment: Immediate referral to a specialist is necessary for prompt diagnosis and treatment with chemotherapy aimed at achieving remission by eradicating leukaemic cells from bone marrow and allowing regeneration of normal marrow. Supportive care includes management of bleeding and infection, and minimizing toxicity of treatment. Bone marrow transplantation or peripheral stem cell transplant may be necessary to reduce the risk of relapse.

Chronic leukaemia

The predominant cell appears mature though the function is abnormal. The most common types are chronic lymphoblastic leukaemia (CLL), often picked up on a routine blood test. Patients are susceptible to infections. Chronic myeloid leukaemia (CML) is divided into chronic phase and accelerated phase (acute transformation to acute leukaemia).

Features: Symptoms include anaemia, pallor, weight loss, sweating, haemorrhage (bruising, purpura), splenomegaly, and, more rarely, gout, retinal haemorrhage, and fever.

Investigations: These include FBC, neutrophil alkaline phosphatase, U&E, bone marrow aspirate, and serum lactate dehydrogenase.

Treatment: Choice of treatment for CLL includes fludarabine and cyclophosphamide; or single agent fludarabine; or chlorambucil and prednisolone; or rituximab. Treatment for CML includes imatinib or dasatinib. Allogenic stem cell transplantation and autologous stem cell transplantation are also a consideration. FBC is monitored; prophylactic antibiotics may be considered.

Nursing support and advice for patients with leukaemia

- Spend time with the patient and family to develop an effective relationship; encourage them to express their fears and feelings about the diagnosis, treatment and prognosis; and answer questions as honestly as possible. Continue this throughout the treatment.
- Provide the patient with written information about the disease and treatment to supplement discussions and provide contacts where they can get additional information and access support groups such as:
  - British Association of Cancer United Patients (BACUP)
  - Leukaemia Research www.lrf.org.uk
  - Leukaemia Care
- Provide supportive care.
  - Provide hygiene and skin care, especially mouth care and prevention of pressure damage.
  - Prevent and detect early signs of infection—observe for fever, take temperature and pulse, ensure aseptic techniques, reverse barrier nursing if required, administer IV antimicrobial agents as prescribed.
  - Detect bleeding—check for signs of bruising, bleeding in the gums, nose bleeds, administering blood or blood product transfusions.
  - Ensure the patient has adequate fluids and nutrition.
  - Help the patient cope with the side effects of treatment, e.g. nausea and vomiting, hair loss, neuropathy.
  - Give prescribed pain relief.
- Ensue the patient has access to specialists in the multidisciplinary team including nurse specialists, dietitians, social workers, and clinical psychologists.
- Make referrals to palliative care specialists, when appropriate.
- If patients are considered for a clinical trial, ensure they have sufficient information to make an informed decision.
- Ensure patients have the chance to consider sperm or egg banking prior to commencement of chemotherapy.

Lymphomas

These are a diverse group of diseases caused by malignant lymphocytes that commonly accumulate in lymph nodes. They may infiltrate organs outside the lymphoid tissue. There are two main types which derive from T-cell or B-cell lineage.

Hodgkin's lymphoma

This is characterized by the presence of a 'Reed–Sternberg cell' which studies suggest is often derived from a B cell. It has a high cure rate especially when it occurs in younger patients and when diagnosed early. Epstein-Barr virus is detected in more than 50% of cases. It is often classified into five subtypes.

Clinical features: There may be no symptoms and the lymphoma is picked up at routine examination. Otherwise, symptoms may include painless swelling of the lymph nodes in the neck, axilla, or groin and enlargement of the liver and spleen. At a later stage, recurrent fever, night sweats, weight loss, anaemia, and severe fatigue may occur. These are known as B symptoms. Very severe itching and pain in the affected nodes on drinking alcohol is less common.

Investigations: These include blood tests that show anaemia, leucocytosis, ESR; chest x-ray; CT scan; bone marrow biopsies; and fine-needle, incisional, or excisional biopsy of affected tissues. Assessment of B symptoms is also important.

Treatment: Radiotherapy for stage I and IIa Hodgkin's disease may be curative. Cyclical combination chemotherapy is used for stage III and IV.

Non-Hodgkin's lymphoma (NHL)

This includes all other types of lymphoma (i.e. all lymphomas without presence of a Reed–Sternberg cell). There are more than 20 subtypes and therefore NHL represents a very diverse group of diseases. The incidence has increased dramatically in the last 20 years.

Risk factors: Contributing factors include acquired or inherited immune deficiencies; organ transplantation; HTLV-1 virus; exposure to radiation, pesticides, herbicides, and chemicals (e.g. benzene, creosote, formaldehyde); and previous treatment with cytotoxic drugs.

Clinical features: These are similar to Hodgkin's lymphoma. Clinical features reflect the spectrum from low grade to high grade disease. Superficial lymphadenopathy is common and is dependent on how aggressive the disease is. Symptoms may progress slowly or rapidly. Involvement of the GI tract is a feature of some subtypes of NHL. B symptoms may be present. The bone marrow may be involved and there may be symptoms of anemia, neutropenia with infections, or thrombocytopenia.

Investigations: These are as above and include cytogenetics in specific cases.

Treatment: This is determined by histology and progression. For low grade, slow growing NHL, the disease is monitored but treatment is not commenced until the patient has symptoms. The aim is palliative rather than curative. For high grade bulky disease with B symptoms, treatment is commenced promptly as these may be aggressive tumours that may become rapidly fatal. Intensive combination chemotherapy and maybe a monoclonal antibody therapy are used to achieve a cure.

Bone marrow and haemopoietic stem cell transplantation (HSCT)

Bone marrow

- Bone marrow transplant has been considered as a treatment for benign conditions, e.g. sickle cell anaemia and polycythemia vera, but is rare. Bone marrow transplants are commonly used for malignant diseases, e.g. leukaemia, myeloma, and lymphoma.
- Recipients are exposed to a range of life-threatening procedures including total body irradiation and high-dose chemotherapy to ablate their own bone marrow. Healthy marrow is then infused to engraft over a period of weeks.
- Types of transplant include:
  - Syngeneic transplants between twins—the bone marrow is identical.
  - Allogeneic transplants—cells are transferred from a donor to the patient. Donors are usually human leucocyte antigen (HLA) compatible siblings or unrelated HLA-matched donors.
  - Autologous transplants—uses the patient's own cells. The cells may be taken when the patient is in remission. It is considered simpler and safer than allogeneic transplant, but there is a risk of relapse of the original disease.
- Risks to patients include potentially fatal infections, haemorrhage, mucositis and parotitis, nausea and vomiting, diarrhoea, alopecia, skin rash, graft versus host disease or graft rejection (in allografts), pulmonary complications, secondary malignancies, psychological problems, reduced quality of life, fear of dying, and survivor guilt.

Haemopoietic stem cell transplantation (HSCT)

HSCT may be used as a treatment for malignant disorders (e.g. lymphoma, leukaemia, myeloma, and occasionally for non-malignant conditions such as beta thalassaemia major). There are two major types of HSCT: autologous and allogeneic transplants. Bone marrow transplantation may also be of low intensity, known as mini-transplantation.

The risks to patients from these procedures include mucositis, vomiting, diarrhoea, skin rashes, infection, bleeding, alopecia, graft versus host disease, and graft rejection. Longer-term consequences include pulmonary complications, secondary malignancies, endocrine dysfunction, and psychosocial/psychosexual problems.

Autologous transplants

These use patient's own haemopoietic stem cells that have been harvested when patient is in remission. It allows the dose of chemotherapy (sometimes with radiotherapy) to be intensified so that chemosensitive disease is potentially eradicated. These doses of treatment also eliminate all normal bone marrow which is then reconstituted by the infusion of the previously harvested stem cells. Autologous transplantation is generally safer and less immunosuppressive than allogeneic transplantation, although the risk of relapse of the original disease remains.

Allogeneic transplants

These use haemopoietic stem cells from a healthy donor. The donor may be a genetically identical twin (syngeneic transplant), an HLA-matched sibling, or an HLA-matched unrelated donor. Allogeneic transplants are more risky to undertake because of the potential for immunological interactions between the immune systems of the host and the donor, leading to either graft rejection or to graft versus host disease. The chances of the original disease relapsing are lower because of the potential for a graft versus tumour effect. Immunosuppressive drugs are used to modulate this interaction between the two immune systems and therefore the risks of serious infections are increased.

Blood transfusion

Principles for the use of blood and blood products

- All organizations should have written policies and procedures that are communicated to staff for the prescribing, cross-matching, sample collection, issue, collection, and administration of blood. They are usually in line with the National Blood Service (NBS) guidance and British Committee for Standards in Haematology (BCSH) guidance.
- Staff should be trained and updated annually to follow these procedures.
- Blood should be prescribed on the treatment sheet and indicated in the patient's notes by the medical practitioner, stating rationale for transfusion.
- Patients should be given written and verbal information about the risks and benefits of the procedure and observations to enable them to provide informed consent.
- A registered practitioner should check the blood for transfusion, check the identity of the patient, check the prescription chart and the compatibility report, and document the details of the transfusion. The checking procedure should be done in accordance with local policy (some organizations operate one person checking procedure in line with NBS guidance, and some organizations continue to use two person checking procedure).
- Observe the patient's blood pressure and pulse at least prior to, after 15 min of, and at the end of the transfusion. The patient must be observed and checked for adverse reactions, e.g. fever, chills, rigors, itching, back or chest pain, dyspnoea, restlessness (📖 Action in the event of an adverse transfusion reaction or incident, p.595). Blood transfusion observation must be recorded in line with local policy.
- Ensure that only blood transfusion administration sets are used, that the rate of transfusion is calculated accurately, that specific instructions are followed (e.g. transfuse through a blood warmer), and that blood is stored at the correct temperature.
- Attach biohazard labels to all high-risk samples and place in a sealed plastic specimen bag.
- Ensure all used bags of blood are disposed of correctly.

Risks of blood transfusion

- Human error and failure to comply with policies, e.g. inaccurately completing samples, inadequate safety checks prior to starting transfusions, collecting the wrong unit of blood, failing to verify the patient's identity at the bedside correctly, and failing to label the sample at the patient's bedside.
- Laboratory errors, e.g. use of incorrect sample, release of wrong unit from the bank.
- Failure to recognize adverse reactions and follow appropriate actions.
- Contamination of blood products, e.g. variant Creutzfeldt–Jakob disease, HIV, hepatitis C (although very rare due to the testing for this at the NBS level).

- Inadequate systems, e.g. out-of-date policies and procedures for checking and administering blood.
- Inadequate communication and education and updating of staff in new procedures.
- Under-reporting of errors and failure to act on incidents, alerts, and errors.

Action in the event of an adverse transfusion reaction or incident

Follow local policy, but general guidance is as follows:
- Observe patient for signs of adverse reactions to blood transfusion, e.g. flushing, urticaria, vomiting, diarrhoea, fever, itching, headache, haemoglobinuria, pain at transfusion site, rigor, severe backache, collapse, or circulatory failure.
- Stop the blood transfusion; take down unit of blood and giving set. Check the unit of blood is the correct blood for the patient, i.e. right blood, right patient. The cannula should be kept *in situ* and the line kept open with 0.9% saline, through a new giving set.
- Notify the doctor immediately and contact a haematologist for advice.
- Record pulse, blood pressure, temperature, and oxygen saturation levels at least hourly.
- Send blood to the laboratory for coagulation screen, FBC, U&Es, LFTs, and a specimen of urine to check for haemoglobinuria.
- IV piriton and hydrocortisone may be given.
- Carefully document all aspects of the event in the patient's notes including the amount of blood transfused and the symptoms of the transfusion reaction.
- Complete an adverse incident form giving the full details of the incident. It should be subsequently investigated to determine the cause and lessons to be learned. 'Near miss' incidents should also be reported. These should be submitted to the Hospital Transfusion Team and Transfusion officer and Blood Bank. Serious incidents should be reported to SHOT (Serious Hazards of Transfusion) — the UK body for reporting incidents involving blood and blood products.

Patient education

Blood disorders may persist over months or years, may be characterized by periods of remission and relapse, may require prolonged periods of treatment, and may affect the quality of the patient's and family's life. Education is required to help promote concordance with the treatment and to enable the individual to manage and take control of their disorder. Education can help the patient have a good quality of life and support the family and patient in managing the disorder. For some patients the prognosis will be poor and the opportunity to discuss reduced life expectancy and death must be provided.

- Explain the disorder, tests and investigations, treatment, and prognosis. Provide written information to supplement this.
- Help patients cope with symptoms, e.g. the need to prioritize activities to conserve energy if they have fatigue and shortness of breath, maintaining a balance between rest and activity. Utilize the vast number of specific charitable organizations such as Leukaemia Research and Myeloma UK. Use assessment tools for monitoring symptoms such as the Functional Assessment of Cancer Therapy (FACT) assessment tool. Inform patients how to access programmes that help patients and family take control.
- Know what complications to watch out for, e.g. signs of bleeding (haematuria, bruising), signs of infection (e.g. fever, sweating), oral problems, signs of DVT, skin irritation; know what action to take; and know what complications to report to the physician/nurse.
- Know first aid measures to take, e.g. for nose bleeds.
- Ensure the patient and family have contact numbers of who to contact in an emergency if they are concerned.
- Avoid triggers, e.g. that give rise to sickle cell crisis or that result in venous thromboembolism.
- Ensure the patient understands impact of food and can adapt this for home use on a daily basis.
- Ensure the patient is able to carry out treatments, e.g. give IV clotting factor, apply anti-embolism stockings correctly.
- Prevent and control infection, e.g. by handwashing; daily hygiene; clean clothing; keeping the mouth clean; using aseptic techniques when dealing with equipment, lines, and dressings; and ensuring food is cooked properly and fruit and vegetables are washed thoroughly.
- Improve understanding of the prescribed medication, the importance of concordance, effects of non-concordance, and side effects, e.g. chemotherapy, anticoagulants, antimicrobials.
- Provide general healthy lifestyle information including exercise, diet, smoking cessation, and reducing alcohol consumption.
- Know where and how to get additional information. 📖 Discharge and continuing care, p.598.
- Advise patients on how to manage hair loss related to chemotherapy, e.g. not perming or colouring the hair for 3–6 months after treatment is finished, using a high-protein shampoo during treatment, and keeping the use of a hair dryer to a minimum.

- Advise patients on specific side effects of chemotherapy, e.g. fatigue, nausea, change of urine colour, etc.
- Know how to access specialist education from members of the multidisciplinary team, e.g. nurse specialist, dietitian, psychologist, haematologist, and oncologist.

Discharge and continuing care

Treatment and follow-up for many patients continues over periods o months and years, and most units will provide an 'open door' policy fo patients to contact them with concerns, advice, and support. Therefore discharge planning needs to focus on continuing care and follow-up Arrangements will vary depending on the patient's condition and treatment plan.

* Ensure the patient and family:
  * have been given sufficient information (📖 Information for patients with haematology disorders, p.599) to manage at home
  * have the contact information of the unit, the GP, and other relevant practitioners
  * have access to members of the multidisciplinary team post-discharge, e.g. dietitian, specialist nurse
  * have appointments made for follow-up care, e.g. attendance at the unit for chemotherapy or radiotherapy unit
  * understand the probable course of treatment, convalescence, and return to activities and work, if appropriate
  * have information about local and national support groups
  * have the necessary supplies of drugs and know where to get further supplies
  * can manage the care they should carry out when at home
  * understand the need to avoid people with infections if they are immunocompromised.
* Check that all arrangements have been made for any aspect of home care and that the patient has relevant contact numbers.
* Arrange for patients with similar conditions who are coping well with the treatment to visit and talk to the patient.
* Ensure that discharge summaries are communicated to colleagues in primary care, e.g. GP and other care sectors as appropriate.

Information for patients with haematology disorders

- Anaemia—bookmark site about anaemia   www.anemia.co.uk
- The Aplastic Anaemia Trust   www.theaat.org.uk
- Bone Marrow Transplantation Support Group   www.bmtsupport.ie
- Cancer BACUP   www.cancerbacup.org.uk
- The Haemophilia Society   www.haemophilia.org.uk
- Leukaemia Research   www.lrf.org.uk
  www.nursing-leukaemia.org.uk
- Children's Leukaemia   www.leukaemia.org.uk
- Lymphoma Association   www.lymphoma.org.uk
- National Institute for Health and Clinical Excellence (NICE)   www.nice.org.uk
- Sickle Cell Society   www.sicklecellsociety.org
- United Kingdom Blood Transfusion and Tissue Transplantation Guidelines   www.transfusionguidelines.org.uk
- United Kingdom Thalassaemia Society   www.ukts.org
- Myeloma UK   www.myeloma.co.uk

Common drugs used for haematological disorders

Common drugs used for haematological disorders are listed in Table 16.1 **All drug doses listed in this table are adult doses and not children's doses**. This table is only to be used as a guide and the current BNF should be consulted for further advice. Nurses should involve themselves only in the administration of medications which fall within their sphere of competence.

Table 16.1 Common drugs used for haematological disorders

Anaemia	Dose	Common side effects
Ferrous sulphate	Prophylaxis: 200 mg daily with or after food Treatment: 200 mg 2–3 times daily with or after food	Gastrointestinal irritation, nausea and epigastric pain are dose related; constipation or diarrhoea
Hydroxocobalamin injection (vitamin B_{12})	Initially 1 mg IM 3 times a week for 2 weeks, then 1 mg IM every 3 months	Nausea, headache, dizziness, fever, hypersensitivity reactions including rash and pruritis; injection site pain; hypokalaemia during initial treatment
Folic acid	Initially 5 mg daily for 4 months, then 5 mg every 1–7 days depending on underlying disease	NB should *never* be given alone for pernicious anaemia or other vitamin B_{12} deficiency states

📖 Table 11.1 Common drugs used for renal and urinary disorders: Erythropoietin, p.392.

Plasma expanders	Dose	Common side effects
Plasma substitutes, e.g. etherified starch	Hexastarch – IV infusion 500–1000 mL, usual daily maximum 1500 mL	Hypersensitivity reactions may occur including, rarely, anaphylactoid reactions; transient increase in bleeding time may occur; other side effects of hexastarch include raised serum amylase and pruritus

Drugs used in neutropenia	Dose	Common side effects
Filgrastim	Dose varies according to condition being treated See BNF	Gastrointestinal disturbances (nausea, vomiting, diarrhoea), anorexia, headache, asthenia, fever, rash, musculoskeletal pain, bone pain, alopecia, injection site reactions, leucocytosis

Drugs used in leukaemia: 📖 Table 25.6 Common drugs used for cancer care, p.854.

Nursing patients with orthopaedic and musculoskeletal trauma problems

Overall aims of nursing care

Orthopaedic and trauma nursing involves the care of patients who have dysfunction of the musculoskeletal system. This dysfunction may be due to a chronic musculoskeletal condition that requires surgery (e.g. osteoarthritis that leads to total hip replacement) or may be due to an injury sustained by accident (e.g. injury occurring during a sport or leisure pursuit). Some of the commonest types of injuries occur due to accidents while working, especially in heavy industry; while traveling, such as road traffic accidents; and while performing do-it-yourself jobs in the home environment. Regardless of the cause of the condition or injury, fundamental principles of nursing care and the overall aims are the same.

• Prevent further damage.
• Promote healing.
• Reduce the risk of complications.
• Maximize independence.
• Promote rehabilitation.

Nursing assessment of patients with orthopaedic and musculoskeletal trauma problems

Whether a patient is entering hospital for a planned (elective) orthopaedic procedure or because they have sustained a musculoskeletal injury nursing assessment issues are similar. In addition to a general nursing assessment (📖 Chapter 3, Individualizing nursing care practice, pp.32–33) perform the following procedures. Assessment of musculoskeletal problems is shown in Fig. 17.1.

- Observe the patient carefully, paying particular attention to how the patient walks or moves about.
- Ask the patient about their condition, especially movement and mobility issues or past trauma.
- Ask the patient to describe characteristics of their pain including its location, nature (e.g. stabbing, aching), and factors that increase (e.g. movement) or relieve the pain (e.g. medication, walking aids, heat/cold therapy). Use a pain assessment tool. 📖 Chapter 23, Nursing patients with pain, pp.794–98.
- Note the appearance of the affected limb or joint. Is there an obvious wound or deformity?
- Evaluate the function of the affected limb or joint, including peripheral neurovascular status. Can the patient still use the arm or leg? How does the function of the affected limb compare with that of the other? What effects might any loss of function have on activities of living?
- Note whether the patient is using any aids for mobilizing, resting, or protecting a damaged limb (e.g. walking sticks, frames, slings, or supports for the upper limb).
- Identify medical conditions that may relate to the current problem, e.g. a bone fracture following a low-impact injury may suggest osteoporosis and requires investigation and treatment.
- Review all medications the patient is taking and determine whether any of the medications may relate to the current problem, e.g. patients on warfarin may bleed into a joint, causing pain and reduced mobility.
- A specialist orthopaedic nurse practitioner, physiotherapist, or physician may assess range of movement of a joint by using a special instrument called a goniometer.
- Review the patient's past history. Previous injury in or near a joint may lead to osteoarthritis in the joint later in life.
- Review the patient's family history. Some musculoskeletal diseases such as rheumatoid arthritis can be inherited.
- Assess the psychosocial effects of the disease or injury. Patients undergoing an orthopaedic operation such as a hip replacement will have lived with their arthritis for many years and may have adjusted to the condition. Patients who have sustained musculoskeletal trauma such as a fractured neck of femur will be facing a situation that they have not had time to adjust to. In both situations the impact of the injury or surgery on the patient's social situation and psychological state must be evaluated. This includes assessment of likely discharge needs.

Assess the patient's knowledge about their injury or orthopaedic condition and surgery.

Consider the age of the patient and the possible changes to the musculoskeletal system due to the effects of chronic disease processes and the fitness/mobility of the patient. Older patients may have decreased activity and range-of-motion restrictions, decreased bone density leading to the greater potential for fractures, metabolic bone disease such as osteoporosis, increased bony prominences leading to the potential for skin breakdown, loss of muscle tone, cartilage degeneration, and posture problems.

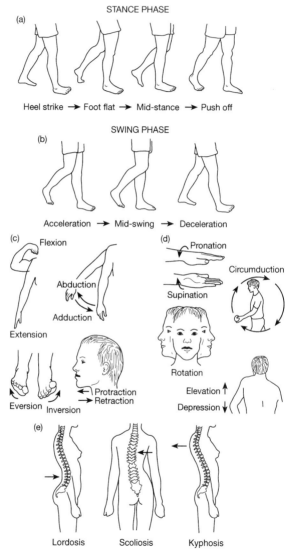

Fig. 17.1 Assessment of musculoskeletal problems.

Common orthopaedic and trauma nursing problems

- Management of pain from joint, bone, muscle injury, or chronic impairment and surgery.
- Impaired mobility leading to potential complications such as pressure ulcer development.
- Maintenance of therapeutic immobilization (i.e. preventing excessive movement of affected limb). This involves properly managing casts, traction, external fixators, and safely moving patients following internal fixation of fractures.
- Potential neurovascular complications including venous thrombo-embolism (VTE), specifically deep vein thrombosis (DVT), and pulmonary embolus (PE).
- Ischaemia of the muscles, e.g. compartment syndrome.
- Infection of surgical wounds, open fractures, or skeletal pin tracks.
- Self-care deficits and limitations in normal activities of daily living.
- Maintenance of usual bowel habits and prevention of constipation due to impaired mobility and medications such as analgesics.
- Body image and self-esteem disturbances due to loss of function, disability, and deformity.
- Lack of knowledge of injury or surgery, leading to patient's inability to contribute to their care and recovery.
- Loss of independence due to reliance on others for help with personal self-care, leading to difficulties in meeting family, social, occupational, and individual obligations in life.
- Social isolation resulting from lack of mobility and activity.
- Mood changes and, eventually, depression due to severe disruption in lifestyle caused by chronic orthopaedic conditions or major trauma.

Diagnostic tests

X-rays are the primary test used to identify fractures, dislocations, and joint disease such as osteoarthritis. Two projections are necessary to ensure that the three dimensional nature of the bone or joint is considered, usually anteroposterior and lateral. Patients should be warned that the x-ray table may be hard and that they must lie still while the x-ray is being taken. If necessary, analgesia can be given before sending a patient to x-ray.

Ultrasound (sound waves) may be used to detect a DVT, a soft tissue lesion such as a muscle fibre tear in the shoulder (rotator cuff tear) an abscess or mass, a joint effusion (collection of fluid), and haematoma.

Computed tomography (CT) scan produces multiple x-rays that a computer uses to produce a three dimensional image of a bone, joint or fracture. Although the scan itself takes only a few minutes, the entire process may take up to 1 hour as the patient has to be carefully positioned.

Magnetic resonance imaging (MRI) uses magnetic fields rather than x-rays to generate an image. MRI can show details that are not visible on x-ray, in particular the spinal column, joint and muscular abnormalities, bone tumours, and soft tissue masses. MRI machines are similar to long narrow tunnels and some patients find them very claustrophobic. The patient must be able to lie still in supine position for up to an hour or more.

Bone scans involve intravenous injection of radio-isotope (technetium) prior to the scan. Bone is scanned for the presence of metastatic disease, tumours, bone infections (osteomyelitis), and other inflammatory changes such as loosening of a hip or knee replacement. The scan is performed in two stages that are several hours apart and patients should be aware of this.

Nerve conduction studies are conducted to identify damage to peripheral nerves, both motor and sensory. Small electrodes are placed on the skin over the muscles being tested and a small electrical current is delivered to the skin, causing the nerves to fire. The electrical signals produced by nerves and muscles are detected by a computer. The stimulator produces only a very small shock that does not cause damage to the body.

Electromyogram (EMG) involves inserting a small needle into a muscle to detect the electrical activity and any muscle or nerve damage. EMG is used to diagnose conditions such as carpal tunnel syndrome.

Arthroscopy involves inserting a small camera device into a joint. It enables diagnosis of the joint problem and biopsy or therapeutic surgery to be performed at the same time.

Laboratory tests

- Biochemical bone profile (serum calcium, phosphate and alkaline phosphatase)
- Serum U&E to assess renal function and FBC to exclude anaemia and infection
- Urine Bence-Jones protein (BJP) and serum protein electrophoresis to exclude myeloma
- Erythrocyte sedimentation rate (ESR) and C-reactive protein (CRP) as markers of inflammation or infection
- Serum creatine kinase (CK) as a marker of muscle inflammation or breakdown

📖 Chapter 39, Common laboratory tests and their interpretation, p.1167.

Musculoskeletal trauma: principles

The most common causes of musculoskeletal trauma are road traffic accidents (RTAs), work related accidents, and sports injuries. Musculoskeletal trauma is one of the primary causes of disability in the UK and around the world. It can range from a simple muscle strain to multiple fractures and soft tissue damage. It may pose a threat to life, place the limb at risk, and interfere with eventual return to full function and activity/mobility.

Initial assessment

Musculoskeletal injuries may not be the priority in terms of immediate treatment, as life-threatening injuries may be present but more hidden elsewhere in the body. Therefore, it is essential that the 'ABC' system is used to assess the patient and life-threatening injuries are systematically ruled out first. Examples of life-threatening complications associated with musculoskeletal traumas include:

- Femoral artery damage with pelvic or femoral fractures
- Contaminated wounds
- Concealed haemorrhage
- VTE (☐ Orthopaedic complications, p.624)
- Fat embolism
- Sepsis, e.g. gangrene, streptococcal sepsis, and tetanus

Principles of fracture treatment

Most patients in hospital with musculoskeletal trauma have sustained a fracture of a bone. Fractures can be classified as closed (i.e. there is no break in the skin) or open (i.e. the skin is broken and the fracture ends may be exposed) (See Fig. 17.2 and Fig. 17.3). Patients often believe fractures and breaks to be different entities, whereas they are the same.

Regardless of which bone is affected, from the smallest finger to the pelvis, the three principles of medical treatment and nursing care are the same.

- *Reduce the fracture* – The bone ends must be as close as possible so that healing can take place. This can be achieved by traction or by open reduction (exposing the fracture in theatre so that the ends can be put together).
- *Maintain position* – A fracture takes 6–12 weeks to heal, depending on its type and position. Throughout this period, the bone ends must be kept in a good position. This can be achieved by traction, a cast, external fixation, or internal fixation.
- *Restore function* – This refers not only to the rehabilitation of the affected limb when a cast or traction is removed, but also to helping the patient to maintain function in joints and limbs not affected by trauma. For example, patients with a below-elbow cast for a wrist fracture should be taught and encouraged to perform exercises to ensure that they retain movement of the elbow and shoulder joints.

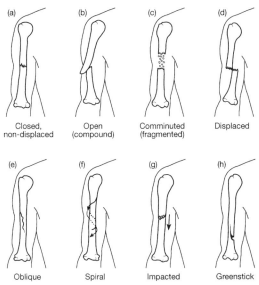

Fig. 17.2 Different types of fracture.

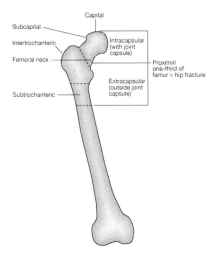

Fig. 17.3 The femur, showing sites of fractures.

Key nursing tasks and interventions for orthopaedic/trauma patients

- On admission, record:
  - Pain assessment
  - Vital signs and oxygen saturation
  - Pressure ulcer prevention score
- Apply anti-embolic stockings and assess/reduce the risk of VTE.
- Take an MRSA screen if joint arthroplasty is being considered; if patient has prior hospital admission; or if patient is high risk or is a nursing home resident (☐ Chapter 20, Nursing patients with infectious diseases, p.695).
- Determine the category for risk of falls and implement appropriate interventions.
- Assess the risk of peripheral neurovascular deterioration by checking skin colour, pulse, and sensation. Reduce risk by encouraging patient to verbalize unusual feelings in traumatized limb.
- Assess for ischaemia of the muscles and possibility of compartment syndrome (☐ Compartment syndrome, p.624).
- Follow relevant integrated care pathway.
- Monitor and manage pain.
- Monitor and manage bowels and bladder function.
- Assess and manage nutrition and hydration.
- Observe and care for surgical wound.
- Encourage mobility and movement—especially if bedbound.
- Encourage deep breathing and coughing, consider an incentive spirometer.
- Assess patient's level of communication, comprehension, and orientation.
- Liaise and reinforce teaching of the physiotherapist on the use of appliances/mobility aids for the patient and family, e.g. crutches, zimmer frame, and wheelchair.
- Liaise with the multidisciplinary team with regard to arrangements for return home or convalescence.

Musculoskeletal trauma: care— traction and casts

Care of patients with traction

Traction occurs when a pulling force is applied to one or more parts of the body, either manually or by the use of skin or skeletal traction (See Fig. 17.4). Counter traction is also necessary, which is usually supplied by the body weight of the patient. Manual traction is used only for short-term traction, such as when manipulating a wrist fracture in the emergency department before applying a cast.

Nursing management for patients with skeletal or skin traction
- Ensure care of the traction equipment.
  - Check at least once per shift, or after a patient has been moved in bed, that the traction cord is running smoothly and that the weights are hanging freely and not touching the floor or the bed.
  - Elevate the foot of the bed to provide counter traction.
- For patients with skin traction, remove the bandaging at least once per day to check integrity of the skin underneath. Incorrect and excessive weight being applied via skin traction (> 5 lb) can cause severe damage to the skin.
- Manual traction (i.e. pulling on the limb) may be necessary while adjusting the traction apparatus. If bandaging has slipped, reapply it immediately or tissue may become damaged.
- Monitor for the complications of DVT or compartment syndrome.
- The patient will be on prolonged bed rest with all the potential problems of immobility such as constipation, pressure sores, increased risk of infection, and boredom. Assess the risk of each of these complications and put a plan of care into place.
- For patients with skeletal traction, properly care for the pin sites to reduce the risk of infection. 📖 Musculoskeletal trauma: care – fixation, p.616.
- Provide pain relief if required.

Care of patients with a cast

Casts may be made of plaster of Paris, which is mouldable but heavy, or they may be made of synthetic materials, which are lighter and dry more quickly. For new fractures, a backslab (a slab applied to the back of the limb and held to it by a crepe bandage) is usually used. This allows for any swelling that may occur immediately after the injury. However, a backslab may still constrict circulation and the use of a backslab does not prevent compartment syndrome. 📖 Chapter 33, Part 1. General principles of first aid for nurses, p.1023.

Nursing management for patients in a cast or backslab
- Check that the cast is not too tight (which can lead to neurovascular problems such as compartment syndrome) or too loose (which may allow the fracture ends to move).
- Check that the ends of the cast are not rough or they may cause skin damage.

- Handle a wet cast with care so as to avoid causing indentations, which can lead to pressure sores beneath the cast. Hold a cast with the palm of the hand and not with the fingers.
- Assess neurovascular status for signs of compartment syndrome or DVT.
- Observe for signs of pressure damage beneath the cast.
  - Localized pain caused by pressure of the supporting slab or cast
  - Pyrexia
  - Staining of the cast with pus or blood (though this is a late sign)
- Check whether the patient is allowed to put weight through a lower limb cast before they walk.
- Ensure that the patient can recognize when a problem with a cast is developing (e.g. it becoming too tight due to swelling) and who to contact if they have been discharged from hospital.
- Instruct the patient not to place objects down inside the cast as they can cause skin damage.
- Instruct the patient not to get a cast wet as it will lose its strength and shape. If a cast becomes wet, instruct the patient not to dry it using an external heat source such as a hairdryer or heater, as the cast will transmit the heat to the skin causing burns.

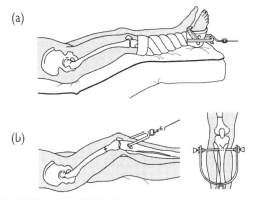

Fig. 17.4 (a) Skin traction; (b) skeletal traction.

Musculoskeletal trauma: care – fixation

Care of patients with external fixation

External fixation involves inserting skeletal pins into the bone on either side of the fracture and holding it in alignment by a scaffold or a ring fixator (See Fig. 17.5). External fixation can be used for a variety of conditions including acute trauma, injuries with severe soft tissue damage that prevents internal fixation, poor tissue condition due to underlying co-morbid pathology, gradual correction of a deformity, etc. External fixators can remain in place from 6 weeks to a year or more, depending on the reason for their use.

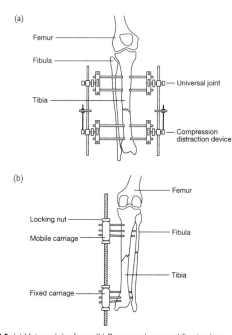

Fig. 17.5 (a) Universal day frame (b) Portsmouth external fixation bar

Nursing management for patients with an external fixator

- Perform postoperative observations. 📖 Chapter 22, Nursing patients requiring perioperative care, pp.762–70.
- Ensure proper care of the pin sites.
  - Keep pin sites clean and dry.
  - Clean pin sites with normal saline and apply a dry gauze dressing around the pin sites (the gauze should not be cut as the fibres may shed into the pin site tract and cause inflammation).
  - If the pin sites are dry with no oozing, no dressing is needed.
  - Note that many surgeons have different protocols. For example some surgeons use a dilute iodine wash for pin care, and then chlorhexidine gauze dressing until the pin sites are mature, and then no covering.
- Monitor the peripheral neurovascular status of the limb. 📖 Musculoskeletal trauma: principles, p.610.
- Ensure the patient can recognize signs and symptoms of potential complications such as compartment syndrome so that they can inform staff if symptoms develop.
- For patients being discharged, ensure that pin site care will continue. Teach patients to perform their own pin site care or arrange for community nursing services.
- Recognize that patients may have body image issues related to the external fixator and provide an opportunity for them to discuss any concerns.

Care of patients with internal fixation

Internal fixation involves the subdermal insertion of nails, plates, wires, screws, or rods to provide stability for a fracture. The advantage is that patients can generally mobilize more quickly than with other forms of fixation and therefore avoid the complications of immobility.

Nursing management for patients after internal fixation

- Ensure recovery from the anaesthetic and surgery. 📖 Chapter 22, Nursing patients requiring perioperative care, p.761.
- Check the operation records for the degree of mobility allowed after internal fixation. For example, some hospitals may have guidelines that allow patients who have had internal fixation of a leg fracture to walk on it before an x-ray has been performed.
- Assess and manage the surgical wound, checking for wound drainage and oozing.
- Assess for the potential problems of peripheral neurovascular damage. 📖 Musculoskeletal trauma: principles, p.610.

Specific musculoskeletal injuries: limb fractures

Shaft of femur fractures (See Fig. 17.3)

The most common cause of femur fracture is road traffic accidents (RTAs). Severe haemorrhage and internal displacement of the bones due to muscle spasm are common. These are sometimes classified as 'complicated' or 'compound' fractures when there is a wound leading down to the site of the fracture, or the bony prominences are piercing the skin. Traditionally treatment was skeletal traction using a Thomas splint, followed by a cast brace or hip spica cast. Today most patients are treated with internal fixation, such as an intramedullary nail which allows early mobilization.

Hip fractures (fractured neck of femur)

- Occur most frequently in the older person, particularly in women with osteoporosis.
- Falls are the most common cause, with impaction or displacement of the fracture.
- The patient is admitted to hospital for immediate bed rest and assessment.
- Surgical intervention is the first choice of treatment within 24 hours.
- Fractures within the joint capsule are treated with a hemi-arthroplasty (half a joint replacement, with removal of the femoral head and replacement with a metal ball and stem) or screws.
- Young patients are treated with internal fixation, often using screws.
- Older patients (50–70 years of age) are often treated with total hip replacement.
- Very elderly or immobile patients are treated with hemi-arthroplasty, which means they are also at risk to dislocation.
- Fractures outside the capsule are fixed with screw and plate (dynamic hip screw).
- If a patient is not fit for surgery, traction or bed rest may be used but these are not ideal for long-term treatment due to the high risk of chest infection, urinary tract infection, and pressure ulcer development.
- Non-operative management of hip fractures is invariably associated with death – only moribund patients are denied surgery. The purpose of surgery is to permit better nursing care and pain control, prevent complications, and enhance recovery.
- After fixation of a hip fracture patients can usually begin full, partial, or non-weight bearing the next day, often without the need for x-ray depending on local protocols. (Usually it is only arthroplasty patients and some patients fitted with a dynamic hip screw who bear their full weight on the affected limb.)
- Care should be taken with patients who have had hip replacements, as all are at risk of dislocation of the prosthesis (the prosthetic head of the femur being prised free from the hip socket). Nurse patients according to local evidence based protocols.

- Patients who have had screws or a screw and plate cannot dislocate and can lie and be moved as they feel comfortable.
- Assess the patient carefully for any pain and encourage to take analgesia as they require.
- General physiotherapy includes deep breathing and appropriate exercises.

Pelvic fractures

Pelvic fractures can result from RTAs, falls, and sport injuries. They can result in large amounts of blood loss internally and damage to internal organs such as the bladder and bowel. Therefore, a full systemic examination needs to be performed. Pelvic fractures may be treated by bed rest alone if stable, or if the fracture is unstable, by external or internal fixation. Complex pelvic fractures are treated in specialist centres.

Wrist and lower arm fractures

Fractures of the wrist and lower arm are the most common fractures seen in the emergency department and usually involve the lower end of the radius within 2.5 cm of the wrist joint (Colles' fracture). It commonly occurs in middle-aged and older women after a fall on an outstretched hand and is a strong predictor of osteoporosis. Patients with this type of fracture may be admitted to hospital if they have another injury such as a fractured neck of femur as well. The fracture is reduced using manual traction and treated in a backslab until the swelling has reduced, then a full below elbow cast for 6–8 weeks. Unstable fractures may require internal or external fixation. All elderly patients who sustain a wrist fracture after a low-impact fall should be investigated for osteoporosis and commenced on appropriate treatment, if found. Chapter 15, Nursing patients with rheumatologic problems and connective tissue disorders, p.550.

Specific musculoskeletal injuries: spinal, muscular, and neurovascular

Spinal injuries

The vertebral column protects the spinal cord. As the spinal cord passes through the spinal column, it branches at each vertebrae from the cervical to the sacral region. Injury or damage to any area can be confined to bony and/or ligament injury or can be accompanied by damage to the cord itself, or the nerve branches leaving it. Spinal cord damage can result from trauma but can also result from poor handling of the patient after initial injury. Fig. 17.6 illustrates whiplash injuries, Fig. 17.7 illustrates compression injuries, and Fig. 17.8 illustrates common spinal cord syndromes.

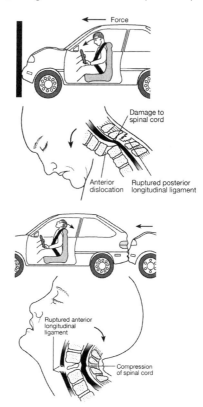

Fig. 17.6 Diagram illustrating whiplash injuries.

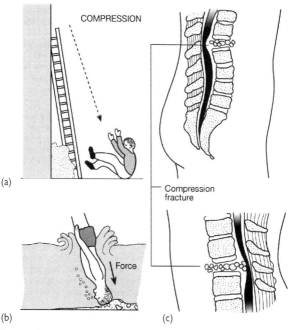

Fig. 17.7 Compression injuries. (a) Hyperflexion injury and (b) hyperextension injury of the cervical spine. (c) Axial loading injury of the cervical spine and the lumbar spine.

Patients with a definite spinal cord injury are transferred to a spinal injuries unit (SIU), but this may take a few days if a bed is not available. All nurses therefore need to understand principles of caring for patients with a suspected or confirmed bony or spinal cord injury.

Incorrect management of a patient with an unstable spine can cause permanent paralysis.

Nursing management for patients with suspected or confirmed spinal damage
- Careful moving and handling of the patient is critical.
  - For a patient with a suspected cervical spine injury, four people are required to turn the patient, including one to stabilize the head and cervical spine.
  - One or two additional nurses are required to perform tasks such as changing the sheet or checking pressure areas whilst the patient is turned.
  - For thoracic and lumbar injuries, three nurses are required to turn a patient.

- Respiratory and cardiovascular monitoring is necessary, as spinal cord injury may lead to breathing difficulties and disruption to the cardiovascular system.
- Patients with a spinal cord injury have the potential to develop other physical problems, such as paralytic ileus, gastric ulceration, and pressure damage. A patient with a spinal cord injury may have a flaccid bowel and bladder; therefore urinary catheterization and manual evacuation of faeces by a suitably qualified practitioner will be necessary.

Spinal cord injury is a life-changing event for both the patient and family. Psychologically patients benefit from consistency in information given and interventions to reduce the effects of sensory deprivation. Nurses should consider the use of mirrors and therapeutic touch to enable patients to remain connected to their environment. Long-term support and adaptation will be necessary and organizations such as the Spinal Injuries Association are vital in this.

Muscle and neurovascular injuries

Trauma such as a sprain can cause muscle or neurovascular damage rather than bony injury. Fractures can also be accompanied by muscle or neurovascular damage.

For muscle injuries the principles of RICE – Rest, Ice, Compression, and Elevation – should be followed in order to control haemorrhage and haematoma, a collection of blood beneath the skin. Tendon and ligament injuries, such as rupture of the Achilles' tendon, may be treated by conservative measures, immobilization in a cast, or by surgical repair of the damage. This repair may well be successful but, due to the formation of scar tissue, may lead to a poor functional outcome.

Nerve injuries may be treated by surgical repair or immobilization. Peripheral nerves are capable of regenerating at a rate of 1–2 mm a day, although there is no guarantee that each nerve cell will heal. The patient may be left with reduced or altered sensation.

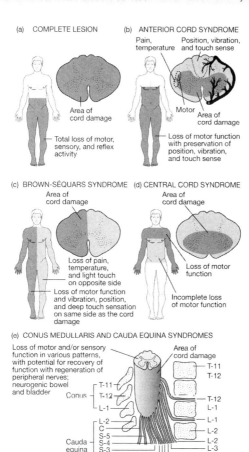

Fig. 17.8 Common spinal cord syndromes.

Orthopaedic complications

Compartment syndrome

Compartment syndrome is a serious situation that can develop when there is increased pressure within one or more compartments (sheaths of inelastic fascia that support and partition muscles, blood vessels and nerves). It can develop pre- or post-admission or postoperatively. Pressure can arise due to bleeding within a compartment or due to external compression, e.g. use of a cast or traction, or use of a tourniquet during surgery. The most common cause is direct or indirect traumatic injury and secondary swelling. Compartment syndrome can also occur in patients with severe oedema, e.g. patients with burns. The most common sites are the lower leg and the forearm. If undetected, compartment syndrome can lead to the complete loss of function of a hand or foot because the nerves and blood vessels within the affected compartment are irreversibly damaged.

The aim of nursing care is risk reduction and early detection.
- Elevate the limb to reduce the risk of swelling.
- Perform regular neurovascular observations on the hands or feet below the injury or surgery. 📖 Nursing assessment, p.604.
- Check for the five 'P's that suggest compartment syndrome:
  - Pain (especially on passive movement, when the nurse rather than the patient moves the foot or hand)
  - Parasthesia
  - Paralysis
  - Pallor
  - Pulselessness (pulses are often present until late in the development of compartment syndrome and their presence may be misleading)

If compartment syndrome is suspected, it is a medical emergency and medical staff must be contacted as soon as possible. Elevation should be stopped as it may exacerbate the condition by further impairing oxygenation of muscle tissue. Any external pressure, such as traction, should be removed. If a patient has a cast in place it should be split down to the skin by a suitably experienced practitioner.

If compartment syndrome occurs the patient may need a fasciotomy, where the inelastic fascia is cut to allow the compartment to expand. Oxygen, IV fluids, preoperative laboratory tests and pre-surgical preparation are first required. The patient may be left with an open wound until the compartment swelling has gone down.

Venous thromboembolism
(deep vein thrombosis and pulmonary embolus)

Venous thromboembolism (VTE) is the umbrella term for thrombi forming within the venous system, primarily deep vein thrombosis (DVT) and its potential complication a pulmonary embolus (PE). A DVT is a blood clot in the deep veins and most frequently occurs in the calf. 📖 Chapter 7, Peripheral venous disease, p.184.

Predisposing factors

- Venous stasis, due to reduced mobility
- Hypercoaguability of the blood. (Blood becomes more viscous or sticky throughout the body following trauma; therefore even patients with an upper limb injury are at risk.)
- Damage to veins

Some patients, such as those who have sustained lower limb injuries, are likely to have all three of these predisposing factors and therefore are at high risk of developing a DVT.

Risk reduction and early detection

The aim of nursing care is risk reduction and early detection.

- Use prevention measures according to local policies.
  - Early mobilization
  - Anti-embolism stockings
  - Subcutaneous heparin injections
  - Intermittent pneumatic compression (calf or foot pump machines)
- Assess signs of DVT
  - Red, hot, swollen calf
  - Pain on passive movement of the foot (the nurse moves the patient's foot up and down)
  - Presence of a DVT is often asymptomatic (📖 Chapter 16, Nursing care of patients with VTE, p.586)

Pulmonary embolism

If a DVT dislodges, it may travel via the circulatory system to the pulmonary circulation leading to a PE. The aim of nursing care is risk reduction and early detection.

- Observe for warning signs:
  - Breathlessness
  - Confusion
  - Chest pain
  - Tachycardia
- If PE is suspected, alert the medical staff immediately as patients will require high level care, probably within an intensive care situation.

Fat embolism

A fat embolism causes similar symptoms to a PE, with the addition of reddish-brown, nonpalpable petechiae (pinpoint sized haemorrhages under the skin) developing over the upper body, particularly in the axillae. It is very rare and usually only seen in patients with tibial or femoral fractures.

The exact cause of fat emboli is disputed but it is likely to occur when fat globules are released from long bones when they are fractured and enter the circulatory system. This can also happen in elective surgery, for example when bones are cut in joint replacement surgery. The care of a patient with suspected or actual fat embolism is the same as that of a patient with a PE.

Orthopaedic conditions

Patients admitted to hospital with orthopaedic conditions may have joint disorders caused by conditions such as osteoarthritis or rheumatoid arthritis, back pain, bony tumours, or bone infections.

Initial assessment

In addition to the general assessment described previously (📖 Nursing assessment of patients with orthopaedic and musculoskeletal trauma problems, p.604), consider the following.

- Patients with a chronic orthopaedic condition have probably been living with it for many years, and will be experienced in managing it themselves. Listen carefully to their history. Ensure that the assessment includes identifying effective pain relieving measures and any adjustments to activities of living they have made.
- Discharge planning begins before the patient is admitted to the ward for planned surgery, on listing for surgery, or at the preoperative assessment clinic. Ward nurses should check that this has taken place and that patients have been fully informed about their surgery and rehabilitation.

Joint replacement for arthritis

When conservative measures no longer control the symptoms of osteoarthritis or rheumatoid arthritis (📖 Chapter 15, Osteoarthritis, p.554 and Rheumatoid arthritis, p.556), joint replacement will be considered. The most commonly replaced joints are the hip and the knee joints. Both types of replacements are very successful with 95% of patients remaining pain free 10 years after surgery.

Hip and knee replacements consist of articulated components that may be metal, plastic, ceramic, or a combination. Younger patients with hip osteoarthritis may undergo hip resurfacing. This involves smoothing rather than removing the femoral head and covering it with a metal cap. The cap articulates with a metal socket.

Nursing management for patients with joint replacement

- Ensure that a full assessment has been made of the patient's home prior to admission, as both hip and knee replacement patients require correct height of bed, chair, and toilet.
- Assess and manage the risks of DVT/PE. 📖 Orthopaedic complications, p.624 and 📖 Chapter 7, Peripheral venous disease, p.184.
- For patients with total hip replacements, ensure that all staff as well as the patient and their carers understand the risk of dislocation and how to reduce this risk. Dislocation means that the ball-shaped head of the femur becomes detached from the hip socket. Patients are instructed not to bend down, not to raise their knee above their hip, and not to cross their legs. Nurses play an important role in ensuring that patients adhere to these instructions.
- Arrange an appropriate discharge. Many hospitals now have early supported discharge schemes, while others have rehabilitation facilities. If a patient is being discharged to their own home, ensure good communication and liaison with the multidisciplinary team to ensure a safe discharge.

Joint replacement is not as successful for some joints, such as the ankle joint. Alternative surgical options for arthritis include arthrodesis (i.e. fusing) of a joint and osteotomy (i.e. cutting a bone to realign the joint), which is used for knee arthritis in young people.

Back pain and back surgery

Back pain affects individuals of all nationalities, all social groups, and all professions. In the 21st century back pain is (along with the common cold) a leading cause of absence from work. The cervical (upper back) and lumbosacral (lower back) vertebrae are the most commonly affected.

Causes

Back pain can arise from stiffness in the inter-vertebral disc between two vertebrae, arthritis (particularly of the facet joints), an acute locked back with severe muscle spasm, a slipped disc, and unstable spinal segment. Pain can range from a dull ache to severe pain with nerve involvement. There are several causes of back pain:

- Trauma and repetitive lifting (most common cause)
- Obesity
- Lack of exercise
- Congenital spinal conditions
- Scoliosis
- Poor posture
- Vascular changes
- Tumours
- Chronic degenerative conditions

Prevention

Many problems associated with acute back pain can be prevented by recognizing causes and taking appropriate action. All patients with back pain should be taught preventative measures.

- Adopt good posture when sitting, standing, and walking.
- Use proper body mechanics when bending, lifting, and sitting.
- Avoid prolonged sitting (especially driving in a car) or standing.
- Participate in a regular exercise programme, especially one promoting back strengthening, such as swimming, tai chi, Pilates, and the Alexander technique.

Patients with acute lower back pain should be taught specific preventative measures.

- Sit as little as possible.
- Place a supportive roll in the small of the back, especially when sitting in a car or lounge chair.
- Avoid knees being above hips when sitting.
- Keep back straight and bend legs when rising from a chair and lifting.
- Use a firm mattress when sleeping.
- Follow physiotherapy advice regarding suitable exercises.
- Avoid forward bending or stooping.

Key nursing interventions for back pain

- Teach patient about common contributing factors, e.g. poor posture, poor lifting technique, wearing high-heeled shoes.
- Encourage limited bed rest.
- Good body positioning and awareness.
- Heat and ice therapy by packs, towels, or showers and baths.
- Check skin condition.
- Diet control and return to appropriate weight.
- Use a variety of pain control measures such as distraction, imagery, and music therapy.
- Follow recommended exercise programme, including back and abdominal exercises.
- Control pain with drug therapy, where appropriate.
- Encourage relaxation with complementary medicine techniques such as massage and aromatherapy.
- Manipulation of the spine by a recognized expert may help.
- Special corsets and cervical lumbar supports may help.

Diagnosis
- History
- Examination
- X-ray
- CT scan
- MRI scan

If the sciatic nerve is compressed, the patient complains of severe pain when raising a straight leg. Local muscle spasms are common. In patients with cervical injury, pain radiates down one arm. When the lumbo-sacral area is involved, pain radiates down the posterior leg and occurs in the middle of the buttock, thigh, or calf. In severe cases, sensory loss, numbness, and loss of bowel and bladder control may occur. This requires an immediate MRI scan and possible surgery to remove the disc pressing on the nerves.

Treatment
- Limited rest (prolonged bed rest is not recommended because it weakens the muscles)
- Appropriate exercise and education
- NSAIDs
- Steroid epidural injections
- Analgesics, muscle relaxants, and antidepressants
- Surgery for severe cases includes laminectomy and spinal fusion

Amputation

Amputation is the removal of a body part, from the finger or toe to a major limb. Lower-extremity amputations are performed much more frequently than upper-extremity amputations (See Fig. 17.9).

Methods used

- Open or guillotine method (which of these methods used depends on the type of prosthesis to be used subsequently)
- Closed or flap method

Causes

- Loss of circulation
- Severe chronic infection
- Bone cancer
- Traumatic accidents, e.g. chain saws, RTAs, or industrial machine (if possible, attempts are made to save the amputated part and replant it, 📖 Musculoskeletal trauma, p.610; Chapter 33, Nursing care of patient emergencies, p.1064.)

Complications

- Haemorrhage
- Infection
- Phantom limb pain
- Severe body image disturbance. 📖 Chapter 24, Nursing patients with body image problems, p.818
- Severe loss and grieving
- Immobility and contractures

Nursing care

- Provide psychological preparation and after-care for the patient.
- Observe the site of the amputation.
- Manage pain.
- Prevent infection.
- Promote ambulation, exercise, and adjustment to a suitable prosthesis.
- Assist patient to adjust to a new lifestyle and adapt to facilities in the home.

Fig. 17.10 illustrates the proper method for wrapping a stump.

Rehabilitation

If a prosthesis is deemed necessary for a patient they will be referred to a specialist centre for assessment and fitting. Following this, the patient will need help from occupational therapists and physiotherapists to regain a suitable level of mobility and adjustment to their new situation. This may include assessment for driving and mobility aids. Assessment by a social worker for invalidity benefit may be necessary; advice regarding re-employment and retraining may also be required.

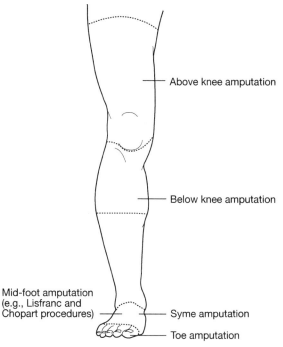

Fig. 17.9 Common levels of lower-extremity amputation.

Above knee amputation

Below knee amputation

Mid-foot amputation
(e.g., Lisfranc and
Chopart procedures)

Syme amputation

Toe amputation

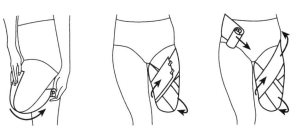

Fig. 17.10 Wrapping a stump.

Other orthopaedic bone disorders

Carpal tunnel syndrome (See Fig. 17.11a)

This is a common condition of the hand, occurring in 2% of men and 3% of women. The median nerve in the wrist becomes compressed causing pain, tingling, and numbness of the fingers. The carpal tunnel is the canal lying between the carpal bones and the flexor retinaculum. Causes include synovitis of the wrist, pregnancy, hypothyroidism, diabetes mellitus, and work. A nerve conduction study is required to confirm diagnosis. Management includes the use of wrist splints to relieve symptoms in mild cases and local steroid injection. If symptoms persist surgical decompression may be required.

Dupuytren's contracture

This is a slowly progressive deformity of the palmar fascia in the hand resulting in flexion of the 4th and/or 5th digit. The condition is more common in men, but its cause is unknown. It is treated surgically.

Ganglion

This is a round cyst-like lesion occurring over a wrist joint or tendon. It is usually removed by minor surgical technique.

Hallux valgus (See Fig. 17.11b)

The common name for hallux valgus is a bunion. The big toe deviates laterally at the metatarsophalangeal joint. It is often congenital, but can occur as a result of arthritis and poorly fitting shoes. Women are affected more than men. It is treated surgically by bunionectomy.

Hallux rigidus (See Fig. 17.11c)

The common name for hallux rigidus is a hammer toe. It sometimes occurs with bunions, resulting in dorsiflexion of any metatarsophalangeal joint with plantar flexion of the adjacent proximal interphalangeal joint. The second toe is most commonly affected. It can be treated with surgery.

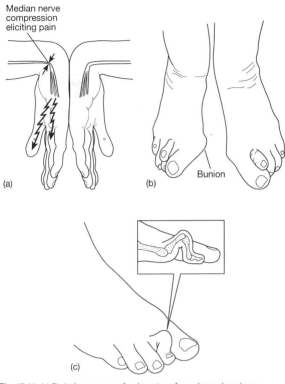

Fig. 17.11 (a) Phalan's manoeuvre for detection of carpal tunnel syndrome. (b) Hallux valgus (bunion). (c) Hammer toe.

Common drugs used in musculoskeletal disorders

Common drugs used for orthopaedic and musculoskeletal disorders are listed in Table 17.1. **All drug doses listed in this table are adult doses and not children's doses.** This table is only to be used as a guide and the current BNF should be consulted for further advice. Nurses should involve themselves only in the administration of medications which fall within their sphere of competence.

Table 17.1 Common drugs used for orthopaedic and musculoskeletal disorders

Anti-inflammatory drugs	Dose	Common side effects
Non-selective non steroidal anti-inflammatory drugs (NSAIDs) (ibuprofen carries lowest risk of adverse gastrointestinal effects, with piroxicam, ketoprofen, indomethacin, naproxen, and diclofenac as intermediate risk)	Ibuprofen – initially 1200–1800 mg daily in 3–4 divided doses after food; increased if necessary to maximum 2400 mg daily; maintenance dose of 600–1200 mg daily may be adequate See BNF for dosages with other NSAIDs	Gastrointestinal discomfort, nausea, diarrhoea and occasionally bleeding and ulceration occur particularly in the elderly; a degree of worsening of asthma may occur; hypersensitivity reactions See BNF for full range of side effects and degree of risk with different NSAIDs
Selective NSAIDs i.e. Cyclo-oxygenase-2 inhibitors (Cox-2s) (as effective as non-selective agents and should only be used instead of a standard NSAID in patients at high risk of developing serious gastrointestinal problems)	Celecoxib – osteoarthritis, 200 mg daily in 1–2 divided doses, increased if necessary to maximum 200 mg twice daily	As above plus flatulence, pharyngitis, sinusitis, insomnia, increased risk of thrombotic events, e.g. myocardial infarction and stroke

Osteoporosis	Dose	Common side effects
Biphosphonates, e.g. alendronic acid, etidronate	Paget's disease of bone: etidronate 5 mg/kg as a single daily dose for up to 6 months Prevention of postmenopausal osteoporosis: alendronic acid 5 mg daily Treatment of postmenopausal osteoporosis: alendronic acid 10 mg daily or 70 mg weekly	Nausea, diarrhoea or constipation, abdominal pain; increased bone pain and risk of fractures with high dose in Paget's disease (discontinue if fractures occur) Oesophageal reactions, abdominal pain and distension, dyspepsia, regurgitation, melaena, diarrhoea or constipation, flatulence, musculoskeletal pain, headache

Drugs for osteomyelitis: 📖 Table 20.1 Common drugs used for infectious diseases: flucloxacillin, p.728 and sodium fusidate, p.729.

Nursing patients with human immunodeficiency virus (HIV)

Introduction

The term 'HIV disease' is used to cover the spectrum of illness (and wellness) of individuals diagnosed with HIV. More than 40 million people are HIV positive and more than half live in Africa (WHO 2004). There are two types of virus that produce similar illnesses; the most common is the retrovirus HIV-1.

The terms acquired immunodeficiency syndrome (AIDS) and human immunodeficiency virus (HIV) were once used interchangeably; now they have been clearly defined. AIDS is one end of a spectrum of disease caused by HIV.

The AIDS epidemic started slowly and it is not clear where it originated. The disease is very common in South Africa where it may have spread because of demographic shifts from rural to urban living and other factors such as increased heterosexual prostitution.

The main modes of HIV transmission are unprotected sexual activity (more heterosexuals acquire the disease now than homosexuals in the UK), blood-to-blood contact (e.g. drug users sharing equipment), infected blood or blood products, and transference from mother to child. In the developing world, increasing numbers of children are being born with HIV. HIV infection cannot be transmitted by touch, other than by contact with bodily fluids. Therefore touching and handling patients without wearing gloves is acceptable and wearing gloves is not a requirement unless handling internal bodily fluids, especially blood. Wearing gloves, washing hands, and avoiding needlestick injuries are important in these instances.

Patients with HIV disease may be admitted to acute, critical, long-term, and hospice settings for reasons other than the effect of their HIV infection and many remain well and are living longer than was anticipated when the disease was initially encountered. Progression of the disease is not common with modern drug therapy, especially since the advent of HAART (highly active antiretroviral therapy).

Key stages of HIV

Acute infection is often asymptomatic.

First stage. During this phase of HIV, influenza or cold-like symptoms with a mild skin rash are the first symptoms to develop, followed by fatigue, sore muscles, mild persistent fevers, and swollen lymph nodes. Once these symptoms have passed the patient has detectable antigens in their blood (this is termed being 'seroconverted'). This is the most infectious period and once this is over the patient may be asymptomatic for some time, sometimes for 10–15 years.

Second stage. This is known as the symptomatic stage, in which the infected person suffers from various symptoms including weight loss.

Final stage or end-stage. This stage of HIV disease can last for up to 10 years because of new drug therapies. Patients can also develop more common illnesses at this stage such as tuberculosis, pneumonia, and a cancer of the skin (Kaposi's sarcoma).

Problems experienced by patients with HIV

Following is a list of the most common signs and symptoms associated with immunosuppression resulting from HIV.

Skin disorders

- Dry skin
- Kaposi's sarcoma (cancer of the blood vessels that shows as pinkish-brown blemishes)
- Yeast infections usually involving the mouth, throat, or vagina, e.g. *Candida*
- Herpes zoster
- Persistent or recalcitrant warts in genital or perianal areas
- Impetigo
- Various skin conditions such as seborrheic dermatitis (skin disease on face and scalp)
- Psoriasis may become worse with the onset of HIV

Mucous membrane problems

- Angular stomatitis (inflammation of the corners of the mouth)
- Ulcers
- Oral hairy leucoplakia (white patches on side of tongue)
- Persistent or recurrent vaginal candidiasis
- Oral candidiasis

Eye problems

- Retinal haemorrhage
- Weeping/discharge

Pulmonary problems

- Chest infection
- Tuberculosis
- Bacterial pneumonia
- Cough

Gut problems

- Anorexia and weight loss
- Diarrhoea
- Hepatomegaly

Night sweats, fever

- Blood problems such as coagulation abnormalities and anaemia

Neurological problems

- Headache
- Sensory problems/peripheral neuropathy

Nursing assessment to establish HIV

Patients with possible HIV infection must be identified as early as possible for treatment purposes and to prevent unwanted transmission of infection. Establish:

- *Health history* – Obtain a full history including primary complaint, reason for seeking medical help, details of present complaint (e.g. duration of symptoms), HIV status, and past medical history.
- *Social history* – Ask about any drug use, smoking, and alcohol habits. If the patient admits to drug taking ask them which drugs they take, how often, how they are administered, and when drugs were last taken. If patient is taking drugs, ask about any needle sharing.
- *Travel history* – Determine whether the patient has had possible exposure to areas of high HIV infection. Has the patient had any blood transfusions abroad? Or any injections?
- *Sexual history* – Use open-ended questions that are straightforward and non-judgemental. Ask the patient whether they are sexually active or have been in the past. Ask them whether they have sex with men, women, or both. Anal sex carries a greater risk of HIV than vaginal or oral sex, and questions should be carefully asked to assess the patient's sexual activities. Number of sexual partners should be obtained. Ask whether condoms are used. Take a history of any sexually transmitted infections.
- *Psychosocial history* – Assess for any signs of depression or other psychological illnesses. Ask patients to describe their methods of coping with stress. Ask patients questions about their family and friends to assess support systems they may have. Explore the implications of HIV on their employment role and future job prospects.

Other assessments:

- Record the patient's vital signs and observe breathing for rate, depth, and sounds.
- Determine whether the patient experiences any coughing; if sputum is produced, collect a sample.
- Assess the patient's skin for any rash, sores, or blemishes.
- Look for signs of weight loss and ask about current food intake. Record patient's weight.
- Carry out a urine dipstick and take a midstream specimen of urine if indicated from urine dipstick.

Nursing problems

The time between diagnosis and being symptomatic varies from patient to patient. As HIV is complex, various nursing problems can be identified at different stages of the disease, but not all patients will necessarily experience all of the problems listed below. Patients experience a variety of emotional responses to their condition and symptoms. Good communication and counselling may help in monitoring and coping with these.

Nutritional problems

Nutritional problems result from the disease process, infection, pain, discomfort in mouth due to ulcers and sores, and nausea.

- Monitor frequency of nausea and inform the physician (if not an independent prescriber) so that anti-emetics can be prescribed.
- Assess the mouth for sores and ulcers, carry out a pain assessment, and inform the physician of the assessments.
- Offer mouth washes and carry out oral care regularly.
- Refer to a dietitian for dietary advice and consider supplements.

Disturbed sleep

Disturbed sleep results from night sweats, medication, diarrhoea, urinary and bowel incontinence, anxiety, and pain.

- Consider night sedation.
- Suggest a warm drink before bedtime, herbal tea, or a high-carbohydrate snack.
- Suggest complementary therapies such as massage.
- Assess pain and, if necessary, identify effective medication.
- Consider the use of antidepressants if there are signs of clinical depression.
- Identify methods to control incontinence and discuss with the patient.
- Suggest ways to reduce sleep disturbance, e.g. creating an environment that will promote sleep by minimizing noise and maintaining adequate room temperature.

Fatigue

Inadequate nutritional intake, respiratory problems, infection, and fever may all affect the energy levels of the patient and lead to tiredness.

- Encourage nutritional intake.
- Support respiratory conditions with oxygen to keep patient comfortable.
- Encourage the patient to exercise as this promotes immunity and helps prevent problems associated with immobility.
- Assess the nature and severity of fatigue.
- Educate and counsel.
- Treat physical causes such as anaemia and mental health problems such as depression.

Fever

Fever is caused by infection.

- Monitor temperature; observe for sweating and chills.
- Offer antipyretic medication.

- Use tepid sponges on the forehead, fans, and cotton sheets for symptom relief.
- Sweating can damage the skin's integrity, so take care to protect it, i.e. regular washing of the skin.
- If the patient is nursed in bed, turn regularly to prevent pressure sores from developing.
- Reduce the room temperature, if possible. Typically, HIV patients do not need to be nursed in a side room, and on the general ward reducing the room temperature may not be possible.
- Encourage oral fluids to prevent dehydration and give regular mouth care.
- Change patient's clothes and bed linen regularly to assist with comfort.

Diarrhoea

May be serious and due to pathogens in the bowel, sexually transmitted infections, inadequate nutrition, and medication side effects. Patients can have >20 stools a day and antidiarrhoea medications can be ineffective. Patients can experience fluid and electrolyte imbalances, sores around the anus, as well as socialization and self-esteem problems.

- Diagnose the cause of diarrhoea if possible, and treat specifically.
- Monitor frequency, quantity, colour, and smell of stools; collect a sample for laboratory testing.
- Administer medication prescribed to treat cause of diarrhoea (if known); administer antidiarrhoea medication, e.g. loperamide.
- Consider dietary intake, e.g. eating little and often, decreasing fat and soluble fibre intake, and increasing insoluble fibre intake. Yoghurt can help if normal gut flora has been altered. 📖 Chapter 8, Nursing patients with nutritional and gastrointestinal problems, p.242.
- Offer barrier cream to protect skin surrounding the anus.

Fluid and electrolyte imbalances

Diarrhoea is the most common cause of this problem. The presence of fever and infection increases the need for fluids.

- Monitor fluid balance and vital signs, and observe the skin for signs of dehydration.
- Inform the physician of the patient's condition.
- Patients may be prescribed IV fluids that may contain potassium; care should be taken to administer such fluids via an electronically controlled giving set, where available.

Incontinence

Urinary incontinence and bowel incontinence are not problems for most patients with HIV. These may occur during the very end stage of the patient's life, however, if the disease progresses to that level.

- Male patients could use external catheters, and this should be discussed with them by the nurse.
- Indwelling catheters should also be considered for the advantage they can offer in protecting the skin and improving patient's confidence and socialization versus the risk of infection that catheters pose upon the body.

- Discuss the options with the patient and provide time for them to come to a decision. 📖 Chapter 8, Nursing patients with nutritional and gastrointestinal needs, p.203 and 📖 Chapter 11, Nursing patients with renal and urological needs, p.328.
- Clothes and bed linen should be kept clean and dry to maximize comfort and dignity, and to protect the skin.

Nausea and vomiting

These can be due to adverse effects of HIV drug treatment.
- Monitor frequency and amount.
- Give anti-emetics intrathecally and ensure vomit bowls are within patient's reach.

Respiratory problems

- Monitor breathing rate, pattern, breath sounds, and secretions.
- Nurse patient in a position that aids breathing and encourages coughing.
- Monitor oxygen saturation levels and provide oxygen if necessary.
- Suction to keep airway clear and give prescribed nebulizers.
- Relaxation exercises may be useful.

Weight loss

This may be associated with HIV or with severe effects of diarrhoea. Wasting creates a vicious cycle of weakness and GI impairment, creating nutritional risks.
- Nutritional supplements or total parenteral nutrition (TPN) may be needed.
- Monitor weight and food intake on a daily basis.
- Refer to dietitian.

Many of these issues can be a part of end-of-life nursing care. 📖 Chapter 26 Nursing patients with palliative care needs, pp.861–83 and 📖 Chapter 27 Nursing the dying patient, pp.885–97.

Psychosocial problems

Four main areas can be identified.

Ineffective coping

When first diagnosed with HIV, emotional response varies from anger towards the person who may have given them the virus to guilt and intense fear for the future. Patients fear the reactions from family, friends and society. They may not know how or who to tell that they have HIV. Nurses can help patients to clarify their options, and support them if they do choose to inform family and friends. Give them information about employment laws if necessary. Anger is a common reaction to the diagnosis and nurses should provide a safe outlet for patients to express their feelings. Nurses should listen and empathize; it may be useful to have the patient write down their feelings. Anger can sometimes be expressed in ways that endanger others, e.g. unprotected sex without informing the partner, hitting or punching others. Nurses should be aware of this and seek advice on how to deal with such problems.

Anxiety and fear

HIV patients face many fears and anxieties, such as isolation, loss of health, financial difficulties, and uncertain futures. Fear and anxiety may affect adherence to treatment, appropriate health behaviours, and sleeping. Positive support systems are vital from family and friends. Patients who do not have this type of support available will require increased support from the health care team. Give details of local support groups (e.g. The Terrence Higgins Trust). Encourage activities to aid relaxation, e.g. reading, listening to music, warm baths, and meditation. Encourage patients to talk to others who also have HIV.

Grieving

This is a normal response. Patients may mourn for a period, and need support to recognize what they still have in terms of life. As the body changes, support from nurses may need to increase to help patients deal with and accept what is happening to them. They may grieve for friends who die from HIV.

Altered thought process

As illness progresses, cognition can be affected, e.g. forgetfulness can occur and be distressing for the patient and family or friends. In some cases AIDS-related dementia may occur. Nurses should use familiar communication and routines with patient. Visual aids and repeated orientation to person, place, and time may be helpful. Support family and friends by explaining what is happening.

Patient education

The nurse's role in patient and family education is a key factor in prevention, acute care, and long-term management of the patient with HIV. Nurses should use a variety of teaching aids, such as leaflets and DVDs. As patients with HIV may not want to keep literature on the virus (in order to protect their privacy), the nurse should ask the patient to repeat back the major points of the teaching session in order to assess learning.

Education should include:
- HIV testing—confidential versus anonymous testing, information regarding waiting period for results, pre- and post-test counselling sessions.
- Correcting myths about HIV including methods of transmission.
- Blood-to-blood or body fluid contact precautions.
- Reducing onward transmission both by horizontal transmission (sexual and sharing needles) and by vertical transmission (mother-to-child).
- Sexual behaviour:
  - Importance of sexual health screening
  - Risk of transmission during sex
  - Importance of disclosure to sexual partners
  - How HIV-negative partners can access post-exposure prophylaxis after sexual exposure, if needed
  - Use of condoms
- Drug use involving needles (if patient is a drug user).
- Maternal transmission—prenatal, during birth, and breastmilk.
- Health promotion and health maintenance—diet, exercise, sleep and rest, and stress management.
- Nutritional information—importance of a healthy diet, foods to avoid.
- Medications used—purpose of these, adverse effects, how medications should be taken (e.g. with food), when medication should be taken, what to do if a dose is missed, and the importance of concordance.
- Importance of regular health screening, e.g. dental examinations, cervical cytology examinations.
- Information about the health care team—whom they may meet, when, where, what each one's role is, and any contact details.
- Role of support groups.
- The need to disclose HIV status to others such as employer, insurers, and building societies.
- Warn against the developments of re-infecting people with other strains of HIV including new drug-resistant strains of HIV (super-infection) and the criminalization of HIV when someone knowingly infects others while hiding their status.

The patient and family should be assessed initially to determine their understanding of HIV as a disease, and given time to ask questions. Teaching sessions should be adjusted for each individual patient in order to meet their specific educational needs. The nurse must show sensitivity when educating HIV patients and their families.

Discharge and continuing care

One of the goals of caring for HIV patients is to care for them in their own home environment. In some cases they may be admitted to a hospital or hospice with exacerbation of their symptoms. There are a variety of networks available to the patient in the community. These include HIV specialist nurses, community dietitians, psychiatric nurses, support groups, social services, and district nurses. Ideally the patient at home should be visited by the same nurse or team of nurses to maintain continuity and enable a relationship of trust to develop.

Referrals should be made early to prevent any delays in discharge. The patient and family should be informed about the referrals that are made, including what they should expect from each network or discipline involved in their treatment and care.

The patient needs to be prepared for discharge, as this may be frightening for them and cause anxiety. Help the patient to gradually become more independent and confident with aspects of self-care, such as administering their own medication. On each drug round ask the patient what medication they are due. This will help them remember what medication to take and when to take it when they are at home. Other measures to help them remember are available from the pharmacist.

Patients at home must be provided with adequate pain management. This may require teaching the patient and their family how to administer injections or use patient controlled analgesic pumps before they are discharged from hospital. All medications should be explained prior to leaving hospital to aid compliance at home.

Outpatient appointments should be arranged before the patient is discharged, and hospital transport booked if it is required.

Common drugs used for patients with HIV

Common drugs used for patients with HIV are listed in Table 18.1. **All drug doses listed in this table are adult doses and not children's doses**. This table is only to be used as a guide and the current BNF should be consulted for further advice. Nurses should involve themselves only in the administration of medications which fall within their sphere of competence.

Table 18.1 Common drugs used for patients with HIV. NB a wide range of drugs exist and many are used in combination

HIV infection	Dose	Common side effects
Nucleoside reverse transcriptase inhibitors		
Zidovudine	500–600 mg daily in 2–3 divided doses	Lactic acidosis with hepatomegaly and hepatic steatosis (discontinue); lipodystrophy syndrome, gastrointestinal disturbances, anorexia, pancreatitis, dyspnoea, cough, headache, insomnia, dizziness, fatigue, blood disorders, myalgia, arthralgia, rash, urticaria and fever; many others (See BNF)
Protease inhibitors		
Nelfinavir	1.25 g twice daily or 750 mg 3 times daily	Gastrointestinal disturbances, hepatic dysfunction, pancreatitis, blood disorders, (anaemia, neutropenia, thrombocytopenia), lipodystrophy syndrome and many more (See BNF)
Non-nucleotide reverse transcriptase inhibitors		
Nevirapine	200 mg once daily for 14 days, then (if no rash present) 200 mg twice daily	Rash common (including Stevens-Johnson syndrome), hepatic disease and reactions and many more (See BNF)
Anaphylaxis		
Adrenaline (epinephrine) injection	Acute anaphylaxis: 500 mcg (0.5 mL) by IM injection (or by SC injection) of 1 in 1000 (1 mg/mL) Self-administration: 300 mcg IM	Anxiety, tremor, tachycardia, arrhythmias, headache, cold extremities, hypertension (risk of cerebral haemorrhage) and pulmonary oedema (on excessive dosage or extreme sensitivity)

Table 18.1 Common drugs used for patients with HIV. NB a wide range of drugs exist and many are used in combination *(continued)*

Anaphylaxis	Dose	Common side effects
Hydrocortisone injection	By IM or slow IV injection or infusion, 100–300 mg, 3–4 times in 24 hours as required	Gastrointestinal, musculoskeletal, endocrine, Cushing's syndrome, neuropsychiatric effects, ophthalmic effects (See BNF for details and more side effects). NB most side effects only apparent after prolonged use

For pegylated interferon alpha: 📖 Table 9.1 Common drugs used for liver and gall bladder disorders: Hepatitis B, p.301.

For selective and non-selective NSAIDs: 📖 Table 17.1 Common drugs used for orthopaedic and musculoskeletal disorders: Anti-inflammatory drugs, p.635.

Drugs used in myeloma: 📖 Table 25.6 Common drugs used for cancer care, p.854.

Nursing patients with reproductive and gynaecological problems

Nursing assessment of women with reproductive problems

Nursing assessment should be holistic and ensure privacy and reassurance about confidentiality because of the sensitive nature of the discussions. In addition to a general nursing assessment (☐ Chapter 3, Individualizing nursing care practice, pp.32–33) perform the following procedures.

Observe the patient
- Genitalia (See Fig. 19.1)—Examination should be performed only by an appropriately trained nurse competent in speculum examination.
  - Observe for lesions, erythema, vulvitis.
  - Note appearance of vaginal walls, cervix.
  - Observe for discharge.
- Breasts—Observe for:
  - Asymmetry
  - Supernumerary or accessory nipples or breasts (rare)
  - Lumps
  - Inverted nipples
  - Discharge
  - Redness and swelling
  - Skin abrasions
  - Dimpling
  - General and periareolar inflammation

Ask the patient about

Nursing history
- Age
- Ability to manage self-care and activities of daily living
- Family support and dependants
- Anxieties, fears, and feelings about problems, potential care, and treatment
- Whether embarrassed to discuss condition
- Willingness to share with other family members
- Coping strategies

Vaginal health
- Vaginal discharge—colour, offensive smell, amount
- Irritation or soreness—onset and duration, previous history, precipitating events
- Use of perfumed soaps or vaginal deodorants

Menstrual history
- Last menstrual period (LMP)
- Details of menstrual cycle—age of onset, menopause (if relevant), frequency, loss, duration
- Problems of dysmenorrhagia, menorrhagia, amenorrhoea, bleeding or spotting between periods, after sexual intercourse or menopause

Sexual history
- Whether sexually active
- New sexual partner(s)
- Use of contraception and condoms
- Genital symptoms in partner
- Dyspareunia

Screening history
- Cervical screening—last date, results
- Breast screening mammography—last date, results

Breast history
- Whether breast self-examination is done
- Breast pain or tenderness
- Cyclical mastalgia
- Changes to shape and contour of breasts
- Discharge, lumps, swelling
- Changes in position and discharge of nipples, redness, skin dimpling
- Family history of breast disease

Obstetric history
- Number of pregnancies, still births, live births, and existing children
- Complications during pregnancy, birth, and afterwards
- Whether breastfed children
- Problems with fertility

General medical history
- Abdominal pain and discomfort
- Urinary symptoms
- Known endocrine or genetic disorders
- Medications used, particularly contraception, antibiotics, hormone replacement therapy (HRT), self-help, or complementary medicines

This assessment should form part of the patient's individual care pathway.

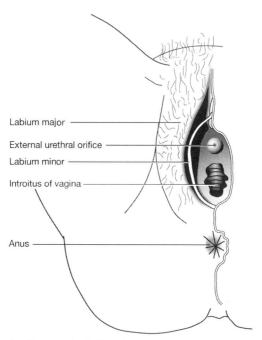

Fig. 19.1 Perineum in female. Taken from Mackinnon P and Morris J (2005). *Oxford textbook of functional anatomy*, vol 2, Fig 6.10-9. Oxford University Press, Oxford. Reproduced with permission from Oxford University Press.

Nursing problems for women with reproductive conditions

Abnormal vaginal discharge

This may be due to foreign body, vaginal or cervical infection, retained tampon, or other gynaecological disorder. Discharge may be increased in volume, offensive, or of changed consistency.

Menstrual problems
- Dysmenorrhoea—painful periods
- Menorrhagia—heavy periods
- Amenorrhoea—absence of periods
- Post-coital (bleeding after intercourse) or intermenstrual bleeding (bleeding between periods)

Urinary problems
- Incontinence—stress or urge incontinence
- Incomplete emptying of bladder

Pain
- Abdominal, pelvic, dyspareunia (painful intercourse), pruritis (vulva and vagina)
- Mastalgia (breast pain and discomfort)—may be cyclical, related to menstrual cycle

Breast problems

Lack of breast awareness and self-examination

Fear and anxiety
- Of tests and examinations, e.g. cervical smear, mammography
- Of positive test results, coping with treatment, and uncertainty about the future
- Of loss of control, opportunities, and choice
- Of changes in lifestyle
- Doubts about reliability of tests (following well-publicized errors)

Misconceptions
- Lack of understanding about normal anatomy and physiology of condition and options for treatment

Other psychological problems
- Loss of libido
- Negative feeling and resentment towards partner
- Embarrassment and unwillingness to discuss problems and treatment
- Lack of self-esteem due to body image and sexuality

Specific tests and investigations for women with gynaecological and breast problems

This topic is intended as an introduction to these tests and procedures many of which will be performed by specialist nurses. See the recommended further reading for more detail.

Genital speculum examination

This is systematic assessment of external and internal genitalia.

- Explain the procedure and obtain consent.
- Ensure privacy, dignity, and confidentiality.
- Ensure patient's bladder is empty and she is supported in lithotomy position.
- Decontaminate hands and wear disposable gloves.
- Examine labia, perineum, and introitus for lesions and erythema (inflammation).
- Use Cusco speculum to view vagina and cervix. Swabs of vaginal walls, cervix, and vaginal vault and a cervical smear can be taken.
- Provide tissue and handwashing for patients.
- Dispose of equipment and wash hands.
- Discuss findings with patient and when results are expected.

Cervical screening

This is performed to detect cervical pre-cancerous changes—cervical intraepithelial neoplasia (CIN) from nuclear abnormalities to dyskaryotic cells (See Fig. 19.2). Preparation and care are as above. Inform patients when to expect results and of possibility of recall for further screening or colposcopy. Giving information on support that is available in cases of positive (abnormal) smear may be helpful in reducing anxiety.

Colposcopy

This is examination of the cervix with an optical magnifying instrument to identify pre-invasive lesions of the cervix and lower genital tract. It can be undertaken by specialist nurses. Colposcopy is indicated for cervical intraepithelial neoplasia (CIN) levels 2 and 3, persistent unsatisfactory smear, post-coital or intermenstrual bleeding, or clinically suspicious cervix. Preparation is as for genital speculum exam (📖 Genital speculum examination, above). Treatment by excision or destruction of the cancer cells may be carried out via colposcopy.

Swabs

- Vaginal pH
- Potassium (KOH tests vaginal discharge; +10% potassium hydroxide produces distinctive smell in bacterial vaginosis)
- Microscopic examination and culture

Breast examination

- Clinical examination—evaluate symmetry, observe for skin dimpling, change of contour; palpate breast tissue using flat hand; check for nodes in neck, axilla, and supraclavicular fossa.
- Mammography—breast is compressed between two plates and an X-ray image is made. Ultrasonography may be used in women under 35.
- Fine-needle aspiration cytology—sample tissue is aspirated from breast; several samples are taken from different directions to determine benign and malignant lesions.
- Core biopsy—small core of breast lump removed using cutting needle.

Laboratory tests

- Serum gonadotrophins (LH, FSH), oestradiol
- Serum prolactin
- Serum FT4 and TSH

 Chapter 39, Common laboratory tests and their interpretation, p.1167.

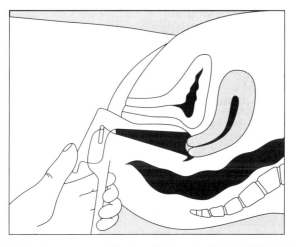

Fig. 19.2 Cervix examination. Taken from Mackinnon P and Morris J (2005). *Oxford textbook of functional anatomy*, vol 2, Fig 6.9.8. Oxford University Press, Oxford. Reproduced with permission from Oxford University Press.

Further information

Kubba A, Gupta S, and Holloway D (2009). *Oxford handbook of women's health nursing*. Oxford University Press, Oxford.

Menstrual problems and endometriosis

Amenorrhoea

Absence of menstruation is normal pre-puberty, during pregnancy and lactation, and after menopause. Primary amenorrhoea is the absence of periods in a patient who has never menstruated and secondary amenorrhoea is the absence of periods for >6 months in women who have previously menstruated. Causes include endocrine problems, hypothalamic disorders, tumours (e.g. craniopharyngioma), excessive weight gain or loss, excessive exercise, psychogenic (e.g. stress), pituitary tumours, ovarian disorders, polycystic syndrome, hypo- and hyperthyroidism, and adrenal disorders. Treatment is based on the cause.

Dysmenorrhoea

Primary dysmenorrhoea occurs when a person has painful menstruation from the onset of menses. Secondary dysmenorrhoea occurs when a person has previously had non-painful periods and may be due to endometriosis or pelvic inflammatory disease. Symptoms include cramping pain in the lower abdomen that radiates to the thighs and back, and may include nausea and vomiting. Patients may be less productive and take time off work. Treatment is with analgesia, NSAIDs, or combined oral contraceptives. Pelvic pathology should be investigated by the doctor and treated accordingly.

Menorrhagia

This is loss of at least 80 mL of blood; usually with clots during each period (normal loss is 35–50 mL). It may be caused by fibroids, congenital abnormalities (e.g. bicornate uterus), pelvic infection, endometriosis, polyps, or clotting disorders. It may have a significant impact on life due to physical discomfort and fatigue, anxiety, and embarrassment about flooding and adequate sanitary protection. Treatment includes NSAIDs and tranexamic acid to reduce menstrual flow; Mirena IUS endometrial ablation; and hysterectomy. 📖 Hysterectomy and pelvic floor repair, p.666.

Premenstrual tension

This refers to body changes occurring prior to period including breast pain and tenderness, bloated feeling, headache, weight gain, irritability, and mood swings. Evening primrose oil, vitamin B_6, diuretics, exercise, and relaxation techniques are helpful.

Endometriosis

This occurs when endometrial tissues grow independently outside the uterine cavity, e.g. in ovary, peritoneum, bowel, bladder, cervix, vagina, and very rarely in brain, bone, muscle, and skin. Symptoms may be mild or severe and are mainly disabling pain, heavy bleeding, painful intercourse, tiredness, depression, and reduced quality of life. Treatment is with NSAIDs, mefenamic acid, hormone therapy, laser therapy to eradicate lesions, and surgical interventions.

Nursing support for women with menstrual problems

The nurse has opportunities to provide information and health promotion to women with menstrual problems in a variety of clinical settings. It is important that the nurse is sensitive and recognizes that the patient may be embarrassed discussing her problems.

- Provide information about menstrual problems and promote ways that patient can help herself.
- Explain some of the symptoms she may experience.
  - For tiredness, advise patient to rest where possible and have blood checked for anaemia.
  - For urinary dysfunction, advise patient to empty bladder regularly.
  - For constipation, advise patient on increasing fluid intake and eating high fibre and healthy diet.
  - For mood swings, help the patient recognize the link with the menstrual cycle, which may make mood swings easier for the patient to cope with.
- Discuss the various treatments and drugs and side effects, and supplement the discussion with written information.
- Provide advice on how patients can relieve and cope with pain.
  - Encourage patient to take pain relief regularly as prescribed and not to wait until pain worsens before taking the next dose.
  - Encourage patient to use heat (e.g. hot water bottle) to relieve stomach cramps. (Care should be taken to prevent burns and scalds.)
  - Reassure patient that her pain is 'real', especially if menstrual problems have been dismissed or if she has been made to feel a fraud about complaining in the past.
  - Reassure patient that if the pain becomes worse further options for treatment are available.
  - Encourage patient to wear a well-fitting bra if breast pain and swelling is a problem. This may need to be a different size than during the rest of the menstrual cycle.
- Consider recommending alternative approaches to care, which may be helpful.
  - Over-the-counter medicines may help relieve symptoms, e.g. evening primrose oil for controlling pain and bloating in premenstrual tension.
  - Vitamin B_6 may help to combat depression associated with cyclical pain.
  - Acupuncture and homeopathy have been helpful for some women. Explain to the patient that scientific trials have not supported these treatments yet.
- Tactfully raise topics that might be embarrassing for the patient, e.g. dyspareunia (painful intercourse). This may be helped by adopting different positions.
- Advise on a generally healthy lifestyle with exercise and healthy diet and desirable weight.

📖 Chapter 5, Health promotion, p.85.

Infertility and early pregnancy problems

Infertility

This is a delay in conception of >1 year and occurs in 1 of 7 couples (See current NICE guidelines). Primary infertility occurs without prior pregnancy; secondary infertility occurs when there has been at least one pregnancy.

- Male factors—low sperm count, impotence, hypospadias. Alcohol consumption, drug misuse, and obesity are also factors.
- Female factors—endometriosis, abnormalities of uterus, blockage of fallopian tubes, ovulatory dysfunction, cervical hostility. Smoking, alcohol consumption, drug misuse, and obesity are also factors.
- Fertility may be impaired in poorly controlled diabetes. Fertility reduces with age. The cause may be unknown or multiple factors may be involved.

Management starts with advice about regular intercourse. Advise males to wear loose clothing and to abstain from hot baths. Advise males and females to stop smoking, reduce alcohol consumption, and reduce weight, if obese.

Investigations include history and examination, semen analysis, assessment of ovulation, tubal patency, cervical compatibility, hormonal tests, and checks for pelvic adhesions.

Treatment depends on cause. For ovulation disorders, clomiphene increases the chance of becoming pregnant. Assisted reproduction includes *in vitro* fertilization.

Abortion

Spontaneous: loss of pregnancy—miscarriage.

Threatened: early spontaneous vaginal bleeding, cervix closed, minimal pain.

Inevitable: pain, bleeding, cervix open. May be complete (uterus empty) or incomplete (retained products of conception).

Missed: no pain, minimal bleeding, cervix closed.

Treatment: evacuation of retained products of conception where necessary.

Termination of pregnancy: allowed up to 24 weeks of pregnancy if there is risk to woman's life or to her existing children's physical or mental health, or if the baby is at serious risk of physical or mental handicap.

Ectopic pregnancy

This occurs when the pregnancy implants outside the uterine cavity, most commonly in the fallopian tube and rarely in the ovary or abdominal cavity. It may present as acute or chronic. A ruptured ectopic pregnancy is an acute emergency and may be life-threatening. Patients present with severe pain in the pelvis and lower abdomen, collapse, and shock due to internal haemorrhage. Immediate fluid replacement and surgery is essential.

Nursing support for patients with early pregnancy loss

- Acknowledge that both partners may be grieving over their loss.
- Understand that people will react in different ways, for instance with:
  - Feelings of physical hurt or assault
  - Feelings that they were robbed
  - Guilt or self-blame
  - Sadness, depression, grief
  - Acceptance – just part of a life event
- Explain that such feelings are normal and to be expected.
- Spend time with the couple, providing empathy and seeking to understand what the loss means to them; let them lead the care required.
- Encourage them to ask questions and provide information as required about the future and further risks to pregnancies. It may be helpful to them if the nurse voices some of the difficult topics about loss that they find hard to discuss.
- Discuss the importance of remembering their loss and give ideas on how others have achieved this, e.g. planting trees or rose bushes, and explain how this has helped them cope with anniversaries. Advise on self help groups, e.g. Miscarriage Support Association.
- Discuss practical issues such as when to resume intercourse and when to try for pregnancy again. This will vary with the individuals, their reaction to the loss, and how they feel.
- Ensure follow-up arrangements with the GP or at a clinic are made.
- Discuss how they will tell family and friends. It may be helpful to recognize that parents and siblings often do not know how to respond and appear to say hurtful things although they are often well meaning.
- Recognize when grieving is becoming abnormal and expert counselling and support is necessary.
- Take folic acid to improve chances in next pregnancy.
- Risk of miscarriage after one miscarriage is slightly increased.

📖 Chapter 27, Nursing the dying patient, p.885.

Gynaecological cancers

Cervical cancer

Often found on routine cervical smears or colposcopy or following post-coital, intermenstrual, or postmenopausal bleeding. Cervical intra-epithelial neoplasia (CIN) describes the range of cell abnormalities—from minor changes of inflammation, viral or pre-cancerous, up to severe dyskaryosis (abnormalities with likely pre-cancerous changes) or cancer. Conservative treatment is with cytology or colposcopy, surveillance for low-grade abnormalities. Excision by diathermy loop excision (DLE) and hysterectomy removes the whole area of abnormality. Cryocautery destroys tissues by freezing. Pain and haemorrhage are risks of treatment. Follow-up checks, e.g. smears and colposcopy, are required annually.

Uterine cancer

Endometrial cancer often presents with postmenopausal bleeding. Risk factors include age, obesity, late menopause, no pregnancies, and diabetes mellitus. Diagnosis is by ultrasound scan and dilation and curettage (D&C) of the uterus. Treatment depends on stage and includes total hysterec-tomy with bilateral salpingo-oophorectomy, radiotherapy, progesterone therapy, and/or chemotherapy. Fig. 19.3 illustrates a coronal section of the uterus.

Ovarian cancer

Approximately 75% of ovarian cancers are not diagnosed until the late stages and survival rate is 20%. Risk factors include increasing age, high fat diet, infertility, use of fertility drugs, and history of the disease in first-degree relatives. It may present with ascites, bloating, abdominal mass, pelvic pain, vaginal bleeding, or cyst noted on scan. Treatment is removal by laparotomy with adjuvant therapy including radiation and chemotherapy.

Vulval cancer

Vulval intraepithelial neoplasia: presents with abnormal appearance and texture of the vulva. Biopsy is required for diagnosis. Treatment includes surgery, cryosurgery, or local chemotherapy.
Vulval carcinoma: usually occurs in patients over 70 and comprises 5% of genital cancers. Most are squamous cell carcinoma of the labia. Most present with chronic pruritis and a lump or ulcer. Simple vulvectomy (removal of labia majora, clitoris, and fourchette) or radical vulvectomy (as above plus labia minora, perineal body and inguinal and femoral nodes, associated lymphatics, and surrounding tissues) is done. This is extremely disfiguring surgery with significant physical, psychological, and emotional effects on patient and partner.

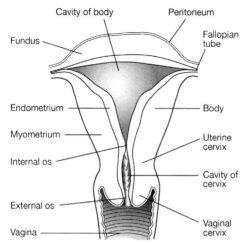

Fig. 19.3 Coronal section of the uterus. Taken from Mackinnon P and Morris J (2005). *Oxford textbook of functional anatomy,* vol 2, Fig 6.9.22. Oxford University Press, Oxford. Reproduced with permission from Oxford University Press.

Hysterectomy and pelvic floor repair

Hysterectomy

Types of hysterectomy

- Subtotal—the body of the uterus only is removed.
- Total—the body and cervix are removed.
- Total + bilateral salpingo-oophorectomy—the fallopian tubes and ovaries are removed.
- Radical or Wertheim's hysterectomy—includes the above plus broad ligament, local lymph nodes and glands, and upper third of the vagina.

Reasons for hysterectomy: cancer, fibroids, abnormal uterine bleeding, pelvic inflammatory disease, endometriosis, and uterine prolapse. An abdominal, vaginal, or laparoscopic hysterectomy may be performed.

Alternatives to hysterectomy

Endometrial ablation for menorrhagia: involves destroying the endometrial lining but preserving the uterus. Advantages include shorter operating time, fewer complications, faster recovery, and less need for analgesia. However, bleeding may continue, though lighter, and there is a risk of repeat surgery.

Arterial embolization of uterine fibroids: involves occluding the vessels that supply the fibroid which shrink and result in considerable post-procedure pain, infection, nausea, and vomiting but conserves the woman's fertility and reduces the risk of blood loss associated with hysterectomy and myomectomy.

Pelvic floor repair

The muscles, fascia, and ligaments of the pelvic floor become weakened and as a result the pelvic organs sag into the vagina. This is caused by stretching in vaginal delivery, reduction in oestrogen at menopause, heavy lifting, straining, coughing, and obesity.

Types of pelvic floor conditions

- Cystocoele—the bladder bulges into the vagina
- Urethrocoele—the urethra bulges into the vagina
- Rectocoele—the rectum bulges into the vagina
- Enterocoele—loops of intestine bulge into the vagina
- Prolapsed uterus
  - 1st degree—cervix remains in the vagina
  - 2nd degree—cervix protrudes from the vagina
  - 3rd degree—procidentia, uterus lies outside the vagina

Symptoms include urinary tract infections, cystitis, stress or urge incontinence, dragging sensation, feeling of 'something coming down', and difficulty in defecation.

Prevention includes good maternity care, physiotherapy, pelvic floor exercises, healthy diet, avoiding obesity and smoking, and managing any precipitating conditions, e.g. constipation, chronic cough.

Management includes ring pessary, which may provide temporary support for patients waiting for surgery or for those unfit for surgery. Surgical options include anterior or posterior colporrhaphy, colposuspension, or hysterectomy.

Role of the nurse

- Ensure the patient understands the reason for the surgery and the consequences and has the opportunity to consider the implications for her sexuality and relationship with her partner. Spend time talking through concerns, answering questions, and accepting how the patient feels.
- Provide details of what the surgery entails, the risks, and the consequences, which will help the patient in giving informed consent.
- Prepare the patient preoperatively as for major abdominal or vaginal surgery. In addition, preoperative preparation specifically requires:
  - Bowel preparation to empty the bowel.
  - Skin preparation. The pubic crown is usually shaved for abdominal surgery as a horizontal incision is usually made above the symphysis pubis.
  - Instruction on what will happen after surgery and what will be expected of the patient. For example, importance of early ambulation, deep breathing, and wearing compression stockings to prevent thrombophlebitis and chest infection; the role of the physiotherapist in ensuring that the patient is able to ambulate and do deep breathing effectively; and that the IV infusion may be in place to maintain hydration until she is taking sufficient oral fluids and diet.
- Monitor the patient postoperatively for:
  - Infection—Take care to use aseptic techniques for wound dressings and catheter care; decontaminate hands before and after contact with the patient; advise patient on how she can help prevent infection.
  - Pain—Give pain relief regularly before the pain becomes severe. An assessment chart will help.
  - Vaginal or wound bleeding—In some operations a vaginal pack may be in place. The patient should remain in bed until this is removed. The patient may also have a drain *in situ*. Drainage should be monitored and the drain removed when drainage is minimal.
  - Bowel sounds—Check that bowel sounds have returned and the patient has passed flatus. Patients should avoid straining and a mild aperient may be required to prevent this.
  - Dehydration—Measure and record the IV infusion and oral intake.
  - Urinary output and signs of bladder distension—Some patients may have a Foley catheter *in situ* and bladder retraining may be required when this is removed.
  - Emotional reactions—Check for signs of anxiety or depression which the patient may describe as 'feeling low'. Encourage the patient to discuss with both the nurse and family members or a patient with a similar operation who has successfully passed this phase. Address any psychosexual concerns following hysterectomy.

Menopause

Definition
This is defined as the end of the last menstrual period; a woman is postmenopausal 1 year after the last period. Onset is usually between 45 and 54 years and is considered premature if it occurs before 40 years. It occurs naturally or as a result of drugs, surgery, or radiotherapy. The impact on a woman's life varies depending on her beliefs and experiences. Many suffer in silence because they are too embarrassed to discuss it or because of lack of sympathy or poor understanding experienced in the past.

Patients' experience
Patients have different experiences in the climacteric (the perimenopausal months or years).
- Changes in the menstrual pattern, e.g. cycle becomes irregular, length between periods shortens or increases, or the amount changes (very heavy or scant loss)
- Painful periods or post-coital bleeding
- Hot flushes that may be associated with palpitations
- Vaginal dryness and atrophy
- Urinary problems, e.g. nocturia, stress and urge incontinence
- Mood changes and anxiety, loss of concentration, and forgetfulness
- Tiredness and lack of energy
- Osteoporosis, i.e. reduction of bone density. (This may not be apparent for many years and may present with fractures, commonly in wrist, spine, and femur.)
- Cardiovascular disease and increase in harmful lipids

Support for patients
- Carefully explain the types of treatments available and their effects and side effects to help the woman choose which is best for her circumstances.
- Offer general lifestyle advice—encourage a healthy diet, exercise, smoking cessation, moderate alcohol intake, and rest and relaxation, which will help the woman's general well-being and enable her to feel positive about herself. Exercise is essential in helping to reduce osteoporosis. Partner support is helpful.
- Discuss hormone replacement therapy (HRT). Oestrogen preparations may improve vasomotor symptoms, urogenital symptoms, and depressed mood, but adverse effects include venous thromboembolitic disease, breast cancer, and endometrial cancer. They may also cause breast tenderness, leg cramps, and vaginal discharge. Progesterone preparations (recommended for a maximum of 5 years) improve vasomotor systems but are usually given in combination with oestrogen; they may give rise to breast pain, fluid retention, irritability, anxiety, and depression.
- Suggest other therapies that may help including vitamin B_6, evening primrose oil, or vaginal lubricants. Acupuncture, aromatherapy, and yoga may also be of benefit.

Gynaecological infections

Vaginal discharges

Bacterial vaginosis

This is a common cause of vaginal discharge with an offensive, often heavy, discharge. It is caused by an increase in bacteria (e.g. *Mycoplasma hominis*, *Gardnerella vaginalis*) following reduction in lactobacilli resulting in alkaline pH in the vagina. It may result in gynaecological complications. Treatment is with metronidazole orally or topically. Advise the patient to avoid alcohol.

Trichomoniasis

This is an infection with a protozoan flagellate *Trichomonas vaginalis*. It produces a frothy grey vaginal discharge and superficial dyspareunia, vulvitis, and vaginitis. It can be transmitted through saunas and jacuzzis or through sexual transmission. Treatment for both partners is with metronidazole.

Candidiasis (thrush)

This is due to *Candida albicans*, a commensal organism in the vagina. It causes vaginal and vulval itching and soreness and irritation of the glans penis in males. It causes increased white cottage-cheese-like discharge and superficial dyspareunia. Treatment is by oral fluconazole or vaginal clotrimazole available as over-the-counter medications. Topical application or ingestion of live yoghurt may be helpful.

Bartholin's cyst and abscess

Bartholin's cysts usually present with a unilateral swelling and range from 2–8 cm in diameter. They may become infected with staphylococci, streptococci, *E. coli*, or occasionally gonococci. Antibiotics should be prescribed, but if an abscess is formed it is drained and marsupialization of the gland carried out. Repeat infections may rarely indicate carcinoma.

Support and advice to patients

- Provide information and education about the infection as the patient may be anxious that it is a sexually transmitted disease. Written information will be helpful.
- Recognize that recurrent infections can have an effect on patient's general well-being and remind patients that seeking medical help is important.
- Advise simple hygiene measures and avoidance of strong detergents and bath oils.
- Advise cleaning from front to back following defecation.
- Suggest wearing loose-fitting cotton underwear.
- Recommend healthy diet and inform that some women find taking oral live yoghurts to be of benefit.

Contraception

The main purpose of contraception is to prevent unplanned and unwanted pregnancies. However, these still occur because of inconsistent or incorrect use of the contraceptive method (i.e. it was not used at the time of sexual activity, the method was ineffective, or the product failed).

Types of contraception

Oral contraceptive pill

- Combined oestrogen and progesterone pill. Side effects include cyclical weight increase, vaginal discharge, breast tenderness, loss of libido, breakthrough bleeding (bleeding between periods), slightly increased risk of CHD and breast and cervical cancer, reduced risk of ovarian and endometrial cancer.
- Progesterone only. May cause menstrual irregularities, increased risk of ectopic pregnancy, slightly increased risk of breast cancer, weight and libido changes.

Injections of progestogens: These may be monthly or 3-monthly injections. Beneficial for women who travel, work shifts, or have difficulty with concordance.

Intrauterine contraceptive devices (IUCDs): These must be inserted by specially trained practitioners and may remain in place for 3–8 years. Complications include menorrhagia, dysmenorrhoea, intermenstrual bleeding, and pelvic infection.

Sterilization: This has few side effects once the surgery has been completed but is deemed irreversible.

Barrier methods: These include diaphragm, condoms, and female sheath. Use of spermicide cream or pessaries give added protection. Diaphragm must initially be fitted by specially trained practitioner and the woman taught how to use on subsequent occasions. It is essential that devices are inserted, removed, and maintained properly.

Role of the nurse

- An assessment is usually performed by a suitably trained nurse in sexual and reproductive health.
- Obtain a history from the patient to determine if there are contra-indications for using specific types of contraception.
- Ensure patient understands menstrual cycle and how pregnancy occurs.
- Ensure the patient understands:
  - How to take or use the contraceptive pill or device safely. Demonstrate or use videos where possible.
  - Possible consequences of non-concordance.
  - What to do if the pill is missed or taken late, i.e. take additional precautions.
  - To check with the doctor or nurse if taking antibiotics and other medications.
  - To take additional precautions for 7 days following vomiting and diarrhoea.
  - What to do if the product has failed, e.g. split condom.
  - Where to obtain emergency contraception and that this should be taken within 72 hours of unprotected sex.
  - How to take care of devices before and after use.

Nursing assessment of men with reproductive disorders

The nurse must ensure privacy, dignity, and confidentiality as the patient is likely to be embarrassed or distressed by the nature of the condition. In addition to a general nursing assessment (📖 Chapter 3, Individualizing nursing care practice, pp.32–33) perform the following procedures.

Observe the patient

- Evaluate reactions to discussing the condition and problems, particularly their willingness, embarrassment, what is said, and what is not said.
- Inspect genitalia for abnormalities:
  - Swelling
  - Cysts
  - Mass in scrotum
  - Absence of testicle
  - Trauma to scrotum or testicle
  - Bleeding or discharge from the penis
  - Redness and inflammation in the groin
  - Fever

Ask the patient about

Nursing history

- Ability to manage self-care and activities of daily living
- Help and support in place at home, dependants at home
- Coping mechanisms and lifestyle
- Feelings about the condition and what it means to him (e.g. relationships, sexuality, fears about treatment and the future)
- How much he understands about the condition and what else he wants to know
- Previous experience of nursing care
- Whether testicular self-examination is performed

Current problems

- Pain or tenderness, swelling, or oedema in the pelvis, scrotum, penis, or perineum
- Change in size or texture of the testicle
- Feelings of heaviness or a dragging sensation in the scrotum
- Related urinary symptoms, e.g. frequency, dysuria, problems with urinary flow, urethral discharge or irritation

Past medical history

- Mumps, particularly at puberty
- Subsequent orchitis
- Undescended or partially descended testicles
- Inguinal hernias
- Previous surgery, e.g. orchidopexy, fixing the scrotal sack by surgery, circumcision
- Drugs, e.g. antihypertensive drugs and antidepressants, which may have an impact on sexual function

Sexual health

- Changes in sexual function, e.g. whether sexually active, loss of libido, erectile disorders, premature ejaculation
- Changes in relationships (e.g. new partners, divorce)
- Changes in life circumstances (e.g. loss of employment)

Men's health

- Men die at a younger age than women, and they are less likely to access health care services or participate in health-promoting behaviours.
- Many men's health problems are preventable and are related to lifestyle, health risk behaviour, and poor use of health services.
- Men are particularly influenced by male socialization and the need to conform to male stereotypic behaviours, e.g. it may be considered unmanly to seek help for minor ailments. Attitudes of 'must keep up with the boys' with rounds of alcoholic drinks may be prevalent.
- Men may have difficulty talking about health and find it embarrassing to do so, especially with other men.
- Many men are not aware of what screening is available and its benefits and do not readily have access to information.

How nurses can help

- Consider establishing services where men are likely to gather, e.g. at sports centres, pubs, etc.
- Find out what is relevant for men in a particular setting.
- Focus on having an 'MOT' (i.e. a general health check) and improving fitness rather than specific screening or disease prevention.
- Use any existing services as opportunities to provide a broader base of information, e.g. vasectomy clinics, workplace, GP practice.
- Women can sometimes be a useful route of ensuring information gets to their partners.
- Ensure anonymity, privacy, and confidentiality.
- Work with the press and media to raise health issues for men and ensure that information about where to get further help locally is included.
- Recognize that drop-in centres are often better attended than those requiring an appointment.
- Ensure that information materials are specifically geared to men, e.g. use fit healthy men as role models.

Nursing problems for men with reproductive conditions

Pain

Pain in the scrotum, penis, lower abdomen, and perineum may range from ache to tenderness to severe pain of sudden onset.

Swelling

Swelling of the scrotum may be due to inflammation from infections of the testes and may be accompanied by redness, or may be due to an excess of fluid in the tunica vaginalis. Swelling of the glans penis may be due to infection or trauma.

Urethral discharge

This may be purulent, blood stained, or serous fluid due to infection and inflammation.

Urinary problems

These include dysuria, retention, and poor flow. May be due to problems of the penis or to other urinary or prostate problems. 📖 Chapter 11, Nursing patients with renal and urological needs, p.327.

Erectile dysfunction

This may be due to lack or loss of sexual desire, failure of sexual arousal, premature ejaculation, inhibited orgasm, or as a result of diabetes.

Anxiety and fear

These may be due to broken relationships. Patients may have anxiety and fear about future health, potential loss of employment and financial worries, relationships and sexual performance, fertility loss, loss of masculinity, surgery, and possible death.

Embarrassment

This may lead to unwillingness to discuss condition with health care professional and partner.

Altered body image

A lack of self-esteem may result from loss of body hair, loss of testicle, and feelings of being unattractive.

Feelings of isolation

These feelings may result from lack of support and feeling alone.

Specific tests and investigations for men with penile and testicular conditions

Physical examination

This will include examining the testicles, scrotum, and penis for abnormalities and the groin, axilla, chest, and neck for signs of metastases.

Blood tests

- Tumour markers (serum β-HCG and α-FP) may be used to identify whether testicular cancer is present and will also help monitor treatment.
- FBC and blood cultures may be done when infections are suspected.

Radiological tests

- Chest radiography is used to determine general fitness of the patient and to identify signs of metastases in suspected cancer.
- CT scan of chest, abdomen, and pelvis is used to stage cancers.
- Ultrasound scan can be used to help identify cause of swollen testicle.

Exploration and biopsy

These may be done to identify cancer.

Swabs

Swabs of urethral discharges may be done for microscopy, culture, and sensitivity and to rule out sexually transmitted infections.

Urine tests

These may be done for microscopy, culture, and sensitivity.

Testicular self-examination

This is a regular inspection and palpation of the testicles to detect any changes that may indicate testicular disorders.

The nurse should recognize that men may:
• Be unaware of the potential benefits of testicular self-examination.
• Be unaware of how to carry it out.
• Be skeptical of the value.
• Forget to do it.
• Be fearful of finding something.

The nurse should teach men to:
• Be aware that it is normal for the testicles to be a different size from each other and that they may hang differently in the scrotal sac.
• Become familiar with the normal weight, consistency, and texture of his testicles. This should include the feel of the epididymis which runs behind the testicle.
• Carry out the test at least once a month.
• Observe himself in a mirror and identify any changes.
• Feel the whole surface of each testicle.
• Roll each testicle between the thumb and forefinger to ensure the surface is free from lumps.
• Report any abnormalities immediately to GP or practice nurse.

The nurse should remember:
• To be sensitive; the patient might be embarrassed.
• To ensure privacy and dignity. Ensure no one can overhear discussions or enter the examination room or area. Appropriate use of a chaperone may need to be considered, however.
• Demonstration as well as instruction—a video might be helpful.
• Leaflets or a video may be helpful as supplementary information.
• Other sources of advice and information.

Conditions affecting the penis

Infections

Balanitis

This is inflammation of the glans penis and foreskin. It occurs at any age but is common in young boys. It is caused by streptococci, coliforms, and *Candida* and can be associated with diabetes. Patients complain of irritation and pain in the penis and of discharge. Treatment is with topical antifungal cream for *Candida* infections or oral antibiotics. Recurrent balanitis may be linked to phimosis and circumcision may be required.

Phimosis

This is the inability to retract the foreskin. It may be congenital or due to recurrent balanitis or trauma. It presents with poor or obstructed urinary flow or spraying; and pain during intercourse in adults. Treatment is by circumcision.

Paraphimosis

This is the inability to pull forward a foreskin that has been retracted, usually due to oedema and congestion in the glans and prepuce. It occurs at any age. Treatment is by manual reduction after applying local anaesthetic jelly as lubricant and to relieve pain. If unsuccessful, surgery may be required to perform dorsal slit in the foreskin or circumcision.

Cancer

Cancer of the penis is relatively rare and is usually squamous cell carcinoma or malignant melanoma. It usually occurs in older men. It presents with an ulcer on the penis and biopsy confirms diagnosis. Treatment is usually by radiotherapy.

Conditions affecting the testicles

Torsion of the testes

There is sudden onset of pain, with a tender swollen scrotum and possible lower abdominal pain, nausea, and vomiting. It is common in adolescents. Emergency surgery is required.

Infections

Orchitis is inflammation of the testes, often by a virus. It causes painful and swollen testes and may follow viral infections, e.g. mumps, rubella. Nurse the patient in bed with scrotal support. Administer analgesia and observe for fever and urinary problems such as dysuria.

Acute epididymitis is inflammation of the epididymis, with bacteria or viruses (*E. coli, Chlamydia*) and may be sexually transmitted. Symptoms include acute scrotal pain, tenderness, redness, and swelling, and a secondary hydrocoele may develop. Nurse patient in bed with scrotal support; administer antibiotics and pain relief.

Impaired fertility is a complication of the above.

Hydrocoele

This is the collection of excess fluid in the tunica vaginalis (serous space in the testis). It causes a cystic swelling in the scrotum that transluminates, but is not usually painful. It may be treated conservatively with a scrotal support, by aspiration which may need to be repeated, or by surgery if malignancy is suspected or the hydrocoele is large. Information and explanation of condition and reassurance are important.

Testicular cancer

This is the most common malignancy in men aged 15–35 years, is not a major cause of death, and is curable if detected early.

- Risk factors include age (20–44), undescended testes, trauma to the testes, mumps, and temperature variation (may be linked to tight clothing). It is more common in professional groups.
- It presents with a painless lump and enlargement of the testicle. The patient may have a dull ache in the lower abdomen and groin or a hydrocoele.
- Treatment and care includes surgery—orchidectomy (a prosthesis may be inserted). The patient's sexual functioning should not be affected and the sperm count may be lower but should still be fertile. A biopsy is taken to indicate whether further treatment is required, e.g. radiotherapy or chemotherapy. The side effects of these should be explained in detail and support and advice provided for each patient on how to cope with these, e.g. skin reactions, vomiting, diarrhoea, and hair loss. In particular, patients should understand that chemotherapy may cause infertility and the opportunities for 'sperm banking' should be explored.

Sexually transmitted infections

Sexually transmitted infections (STIs) require standard infection control precautions to be taken to minimize the risk of transmission of infections.

Chlamydia

This is a major cause of infertility in women; it affects the endo-cervix, urethra, rectum, eye, and pharynx. Approximately 80% may be asymptomatic or it may cause vaginal discharge, post-coital or intermenstrual bleeding, or pelvic inflammatory disease. It can cause reactive arthritis (Reiter's syndrome). Most males (60%) are usually asymptomatic but may have urethritis, dysuria, and penile discharge. Mother-to-baby transmission causes conjunctivitis, pneumonia, and otitis media in neonates. Treatment is with azithromycin or erythromycin in pregnancy. All contacts should be treated.

Gonorrhoea

This is caused by *Neisseria gonorrhea*. It can also be spread from mother to baby. Males may have urethritis with purulent yellow/green urethral discharge, meatal oedema, and dysuria; it can affect the rectum, urethra, and throat. Females may be asymptomatic or have purulent vaginal discharge, frequency or ano-rectal pain, endometritis, and salpingitis. Patients may have fever, malaise, and myalgia. Antimicrobials are used dependent on local antibiotic resistance patterns, currently ceftiaxone and cefixime.

Syphilis

This presents with a minor early illness (painless chancre at site of contact, followed 4–6 weeks later by fever, rash, swollen lymph nodes) and a more serious illness which develops after a variable latent period (involves cardiovascular and nervous systems). It is caused by *Treponema pallidum*, a spirochaete. Long-acting penicillin, e.g. IM benzathine benzyl-penicillin, is required with follow up over 2 years. The incidence is rising.

Genital herpes

This is caused by the herpes simplex virus (HSV). It causes multiple painful genital blisters and ulcers. The first attack is most severe. Most infections are with visible ulcers but viral shedding is possible. Treatment is by oral antiviral drugs, e.g. valaciclovir. Condoms may reduce transmission. Mother-to-baby transmission occurs; if active lesions are evident, caesarean section is performed.

Partner notification

This is essential for all sexually transmitted diseases as a large percentage of people with an STI do not have signs or symptoms. Sexual partners are informed of their exposure to infection by patient referral, provider referral, and contact referral. Partners must be treated simultaneously to prevent re-infection.

Sexual health

- Use all available opportunities to raise awareness about sexual health, e.g. antenatal clinics, outpatient clinics, GP surgery, and community health clinics.
- Provide information for patients about their condition and check their understanding. Up-to-date leaflets may be helpful.
- Encourage the patient to make and keep appointments with sexual health or genitourinary medicine (GUM) clinics. Provide information on locations, telephone numbers, opening times, and referrals to staff and services. (Most centres have genitourinary specialists, specialist nurses, sexual health advisers, counsellors, and HIV specialists.) If the patient refuses to attend, encourage them to visit their GP instead.
- Explain how confidentiality, privacy, and dignity are maintained at the clinics.
- Advise to recommend treatment and screening for all sexual partners.
- Explain about contact tracing and how and why this is undertaken by the GUM clinic.
- Explain that sexual abstinence is required during treatment for all partners to prevent re-infection.
- Promote safe sex by raising awareness of risk factors for sexually transmitted diseases (age <25, new sexual partner, two or more sexual partners in last 12 months and non-barrier method of contraception, casual holiday relationships, and risky situations arising due to the consumption of excess alcohol or drugs).
- Work with schools and other youth groups to set up sex and relationship education for young people to focus on:
  - preventing sexually transmitted diseases
  - reducing unplanned and unwanted pregnancy
  - learning about sex, sexuality, emotions, relationships, and sexual health
  - developing confidence and self-esteem
  - behaving responsibly in sexual and personal relationships
  - having sufficient skills to protect themselves
  - ensuring access to confidential advice and support
  - ensuring referrals are made to specialist nurses, psychologists, and doctors for patients with erectile dysfunction, or who need sexual counselling or sexual therapy
  - ensuring patients understand about effective contraception.
- Advise on hygiene measures.
  - Avoid strong detergents and perfumed soaps.
  - Keep vulval area clean but avoid vaginal douching.
  - Wear loose cotton underwear and avoid tight restrictive clothing.
  - Do not share towels.
  - Do not share sex toys.

Benign breast disorders

Benign breast conditions cause stress and anxiety to women, particularly because they are difficult to differentiate from cancer.

- *Congenital conditions* include breast asymmetry, supernumerary or accessory nipples or breasts (rare). These rarely require treatment but reassurance and advice and support are often needed.
- *Juvenile hypertrophy* refers to breast enlargement before puberty and is common. Exaggerated growth causing large breasts may require reduction mammoplasty to reduce embarrassment and improve quality of life.
- *Fibroadenomas* are benign tumours that develop in lobules and are affected by hormonal changes as with the rest of the breast. Determine whether the fibroadenomas need to be removed.
- *Mastalgia* is breast pain. It is sometimes linked to lumpiness and may be cyclical, linked to menstrual cycle with tenderness, heaviness, and fullness for 3–7 days or longer before menstruation. It can significantly affect quality of life. Evening primrose oil and a well-fitting bra may be helpful. Non-cyclical mastalgia may occur over decades and be related to the chest wall and ribs. It may also be linked to periductal mastitis, but the cause is often unknown and may cease after pregnancy or menopause.
- *Nodularity* that is generalized is common before menopause. Focal nodularity is a common cause of breast lumps but is rarely associated with cancer.
- *Cystic disease* is common in perimenopausal women. Local areas of excessive fibrosis or sclerosis develop and should be investigated as the appearance is similar to cancer.
- *Breast infections* due to lactation during the early weeks of breast feeding are due to poor hygiene, cracked nipples, and skin abrasions. They result in tender painful breasts and sometimes abscesses occur. Antibiotics, good hygiene, and possible drainage of abscess are required. Non-lactating periareolar infections and abscess may also occur.

In males

Gynaecomastia refers to the growth of breast tissue in males. It tends to resolve spontaneously. In males 50–80 years old it may be due to hormonal changes or drug therapy.

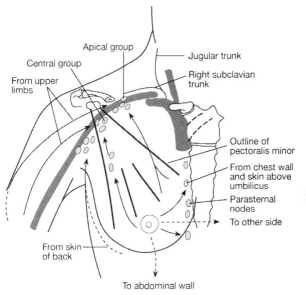

Fig. 19.4 Lymphatic drainage of breast to axillary and parasternal (internal thoracic) nodes

Breast cancer

Female risk factors

- Age (most common after menopause)
- Early onset menstruation (before 11 years)
- Late menopause (55+ years)
- First child born at 35+ years or no children
- Small risk with contraceptive pill and HRT
- Genetic predisposition

Presentation and diagnosis

- Breast pain
- Breast lump detected by self-examination, clinical examination or mammography
- Confirmed by needle biopsy. 📖 Specific tests and investigations for women with gynaecological and breast problems, p.658

Classification

Classified as cancer *in situ* (noninvasive) or invasive cancer spread outside the basement membrane into surrounding tissue. Local lymphatic and vascular involvement indicates poorer prognosis (See Fig. 19.4). Extent of disease is measured in TNM system (i.e. tumour, node, metastases).

Treatment

Includes surgery, radiotherapy, chemotherapy, hormone therapy, and combinations.

For local disease: Breast conservation (excision of tumour and margin of normal tissue) or mastectomy and radiotherapy. Presence or absence of axillary lymph nodes and number of nodes involved determines treatment choice. Radiotherapy, usually over 3–5-week period, results in mild erythema, skin desquamation and infection, lymphoedema, and tiredness.

Chemotherapy: Systemic treatment either before surgery (neo-adjuvant) or after surgery (adjuvant) improves survival. Combinations of agents are more effective than single agents. Side effects include hair loss, fatigue, lethargy, nausea, vomiting, and loss of fertility.

Hormone therapy: Most breast cancers are oestrogen-positive tumours; tamoxifen, an anti-oestrogen drug, is given usually 20 mg daily for 5 years. Side effects include hot flushes, night sweats, altered libido, vaginal dryness, and weight gain.

Oophorectomy: Beneficial in women <50 and can be achieved by surgery, radiation, or hormone-induced menopause.

Male breast cancer

Similar to female breast cancer. Klinefelter's syndrome, hormonal imbalance, and gynaecomastia increase the risk.

Prevention and early detection of breast cancer

Whenever opportunities arise, e.g. in family planning clinics, antenatal and postnatal clinics, outpatient clinic, day surgery, and surgical wards, nurses and midwives should take measures to prevent and detect breast cancer.

- Raise awareness of breast cancer, risk factors, and early signs of the disease.
- Teach breast awareness.
  - Regularly observe the breasts in mirror when dressing or washing with hands by the sides then arms above the head.
  - Be aware of what is normal for you, shape and contour of breast, changes during the menstrual cycle, direction and position of the nipples.
  - Teach patients what to look for and instruct them to report changes without delay.
    — Changes in shape and contour, and differences between breasts
    — Lump in breast and axilla
    — Areas of thickening
    — Dimpling and puckering of skin
    — Alteration in position or direction of the nipple
    — Changes in skin colour
    — Discharge from the nipple
    — Pain or discomfort in breast (not normally experienced during menstrual cycle)
- Provide information for patients and families.
- Encourage participation in screening programme and how to access.
- Inform patients of family history clinics.
- Suggest genetic counselling for high-risk individuals.
- Consider possible bilateral subcutaneous mastectomy.
- Use opportunities to discuss concerns with women.
- Ensure there is information for women from different ethnic groups.
- Ensure there is information for men.
- Provide further sources of information.
  - www.breastcare.co.uk; www.breastcancercare.org.uk

Role of the nurse in caring for patients with breast cancer

- Raise public awareness of the importance of risk factors, early detection, and treatment.
- Understand types of treatment, risks, benefits, and side effects. Be prepared to discuss with patients.
- Provide patients with written information.
- Ensure patients have early access to specialist breast care nurses who can provide more detailed information regarding treatment plans, prognosis, and options for breast prosthesis or reconstruction.
- Understand the psychological effects of loss of health and confidence, changes to body and self image, anxiety about sexuality, and future survival.
- Be approachable, sensitive, and supportive to patients and their relatives. Recognize when patients are anxious or depressed, and encourage them to discuss their feelings.
- Help patients discuss their feelings with family and friends who can provide practical help, provide emotional support, and help them come to terms with their condition.
- Ensure access to support groups.
- Ensure patients are successfully coping during or after treatment.
- Encourage patients to take the lead in decision making.
- Ensure patients have access to physiotherapy, particularly following mastectomy and axillary node dissection, and have access to lymphoedema specialist, if necessary.
- Ensure patients who are undergoing radiotherapy are advised about skin care, dressing, and the help and support needed when experiencing fatigue.
- Provide practical advice to boost morale, e.g. using hats and wigs when hair loss occurs, consulting image advisors and stylists for appearance.
- Discuss prostheses, cosmetic effects, and living with a mastectomy.

Patient education for reproductive disorders

Psychological and emotional problems are inextricably linked to the patient's physical condition and should influence the way information and education is provided.

- Use a variety of opportunities (e.g. in the ward, outpatient clinic, day case, patient's home, or workplace) to provide information about the risk factors of relevant conditions, breast awareness, testicular self-examination, screening programmes, and sexual and reproductive health. Encourage attendance at GP, and community well woman/man clinics.
- Use leaflets, videos, models, and posters to supplement information and raise awareness.
- Spend time listening to patients to learn about:
  - Myths and misconceptions they may have about reproductive conditions, conception, contraception, and sexually transmitted diseases (e.g. belief that cervical screening is unnecessary in post-menopausal women, sexually inactive women, or virgins).
  - Fears and anxieties (e.g. that they will be viewed as promiscuous or that their sexual preferences will be made known to family members) or concerns relating to self-image, sexual attractiveness, and value in family and relationships.
  - Any negative feelings they may have about themselves or their partners.
- Where appropriate encourage both partners to be involved in education and discussion.
- Ensure patient understands:
  - Preoperative care and has sufficient information to give informed consent.
  - Effects of surgery and how these can be managed (e.g. tiredness, hot flushes, weight gain, and digestive disturbances post-hysterectomy), effects of orchidectomy, and effects of chemotherapy and radiotherapy on fertility following testicular cancer.
  - Any side effects or complications of treatment and what to do if these arise, e.g. vaginal bleeding, urethral discharge.
  - When to resume usual activities including sexual activities; any precautions that should be taken; and that adjustments and full recovery may take weeks, months, or even longer depending on the operation.
- For some patients it will be helpful to discuss with someone who has successfully recovered or is coping with the condition.

Discharge and continuity of care for patients with reproductive disorders

- Recognize that some patients may be reluctant for family members and friends to have information about their condition and admission because of the sensitive and personal nature of the disorder.
- Check that the patient has appropriate knowledge of their condition, that sufficient information has been provided for patients to continue care at home, and that sufficient supplies of equipment and dressings have been provided or that patients know where to obtain them.
- Explain possible complications that may develop, e.g. urinary infections, hot flushes, weight gain following hysterectomy.
- Check that the patient understands the amount and type of activities they are permitted to do, how much rest to have, when it is likely they can start work again, and when they can resume sexual activity.
- Encourage the patient to incorporate behaviours that will reduce the risk or recurrence, e.g. ensuring they have effective contraception for their needs, using barrier methods of contraception to reduce risk of STI, and maintaining a healthy diet.
- Ensure they have information on how to manage their own condition on a longer-term basis and have contacts for organizations that will provide help and support.
- Emphasize the importance of using medications properly for reproductive conditions and ensure that the patient understands the purpose, side effects, dose and times, and effects of non-concordance for each of the drugs and where to get further supplies.
- Arrange community nursing and social services support well in advance of discharge, if needed, and provide contact details of relevant people.
- Arrange continuing support from specialists such as breast care nurses and sexual health advisers, if necessary.
- Arrange follow-up appointments with GP, outpatient clinic, GUM clinic, and well man/woman clinics as appropriate.
- Provide written information for patients to take with them.

Caring for patients with reproductive disorders—sources of information

- Testicular Cancer Resource Centre — www.tcrc.acor.org
- Testicular Cancer (Cancer Research UK) — www.cancerhelp.org.uk
- Cancer BACUP — www.cancerbacup.org.uk
- STI Online (Sexually Transmitted Infections) — http://www.sti.bmjjournals.com
- Family Planning Association (FPA) — www.fpa.org.uk
- Faculty of Family Planning and Reproductive Health — www.ffprhc.org.uk
- Infertility Network UK — www.infertilitynetworkuk.com
- Gynaecological Cancers UK — www.ukdirectory.co.uk
- Ovarian cancer and uterine cancer — www.patient.co.uk
- Marie Stopes International — www.mariestopes.org.uk
- Breast Cancer Care — www.breastcancercare.org.uk
- British Gynaecological Cancer Society — www.bgcs.org.uk

Common drugs used in women with reproductive problems

Common drugs used in women with reproductive disorders are listed in Table 19.1. **All drug doses listed in this table are adult doses and not children's doses**. This table is only to be used as a guide and the current BNF should be consulted for further advice. Nurses should involve themselves only in the administration of medications which fall within their sphere of competence.

Table 19.1 Common drugs used in women with reproductive problems

Anti-oestrogens	Dose	Common side effects
Clomifene	50 mg daily for 5 days, starting within about 5 days of menstruation; second course of 100 mg daily for 5 days may be given in absence of ovulation; three courses should constitute an adequate therapeutic trial	Visual disturbances or ovarian hyperstimulation—withdraw; hot flushes, abdominal discomfort; other side effects occasional (See BNF)
Hormone replacement therapy (HRT)	**Dose**	**Common side effects**
Oestrogens for HRT	See specific product	(See BNF for risks of long-term use) Nausea and vomiting, abdominal cramps, weight changes, bloating, breast enlargement and tenderness, premenstrual-like syndrome, fluid retention, cholestatic jaundice, altered lipids, mood changes, depression, headache, migraine, dizziness, leg cramps (NB rule out deep vein thrombosis), and other side effects (See BNF)

Table 19.1 Common drugs used in women with reproductive problems *(continued)*

Contraception/ menstrual regulation	Dose	Common side effects
Combined oral contraceptives	Low strength (See BNF) – 1 tablet daily for 21 days, then 7 tablet free days and repeat Standard strength (See BNF) – NB dose is dependent on product used; packs may include a tablet-free interval with placebo tablets or colour-coded tablets taken sequentially	Nausea, vomiting, headache, breast tenderness, change in body weight, fluid retention, thrombosis, changes in libido, depression, chorea, skin reactions, chloasma, hypertension, contact lenses may irritate, impairment of liver function, hepatic tumours, reduced menstrual loss, 'spotting' in early cycles, absence of withdrawal bleeding

Intra-uterine progesterone only device for contraception and menorrhagia	Dose	Common side effects
Mirena®	Insert into uterine cavity within 7 days on menstruation (anytime if replacement) or immediately after 1st trimester termination by curettage; postpartum insertions should be delayed until 6 weeks after delivery; effective for 5 years Prevention of endometrial hyperplasia during oestrogen replacement therapy: insert during last days of menstruation or withdrawal bleeding or anytime if amenorrhoeic; effective 4 years	Nausea, vomiting, headache, nervousness, acne, dizziness, breast discomfort, depression, skin disorders, disturbances of appetite, weight changes, changes in libido, abdominal pain, peripheral oedema, nervousness, salpingitis and pelvic inflammatory disease, pelvic pain, back pain

Table 19.1 Common drugs used in women with reproductive problems *(continued)*

Induction of abortion	Dose	Common side effects
Gemeprost	Dependent on stage of pregnancy (See BNF)	Vaginal bleeding and uterine pain, nausea, vomiting or diarrhoea; headache, muscle weakness, dizziness, flushing, chills, backache, dyspnoea, chest pain, palpitation and mild pyrexia; uterine rupture reported (most common in multiparas or if history of uterine surgery or if given with IV oxytocics); also reported severe hypotension, coronary artery spasm, and myocardial infarction

Common drugs used in men with reproductive problems

Common drugs used in men with reproductive disorders are listed in Table 19.2. **All drug doses listed in this table are adult doses and not children's doses**. This table is only to be used as a guide and the current BNF should be consulted for further advice. Nurses should involve themselves only in the administration of medications which fall within their sphere of competence.

Table 19.2 Common drugs used in men with reproductive problems

Drugs in prostatic disease: 📖 Table 11.1 Common drugs used for renal and urinary disorders, p.392.

Drugs for erectile dysfunction	Dose	Common side effects
Alprostadil	By intracavernosal injection – dose varies dependent upon response and product used (See BNF)	Penile pain, priapism, reactions at injection site and many more side effects (See BNF)
Sildenafil	Adult over 18 years – initially 50 mg 1 hour before sexual activity; subsequent doses adjusted according to response (25–100 mg as a single dose as needed); maximum 1 dose in 24 hours	Dyspepsia, vomiting, headache, flushing, dizziness, myalgia, visual disturbances, raised intra-ocular pressure, hypersensitivity reactions, priapism, painful red eyes, and nasal congestion; serious cardiovascular events reported

Common drugs used for breast conditions

Common drugs used for breast conditions are listed in Table 19.3. **All drug doses listed in this table are adult doses and not children's doses**. This table is only to be used as a guide and the current BNF should be consulted for further advice. Nurses should involve themselves only in the administration of medications which fall within their sphere of competence.

Table 19.3 Common drugs used for breast conditions

Drug	Dose	Common side effects
Tamoxifen and anastrazole: 📖 Table 25.6 Common drugs used for cancer care, p.854.		
Danazol	Severe pain and tenderness in benign fibrocystic breast disease not responding to other treatments: 300 mg daily in divided dose usually for 3–6 months	Nausea, dizziness, skin reactions, photosensitivity and exfoliative dermatitis, fever, backache, nervousness, mood changes, anxiety, changes in libido, vertigo, fatigue, epigastric and pleuritic pain, weight gain, menstrual irregularities, vaginal dryness and irritation, flushing and reduction in breast size, androgenic effects, thrombotic events and many more side effects (See BNF)
NSAIDs often used to treat pain/inflammation in all the above: 📖 Table 17.1 Common drugs used for orthopaedic and musculoskeletal disorders: Anti-inflammatory drugs, p.634.		
Drugs used in HIV: 📖 Table 18.1 Common drugs used for patients with HIV, p.649.		
Drugs used in infectious diseases: 📖 Common drugs used for infectious diseases, p.728.		
Drugs used in cancers: 📖 Table 25.6 Common drugs used for cancer care, p.854.		

Nursing patients with infectious diseases

Nursing assessment of patients with infectious diseases

A general nursing assessment of the patient (📖 Chapter 3, Individualizing nursing care practice, pp.32–33) is required in addition to the specific areas indicated below. The aim is to elicit information that will lead to a diagnosis and treatment of the infectious disease and to enable development of a nursing care plan. Specific tests and investigations will support this. 📖 Specific tests and investigations, p.698.

Observe the patient

- Dehydration—dry mouth, lips, inelastic skin, low urine output, concentrated urine
- Fever—pyrexia, flushed skin, tachycardia, bradycardia, sweating, chills, and shivering
- Chest infections—dyspnoea, shallow breathing, cough, sputum (thick purulent, bloodstained)
- Vomiting—amount, colour, consistency, smell
- Diarrhoea—consistency, amount, frequency, smell, presence of mucus, blood, and any associated pain
- Skin—wounds (infected or inflamed), ulcers, rashes (pustules, macular, papular), petechial (meningitis), abscesses, signs of scratching, bruising, needle tracks
- Specific infections—e.g. jaundice (dark urine, pale stools), meningitis (neck stiffness and/or rash)
- Changes in conscious level, drowsiness, and confusion

Ask the patient about

- Relevant history
  - Episodes of malaise, aches and pains, anorexia and lassitude, headache, vomiting, diarrhoea, chills, rigors, thirst
  - Animal contacts, insect bites
  - Recent wounds, e.g. lacerations, chronic wounds, or leg ulcers
- Pre-existing diseases, e.g. diabetes, cancer, emotional problems, immunosuppressive illness
- Contact with infection—onset, severity, and duration of symptoms
- Vaccination/immunization history
- Lifestyle—IV drug use, sexual history and habits (if appropriate), travel abroad including stopovers, possibility of food/water contamination, water sports, basic hygiene
- Drugs prescribed and taken
- Recent admissions to hospital or other medical treatment—to identify previous infections or possible exposure

Nursing problems

Raised body temperature

May be accompanied by flushed warm skin, sweating, tachycardia, chills and rigors, raised respiratory rate.

Disturbed body image

May result from skin rashes, bruising, jaundice, isolation nursing.

Diarrhoea

Loose semi-solid or liquid stools that are passed at more frequent intervals than normal for the patient.

Vomiting

A common symptom, particularly of faeco-oral infections.

Fatigue

Generalized aches and pains, listlessness.

Dehydration

Results from sweating, low fluid intake, increased urine output. Presents with dry mouth and lips, inelastic skin, concentrated low output of urine.

Impaired breathing

Breathing may be rapid, shallow, painful, and result in restlessness and cyanosis.

Altered consciousness level

May be anywhere in the range from slight drowsiness and confusion to coma. Consider objectively measuring this using a scale such as the Glasgow Coma Scale. 📖 Chapter 13, p.475.

Feelings of isolation

May occur particularly if the patient is being barrier nursed or is in isolation.

Risk of spread of infection

Will depend on cause of infectious disease and mode of transmission, e.g. faeces, blood, respiratory secretions.

Skin rash or wound

Skin rashes may be macular, papular, pustular, or petechial. Wounds may become infected and inflamed.

Specific tests and investigations

General principles
- Explain and discuss the procedures with the patient.
- Ensure privacy and dignity.
- Prevent contamination of the specimen.
  - Wash hands with soap and water or by using an alcoholic hand rub/gel. Wear sterile gloves as appropriate.
  - Clean area, if relevant, to prevent contamination with surrounding flora.
- Use appropriate correctly labelled leak-proof containers and self-sealing plastic bags for transporting specimens. Ensure the form is fully completed with patient details, date, and sample site of the specimen.
- Use biohazard labels when appropriate, e.g. blood and body fluid, infections (e.g. hepatitis B or HIV infections).
- Dispatch to laboratory promptly.
- Recognize that tests to be used in conjunction with clinical signs as false positives or negatives may occur with some tests.

Laboratory tests
- Blood cultures should be taken when signs of infection are present. Use special culture bottles and pay rigorous attention to aseptic technique to prevent contamination.
- FBC, CRP, ESR, U&E, LFTs, and serum for virology, blood film for malaria.
- Hepatitis serology—hepatitis A, B, and C.

Body fluids
- *Urine:* midstream specimen or catheter specimen for microscopy, culture, and sensitivity. Dipstick urinalysis to indicate bilirubin, blood, protein, and infection.
- *Faeces:* for microscopy and culture, ova, cysts, parasites, viruses, and *Clostridium difficile* toxin.
- *Sputum:* microscopy, culture, and sensitivity and acid fast bacilli (AFBs).
- *Cerebrospinal fluid (CSF):* cloudy CSF may indicate infection; bloodstained CSF usually indicates a traumatic tap.

Swabs
Swabs for culture can be taken from any body site and may include eyes, ears, nose, throat, skin, wounds, groin, axilla, perineum, IV sites, drain sites, vagina, penis.

Tuberculin skin tests
Tuberculin skin tests include Mantoux and Heaf tests. Strong positive tests may indicate active infection.

Blood-borne and droplet infections

Blood-borne infections

Hepatitis B and C

These are viral infections that can be transmitted by blood or body fluids. Infection is usually chronic. Patients may be asymptomatic or may present with flu-like illness or, in more severe acute cases, with abdominal pain and/or jaundice. Nursing care is based on symptoms. Infection may lead to cirrhosis, liver carcinoma, or liver disease. Treatment may include an antiviral agent such as interferon or ribavirin.

Human immunodeficiency viruses

Includes HIV1 and HIV2. 📖 Chapter 18, Nursing patients with human immunodeficiency virus, p.637.

Droplet infections

Pulmonary tuberculosis

This is caused by *Mycobacterium tuberculosis*. Patients may be asymptomatic or may present with fever, malaise, sweating, anorexia, weight loss, and cough with sputum which may be bloodstained.

Management
- Isolation is recommended for patients with smear-positive sputum (indicates the presence of acid-fast bacilli).
- Nurse patients with confirmed pulmonary tuberculosis in a negative pressure side room, if available.
- Use particle filtration respirator (PFR) masks when caring for patients with confirmed or suspected pulmonary tuberculosis, especially during aerosol producing activities.
- Segregate suspected cases from immunosuppressed and HIV antibody positive individuals.
- Most patients with fully sensitive organisms are non-infectious after 2 weeks, treatment.
- Notify Consultant in Communicable Disease Control (CCDC) of cases for tracing of contacts. Staff contacts will be checked by occupational health (OH) departments.
- Only staff immune to tuberculosis should attend patients.

Care and treatment
The focus of care is on managing symptoms and providing psychological support during isolation. Education is required for medication concordance and to inform patients of potential side effects. Teach patients how to reduce dissemination of infected droplets and to securely fasten sputum pots before disposal. Treatment includes a combination of antibiotics (may include rifampicin, isoniazid, pyrazinamide, and ethambutol).

Influenza

Influenza is a common viral infection. Viral mutations result in new strains. Patients present with fever, headache, malaise, weakness, nausea, and vomiting. Standard barrier precautions are required for 5 days. Complications include pneumonia, bronchitis, and sinusitis. Care includes bed rest and is based on symptoms.

Pneumonia

Streptococcus pneumoniae is the most common cause of pneumonia. Patients present with fever, rigors, anorexia, dyspnoea, cough, occasional haemoptysis, and pleuritic chest pain. Nursing care includes bed rest, fluids, observation of respiration, temperature, and pulse. Antibiotics, analgesics, and oxygen are usually prescribed.

Faeco-oral infections

Bacteria

Mode of transmission may be via food, e.g. *Salmonella*, *Campylobacter*, or person to person, e.g. *Shigella*, *Clostridium difficile* (*C. difficile*). Diarrhoea nausea and vomiting, fever and malaise are common symptoms.

C. difficile, an anaerobic bacterium, is the most important cause of health care associated diarrhoea. It rarely causes problems in the healthy adult but certain antibiotics may disturb the normal bacterial population of the intestine causing the *C. difficile* bacteria to multiply rapidly, produce toxin, and cause illness. *C. difficile* can cause mild to severe disease and may in some cases lead to a pseudomembranous colitis (severe inflammation of the bowel) and toxic megacolon. Transmission occurs via the hands of health care workers who have come into contact with an infected patient or their environment. Spores are produced which can survive in the environment for long periods. Handwashing with soap and water, and environmental cleaning with a disinfectant containing bleach, along with isolation, are important in the management of any patient with *C. difficile* infection. Care focuses on the management of symptoms and specific antibiotics according to local policy. All hospitals undertake mandatory surveillance of *C. difficile*.

Viruses

Mode of transmission may be through vomit and faeces via the hands of carers, surfaces, equipment, or occasionally by aerosols (e.g. small round structure viruses such as Norovirus). Viruses may spread rapidly through wards affecting patients and staff, and sometimes ward closures are essential to control transmission. Diarrhoea, vomiting, fever, and malaise are common symptoms.

Hepatitis A and E are transmitted via the faeco-oral route and may result in fever, malaise, anorexia, nausea, and sometimes jaundice. Care focuses on symptoms and avoidance of alcohol. Immunization for hepatitis A is available.

Parasites

Risk of transmission in hospital is low (e.g. *Giardia*, *Cryptosporidium*). Abdominal bloating, explosive diarrhoea, and lassitude are common symptoms.

Precautions

- Single room with own toilet facilities is advisable, especially if the patient has explosive diarrhoea or if a viral cause is suspected.
- Gloves and aprons should be worn for contact with infected material.
- Separate toilet and washing facilities, if possible, and decontaminate after use with detergent and hot water.
- Handwashing is essential by staff after contact with patients or bed linen; by patients after using the commode or toilet; by mothers changing nappies; and by visitors to patients on entering and leaving the clinical area.
- Staff that are nursing patients with GI infections should not care for immunosuppressed patients or prepare feeds.

- Staff with diarrhoea should report to Occupational Health (OH) department and should not work until having formed stools for 48 hours.
- Precautions should continue until diarrhoea has ceased for 48 hours and the patient has passed a formed stool.

Infections with resistant organisms

Infections caused by multiple resistant bacteria can cause serious problems in hospital because of limited antimicrobial therapy. Precautions to prevent cross-infection are required. Guidance from Infection Prevention and Control Team (IPCT) is essential.

Meticillin resistant *Staphylococcus aureus* (MRSA)

This can cause wound infections, pneumonia, septicaemia, and death. It is commonly carried as a skin commensal and may be found in the nose, perineum, groin, and axillae. Its mode of transmission is through direct contact, airborne methods and heavy environmental contamination. It requires barrier nursing and preventative measures (☐ Specific precautions for patients with MRSA, p.705). All hospitals are required to take part in the Department of Health mandatory MRSA bacteraemia surveillance scheme.

Antibiotic resistant gram-negative bacilli

Gram-negative bacteria normally inhabit the gut of humans but can survive in moist areas both intrinsically (in the body) and extrinsically (in the environment). There has in recent years been an increase in the number of gram-negative bacteria that are resistant to antibiotics (e.g. *Acinetobacter*, *E. coli* and *Klebsiella* sp.). Strict handwashing, use of personal protective equipment, and effective cleaning is essential in reducing transmission of these organisms.

Vancomycin Resistant Enterococci (VRE)

Enterococci are part of the normal flora of the bowel in humans and rarely cause infection. Vancomycin resistant enterococci are resistant to some antibiotics and when they do cause serious infection they present a therapeutic challenge. Some patient groups are commonly colonized but do not demonstrate any ill effects. Infection control precautions will vary according to the clinical context and care setting in which the patient is being managed.

Specific precautions for patients with MRSA

Screening

High-risk admissions

Refer to local policy but likely to include:

- Swabs of skin lesions, IV sites, nose, groin, and sputum and catheter urine should be taken as appropriate on:
  - Previous MRSA carriers
  - Nursing or residential home residents
  - Patients who have had a previous hospital admission

Preoperative and pre-admission screening

Early detection of MRSA in patients undergoing surgery and invasive procedures or who are admitted to intensive care units will assist in limiting dissemination in acute wards, e.g. orthopaedics, cardiothoracic, neurosurgery, and general surgery. Consider screening staff during outbreaks.

Early review of patients re-admitted

Patients should be identified to the ICT to ensure controls and prevention measures are in place.

Isolation of patients

Infected patients, carriers, and high-risk patients should be nursed in a side room with standard barrier procedures. Transfer to other areas should be restricted as much as possible.

Treatment

See local policy but likely to include:

- Seeking advice from ICT.
- Covering lesions with impermeable dressings.
- Using mupirocin cream for nasal carriage of MRSA. Seek advice from ICT in persistent carriage.
- Washing patients with chlorhexidine daily for 5 days. Apply chlorhexidine powder to groin and axillae. Change nightwear and bed linen daily.
- Re-swabbing sites 2 days after treatment has been discontinued.
- Serious infections may require vancomycin or alternative which must be discussed with microbiologist.

Education of staff

Staff training including annual updates will ensure that knowledge and skills regarding prevention, control, and antibiotic use is current.

Identify hotspot areas

Target prevention measures at specific areas.

Discharge arrangements

MRSA carriers should be discharged home as soon as possible. Arrangements for continuing treatment must be made. Carriers should be identified in health record.

Infestations

Scabies

📖 Chapter 12, Skin infections and infestations, p.410

Scabies is characterized by a widespread itchy rash caused by an allergic reaction to the scabies mite. It is spread by prolonged direct contact and usually presents with severe itching on hands, arms, legs, trunk, inner thighs, and axillae 1–8 weeks after contact. Skin excoriations and secondary infections result from scratching. Treatment is with a scabicide, e.g. malathion or permethrin. It is essential to follow instructions for application and repeat treatments.

Prevention and management of outbreaks
- Contact the ICT for advice.
- Institute treatment and barrier precautions immediately and continue for 24 hours after treatment.
- Identify staff involved in close contact and provide with treatment, if appropriate.
- Avoid direct skin contact and wear gloves and aprons, especially while administering treatment.
- Assess the risk of secondary cases among other patients. Consider prophylactic treatment as appropriate.
- Provide information to patients and family about treatment and mode of transmission.

Fleas

Pest control officers should be contacted. Clothing and bed linen must be washed at temperatures >60°C. If carpets are present these must be vacuumed daily.

Head lice

This is usually found on the scalp but may also occur in the axillae, beard, and eyebrows. It may be asymptomatic or present with itchy scalp. It is spread due to close contact, e.g. children at school or nursery. Apply insecticides, e.g. malathion, phenothrin, or permethrin according to instructions; may be used in conjunction with a fine tooth comb to remove lice. An alternative insecticide can be used for re-infestation. Treatment of recent contacts is necessary to prevent re-infestation.

Intestinal parasites

Threadworm (*Enterobius vermicularis*) is common in children in the UK. It causes anal irritation and itching. Spread is by close contact between children and poor hand hygiene. Treatment of the whole family with mebendazole is necessary. Hygiene is essential to prevent re-infection.

Schistosomiasis (bilharzia) is caused by a fluke that penetrates the skin while swimming or paddling in infected waters. It is not present in the UK but may be seen in travellers returning from endemic areas. Symptoms may include fever, urticaria, diarrhoea, hepatomegaly, splenomegaly, and renal problems. Usual treatment is praziquantel.

Serious rare infections

It is the responsibility of the medical staff to inform the Health Protection Agency of any diseases notifiable (to Local Authority Proper Officers) under the Public Health (Infectious Diseases) Regulations 1988 Act (in the UK – different requirements will apply in other countries).

Diphtheria

This is caused by the toxin of *Corynebacterium diphtheriae* and is an acute infectious disease that usually affects the upper respiratory tract. Symptoms can include fever, tonsillitis, and pharyngitis which can sometimes lead to respiratory obstruction in severe cases. Respiratory tract secretions are infectious and the disease can be transmitted by close face-to-face contact. Requires strict isolation until pathogen is eradicated (up to 4 weeks). Treatment is with antitoxin and IV erythromycin. Prevention is by vaccination.

Rabies

Rabies is an acute viral infection that is usually transmitted through saliva via the bite of an infected animal (usually dogs). It may present with headache, malaise, abnormal behaviour, agitation, and fever. Treatment focuses on symptom control and by keeping the wound clean, vaccination, and human rabies immunoglobulin. However, rabies is almost always fatal. Patients must be strictly isolated as the respiratory secretions may contain the virus.

Viral haemorrhagic fevers

These include Lassa fever, Ebola, and Marburg virus. Symptoms vary according to the type of virus but initial symptoms may include headache, fever, nausea, myalgia, and dehydration followed by bleeding. Treatment is based on symptoms and strict isolation is essential.

Creutzfeldt–Jakob disease (CJD)

CJD is a rare progressive degenerative brain disease that is ultimately fatal. A new variant of the disease known as variant CJD (vCJD) is linked to exposure to bovine spongiform encephalopathy (BSE). It causes brain degeneration with dementia, personality change, psychiatric symptoms, and cognitive and motor impairment. Care focuses on alleviating symptoms and providing psychological and social support to the patient and family.

Legionnaires' disease

This is caused by the bacteria *Legionella pneumophila* which is widely found in the environment and has been associated with hot water systems and air conditioning cooling towers. Early symptoms include an influenza-like illness, anorexia, diarrhoea, and vomiting, and these symptoms frequently lead to pneumonia. Treatment is usually with erythromycin. It may spread through communities until the source is found. No specific infection control precautions are required.

Cholera

This is caused by the Gram-negative bacteria *Vibrio cholerae*. It presents with profuse watery diarrhoea, fever, vomiting, and rapid dehydration. Transmission is via contaminated food and water. Treatment includes barrier nursing, replacement of fluids (IV or oral rehydration fluids), and antibiotic therapy.

Influenza

Commonly referred to as 'flu is a common cause of respiratory tract infections in humans. It is caused by an RNA virus of the family *Orthomyxoviridiae*. There are 3 types: influenza A, influenza B, and influenza C. The virus has surface glycoproteins called haemagglutinin (H) and neuraminidase (N) that gradually change over time and are used to classify the virus into subtypes e.g. H1N1.

Epidemiology

- Transmitted by an aerosol action/droplet effect or contact with fomites from infected persons, birds, or animals
- Outbreaks of seasonal influenza typically occur over the winter months and are associated with increased rates of pneumonia and death
- Attack rates are highest in the young, those with pre-existing medical conditions (e.g. cardiovascular, respiratory, or renal disease, diabetes mellitus, immunodeficiency), and the elderly
- Epidemics are confined to a single location e.g. town or country and usually occur in winter
- Pandemics are severe outbreaks caused by influenza A that rapidly spread to all parts of the world. Pandemics are associated with emergence of a new influenza virus. Three pandemics occurred in the 20th century (1918, 1957, and 1964) and killed millions of people. Like many other countries the UK has developed a pandemic preparedness plan.

Clinical features

- Influenza syndrome – fever, chills, headache, malaise, muscle pains, sore throat, cough, nasal discharge
- Respiratory complications – viral pneumonia, secondary bacterial pneumonia
- Complications – myositis, myocarditis, pericarditis, toxic shock syndrome, encephalitis, Guillain-Barré syndrome
- Severe disease is more common in the elderly, immunocompromised and those with underlying medical conditions.

Diagnosis

- Diagnosis is usually clinical. Laboratory confirmation may be by antigen detection tests, PCR, viral culture, or serology.

Treatment

- Treatment is usually symptomatic e.g maintain fluid intake, antipyretics, analgesics, decongestants
- Antivirals such as oseltamivir and zanamavir are recommended for the treatment of patients deemed to be 'at risk' – see NICE guidelines www.nice.org.uk

Nursing care

- The nursing care is also symptomatic and involves bed rest, encouraging fluids and good nutrition, administering appropriate drugs and analgesics, and monitoring the patient's progress carefully. Patients should be isolated and kept away from public places such as schools, entertainment centres, and places where vulnerable people are present. Good hand hygiene and careful disposal of materials such as tissues is essential.

Prevention
- Annual vaccination is recommended for certain groups e.g. age >65 years, patients with cardiac, respiratory, and renal disease, diabetes mellitus, immunocompromised patients
- Antivirals e.g. oseltamivir are recommended for post-exposure prophylaxis of 'at risk' patients or after contact with patients who have avian influenza H5N1 or swine origin influenza H1N1 (see below).

Recent important outbreaks
- Avian influenza H5N1 has been around since the 1950s. In 1997 an outbreak in poultry in Hong Kong resulted in 18 human infections and 6 deaths. Since 2003 numerous human H5N1 cases have been associated with exposure to poultry in southeast Asia. By May 2009 there had been 429 cases and 262 deaths
- Swine-origin influenza H1N1 was reported in Mexico and the United States in April 2009.

Further information

NHS Direct England– 0845 4647
NHS Direct Scotland- 08454 24 24 24
NHS Direct Wales- 0845 4647
NHS Direct Northern Ireland-08000514 142
Health Protection Agency website http://www.hpa.org.uk/webw/HPAweb&Page&HPAwebAutoList Name/Page/1202115586990?p=1202115586990
Department of Health http://www.dh.gov.uk/en/Publichealth/Flu/index.htm
World Health Organisation website http://www.who.int/topics/influenza/en/

Prevention of infection

Health care associated infections (HCAI)

These are infections acquired by patients as a consequence of their care and treatment, and can be life-threatening. Reasons for the growth in the number of patients with HCAIs may include:

- Increase in patients with serious illnesses that heighten susceptibility to infection.
- Control and prevention of infection measures not being implemented rigorously.
- Antibiotic resistance makes treatment of infections difficult.
- Emergence of new strains of multi-resistant bacteria (MRSA, VRE, penicillin-resistant *Streptococcus pneumoniae*).
- Use of medical devices—urinary catheters and intravenous access devices.
- Organizational arrangements—high bed occupancy, movement of patients, low staff-to-patient ratios, low numbers of single rooms and isolation facilities. 📖 Isolation/barrier nursing, p.718.
- Lack of information on infections available to clinical staff.

Procedures to substantially reduce HCAI

- Ensure there are high standards of hygiene in clinical practice, e.g. hand decontamination (📖 Hand decontamination, p.712), aseptic techniques (📖 Aseptic technique, p.714), use of personal protective clothing, and adoption of standard precautions.
- Increase surveillance for HCAI to provide information for instituting prevention and control measures, e.g. blood stream infections including MRSA, surgical site infections, *C. difficile* associated disease, serious incidents, and post-discharge infections.
- Reduce infection risks from medical devices by implementing policies to control the use of devices, ensuring staff are competent in the use of the device, and ensuring devices are effectively decontaminated or disposed of following use. 📖 Decontamination, p.719.
- Improve organizational arrangements to ensure hospitals are clean, facilities are available to isolate patients, waste is handled safely, ventilation and decontamination facilities are available, and policies and procedures to support infection prevention and control are in place. 📖 Involving patients and public in infection control and prevention, p.720 and 📖 Patient education for infection control and prevention, p.722.
- Ensure prudent and appropriate use of antibiotics. 📖 Antimicrobial resistance, p.723.

Hand decontamination

Contaminated hands are a major cause of preventable HCAI; therefore hands must be decontaminated before and after every episode of contact with patients.

Methods of hand decontamination

Handwashing with soap and water

Effective in removing dirt or soiling and transient micro-organisms and is essential:

- When hands are soiled
- Before and after shifts
- After removing gloves
- Before and after all patient contact
- Before handling food and administering all medications
- After using the toilet and following contact with contaminated sources and soiled equipment
- After changing bed linen
- Before visiting other wards and departments

Using alcohol hand gel

Use on clean hands as an alternative to repeated handwashing if a hand wash basin is not immediately available. It is not a cleansing agent; visible dirt should be removed with soap and water.

Technique

- Wristwatches prevent effective handwashing and should not be worn for direct care of patients.
- Rings other than wedding bands should not be worn. Dry hands well with paper towels and use emollient cream to prevent skin from drying.
- Nail varnish and false nails should not be worn.
- All surfaces of hands must be covered during every handwash. Hands should be washed under running water for 10–15 seconds with particular attention paid to finger tips, thumbs, and between fingers (See Fig. 20.1).
- Ensure concordance with policies (e.g. 'bare below the elbows').

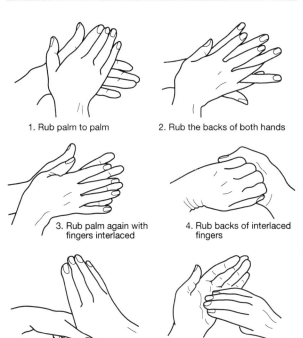

1. Rub palm to palm

2. Rub the backs of both hands

3. Rub palm again with fingers interlaced

4. Rub backs of interlaced fingers

5. Remember to wash both thumbs

6. Rub both palms with fingertips

7. Wash hands under running water using soap. Rinse and dry thoroughly

Fig. 20.1 Hand decontamination. Technique based on procedure described by Aycliffe GAJ, Babb JR, Quoraishi AH (1978). 'A test for "hygienic" hand disinfection'. *J Clin Path*, **31**, 923-8. Reproduced with permission from the BMJ Publishing Group.

Aseptic technique

This is a technique used to prevent contamination of wounds and other sites by organisms that may cause infection and should be used for any procedure where the body's defences are breached, e.g. insertion of IV cannulae urinary catheters, vascular access devices, and respiratory support.

Key principles to achieve asepsis

- *Hand decontamination:* 📖 Hand decontamination, p.713.
- *Non-touch technique:* Disposable sterile gloves are available in latex and synthetic materials. Some individuals are allergic to latex and others to powdered gloves. Nurses should be aware of these problems and a selection of suitable gloves should be made available in the workplace.
- *Use of sterile equipment:* Dressing packs, sterile instruments, and medical devices must meet the Conformité Européene (CE) requirements and be marked as such. Dressing trolleys should be cleaned daily with detergent and dried with paper towels and then wiped with chlorhexidine in 70% ethanol before use. They should not be used for anything else.
- *Personal protective equipment*: Face masks and eye protection should be used where there is a risk of blood, body fluids, or chemical splashing into the face and eyes. Washable shoes should be worn in operating theatres.
- *Environmental cleanliness:* Patient areas should be visibly clean and free from dust before an aseptic technique. This requires effective cleaning standards, waste management procedures, pest control measures, and clean laundry.
- *Airborne contamination:* Aseptic techniques should be undertaken at least 30 minutes after bed making and cleaning, and clean wounds should be dressed first.
- *Patient hygiene:* Patients should be advised to shower or bath to reduce skin flora, to wash hands before and after eating and going to the toilet, and to refrain from touching wounds and dressings.

Reducing environmental transmission of infection

Nurses have a role to play in managing the environment effectively to reduce the spread of infection.

Factors that contribute to the spread of infection

- High occupancy rates—may result in lack of cleaning and preparation of the patient's bed area and associated equipment used between patients
- Low nursing staff-to-patient ratios—may result in patients' hygiene needs not being met and lack of time to give required information and instruction on prevention of spread and hand hygiene
- Frequent transfers of patients between bays and between wards
- Lack of facilities to wash and dry hands for both patients and staff
- Insufficient single rooms for isolation
- Poor waste management
- Insufficient levels of cleaning

Actions that can reduce the spread of infection

- Follow clear bed management policies that ensure patients with infections or who are high risk of acquiring infections (determined locally) are priorities for single rooms. Seek advice from IPCT if single rooms are not available.
- Work in partnership with bed managers to ensure patients with known infections are not transferred unnecessarily to other wards.
- Ensure staff from other departments (e.g. x-ray, physiotherapy) are aware of a patient's infection status if the patient has to go for a test or treatment so that safeguards can be taken.
- Ensure patients bathe or shower daily, wear clean clothing, and have access to handwashing facilities as required.
- Ensure linen is changed daily, especially for patients known to have infections.
- Ensure waste management and linen disposal policies are followed.
- Work in partnership with cleaners to ensure the patient's immediate environment, bed, and equipment are free from unnecessary items and are cleaned daily. Report insufficient cleaning levels to matron or senior nurse.
- Ensure that single-use items are not reused and that any reusable equipment is not used until it has been decontaminated. Carry out checks to ensure that there is adequate cleaning of environmental surfaces, bed, bed rails, and other frequently touched surfaces.
- Ensure facilities are available for hand decontamination and that staff use them appropriately.
- Ensure staff wear a clean uniform daily.
- Ensure visitors assist in keeping the environment clean. 📖 Ten points for visitors, p.721.

Cleanliness and infection control

Cleanliness is an important factor in preventing health care acquired infections and the performance of health care organizations in achieving cleanliness standards is monitored annually.

Aims

The hospital environment must be visibly clean; free from dust, dirt, and spillage from blood and body substances; and acceptable to patients, visitors, and staff. In addition it should smell fresh and have no unpleasant odours. This applies to:

- All patient equipment, e.g. commodes, drip stands, hoists, etc., which should be cleaned after every use
- Vents, ducts, and filters, e.g. attached to ultra-clean theatre canopies
- External and internal features, e.g. entrances, stairs, walls, ceilings, and high and low surfaces
- Windows and doors including frames, vents, and jambs
- Floors including edges, skirting boards, and corners
- Furnishings and fixtures including beds, lockers, general furniture, tables, waste bins, curtains, and blinds
- Kitchens and kitchen appliances and equipment
- Toilets and bathrooms and fittings, e.g. sinks, baths, toilets, showers, mirrors, and rails

Role of nurses

Matrons have overall responsibility for cleanliness (□ Matrons' charter commitments, p.717). NHS organizations are required to review their current practice against these commitments, and take the necessary steps to develop services to meet the spirit of the Matron's Charter. Nurses have responsibilities to ensure cleanliness.

- Agree cleaning standards for your area and ensure staff understand what these are and their responsibilities.
- Make sure that standards are met.
- Raise concerns with matrons when standards are not met.
- Keep lists of items to be cleaned by domestic staff and by nursing staff up to date.
- Work with local cleaning staff to help them fulfill their roles.
- Make sure cleaning materials are available at all times and staff know which ones to use.
- Ensure all staff work tidily and clean up after themselves.
- Listen to patients and act on their concerns about cleanliness.
- Keep the immediate patient environment tidy.
- Ensure requirements for safe disposal of waste, infected linen, food hygiene, and pest control are followed.
- Ensure special arrangements for cleaning rooms and areas occupied by infected patients are followed and terminal cleaning is completed before a further patient is admitted.

Matrons' charter commitments

Keeping the NHS clean is everybody's responsibility.
1. The patient's environment will be well-maintained, clean, and safe.
2. Matrons will establish a cleanliness culture across their units.
3. Cleaning staff will be recognized for the important work they do. Matrons will make sure they feel part of the ward team.
4. Specific roles and responsibilities for cleaning will be clear.
5. Cleaning routines will be clear, agreed, and well publicized.
6. Patients will have a part to play in monitoring and reporting on standards of cleanliness.
7. All staff working in health care will receive education in infection control.
8. Nurses and infection control teams will be involved in drawing up cleaning contracts and matrons have authority and power to withhold payment.
9. Sufficient resources will be dedicated to keeping hospitals clean.

Department of Health (2004). *A matron's charter: an action plan for cleaner hospitals.* www.dh.gov.uk. Reproduced with permission.

Isolation/barrier nursing

Definitions
Spread of infection is prevented by isolation or other barrier procedures.

Source isolation minimizes the risk of spreading infection from an infected person to others and is achieved through:
- *Standard barrier precautions* which apply when spread is by the airborne route, droplets, or direct contact, e.g. MRSA, meningococcal meningitis, pulmonary tuberculosis, scabies, measles, mumps, chickenpox.
- *Blood/body substance precautions* to prevent transmission of blood-borne infections, e.g. hepatitis B and C, CJD, or enteric organisms by faeco-oral route, e.g. *Salmonella*, *C. difficile*, hepatitis A and E.
- *Strict isolation* which applies to serious infections, e.g. diphtheria, rabies, plague. Patients are commonly transferred to infectious diseases unit.

Protective isolation or reverse barrier nursing is done to protect patients who are at special risk of getting infections, e.g. immunodeficient states, severe burns.

General management principles
- Notify the IPCT immediately for support and advice.
- Follow guidance in local infection control policies.
- Instruct all visitors that they must report to the nurse in charge before visiting.
- Notify domestic services when isolation nursing is instituted.
- Ensure terminal cleaning and decontamination of equipment will be carried out when isolation ceases.
- Consider where single-use or single-patient-use items can be employed.

Standard barrier precautions
- Use a single room and ensure that specific instructions for patients, visitors, and staff are displayed outside while maintaining patient confidentiality. Reinforce with verbal and written instructions as necessary.
- Use disposable gloves and aprons for procedures with direct contact with the patient or bed linen. Wear a mask if the risk of transmission via droplet or respiratory route is suspected.
- Wash hands or apply alcohol hand rub/gel before entering and leaving the room.
- Provide special facilities for disposal of waste and linen as well as bags and containers labelled according to local policy.
- Use biohazard labels for laboratory specimens, e.g. blood/body fluid specimens.

Strict isolation
Follow the above plus:
- Use disposable gowns and masks (high-efficiency filter type).
- Use disposable cutlery and crockery.

Decontamination

Definition
Decontamination involves the processes of cleaning, disinfecting, and sterilizing.

Methods of decontamination
Cleaning with soap or detergent and water removes most micro-organisms and materials from surfaces and should be undertaken as soon as possible after use. Warm water is easier for cleaning and brushes or cloths used should be single use. Rinse the equipment with clean water before drying which is essential to prevent growth of any organisms that persist. This process may be done manually or by an automated system and a designated area should be used. Personal protective equipment must be worn. Cleaning is essential before disinfection or sterilization.

Disinfection uses chemical agents or heat to reduce the number of organisms. Chemical disinfection is less reliable than heat but is necessary for heat-sensitive equipment. For chemical disinfection to be effective:
- Always check the label and follow the instructions.
- Ensure the correct disinfectant and concentration is used for the specific task.
- Ensure the disinfectant is not out of date.
- Allow sufficient time for the process to take place.
- Ensure equipment is free of materials, e.g. organic matter, which may neutralize the disinfectant.

Correct personal protective equipment should be used and COSHH regulations followed.

Sterilization is the process that makes items free from all microbes including spores and viruses. This is done by autoclaving or low-temperature steam. Chemicals with sporicidal properties may sterilize but require 3 hours to destroy spore-bearing bacteria and the chemical may have harmful effects on staff.

Visual inspection of equipment at the end of the process is essential to check for dryness, cleanliness, and signs of damage to the item.

Single-use items of equipment
Many pieces of equipment (e.g. endotracheal tubes, cannulae, syringes, and needles) are identified as single use. They should be disposed of after use and decontamination for further use must not be attempted.

Responsibilities
Users of equipment are responsible for ensuring equipment is cleaned and decontaminated before and after use and before submission to service repair departments.

Involving patients and public in infection control and prevention

Nurses should encourage patients, visitors, and members of the public to work in partnership with them to reduce infection rates in health care organizations. Basic information on the spread and methods of prevention of infection is necessary as a starting point. 📖 Prevention of infection, p.710.

Ways of involvement

Assisting in the development of patient information

Patients can be asked about the usefulness of information given to them, what additions would have been helpful, and whether a different format would have been better. They can contribute by reading materials during the development stage to ensure it meets patients' needs.

Giving feedback

Surveys, meetings, discussions, interviews, comments, suggestions, and complaints can be used to get feedback on:

- Cleanliness of the environment and equipment such as beds and lockers
- Cleanliness of facilities such as toilets, bathrooms, and commodes, and availability of soap and towels
- Opportunities for hygiene, e.g. daily bath/shower, handwashing before food, after using toilet or using the bedpan
- Whether they have been shown how to wash hands thoroughly
- Whether they are confident that staff are using infection prevention and control measures such as handwashing and are cleaning equipment

Patients and visitors can alert staff to problems and report something that may be out of place (e.g. empty soap or gel dispensers), concerns about other visitors' behaviour (e.g. sitting on beds) or staff practices (e.g. failure to wash hands before procedures). Feedback can help staff target where more effort, training, and monitoring is needed.

Participating in audit and monitoring

Members of the public or past patients may be involved in cleanliness audits alongside more experienced staff. They have the advantage of looking at things from a different perspective and they may be able to suggest different ways of doing things.

Ten points for visitors

Several polices for visitors can help reduce the risk of infection in the area.

- Adhere to visiting times to allow time for care and treatment, ward cleaning, and patients' rest periods.
- Limit the number of visitors as directed by staff.
- Keep children under control and do not let them wander away from the vicinity of the patient being visited.
- Do not visit if you have signs of infection, e.g. cough, cold or sore throat, diarrhoea and vomiting. Cover all cuts and wounds. Ask staff for advice.
- Use hand gel before entering and leaving the ward and following instructions on how to use it.
- Use chairs provided—do not sit on the beds.
- Do not sharing belongings with other patients, e.g. blankets, combs.
- Follow any special infection control measures, e.g. barrier or isolation precautions. Ask for advice.
- Alert staff to any problems and reporting something which is out of place, e.g. empty soap dispensers.
- Always wash your hands after using the toilet and before eating.

Patient education for infection control and prevention

Patients are often anxious about hospital infections they have heard about through the media. Information can help them understand the reality and contribute to prevention and control measures.

Pre-admission information
- Infection rates for the hospital and speciality
- Measures being taken to reduce infections, e.g. restrictions on visiting, surveillance, and treatment and screening measures
- Specific information on types of infections, e.g. MRSA
- Patients' and visitors' responsibilities

Education for all patients
This should be aimed at achieving the following outcomes:
- Demonstrate effective handwashing techniques—as a minimum before meals and after using toilet.
- Do not share equipment or belongings.
- Change nightwear frequently and ask visitors to follow instructions for removal and washing.
- Dispose of potentially infectious materials safely, e.g. tissues.
- Report poor hygiene and cleanliness, e.g. dirty toilets and basins, poor handwashing.
- Leave dressings intact and report wet or seeping dressings and any redness, soreness, or swelling around the wound immediately.
- Report any unusual symptoms, e.g. rashes, diarrhoea.

Education for patients with existing infections
Focus on achieving the following outcomes in addition to the above:
- Have a daily bath and change of nightwear and bed linen daily.
- Follow medication and treatment as prescribed, e.g. antibiotics, chlorhexidine skin washes.
- Understand the special care of tubes or drains, e.g. catheters, IV infusion sites.
- Adhere to specific measures such as barrier and isolation precautions.
- Understand the specific infection they have, how it may be transmitted, and how this can be prevented.
- Understand why protective clothing may need to be worn by staff and visitors.
- Understand how to dispose of infectious body fluids.

Antimicrobial resistance

Definitions

Antimicrobial resistance is the ability of a micro-organism (bacteria, fungi, viruses, or protozoa) to withstand a microbial agent.

Antimicrobial agents are antibiotics that kill or inhibit growth of microbial pathogens, antibacterial drugs, and antiviral and antifungal agents.

Multi-resistance occurs when a micro-organism is resistant to two or more antimicrobial agents.

Threats to health

- Unnecessary use of antibiotics exacerbates resistance and may also give rise to adverse effects.
- Many patients believe that antibiotics will cure all infections and decisions to prescribe are influenced by patient's expectations.
- MRSA is a major problem in the UK; other problems include *Streptococcus pneumoniae* and enterococci.
- Resistance is emerging in viruses and fungi as well as bacteria.
- Multi-drug resistance may lead to some conditions becoming untreatable.
- Antimicrobial resistance increases clinical complications and increases the length of hospital stay, use of antimicrobial agents, morbidity, mortality, and cost.
- Alternative drugs may be more toxic, expensive, and less effective.
- Resistance is greatest in countries and units where use is heaviest and concordance is poor.
- Development of new antibiotics is slow, expensive, and cannot be guaranteed.

Best practice in reducing resistance

- Do not prescribe antibiotics for simple coughs and colds and viral sore throats.
- Use antibiotics only after a treatable infection has been recognized or there is high degree of suspicion of infection.
- Use local prescribing guidelines to support prudent use of antibiotics.
- Administer antibiotics as prescribed and discontinue when the course is completed.
- Educate patients to ensure they understand:
  - the correct use, benefits, and disadvantages of antimicrobials
  - to take antimicrobials over the prescribed period at the correct dose
  - not to take antimicrobials prescribed for other people.
- Educate student nurses and junior staff about use of antimicrobial agents.
- Support the IPCT in undertaking surveillance of resistant organisms.

Nursing interventions

Physical problems

Risk of spread of infection

Seek advice from IPCT. Instigate strict isolation, standard barrier precautions, and/or blood/body precautions as appropriate. Apply strict handwashing, equipment decontamination measures, aseptic techniques, and cleanliness standards. Administer prescribed antibiotics or other medications.

Raised body temperature

Keep patient clean and comfortable; apply tepid sponges if required. Record temperature, pulse, and respiration 4-hourly or more often, if necessary. Change sheets often; use fan. Administer antipyretics if prescribed.

Diarrhoea

Observe and record the amount, colour, frequency, and consistency. Note smell and presence of blood, pus, and mucus. Nurse the patient in a single room with en suite facilities if possible. If not, nurse near to toilet and ensure thorough cleaning after each use. Keep patient clean if not able to provide self-care and maintain skin integrity if incontinent. Encourage handwashing after using toilet. Collect specimens as required.

Vomiting

Observe and record amount, colour, consistency, and frequency, and note presence of blood or other contents. Provide vomit bowls and remove after use. Keep mouth clean with mouth wash or oral care after vomiting.

Fatigue

Encourage bed or chair rest as necessary. Ensure position is comfortable; support with pillows. Administer prescribed analgesia.

Dehydration

Oral fluids if possible: water, fruit juices, or squashes. IV fluids if prescribed; may need NG tube if poor oral intake persists. Record intake and urine output and weight. Keep mouth clean.

Skin rash and wounds

Discourage scratching and touching. Keep patient's nails short. Apply medication topically as prescribed and use aseptic technique for dressings. Observe for change in condition.

Changes in breathing

Observe and record respiratory rate and depth and oxygen saturation levels; note any pain on breathing. Observe for pallor, cyanosis, and restlessness.

Altered conscious level

Nursing problems, p.697.

Psychosocial problems

Disturbed body image

It is important not to show any distaste or discomfort at the patient's appearance or symptoms. Encourage the patient to talk about how they feel. Explanations about the course of the infectious disease and the impact of the planned treatment will be helpful. The impact on relationships with family and friends may be of concern and should be explored. Explanations to family and how they can support are essential.

Feelings of isolation

This is especially likely if patient is in strict isolation. Communication to maintain the patient's identity is important. Discuss home life, family, pets, hobbies, and interests. Ensure patients have as many choices as possible to ensure they feel in control of their care and treatment and that they have sufficient information to make decisions.

Ensure patients are orientated to time and place by providing clocks newspapers, radios, TV, etc. It also helps if patients have view of the outside. Keep patients occupied with books, games, or other activities to prevent boredom.

Guilt and anxiety

May be related to how patients perceive they have acquired the infection or if the infection has spread to others. Explanations to dispel any myths are essential. Providing time to listen, answer questions, and give information on preventing and controlling further spread will be helpful.

Patient education

Education for patients with infectious diseases needs to be tailored to the individual, the specific condition, and the ability and readiness of the patient to learn.

Nature and course of infectious disease
Patients need to understand the infectious condition, likely sources, how they acquired it, how they are likely to progress, the timescales, and the prognosis.

Treatment and care
This includes drug treatment plus the duration and any side effects; tests and procedures and how they will be prepared for them and the after effects; information about the physical and psychological problems and the nursing interventions and how this will continue following discharge. The importance of following treatment regimens should also be stressed.

Prevention of spread
This includes the isolation and barrier precautions that are in place and why, and the patient's role and responsibilities in this. General measures to reduce the transmission of infection in the environment and teaching patients how and when to wash their hands are important.

Vaccination and immunization
Many infectious diseases can be prevented by vaccination and immunization. Details of these should be given to patients and information on how and where they can obtain advice in future.

General prevention
📖 Prevention of infection, p.710.

Prevention of travel-related illness
Advice should be sought prior to travel from GP or recognized travel centre including vaccination and immunization recommended and required in the area of travel and information on other prophylactic treatments such as anti-malaria treatment. General advice on prevention of diarrhoea and gastroenteritis by drinking bottled water or boiling, chlorinating, or filtering water and not eating raw uncooked foods unless peeled can be given.

Lifestyle issues
Information on the consequences of using IV drugs, sharing needles, unprotected casual sex, and tattooing should be provided. A non-judgemental approach is essential.

Discharge and continuing care

Principles

- Begin planning discharge early, as soon as possible after admission, and work with patient and/or relatives.
- Seek guidance and advice from IPCT early.
- Ensure good liaison with community IPCT and that relevant information is shared.
- Ensure patient has had tailored education relevant to needs. 📖 Patient education, p.726.
- Check that the patient has the correct drugs and understands how and when to take these, the importance of completing the prescribed course, how to obtain further prescriptions, and what to do if side effects are experienced.
- Arrange for follow-up as required, either by GP or outpatient appointment.
- Check the patient has instructions for the disposal of infectious materials following discharge (e.g. tissues), for dealing with infected laundry, and for prevention of spread for chronic carriers (e.g. food handling).
- Check the patient has any dressings or other equipment needed.
- Prepare a written nursing discharge summary that highlights:
  - Care and treatment received
  - Care and treatment to be continued, arrangements made, and with whom
  - Education and information given to patient and level of understanding
  - Patient's understanding of infection and transmission
  - Drugs and any side effects experienced, and any problems with concordance
- Ensure that patients are aware of possible complications and what to do if these or original symptoms recur.
- Check the patient knows who to contact if there are problems.

Common drugs used for infectious diseases

Common drugs used for infectious diseases are listed in Table 20.1. **All drug doses listed in this table are adult doses and not children's doses**. This table is only to be used as a guide and the current BNF should be consulted for further advice. Nurses should involve themselves only in the administration of medications which fall within their sphere of competence.

Table 20.1 Common drugs used for infectious diseases

NB antibiotics should always be given at regular intervals and the prescribed course completed

Penicillins	Dose	Common side effects
Various products including narrow spectrum agents, e.g. benzylpenicillin (injection only), penicillin V (oral only); broad spectrum agents, e.g. amoxicillin, co-amoxiclav; penicillinase resistant penicillins, e.g. flucloxacillin; antipseudomonal penicillins, e.g. piperacillin, ticarcillin	For dose see BNF under each product NB when taken by mouth dose should be given half to 1 hour before food or on an empty stomach	Hypersensitivity (rash, urticaria, fever, joint pains, angioedema, serum sickness reaction, and anaphylaxis which can be fatal); diarrhoea may frequently occur and is more common with broad spectrum antibiotics; CNS toxicity including convulsions (especially with high doses or in severe renal impairment), interstitial nephritis, haemolytic anaemia, leucopenia, thrombocytopenia and coagulation disorders; may also cause antibiotic associated colitis

Cephalosporins	Dose	Common side effects
Various products including 1st generation agents, e.g. cefalexin; 2nd generation agents, e.g. cefuroxime; and 3rd generation agents, e.g. cefotaxime, ceftazidime, ceftriaxone	For dose see BNF under each product NB 1st generation agents should be given half to 1 hour before food or on an empty stomach; 2nd generation agents when given orally should be taken with or after food to minimize gastric irritation	Hypersensitivity and allergic reactions (approx 10% of penicillin allergic patients are allergic to cefalosporins); diarrhoea (though rarely antibiotic associated colitis); nausea and vomiting, abdominal discomfort, headache, liver enzyme disturbance, transient hepatitis, cholestatic jaundice, erythema multiforme

Table 20.1 Common drugs used for infectious diseases *(continued)*

Tetracyclines	Dose	Common side effects
Various products including tetracycline, demeclocycline (also used in inappropriate ADH secretion), and doxycycline	For dose see BNF under each product and for condition being treated NB patients should not take milk, indigestion remedies or medicines containing iron or zinc at the same time of day as this medicine	Nausea and vomiting, diarrhoea (antibiotic associated colitis reported occasionally), dysphagia, oesophageal irritation

Aminoglycosides	Dose	Common side effects
Various products including gentamicin, amikacin, netilmicin, and tobramycin	For dose see BNF under each product and for condition being treated NB all given by injection except neomycin which is given orally but poorly absorbed (used for bowel sterilization or hepatic coma)	Vestibular damage, auditory damage and nephrotoxicity NB these are dose related and occur most commonly in the elderly or patients with renal impairment

Macrolides	Dose	Common side effects
Various products including erythromycin, azithromycin, and clarithromycin	For dose see BNF under each product and for condition being treated	Nausea, vomiting, abdominal discomfort, diarrhoea (antibiotic associated colitis reported), reversible hearing loss after large doses, cholestatic jaundice, myasthenia-like syndrome and others (See BNF and under each product)

Other antibacterials	Dose	Common side effects
Sodium fusidate	500 mg every 8 hours (doubled for severe infections) Skin infections – 250 mg every 12 hours for 5–10 days	Nausea, vomiting, reversible jaundice, especially after high doses (withdraw if persistent); rarely hypersensitivity reactions

Table 20.1 Common drugs used for infectious diseases *(continued)*

Other antibacterials	Dose	Common side effects
Vancomycin	Antibiotic associated colitis – by mouth (since not significantly absorbed) 125 mg every 6 hours for 7–10 days Use parenterally for systemic infections (See BNF for dose details)	After parenteral administration – nephrotoxicity (including renal failure and interstitial nephritis), ototoxicity (discontinue if tinnitus occurs), blood disorders including neutropenia (usually after 1 week or cumulative dose of 25 g), nausea, fever, chills, eosinophilia, anaphylaxis, rashes, phlebitis, on rapid infusion severe hypotension including shock and cardiac arrest, and many more side effects (See BNF)
Trimethoprim	Acute infections: 200 mg every 12 hours (3 days duration may be sufficient for urinary tract infection in women) Chronic infections and prophylaxis: 100 mg at night	Gastrointestinal disturbances including nausea and vomiting, pruritus, rashes, hyperkalaemia, depression of haematopoiesis
Metronidazole	For dose see BNF for condition being treated	Disulfiram reaction occurs when patients also take alcohol; nausea, vomiting, unpleasant taste, furred tongue, oral mucositis, anorexia, gastrointestinal disturbances, rashes
Quinolones, e.g. ciprofloxaxin, levofloxacin	For dose see BNF under each product and for condition being treated	Nausea, vomiting, dyspepsia, abdominal pain, diarrhoea, headache, dizziness, sleep disorders, rash and pruritus; tendon inflammation and damage also reported particularly in elderly and those taking corticosteroids (See BNF for other side effects)

Drugs used to treat MRSA infections: 📖 **Table 12.1 Common drugs used for dermatologic conditions: Mupirocin, p.432.**

Antifungals	Dose	Common side effects
Amphotericin and nystatin (neither agent is absorbed by mouth)	Dose varies for drug, formulation and condition being treated (See BNF for details)	Few side effects and generally mild, e.g. mild gastrointestinal disturbances, some nausea

Table 20.1 Common drugs used for infectious diseases *(continued)*

Antifungals	Dose	Common side effects
Fluconazole	Dose varies according to condition being treated (See BNF for details)	Nausea, abdominal discomfort, diarrhoea, flatulence, headache, rash (discontinue – or monitor closely if infection is invasive or systemic)

Parasiticidal preparations 📖 Table 12.1 Common drugs used for dermatologic conditions: Carbaryl and permethrin, p.432.

Antivirals	Dose	Common side effects
(📖 Table 18.1 Common drugs used for patients with HIV, p.649)		
Aciclovir	Dose varies according to condition being treated (See BNF for details)	Nausea, vomiting, abdominal pain, diarrhoea, headache, fatigue, rash, urticaria, pruritus, photosensitivity

Vaccines	Dose	Common side effects
Tetanus	See BNF for dosage schedule according to age, primary or secondary immunization, and interval between doses	Local reactions (redness, pain, swelling at injection site) may persist for several days; incidence increases with age and according to the number of previous doses; other reactions are uncommon (See BNF for details)
Pneumococcal	Given to at-risk patients 2 weeks before surgery (or chemotherapy) (See BNF for dose, frequency and choice of vaccine)	Patients should be given advice about increased risk of pneumococcal infection
Cholera NB food, drink and other oral medicines should be avoided 1 hour before and after vaccination	Two doses separated by an interval of 1 week; booster dose can be given after 2 years	Diarrhoea, abdominal pain, headache

Nursing specific groups of people

Nursing patients with intimate and sensitive care needs

Introduction

Intimate nursing care concerns the very personal and private aspects of a person's life including biological, psychological, emotional, social, and spiritual aspects of care. The philosophical concept of holism is vital in this sphere of nursing, as nurses must recognize that the whole is greater than the sum of its parts. Nursing is more than just caring or treating the person's disease, symptoms, and health problems.

The word 'holistic' derives from the Greek word 'holos' meaning whole. The patient is more than a physical being. A view of the whole person is required in nursing, and in some situations the very innermost aspects of this whole will assert themselves or emerge in physical, behavioural, and emotionally expressive ways.

The ability of the professional nurse to care for a patient's intimate and sensitive needs depends on an in-depth understanding, confidence, and realization of self. Nurses who are confident with the intimate aspects of their own lives will find it easier to care for patients with very intimate needs. Self-reflection and talking through these aspects of nursing with mentors and clinical supervisors can help nurses achieve these goals. Self-scrutiny also demands an attitude of acceptance and non-judgement. Understanding some of the key concepts surrounding caring for people is also helpful. 📖 Particularly sensitive nursing care needs, p.737.

It is important for patients to sense that the nurse is *honest* and *genuine* in their intentions towards helping them; and that the nurse is *empathic* and *understanding*. *Respect* for the patient as a person with individual needs, some of which may need very sensitive handling, is paramount. 📖 Chapter 3, Interviewing tips and communication skills, p.34.

Particularly sensitive nursing care needs

Physical
- Performing a catheterization
- Performing a rectal examination
- Giving suppositories and enemas
- Digital removal of faeces
- Applying dressings to the genital region and anus
- Caring for a patient's stoma
- Inserting vaginal pessaries
- Washing patient's genitalia
- Caring for the male patient's foreskin
- Caring for the female patient's breasts
- Caring for female patients during menstruation
- Shaving the pubic region for surgery

Psychosocial
- Caring for people who are embarrassed for various individual reasons
- Caring for people's emotional needs
- Caring for people who
  - are fearful, lonely, or confused
  - cannot maintain their privacy
  - have communication difficulties (speech difficulties, illiteracy, language barriers)
  - have cognitive problems or dementia
  - have been abused
- Caring for the patient's sexuality and sexual expression
- Caring for the dying

Key interventions

- Allocate an individual nurse.
- Build up a rapport and a personal relationship.
- Talk, discuss fears, and listen to the patient.
- Develop an individualized care plan.
- Closely monitor progress and evaluate effect of care.
- Involve specialists, such as the Mental Healthcare nurse.
- Liaise with the patient's family.

Patients with self-esteem disturbance

Self-esteem relates to how worthwhile and confident patients feel about themselves. Self-esteem disturbances are revealed when patients express a negative perception about themselves or their personal capabilities.

Signs
- Patient feels inferior, worthless, no good, or inadequate.
- Patient conveys a sense of detachment from the real world, e.g. nobody appreciates them or their work.
- Patient feels unloved, upset, dissatisfied, and unhappy. They may feel they have lost control of their lives, feel they have nothing to be proud of, feel that nothing ever goes right, and have contempt for themselves.
- All of the patient's verbalizations express negative feelings.
- Depressed people often have low self-esteem.

Symptoms
- Anorexia, obesity, sexual problems, and relationship difficulties.

Nursing management
- Keep a non-judgemental empathic attitude.
- Listen actively.
- Recognize the patient's past experiences and achievements.
- Discourage repeated negative conversations about past problems and failures.
- Encourage patient to get involved with activities that are satisfying and rewarding.
- Use positive language.
- Help the patient set new goals to improve their lifestyle.
- Increase opportunities for social interaction.
- Encourage positive body image and appearance-enhancing activities, e.g. make-up, hairstyle, smart dressing, and exercise.
- Suggest use of complementary therapies such as massage and aromatherapy.
- Find out about the patient's family/social network.

Patients suffering from social isolation

Social isolation is a lack of contact with other people because of problems in communication or loneliness. It is a subjective state that exists whenever the person says it does or perceives it as imposed by others. It includes aloneness, loneliness, deprivation, and unhappiness. Patients may also feel stigmatized.

Causes

It may involve loss of a spouse or partner, job, social role, social support, and lack of purpose in life. Some patients feel that their illness or chronic health condition is the cause. Older adults living in nursing homes sometimes become isolated and lose contact with the outside world, their family, and previous friends.

Nursing management

- Actively listen to the patient.
- Explore reasons for isolation and try to reduce them.
- Promote and encourage ways the patient can feel more involved and part of the community.
- Identify the need for assistive or prosthetic devices that can improve the patient's appearance or function.
- Suggest appropriate social institutions and voluntary organizations that help vulnerable and isolated people.

Patients who are fearful

Fear is the emotion of pain or uneasiness caused by the sense of impending danger or by the prospect of some possible harm; apprehension or dread of something that will or may happen in the future (after the Oxford English Dictionary). Hospitalized patients who are separated from their support systems and close family friends are vulnerable.

Causes

Medical jargon and the hospital environment may contribute to a patient's fear. Language barriers may make matters worse, as may sensory impairments such as blindness, diminished hearing, and deafness. In health care and nursing situations this may be pain, suffering, a forthcoming operation, the outcome of test results or treatment, and the effects of treatment or chronic illness. Fear occurs more commonly with life-threatening illnesses and conditions. A phobia is an extreme or irrational fear or dread aroused by a particular object or circumstance. This is exaggerated and often disabling as individuals try to avoid the situation, e.g. fear of needles.

Nursing management

- Encourage the patient to express their fears and find out how their fears impinge on their lifestyle.
- Discuss ways the patient can cope with the situation.
- Help the patient learn to problem solve in a systematic way.
- Teach the patient and involve them in their health care so they have a good understanding and knowledge of what is happening. Try to decrease the fear of the unknown.
- Liaise with relevant health care professionals to help patients overcome their fears.

Patients suffering from hopelessness

Hopelessness is a feeling of despair and discouragement; it is a thought process in which patients expect nothing from themselves or others. Hopes are fluid, transient, and intermittent. The number of difficult life events and the ability to cope with them may be a factor in someone experiencing hopelessness. Hopelessness may affect the immune system; is often closely linked to depression and suicidal thoughts; and can lead to self-mutilating behaviour.

Causes
- Unresolved losses and failure to come to terms with past tragic or difficult events
- Poor mental health
- Poor social situation
- Physical frailty, chronic illness, pain, and cancer

Nursing management
- Encourage the patient to talk and express their feelings.
- Explore activities that may instill hope in patients, e.g. contacting old friends and family and rekindling relationships with others.
- Develop links with past, present, and possible future goals.
- Encourage the patient to make decisions and participate in their health care—this may help them gain control and develop assertiveness.
- Teach the patient to increase knowledge and competence.
- Refer, if necessary, to mental health services or relevant counsellors.
- Provide physical and emotional comfort.

Patients with confusion

Anyone can experience confusion; it is not just restricted to those with cognitive problems or memory loss. Confusion is a disordered or disorganized state where the mind becomes mixed-up or perplexed. It takes time for patients to adapt to the disruptive influence but they eventually come to terms with the changes. Confusion is usually transitory and not permanent (delirium). In some conditions, such as dementia, confusion becomes a chronic state. 📖 Chapter 28, Nursing the older person, pp.916–18.

Causes

Admission to hospital and frequent shifts of position on a ward or unit may cause patients to become confused. Unfamiliar environmental activities and changes, particularly in treatment and care regimens, may be a cause.

Nursing management

- Listen actively to what the patient is saying.
- Observe their behaviour carefully.
- Use methods of reorientation to help the patient adjust to the confusion:
- Provide empathy and understanding.
- Talk to the patient and explore ways of helping them avoid the frustrations which confusion may bring.
- Stick to one subject per conversation as too much information causes problems.
- Ensure the topic is relevant.
- Encourage the patient to talk.
- Never use phrases such as 'Don't you remember?'
- Use memory aids such as calendars, diaries, and picture aids, e.g. photographs.
- Encourage the patient to use a notepad and pen.
- Write things down for them.
- Encourage other health care professionals and visitors to participate in the reorientation process.
- Focus on providing meaningful information, as it is always more easily remembered.
- Consider health and safety issues and remove or replace hazards and dangers in the environment. (Beware of bed rails/cot sides and devices that may restrict the movement of the person.)
- Build on past memory and use pictures, music, and recollections of previous life experiences.
- Use verbal reminders such as offering a glass of water to drink.
- Use alarms or other audible reminders such as setting an alarm clock.
- Power of attorney may need to be established where the patient suffers frequent attacks of confusion.
- Chronic confusion requires additional long-term strategies.

Patients with fatigue

Fatigue, a common complaint with many illnesses, relates to tiredness, weariness, and exhaustion. It may result from the physical or psychological processes involved with regard to health/illness changes. Chronic fatigue syndrome (CFS) was formally defined in the literature in 1988 to describe a syndrome of disabling fatigue lasting longer than 6 months and associated with a variable number of physical and psychological symptoms. (WHO 2000).

Causes
- Physical effects of ill health or a medical condition, such as thyroid problems or anaemia
- Mental stress of coping with a health concern or problem
- Severe and repeated stress
- Lack of appropriate food
- Various medications may exacerbate the feeling of tiredness
- Medical conditions, e.g. anaemia and metabolic disturbances

Nursing management
- Explore the relationship between fatigue and infection, trauma, or physical illness.
- Assess nutritional factors and eating habits.
- Determine whether there is an inflammatory, degenerative, or viral link.
- Assess the presence of emotional distress and stressors such as social relationships and other life stressors.
- Consider using special stress assessment tools, e.g. the life events questionnaire.
- Encourage the patient to talk about their feelings. Write these down and use them in evaluating the patient's progress.
- Teach the patient realistic and practical ways to conserve their energy.
- Encourage regular rest periods.
- Recognize that some patients find it hard to ask for help.
- Encourage planned and programmed exercise, which may help some patients to build up endurance.
- Encourage the patient to gain a sense of control in their lives.
- Discuss sleep patterns – encourage a regular sleep routine and avoid daytime naps.

Further information
World Health Organization: www.who.org

Basic counselling tips (through the therapeutic relationship)

Establish rapport

- Encourage the person to speak freely.
- Use active and accurate listening skills.
- Use questions and open-ended prompts.
- Reflect back meaning and feelings.
- Do not give well-intentioned advice.
- Use open-ended questions.
- Maintain eye contact, if appropriate.
- Make the person feel at ease.
- Be aware of own feelings, thoughts, and body posture.

Develop the relationship

- Continue to encourage the person to speak freely and ventilate their feelings.
- Use appropriate prompts and nods of understanding.
- Encourage the person to think about their problem.
- Challenge the person to examine their behaviour and attitudes.

Develop a more in-depth realization and understanding of the person's problem and move towards decisions

- Help the person verbalize their feelings and actions.

Decision-making stage

- Encourage positive decision-making.
- Teach patients to evaluate the pros and cons of each possible alternative.
- Let the patient make the decision; do not make it for them.

Summarize the counselling

- Evaluate what has been said and summarize your understanding of the person's problem.
- Sum up main points.
- Assess the need for further help, advice, and counselling sessions.
- End the encounter—do not let it drag on.

Note

Successful counselling depends on helping the person make their own decisions and motivating the person to take responsibility for their decisions.

Sexuality and sexual expression

Sexuality is a lifelong characteristic that defines the maleness or femaleness of each person. It is a complex phenomenon that involves biological, psychosocial, and cultural aspects. Sexuality does not necessarily involve sexual behaviour. WHO (1975) defined sexual health as the 'integration of the somatic, emotional, intellectual, and social aspects of sexual being in ways that are positively enriching and that enhance personality, communication, and love'.

All individuals are sexual beings, whether or not they have physical sexual relations. Society tends to associate youth, beauty, and physical agility with sexuality. However, being old or disabled does not diminish human sexuality. The person within a human being does not fundamentally change. Although the hair is grey, the skin is wrinkled, and the body lacks agility, the person inside has feelings and longing for love and affection.

The need to love and be loved is a basic psychosocial and emotional need. It is closely linked to *self-esteem*, which is how one feels about oneself (🕮 Chapter 24, Nursing patients with body image problems, p.814). As people age it becomes increasingly more difficult to be loved and have people to love. Families change, children grow up and move away, and partners may move on. Relationships that provided love, affection, and friendship may be lost through death and geographic distance.

Unless nurses can accept their own sexuality and are comfortable with their own behaviour, it will be difficult to convey sexual comfort to patients. Nurses therefore need to reflect on their own attitudes.

Nursing interventions

The EX-PLISSIT model (Taylor and Davis, 2006) may be useful in guiding nursing interventions.

- Enable patients to voice their sexual needs and concerns—give them 'permission' to talk about their issues.
- Provide information about the effects of illness, medication, or treatment on sexual function.
- Refer patients for specialist help, if necessary, particularly if they have suffered sexual abuse.

Further information

Taylor B and Davis S (2006). 'Using the PLISSIT model to address sexual healthcare needs'. *Nurs Stand*, **21**(11), 35–40.

Key points when assessing sexuality

- Provide privacy, which is absolutely essential.
- Reassure the patient of confidentiality.
- Do not overreact to what you are told.
- Use language the patient understands but avoid slang and technical terms.
- Avoid ambiguity. If necessary, clarify the terms the patient uses.
- Progress from less sensitive to most sensitive issues.
- Whatever your attitudes, do not influence the interview.
- Give patients time to express themselves.
- A useful starting question is: 'Has anything (e.g. illness, heart attack, surgery) interfered with or changed the way you feel about yourself?' This can be followed by: 'Has this affected your ability to function sexually?' Many patients will soon open up without further prompting and questioning.
- Sum up the patient's concerns at the end of the assessment, offer relevant teaching or advice, and offer further help, if necessary.

Forms of sexual expression

Sexual expression takes many forms:
- Gentle touching or holding hands
- Tender communications
- Making rude remarks or sexual innuendos
- Reading or viewing sexually explicit material
- Telling 'dirty' jokes or stories
- Exposing genitals
- Genital caressing
- Masturbation (self-stimulation)
- Genital decoration (piercings)

Older people of all ages may still be interested in and capable of a real sexual expression or experience. In residential nursing situations it may be very difficult for older people to continue with sexual activity, especially in some care settings, although some may provide privacy for sexual activity. It is important not to encourage activities by patients that are not reciprocated by others, in whatever setting.

Patients with severe physical limitations can have successful sexual experiences if nurses can be open, mature, and understanding of human sexual needs. Masturbation is now considered a very healthy activity and is one enjoyed by both sexes. It is a common way of gaining comfort when stressed and when other sexual opportunities are not available. The nurse may feel uncomfortable if they notice such an activity but should not interfere. Instead, treat the situation calmly, draw curtains to provide privacy, or move the patient to a more private area. Do not criticize or make fun.

Factors that may affect sexual function
- Hospitalization
- Menopause
- Chronic illnesses
  - Diabetes mellitus
  - Cardiac disease
  - Hypertensive vascular disease
  - Chronic renal failure
  - Multiple sclerosis
- Surgery, severe trauma, loss of a body part, or other medical conditions
  - Mastectomy or hysterectomy
  - Male reproductive surgery including prostatectomy
  - Stoma (ileostomy and colostomy)
  - Spinal cord injury
  - Urinary and/or faecal incontinence
  - Prior sexual assault
  - Trauma or, in some cultures, mutilation of the genitalia in women
  - Rape victims
  - Certain types of drugs or medications

Tips for patients who are recovering from a health problem and wish to continue their sexual function

- Discuss things carefully with your partner.
- Be prepared to make some adaptations and adjustments.
- Explore positions that minimize your energy or adapt to your situation.
- Do not drink alcohol or eat too much beforehand.
- Choose a relaxed time for sexual activity.
- Think carefully about the temperature of the room.
- Try to avoid rushed situations.
- Allow yourself plenty of time to rest afterwards.
- Remember that some effects following surgery and illness are so personal that nobody can really prepare you for them.
- Discuss any specific details with the surgeon or physician in charge of your case.
- Consult a sexual counsellor for further advice and help.

Care of the patient suffering from sexual abuse

Sexual abuse is the improper use of power by one individual over another for the purposes of sexual pleasure. The British Sexual Offences Act 2003 defines the following:

- **Rape** is non-consented penetration of mouth, vagina, or anus by a penis.
- **Sexual assault** is the act of sexual touching without consent.
- **Sexual assault by penetration** involves the insertion of object or body parts other than the penis into the vagina or anus (previously indecent assault).
- Children under 16 cannot legally consent to sexual activity and therefore do not need proof of consent. There is no defence in mistaken belief of age.

The victim is often tormented and subjected to sexual interference or intimidation. Victims are not chosen because of their physical appearance or attractiveness, but their vulnerability. They can be infants, children, men, women, the elderly, the physically disabled, and those with mental health problems and learning disabilities.

The physical, psychological, and emotional consequences can be enormous and far reaching. Many victims are reluctant to report the abuse because it often involves another member of the family, a close friend, or someone of high status in the community. Victims themselves believe that they are somehow responsible for the abuse. Years later, something may trigger or encourage the person to talk about their ordeal. Sometimes it never is revealed. Sexual abuse may lead to self-mutilating behaviour.

Sexual assault

Sexual assault is a form of aggression, violence, or deception in which sex is the weapon over a non-consenting individual. Rape is forced sexual inter-course. In the acute aftermath of rape, the role of the nurse is to assess the extent of injury, collect forensic evidence, and address the victim's concerns about pregnancy, sexually transmitted diseases, and AIDS. Sexual assault can also be touching another person's genital area without their consent.

The victim may suffer a range of reactions:
- Intense guilt or shame
- Self-blame
- Anger
- Denial
- Fear of retaliation from perpetrator
- Use of drugs or alcohol before a rape
- Fear of not being believed
- Hysteria and isolation

The patient may want to wash and bathe themselves several times, but will still complain of feeling dirty.

Nursing interventions

Providing adequate nursing care for rape victims requires a team approach.

Some key interventions for patients who have suffered sexual abuse

- Have a supportive person of the patient's choice present.
- Provide a room where the patient can talk in confidence and privacy.
- Provide reassurance, unconditional positive regard, and empathetic listening.
- Provide a prompt physical assessment and treatment of injuries and, if needed, a safe haven.
- Encourage the patient to talk about their experiences.
- Discuss with patient possible psychological effects, injuries, and diseases.
- Do not overreact or be judgemental.
- Record the key aspects of your conversation carefully and ask the patient to verify them.
- Warn the patient not to tell you things that they do not want you to pass on. Inform them that you will have to refer to others to ensure the best possible outcomes for them.
- Try not to be embarrassed or uncomfortable when listening to the patient.
- Refer the patient to other expert help, if necessary and desirable.
- Refer to social services, if relevant.

Culturally sensitive nursing care

- Culturally sensitive care refers to the provision of nursing care across cultural boundaries that take into account the context in which the patient lives as well as the situations in which the patient's health problems arise.
- Nurses providing care to patients from other backgrounds must be aware of and sensitive to their own unique heritage and health traditions and to the patient's sociocultural background.
- Careful listening and questioning can help the nurse understand the patient's cultural, ethnic, and religious values and health care beliefs.
- Transcultural nursing is an effort by nurses from all cultural backgrounds to come together and define concepts that enable them to develop the knowledge and skills needed to provide culturally sensitive care.
- There is a wide range of health and illness definitions, beliefs, and practices, not only among different ethnic groups but also within them. The following pages summarize characteristics of different cultural and religious groups, including their values and practices. It is important, however, for the nurse to assess each patient, whatever their background, as an individual.
- Two key population factors have contributed to the need for nurses to practise culturally sensitive care. The first is the profound shift in demographics of the population; the second is the outcome of the enormous wave of immigration that has occurred in the UK over the past 50 years.
- Nurses must understand that patients have differing world views and interpretations concerning health and illness that are based on their unique sociocultural and religious beliefs.
- The nurse who becomes skilful in culturally sensitive care can appreciate the total diversity of our society and strive to meet the needs of each patient.
- Factors that affect the delivery of culturally sensitive care include language barriers, poverty, prejudices, and fear of strangers.

Culture is the socially inherited or learned set of guidelines for a social group that are transmitted from one generation to the next. It influences our whole behaviour and lifestyle.

Ethnicity is a cultural group's sense of identification with its common social and cultural heritage. It includes nationality, race, language, religion, food preferences, and folklore.

Religion is the belief in divine or superhuman powers to be obeyed and worshipped.

Socialization is the process of learning a culture which usually starts in childhood and influences our lifestyle.

Communication is the key to understanding how different cultures behave and express their characteristics. Therefore nurses should be aware of the factors, both verbal and non-verbal, which make up the individual's culture.

Culturally sensitive assessment factors

When assessing patients from different cultural backgrounds the nurse should take into consideration such factors as skin colour (pallor causes black skin to appear ashen grey and brown skin to appear yellow-brown), nutrition and eating customs (these often carry emotional and social significance), and reactions to pain, illness, and the disease itself.

- Determine the needs of the patient who does not speak the nurse's language and provide official competent interpreters.
- Be aware of the patient's territory and ask permission before carrying out nursing interventions and physical examinations.
- Be aware of permissible touch and eye contact.
- Involve the patient's family and relevant community carers from their culture.

Ask patients about:
- Religious preference
- Ethnic background
- Beliefs about the nature of their health problem
- Usual health care practices
- Membership of religious institutions
- Practices relating to their religion
- Nutritional preferences
- Preparation of foods
- Participation in ethnic activities
- Their native language

Nursing, religion, and spiritual needs

The word 'religion' is derived, from the Latin 'religio.' 'Relegare' means to gather or read again and 'religare' refers to a bond. Religious expression is important to people because it brings meaning to their experience of being alive. It may also help structure their way of living by giving them purpose and direction and a moral code to abide by.

The Dalai Lama once said that throughout his journeys and visits to many people he has found that there are many faiths and other cultures capable of enabling individuals to lead constructive and satisfying lives; whether or not a person is a religious believer does not matter much; far more important is that they are a good human being.

Patients should be asked whether religion is important to them and whether they would like to participate in any aspects of it while in hospital. If the patient is unable to give the necessary information, then family members should be asked. If this is not possible, consult with someone from the patient's local religious community.

Allow people to define their own needs. There is a wide variety of interpretation and degree of strictness in observance of cultural traditions and religions. Each person must be assessed according to their own expressed needs within the context of their cultural norms and values.

Religion can be a highly organized cultural group expression of the experience of being fully alive, of being human, and of living and dying. There are close associations between spiritual experiences and religion. It is possible to have spiritual experiences without being religious or following a particular faith.

Religions, with their symbols, scriptures, artefacts, and sacraments, often express something that helps some people give purpose to their lives and a context in which to understand them.

A nurse's keen understanding of a patient's religious and spiritual requirements is very important, particularly as nurses are key workers who interact with patients more frequently than any other health care professional on the wards.

Nursing and different religious needs

Patients from different religions can have specific requirements and practices that they follow, which nurses need to be aware of. In all cases nurses should ask the individual and not make assumptions. Christianity, the most prevalent religion in the UK, has few strictures that pertain in a hospital setting, but Roman Catholics, notably, may request a priest to deliver last rites. Most hospitals will have a chaplaincy. Chaplains, although usually Christian, can help provide contact with other faith leaders. Many hospitals also have a special area allocated to the practice of religious observance, including prayer rooms for Muslims. If nurses need further help and advice they should contact their hospital chaplain, or the chaplain's representative.

Muslims

- Pray five times a day, which involves standing, bowing, and prostration. When a person is ill, prayer can be performed lying down or sitting up providing the chair or bed is facing Mecca.
- Fast during the month of Ramadan; the fast is broken each day at sunset.
- If ill, are exempt from fasting during Ramadan, but some may still wish to fast and even refuse medication during the fasting period.
- Prefer to be cared for by someone of the same sex.
- Perform ritualistic cleansing; the nurse should discuss this with the patient.
  - Ghusal: complete body wash with clean water.
  - Wusu: partial wash with clean water, performed before offering prayers.
- Wash their genitals with running water after using the toilet.
- Prefer immediate family to be consulted about treatment decisions.
- Circumcise male infants, and in Africa, Asia, and the Middle East some female genital mutilation takes place.
- Eat with their right hand and consider it rude to be handed anything in the left hand.
- Consider sickness and suffering to be a form of purification or recompense for wrong deeds.
- When dying, declare their faith and are comforted by a recital from the Quran.
- Observe the following rituals on the dead body:
  - Close the eyes and mouth.
  - Straighten the body and limbs.
  - Turn the head towards the right shoulder, facing Mecca.
  - Do not wash the body, but cover it with a plain sheet.
  - A complete Ghusal is carried out by the family as soon as possible.

Some Muslims may request that a non-Muslim does not touch the body. Use disposable gloves in this case.

Further information

www.islamicity.com

Jews

There are two main types: orthodox and non-orthodox.

- It is inappropriate for a man to shake a woman's hand and vice versa.
- Some may prefer a nurse of the same sex.
- Most men and boys cover their heads with a small skullcap known as the 'kippah'.
- Some orthodox women wear a wig called the 'shaytel' to symbolize marriage; if necessary, it can be removed in an emergency.
- Strict Jews eat Kosher food, i.e. food that is fit to be eaten in accordance with Jewish law. Laws on food state that pork and shellfish cannot be eaten and that meat and milk cannot be cooked or eaten together. Hospital plates and cutlery cannot be used.
- Circumcision usually takes place when a male is 8 days old; the child is given his name at this time.
- Abortion is allowed if the pregnancy threatens the mother's health.
- If someone is certified as brainstem dead, a rabbi should be consulted before life support is withdrawn.
- Judaism does not allow a post-mortem to take place, and the rabbi should be contacted if a body is referred to the coroner.
- Contacting the dead patient's rabbi is important as soon as death has occurred. It is essential that the eyes and mouth are closed; tape should be used if necessary to ensure this happens. The body should be laid flat, with hands open and arms parallel and close to the body. Legs should be straight. The Jewish Burial Society will prepare the body for burial.
- Burial takes place as soon as possible after death.

Further information

United Synagogue Burial Society. Tel: 020 8343 3456.
Jewish Community Information. Tel: 020 7543 5421.

Hindus

- Bodily discharges are seen as impure substances.
- Some are meticulous about personal hygiene.
- Hindu women are traditionally regarded as unclean during menstruation.
- Termination of pregnancy is disapproved of as it breaks the cycle of birth and rebirth (karma).
- Usually eat a vegetarian diet as this is an indication of spirituality.
- Will not eat beef or pork; the cow is a sacred animal.
- Women often fast and say special prayers for the recovery of the sick.
- Some foods are classified as 'hot' or 'cold' based on the way they affect the body. 'Hot' foods are salty, sour, or high in animal protein. 'Cold' foods are sweet or bitter and are believed to cool the body.
- Illness may be thought to be a punishment for bad behaviour.
- Family elders, rather than the patient, may make all decisions relating to treatment.
- Relatives sometimes place blessed items of jewellery on a black string around a patient's neck, arm, or body. These are believed to help protect the patient and should not be removed.
- Illness may be explained in terms of sorcery and evil spirits.

- Family members like to stay near the bedside of the patient if they are dying. There is a preference for the eldest son to be present before, during, and after death.
- A Hindu priest (pandit) may also be present when a patient is dying. Holy water is sprinkled over the person, and the dying person is placed on the floor symbolizing closeness to 'mother earth'.
- At death some Hindus are very strict about who touches the body; the family usually washes and prepares the body for cremation.
- A death is registered as soon as possible and cremation takes place within 24 hours.
- Prefer a shower to a bath.
- Some are unwilling to sign a consent form without first consulting their husband or father.

Further information

www.religioustolerance.org/hinduism.htm

Sikhs

- Wear a symbolic dress, known as the 5Ks. Nurses should not touch these items without washing their hands and without seeking permission. These items are mandatory and therefore Sikhs would want to keep them on while they are in hospital.
  - Kesh: uncut hair for both men and women symbolizes saintly qualities and a nature-loving disposition, including the beard for men.
  - Kara: a steel bangle, worn around the right wrist, symbolizes strength and restraint.
  - Kangha: a small 3–4 cm wooden comb symbolizes cleanliness worn in the hair.
  - Kirpan: a short dagger or sword, worn in a cotton body belt under clothes, represents the duty and right to take up arms to defend the weak and meek and destroy evil.
  - Kaccha: unisex undershorts with a drawstring waist representing chastity/sexual morality.
- Consider removing the turban without permission an insult, except in an emergency.
- Do not approve of termination of pregnancy.
- Prefer a nurse or doctor of the same sex.
- Have a high regard for personal hygiene—showering is preferred to bathing.
- Douche with water after using the toilet.
- Adhere to certain dietary habits, which vary from not eating beef, eggs, or fish to vegetarianism. The cow is a sacred animal.
- When the patient is dying, may give holy water to drink or may sprinkle it around the patient. Reciting passages from Guru Granth Sahib may be of comfort and someone may do this for the patient.
- Permit non-Sikhs to care for the dead body but do not permit them to interfere with the 5Ks.
- Care should be taken to see that the mouth and eyes are closed and that a peaceful expression is on the face.
- Cremation takes place as soon as possible.

Further information

Gateway to Sikhism: www.allaboutsikhs.com

Buddhists

- Wear distinguishing robes.
- Require contact from Buddhist chaplain/elder.
- Require a chaperone if patient is of opposite sex to you.
- Usually eat a vegetarian or vegan diet.
- May refuse food after 12 noon.
- May refuse opioids/sedatives/tranquillizers as these can impair awareness and consciousness.
- Need time and space for meditation.
- Need to wash before meditation and after using the toilet.
- May see anxiety and phobic disorders arising from a violation of an ethical way of life.
- If dying, may request a monk or nun to be present to chant them to rebirth.

Further information

The Buddhist Society, 58 Eccleston Square, London SW1V 1PH.
Tel: 0207 834 5858

Jehovah's Witnesses

- Forbid abortion.
- Refuse all blood transfusions. They may also refuse red cells, white cells, plasma, and platelets. However, some may be willing to receive fractions of these components such as albumin, clotting factors, immunoglobulins, interferon, and haemoglobin-based oxygen carriers. Ask the patient about what is permissible for them, and if consent is given for a transfusion, confidentiality must be upheld, i.e. no family member must know this has taken place.
- If baptized, often carry an advanced medical directive card instructing health professionals not to give blood products to them. This directive can only be rescinded in writing.

Further information

Hospital Information Services for Jehovah's Witnesses: IBSA House, The Ridgeway, London NW7 1RN. Tel: 020 8906 2211

Nursing patients requiring perioperative care

Preoperative assessment: principles

Purpose

- Determine the patient's fitness for operation and reduce cancellations.
- Identify risks to the patient and the best ways of managing them.
- Identify physical, psychological, and educational needs of the patient.
- Determine that the right patient has the right operation
- Plan pre- and postoperative care that the patient will require.
- Plan for discharge and continuing care.

Assessment may begin several weeks prior to the planned surgery to ensure that the patient is fit and well informed. Proper assessment reduces the chance that the surgery will be cancelled. It may take place in a specific clinic in a hospital or community setting.

Key areas for preoperative assessment

Nurses may be responsible for the initial clerking and/or examining the patient and will liaise with surgeons, anaesthetists, and therapists as necessary. This includes gathering information about:

Present complaint – history and any changes since listed for surgery, e.g. change in symptoms

Past medical history – medical conditions including cardiovascular disease (e.g. myocardial infarction, angina, hypertension, deep vein thrombosis/pulmonary embolism), respiratory disease (e.g. asthma, infections, TB, COPD), diabetes, neurological conditions (e.g. CVA/TIA), and other conditions (e.g. sickle cell disease); past surgery involving metal pins and plates that can cause burns if diathermy is used; presence of a pacemaker; previous difficulties with anaesthetics (e.g. intubation, ability to lie flat, problems of nausea and vomiting); relevant family history (e.g. heart disease, stroke, cancer); systematic review and examination of the patient.

Allergies – to certain medications or materials used in surgery (e.g. latex, antibiotics, tapes to secure dressings) and symptoms associated with the allergic response

Medication – details of medications that may have an impact on surgery and essential medications that will be required pre- and postoperatively

Observations – blood pressure, pulse, respirations, weight, height, BMI. Patients with BMI >30 may require referral for weight loss prior to undergoing non-urgent surgery.

Investigations – may include blood for U&E, FBC, ESR/CRP, INR, G&S/X match, fasting glucose, sickle cell; x-rays; screening for infections, e.g. MRSA; thromboprophylaxis risk assessment.

Knowledge and understanding of condition – level of patient's understanding of risks and consequences of surgery; the journey through anaesthetic room, theatre, and recovery; pre- and postoperative care; future and discharge arrangements. The education programme (i.e. what the patient wants and needs to know) should be planned.

Pain – details of any pre-existing chronic pain that may affect postoperative pain management. A pain score may be taken as baseline.

A more detailed assessment will also be required dictated by the patient's clinical condition, e.g. when undergoing ophthalmology surgery, orthopaedic surgery, etc. A summary of the assessment and plan for further action should be made.

Preoperative assessment: practice

A comprehensive physical examination, health history, and assessment are essential if rehabilitation to former health levels is to be achieved postoperatively. The baseline of information helps the nurse anticipate the patient's needs. 📖 Chapter 3, Individualizing nursing care practice, pp.32–33.

A baseline of information should include:

- *Vital signs:* blood pressure, pulse, temperature, respiratory rate.
- *Weight:* to assist in medication dosage and also in nutritional assessment. 📖 below.
- *Urinalysis:* to identify infection or underlying disease such as diabetes.
- *Respiratory assessment:* in addition to respiratory rate, assess whether the patient can walk a short distance without becoming breathless, speak sentences without difficulty, and lie flat without becoming breathless.
- *Mobility level:* assess ability to assist in transfers and to plan for prevention of postoperative complications, to get in and out of bed, move in bed, roll over, and walk to the toilet.
- *Nutritional status:* important as patient may be fasting or have restricted nutritional support for a period. Undertake Malnutrition and Universal Screening Tool (MUST) assessment and look for signs of poor nutritional status (e.g. recent weight loss); ask about normal diet, fluid intake, and appetite; identify likes and dislikes or any nutritional supplements taken; and undertake oral examination to identify mouth and gum infections, dental caries, or ill-fitting dentures. Check skin for elasticity, dry mucosa, and fluid intake and urine output to detect dehydration.
- *Elimination patterns:* normal bowel pattern, problems with urine output and flow.
- *Communication aids:* visual and hearing impairments that cause difficulty in communicating information and instructions, or that lead to disorientation during transfer to theatre and postoperatively. Note use of spectacles and hearing aids and their care and maintenance. Note conditions such as stroke which cause communication and comprehension difficulties.
- *Skin assessment:* including skin colour, circulatory problems, or oedema; existing pressure damage or risk of pressure damage; state of general hygiene; skin rashes, fungal infections, or ulcers.
- *Ability to self-care:* ability to undertake own hygiene and grooming; to dress and undress; and to take own medicines.
- *Sleeping and rest:* normal sleep patterns and anything the patient does to help sleep and rest.
- *Psychological and spiritual assessment:* particular aspects of the surgery, recovery period, or return home that are causing concern or worry. Find out whether there is anything that helps the patient cope with such anxiety.
- *Home and social circumstances:* including a detailed social history to start the discharge planning process including suitability of home, adaptations needed, support from family and friends, and access to telephone and transport.

Preoperative preparation

Preoperative visit

Aim is to supplement the care given by ward staff and to reassure the patient.

Theatre staff can inform patients about the processes in the anaesthetic room, theatre, and recovery and inform them about time schedules. They can answer patient's questions and develop a relationship with them.

Specialist professionals include specialist nurses and therapists who can prepare patients for the operation and instruct them in what they will need to do afterwards when the results and the need for further treatment will be known (e.g. stoma care, exercises).

Surgeon and anaesthetist can answer any questions, discuss concerns, reinforce information already given, and confirm consent to operation.

Expert patients (i.e. those who have had similar surgery) can explain consequences and progress from a patient's perspective.

Patient safety

Follow local policy.

Preoperative fasting

Aim is to avoid excessive periods of fasting and minimize risk of pulmonary aspiration of gastric contents. Follow the anaesthetist's instructions. General guidelines will include:

- Do not eat or drink immediately prior to anaesthesia.
- Adhere to minimum fasting periods:
  - 6 hours for solid food or infant formula or other milk
  - 4 hours for breast milk (for babies)
  - 2 hours for non-particulate or non-carbonate fluids
  - 2 hours for chewing gum
- No alcohol consumption within 12 hours prior to operation.
- Take prescribed medication unless otherwise instructed to do so by the anaesthetist.
- Consider IV fluids if patient is dehydrated.

Other checks and tests

- Identity band – Ensure the patient is wearing two identity bands with the correct name and unique hospital or NHS number. Details must match the patient's record, consent form, and theatre list. The band should not be placed on limbs that are undergoing surgery. Follow local policy for identifying allergies.
- Pregnancy test – All females 12–55 years should be offered a pregnancy test. If positive, notify operating surgeon immediately.
- Clothing – Ensure the patient is wearing correct theatre attire and has had a bath or shower. Ensure the patient's privacy and dignity as operating gowns may expose them. Check that patient is wearing appropriate compression hosiery based on risk assessment by medical staff.

- Site for surgery must be marked with indelible ink on patient's skin and must be checked with patient, consent form, and operating list. Follow organization's policy. The site should also be prepared according to the organization's guidelines and based on best practice.
- Note infections, allergies, and observations on the checklist.
- Ensure all documentation accompanies the patient.
- Ensure the patient's property is stored safely.
- Remove cosmetics, nail varnish, and jewellery. Exceptions are wedding rings that may be securely taped over.
- Hearing aids, dentures, and other prosthesis may remain in place until anaesthetic room. These must be stored safely on removal.
- Ensure specific preparation, e.g. bowel and skin preparation, has been completed.
- Complete check list (See Table 22.1).

Table 22.1 Preoperative checklist—an example

Check	Tick when complete	Signature	Comments
Patient's name and details against consent and theatre list			
Identity bracelet x2 different limbs			
Pregnancy status for females 12–55 years			
Consent form signed			
Correct health record and prescription sheet			
Correct investigation results			
Correct x-rays			
Allergies noted			
Site prepared			
Site marked			
Clothing removed/in theatre gown			
Prosthesis or metal work			
Pacemaker or defibrillator			
Denture removed/crowns noted			
Spectacles/contact lenses removed			
Hearing aid removed			
Bladder emptied			
Premedication given			
Checked nil by mouth for agreed period			
Infection control issues			
Temperature			
Pulse			
Respiratory rate			
Blood pressure			
Blood glucose			
Other special circumstances			

Preoperative education

Fear and anxiety about surgery causes stress which results in physiological imbalance and delays recovery. Patients often fear pain, disfigurement, dependence, the effects of anaesthetic, and loss of life. Education can help to reduce anxiety and improve postoperative results, e.g. quicker recovery, reduced analgesia requirements, reduced nausea, psychological comfort.

Purpose

Patients should be provided with information and explanations about the surgery and pre- and postoperative care.
- Reduce fears and anxiety, develop a confident frame of mind, and increase psychological comfort.
- Ensure patients can give informed consent. 📖 Chapter 30, Consent to treatment, p.976.
- Gain patient's cooperation and participation in pre- and postoperative care and concordance with treatment.
- Ensure accurate expectations of surgery, pre- and postoperative care, and recovery.
- Familiarize the patient with the postoperative environment and demonstrate and practise postoperative exercises and treatment.

Key points in preoperative education

- Patients' ability to understand depends on the communication and education skills of the health care professional.
- Individual assessment of anxieties and need for information is essential.
- Information that is given following admission is not retained as well as information that is given prior to admission. Information should be provided at pre-admission assessment clinics and supplemented by written materials when the patient is not as anxious.
- Listening to patients' anxieties and answering their questions is as important as giving verbal information and instructions.
- Information needs to be reinforced to ensure retention. Ward nurses, visiting theatre staff, specialists, and medical staff need to provide a consistent message and work together to prevent information overload.
- Preoperative education must be built into the patient's care plan. It should not be an add-on extra that is given if time allows.
- Pictures, diagrams, models, or demonstration of equipment may help the patient's understanding.
- Include the family members, if the patient wishes.
- Use a checklist to ensure coverage of information (See Table 22.2).

Table 22.2 Preoperative teaching checklist. (This is to guide the nurse in teaching patients to ensure they understand what is happening to them pre- and postoperatively.)

Subject	Completed by	Date
Purpose of teaching		
Preoperative period		
Simple related anatomy and physiology, e.g. function and structure of the heart for patients undergoing cardiac surgery; structure of knee joint for patients having knee replacement		
Surgery and risks/benefits		
Special tests and investigations. Bloods, radiological examination, ECG, and lung function tests		
Preoperative skin preparation. Shower/bath, specific preparation, shave/clippers, theatre clothing, removal of jewellery and aids (e.g. spectacles)		
Preoperative fasting 🕮 Preoperative fasting, p.764		
Storage of property and valuables		
Special preparation, e.g. enemas, catheters		
Safety measures Checks on patient details and rationale		
Preoperative medications Regular medications, premedication		
Surgery		
Planned time and duration		
Anaesthetic, theatre, and recovery environment		
Anaesthesia		
IVs and drainage tubes		
Incision, dressing, and sutures		
Postoperative (first 24 hours)		
Recovery room environment and staff		
IVs, drainage tubes, and oxygen		
Transfer and postoperative environment (intensive care/high dependency)		
Outcome of surgery		
Frequency of observations and tests		
Special exercises and pressure relief		
Pain relief and other medications		
Wound care and stitches		
Equipment and treatment		
Activity and ambulation		
Visiting		
Operation-specific instructions		

Consent to treatment

Definition

Consent is a patient's agreement for a health professional to provide care and treatment. It may be given orally, in writing, or non-verbally. For consent to be valid it must be given voluntarily (freely without pressure or undue influence) by an appropriately informed person (one who understands in broad terms the nature and purpose of the procedure) who has the capacity (ability to comprehend and retain information) to understand the intervention in question. Competent adults are entitled to refuse treatment even when it would benefit their health, including pregnant women who may refuse treatment even if the action would be detrimental to the fetus.

Capacity

Having mental capacity means that a person is able to make their own decisions. According to the Mental Capacity Act (2005) a person is unable to make a particular decision if they cannot understand the information given to them, retain it long enough to be able to make the decision, weigh up the information to make the decision, and then communicate it. 📖 Chapter 30, Criteria for assessing capacity to give informed consent, p.976 and 📖 Chapter 30, Principles of the Mental Capacity Act, p.976.

Sufficient information for 'informed consent'

Patients must be provided with clear information about the nature and purpose of the procedure. They should be given information about the following:
- Anaesthesia. Patients should be given an opportunity to discuss it with an anaesthetist unless in an emergency situation.
- Any intended benefits of the procedure, any serious or frequently occurring risks, any alternative treatment, and the risk of doing nothing.
- The possibility of tissue samples being removed and retained.
- Additional procedures that may be undertaken if they become necessary during treatment.
- Video or photography that is being taken for teaching or research purposes.

The patient can consent or refuse the above or specify which they agree to or refuse permission for. The patient is usually informed that there is no guarantee that a particular person will perform the procedure. Patients should be encouraged to ask questions, e.g. about the treatment itself or the impact on their future lifestyle. They should also be informed that they may change their minds and withdraw consent at any time. All information given should be documented.

Other points

- The professional carrying out the treatment is responsible for ensuring consent is given, before it begins. Consent can also be obtained by staff who are capable of doing the procedure, or who have been specially trained and assessed.

- Consent should be sought well in advance, with the clinician checking that the patient still consents before the procedure starts.
- Follow local policies and procedures.

Further information

Policy and guidance on consent can be found at www.dh/gov.uk/consent

Anaesthestic room care

Reception and handover
- Local guidelines should be followed when sending for patients and during their handover at theatre reception. The underlying condition should be a deciding factor in the grade and experience of the person accompanying the patient.
- The ward nurse should hand over the patient to the nurse or practitioner and ensure that all records, results, and x-rays are available. During the handover the correct patient is identified with the relevant records and documents, and these are checked against the operating list and identity bands. The consent form should be checked to ensure it has been signed.
- The patient must not be left alone. Effective communication with the patient is essential to ensure they know what is happening.
- Any important information that is relevant to the operative procedure should be highlighted and reinforced, e.g. if patient has crowns or back problems, or is diabetic.

Anaesthetic induction
At least two staff should be present at anaesthetic induction, e.g. the anaesthetist and a trained assistant (operating department practitioner or nurse) to help the anaesthetist administer the anaesthetic. Additional staff may be required to assist with transferring or positioning the patient or to act as a chaperone.

Safety checks
- Ensure availability, safety, and readiness of equipment and medications needed for anaesthetic and patient monitoring, e.g. supplies of medical gases, endotracheal intubation equipment, masks, syringes, etc. Perform regular checks to ensure the equipment has been maintained.
- Ensure availability of IV infusion fluids or blood for transfusion.
- Check that patient, type of procedure, and side and site of operation are correctly identified and correspond with health records, hospital number, theatre list, and consent form. Check that prosthesis, dentures, etc. have been removed.
- Check records for allergies, e.g. to plaster, latex, medications.
- Ensure staff are familiar with the use of equipment and procedures to ensure safety.
- Ensure staff are up to date in the management of critical events such as cardiac and respiratory arrest.
- Ensure staff practise good personal hygiene, use personal protective clothing provided, and follow procedures to minimize risks, e.g. of needle stick injuries, cross-infection.

Lifting and transfer

- Care should be taken during lifting and transferring sedated and anaesthetized patients between trolley and operating tables. A sufficient number of people must be available to lift patients safely and sufficient rollers, slide sheets, or variable-height trolleys must be available to move patients safely.
- When positioning patients ensure that they are protected from pressure damage and damage to nerves and that tubes and drains are not disconnected.

Care in the operating theatre

The role of operating department personnel includes patient management, scrub, and circulating duties.

Appearance

Have a high standard of personal hygiene. Wear appropriate theatre clothing, theatre scrubs, caps that cover hair, and antistatic rubber-soled shoes. Do not wear jewellery. Wear masks that fit securely and are not worn around the neck.

Positioning the patient

Position the patient to ensure good access to the operation site without hindering respiration, circulation, or causing damage to blood vessels and nerves and to ensure there is good lighting. Staff should be accustomed to adjusting theatre tables and lighting. Care should be taken to ensure that any lines or tubes are not obstructed.

Aseptic technique

• Ensure all instruments used in the operation are sterile and kept separate from non-sterile instruments.
• Follow correct sterile scrubbing, gowning, and glove procedures.
• Prepare patient's skin using aseptic solutions to remove dirt and bacteria. Use sterile drapes to provide a safe barrier between sterile and non-sterile parts of the body to prevent cross-infection.

Surgical equipment

Scrub and circulating nurses count the instruments, swabs, needles, and tapes to be used before, during, and after surgery. Pay particular attention to detachable parts, e.g. blades and screws. Inform surgeon of the count and sign as correct. Follow local procedures for checking and recounting if initial count is incorrect. Ensure patient tracking procedure of theatre trays and instruments is followed. Check that diathermy is working properly and the pad is placed safely. Check for and report signs of redness.

Specimens

Ensure that specimens are placed in appropriate containers, that solutions are clearly labelled with patient's details, and that pathology forms are sent to the laboratory.

Hazardous substances

• Be aware of hazardous substances in the operating theatre environment; work to agreed safe practices; use personal protective clothing to prevent or control exposure.
• Check special procedures for patients with infections such as MRSA and blood-borne infections such as hepatitis B and HIV.

Risks in the operating theatre

Untoward events and near misses (no-one injured but risk of injury identified) should be recorded and action taken to minimize risk in future.

- Incorrect patient, operation, site, or side
- Lack of consent or consent does not adequately cover the procedure
- Medication or transfusion errors
- Patient injury due to:
  - Incorrect positioning
  - Poor moving and handling techniques
  - Improper preparation or use of faulty equipment
- Staff injury due to failure to follow agreed procedures or to wear personal protective clothing, e.g. needlestick injuries or exposure to hazardous substances
- Retained swabs or instruments
- Cardiorespiratory arrest
- Failure of medical gas supply—failure to check supplies and have no back-up facility or unplanned disconnection of equipment
- Loss or damage to specimens

Postoperative care: physical

Recovery room

Prepare the equipment and environment to cope with any critical event, e.g. cardiorespiratory arrest and haemorrhage. Prepare the bed area with a special mattress, emergency equipment, oxygen tubing and masks, monitoring equipment for vital signs and oxygen saturation, gas cylinders as a back-up to piped gases, suction equipment, appropriately sized catheters, and infusions and catheter stands as appropriate. The aim is to minimize the risks of the anaesthetic and surgery and promote recovery to an optimal state of health. Focus care on providing a safe environment, monitoring the patient's condition, and preventing and minimizing complications.

The patient should be physiologically stable on departure from the operating theatre and should be observed on a one-to-one basis until regaining airway control, cardiovascular stability, and the ability to communicate. The frequency of observations depends on the patient's condition and stage of recovery. An Early Warning Scoring system may be used to ensure medical staff are notified of a patient's deteriorating condition.

Postoperative risks and management

- *Poor handover:* It is essential that detailed handover occurs between theatre and recovery areas and the ward area.
- *Obstruction of airway:* Observe respiratory rate and depth and colour for peripheral and central cyanosis. Monitor haemoglobin oxygen saturation and oxygen administration. Nurse in the lateral recovery position until patient is fully conscious. Keep airway tube handy.
- *Haemorrhage:* Reactive haemorrhage occurs when blood pressure rises. Observe for tachycardia and low blood pressure, signs of shock (cold clammy skin, weak thready pulse); check wounds and drains for blood loss. Supplement clinical observations with a minimum of pulse oximetry and non-invasive blood pressure monitoring.
- *Hypothermia:* Observe for low core temperature, shivering. Ensure adequate bedding is available.
- *Pressure damage:* Use special mattresses until patient is mobile.
  📖 Pressure ulcers: assessment and prevention, p.424.
- *Pain:* 📖 Postoperative pain management, p.780.
- *Infection:* of wounds, urinary tract, chest, and infusion and drain sites is common. Observe for site redness, inflammation, pyrexia, pain, and discomfort. Prevent by using aseptic technique, encouraging deep breathing and expectoration, keeping wounds covered, and encouraging fluids if no contraindication.
- *Drains, catheters:* Attach to closed system of drainage. Observe and record amount and type of drainage for signs of infection and obstruction.
- *Risk of immobility:* e.g. deep vein thrombosis, joint stiffness, chest infection. Encourage early mobilization, deep breathing, coughing, and moving around bed. Anti-embolism stockings and anticoagulation may be prescribed. Observe peripheral circulation.

- *Nausea and vomiting:* Observe and record amount, frequency, type, and content. Support patient during episode and change vomit bowls after use. Give mouth care and washes, and anti-emetics as prescribed. Introduce fluids and food gradually and record intake and output.
- *Infusions and transfusions:* Follow checking procedures; calculate rate; record amounts; check site for infection and blockage; monitor temperature and blood pressure.
- *Renal failure:* Observe for anuria, oliguria, and retention of urine.
- *Medications required:* Ensure these are administered as prescribed.

Handover to ward staff

Local criteria should be followed when transferring the patient from recovery to general ward areas and the patient should be accompanied by relevant experienced staff. The anaesthetic record, recovery observation charts, and prescription sheet should accompany the patient. Full clinical details and a report of specific equipment and treatments must be relayed to the ward nurse.

Postoperative care: psychological

The period after surgery is focused on recovery and adaptation to the new life situation, which may be temporary or permanent. Recovery and adaptation is influenced by patient's fears, worries, and social circumstances. Specific factors that affect recovery and adaptation include:

- Anxiety about postoperative pain
- Diagnosis and prognosis, e.g. cancer, life-threatening results
- Competence of surgical team and nursing care
- Fear of complications, threat of new episodes, or impact of further treatment
- Premature discharge
- Availability of continuing care and family involvement
- Ability to cope with daily living in hospital and following discharge
- Ability to accept and manage changes in body image, e.g. stoma, amputation, mastectomy
- Reactions of family members and those close to patient
- Effects on work, social and family life

Identifying problems

Patients may appear worried, listless, apathetic, depressed, tearful, or withdrawn. They can be reluctant to participate in and discuss their care, or they may ignore the affected part of the body or the wound. Alternatively they may be offhand, abrupt, angry, aggressive, or may complain about trivial issues. They may be very demanding, may seek reassurance, or have interrupted sleep patterns. Acute confusion may affect elderly people with no previous history, and post-anaesthetic depression may occur 7–10 days postoperatively when patient has left the hospital.

Helping patients cope

- Spend time with patient on one-to-one basis and encourage discussion about anxieties.
- Determine whether any additional major life events or crises are happening.
- Assess normal coping mechanisms and support networks, e.g. family members, friends, hobbies, and involve these if possible.
- Ensure patient has sufficient information to understand the operation, treatment, and care plan.
- Arrange discussions with relevant specialists, e.g. nurse specialist, therapist, social worker, discharge coordinator, and medical staff.
- Obtain information and contacts from support groups, e.g. local cancer support groups, stoma and ileostomy groups.
- Offer patients an opportunity to talk with patients who have successfully recovered and adapted following similar operations.
- Ensure the environment is conducive to recovery, e.g. quiet and calm, where patients can see and be seen by nurses.
- Ensure patient's anxieties are not trivialized.
- Consider whether group support from other patients on ward is helpful.
- Older people may be more vulnerable following surgery and should be carefully assessed and prepared for discharge with appropriate support.

Postoperative pain management

Most patients report pain after surgery. Poor pain management increases morbidity, delays discharge and healing, and increases complication rates and anxiety. Unrelieved pain can cause sleep disturbances that reduce quality of life. It can also be costly because it leads to a longer length of stay.

Factors influencing pain

- *Patient's expectations:* patients expect to have pain after surgery; some are resigned to having pain and tolerate it, are reluctant to take medication, will wait until pain is severe, or do not wish to complain and do not report it at all.
- *Patient's characteristics:* age, culture, and previous experiences of pain.
- *Lack of information* about availability of pain relief affects expectations and increases anxiety, which increases pain.
- *Lack of knowledge* of clinical staff about pain management, its effects on recovery and quality of life, and methods of pain relief. There may be misconceptions about addiction to medication, risks of overdose, or responses to pain of people from different ethnic groups, cultures, and ages.
- *Organizational factors* such as lack of pain management protocols, lack of training and development of staff, and increased workloads lead to poor pain assessment, over-reliance on patient-controlled analgesia equipment, and under-use of non-pharmacological methods of pain relief.

Principles of postoperative pain management

An important aim of postoperative pain management is to facilitate the patient's recovery and restoration of function. It is important that the pain is assessed on an individual basis, is recorded, and involves the patient where possible. Some people (e.g. older people) are more vulnerable to pain but may not seek help due to previous attitudes and culture.

Postoperative pain management usually follows local protocols that have been created by a team of anaesthetists, surgeons, recovery and ward based staff together with input from pharmacy and therapists. The organization may have an acute pain team for referring problems and educating ward teams on providing pain relief.

- *Assessment:* Use a pain assessment tool, e.g. 0–10 scale (10 excruciating pain—0 no pain) or a verbal rating scale (no pain, mild pain, moderate pain, severe pain). The patient should be the prime assessor of their pain. Assess onset, duration, and location of pain, and any precipitating or aggravating factors. Observe behaviour for agitation, crying, groaning, grimacing, or restlessness. 🕮 Pain assessment tools, p.796.
- *Pain medication:* Medication choice and doses should be tailored to the individual and based on the severity and type of pain. The World Health Organization's Analgesic Ladder (1996), originally developed for cancer pain, can be applied to medication choice for postoperative pain (i.e. increasing levels of pain are treated with stronger analgesics: Step 1 uses non-opioids, Step 2 uses weak opioids, and Step 3 uses strong opioids). Because postoperative pain begins at a high intensity

and improves over time, analgesia may be initiated at a higher rung and stepped down as pain improves. Analgesia may be given via several routes: oral, intramuscular, intravenous, epidural, regional, spinal, or patient-controlled analgesia (PCA). A PCA pump enables self-medication of analgesia in synchrony with patient's pain rhythm, and is more effective than bolus injections. Patients must have adequate oral analgesia when pump is discontinued.

- *Non-pharmacological approaches:* These are useful in enhancing pain relieving medication and in diverting attention from pain to an alternative sensory experience. These approaches include repositioning, massage, prayer, distraction, relaxation, and music.
- *Education interventions:* Increased knowledge of pain control and expectation of pain relief leads to assertiveness in demanding relief. Information about the surgery, care, and treatment will reduce anxiety and pain.

Further information

World Health Organization (1996). *Cancer pain relief*, 2nd edn. WHO, Geneva.

Postoperative education

Postoperative education should be a continuation and reinforcement of preoperative education and should be directed at the patient and family as necessary.

Purpose
- Prepare patients and their family for discharge.
- Enable patients to take responsibility for their own care, e.g. manage their own stoma.
- Help patients understand their journey to recovery from reduction of symptoms to resumption of usual activities and return of energy and strength.
- Reduce anxiety and promote self-esteem.
- Help the family provide appropriate levels of support.

Key points in postoperative education
- Ensure education is individualized and geared to the patient's level of perception, understanding, language, and cultural needs, i.e. what the patient wants and needs to know.
- Make instructions specific, e.g. 'rest when tired' rather than 'take it easy'.
- Some patients may have difficulty reading or following detailed written guidelines; others may need an interpreter or help from a carer, advocate, close friend, or relative.
- Find out what makes the patient anxious, e.g. doing something that may harm them.
- Incorporate education into a day-to-day care plan; do not view it as an additional ad hoc add-on.
- Include the following areas as a minimum:
  - Food and drink—Explain that fluids and then food are introduced slowly as anaesthetic and pain medication slow gastric emptying. Advise the patient to have small portions frequently and that good nutrition is essential for healing postoperatively. Advise on special diets and involve dietitian and specialist nutrition nurse if relevant.
  - Bowel movements—Explain that constipation is common after surgery because of anaesthesia, bed rest, and medication. Advise on prevention, e.g. increase fluids and use bulk-type laxatives unless contraindicated.
  - Wound care—Address concerns about wound strength, infection prevention, when sutures/staples will be removed, and how to dress and support wound, if relevant.
  - Exercise and lifting—Advise on restrictions, explain what is meant by lifting and moving 'heavy weights', and what is meant by not performing 'strenuous activities' and for how long.
  - Pain—Describe the diminishing nature of wound pain, give information on analgesia and avoidance of activities that increase pain.
  - Bathing—Advise on showering and bathing, particularly if wound should not get wet.

- Daily activities—Advise patient on why activities such as driving, returning to work, and resuming sexual activity may be restricted and for how long. Inform patient on when these activities can be resumed.
- Medications—Ensure the patient knows what medicines to take and when, what they are for, what side effects to expect, whether repeat prescriptions are required, and where to obtain these.

Care of surgical wounds

The management of surgical wound usually follows local protocols created by a team of surgeons, ward nurses, pharmacists, and infection control and tissue viability specialists.

Assessment

The goal is to ensure that the patient and wound are treated appropriately. Assess the patient and wound for:

- Signs of infection including pyrexia, redness, tenderness, or swelling around wound site.
- Presence of wound drain, e.g. type of drain and colour, consistency, and amount of exudates produced.
- Closure method to identify dressing and wound management needed.
- Location—Determine whether it will impede movement or increase risk of contamination, e.g. perineal wounds.
- Postoperative pain—This must be assessed and controlled.
  📖 Postoperative pain management, p.780.
- Patient's perceptions of wound to determine any problems with acceptance of changes to body image, anxieties, and worries.
- Nutritional status—Malnutrition will impede wound healing; obesity may delay healing and also reduce mobility. Check for dehydration.
- Conditions that may impede wound healing, e.g. diabetes.

Principles of wound management

- Use aseptic technique when changing dressings. Take a wound swab if there are signs of infection.
- Use techniques and choose a dressing to prevent wound trauma.
- Involve the patient, discuss the choice of dressing, and explain processes.
- Use analgesia before a dressing change, if required.
- Use appropriate dressings to address individual needs and promote wound healing. Check local wound formulary. Dressing should:
  - Be absorbent and retain exudate
  - Not fall apart when wet with exudates
  - Be comfortable for the patient
  - Be non-adherent and non-toxic from chemical fibres in dressing
  - Permit bathing if possible
  - Prevent cross-infection
  - Minimize pain and trauma at dressing change
  - Not require frequent or unnecessary changes. Dressings may not be required after 24–48 hours.
- Drains should be checked for signs of infection. Drainage should be measured and recorded. Use closed system of drainage. Drains are removed according to protocols or surgeon's directions.
- Seek advice from tissue viability nurse if necessary.
- Make a record of observations and changes to wound to evaluate healing.
- Observe for complications. 📖 Surgical wound healing and complications, p.785.
- Sutures/staples are usually removed between 7 and 10 days depending on the location. May be left longer if on moving body parts (e.g. joints) or if patient has impaired ability to heal (e.g. immunosuppressed patients).

• Provide information about the wound and address patient concerns (☐ Discharge and continuing care after surgery, p.786). Involve the patient and their carer as appropriate in their wound care and explain the importance of asepsis and infection prevention.

Surgical wound healing and complications

Healing process

• *Healing by primary intent:* The aim is to align the skin edges of the wound by sutures, clips, staples, or tape to promote complete healing without complications.
• *Healing by secondary intent:* The wound is left open and heals by granulation, contraction, and epithelialization. Used if there is considerable tissue loss, incision is shallow but has large surface area, or if drainage of abscess or pus is required.

Phases of healing

• *Inflammatory phase:* The formation of a blood clot joins the wound edges loosely and stimulates an inflammatory response, swelling, heat, redness, and pain, which starts healing and repair. This requires energy and nutrition (0–4 days).
• *Regenerative phase:* Granulation tissue starts the process of wound contraction. Little is seen in wounds healing by primary intent but this can be seen in wounds healing by secondary intent. A new capillary network is formed. The length of stage is variable but is about 24 days in wounds healing by primary intent.
• *Epithelialization:* The wound is covered by epithelial cells which migrate across the wound surface or along the suture line. Variable time span from 2 days in closed wounds.
• *Maturation phase:* The wound becomes less vascularized, scar tissues become comparable to normal tissue, and tensile strength increases.

Complications

• *Haemorrhage:* may occur during surgery or up to 10 days after. Primary and intermediary haemorrhage (during surgery and within the first 24 hours) is due to poor surgical technique. Secondary haemorrhage at 7–10 days is usually due to infection.
• *Infection:* increased risks if environment is poor (inadequate ventilation and poor standards of asepsis in theatre), if patient is older, obese, has diabetes, or takes steroids or immunosuppressive medications. The type of surgery, poor surgical technique, and location of drains are also factors.
• *Dehiscence:* breaking down or splitting of wound healing by first intent—contributing factors are increased age and poor surgical technique.
• *Sinus formation:* track from abscess to body surface.
• *Fistula:* abnormal track from one viscus to another, e.g. recto-vaginal.
• *Scarring:* hypertrophic scar (excessive collagen deposits cause thick scar). Keloids may occur months after surgery and are more common in 10–30 year-olds.

Discharge and continuing care after surgery

- Plan discharge from admission and, where possible, give patients an expected date of discharge.
- Patients may feel vulnerable and apprehensive when discharged from the security of the hospital.
- Specific preparation and arrangements for discharge should occur in addition to postoperative education. 📖 Postoperative education, p.782.
- Plan with the patient and in consultation with family and carers as appropriate.
- Older people and others with complex needs may be particularly vulnerable to rapid or unexpected discharge.

Support systems: The amount of help needed determines the support systems required. This may be provided solely by family and friends or, if patient has complex needs, a care package of social and health care may be necessary or a period of convalescence in a nursing or residential home. Ensure agencies are contacted and provided with details. Visits by discharge coordinators and liaison staff prior to discharge will help to ensure a smooth transfer out of hospital.

Discharge summaries and information: Ensure written information about the patient's nursing care and progress is given to community staff before discharge. Patients and carers should also have written information and a discharge checklist will help to ensure every aspect has been covered.

Convalescence: Explain that periods of fatigue and tiredness are to be expected during the first month after surgery at least. In addition ability to make decisions may be affected due to anxiety and lack of concentration and should be deferred if possible.

Wound care: Ensure arrangements are made to have the wound checked, redressed, and sutures/clips removed (return to hospital, GP practice or in own home). In addition check that the patient has sufficient dressings. Give instructions about the normal appearance and sensations of the wound and complications, e.g. signs of infection, increased pain, and advise to seek help from the GP or practice nurse.

Activity on return home: Advise the patient on why activities such as driving, housework, hobbies, returning to work, and resuming sexual activity may be restricted and for how long. An indication of when the activities can be resumed will be helpful.

Exercises: Special exercises may be taught to strengthen areas affected by the operation. Ensure the patient is able to do these, can gradually increase as strength and stamina return, and has written instructions.

Medication: Ensure the patient has a supply of medications and understands what they are for, what side effects to expect, whether repeat prescriptions are required, and where to obtain them.

Contact information: Ensure the patient has key contact names and telephone numbers for community nurse, social worker, GP, ward/hospital, nurse specialist, and when they can contact them.

Follow-up arrangements: Arrange appointments to see consultant, nurse, GP for continuing care.

Nursing patients with pain

Definition and overview of pain

The International Association for the Study of Pain defines pain as 'an unpleasant sensory and emotional experience associated with actual or potential tissue damage or described in terms of such damage'. Some pain is protective and acts as an early warning sign to alert the individual that tissue damage is occurring or is about to occur. However, pain can also be experienced when there is no evidence of tissue damage.

Margo McCaffery in 1968 defined pain as 'whatever the individual patient says it is'; it is a personal and subjective multidimensional experience. A patient's perception and response to pain varies according to various psychological, physiological, social, and cultural factors:

- Emotional state
- Genetic background
- Personality
- Motor activity and sensory inputs
- Fitness level
- Age
- Culture
- Socioeconomic class
- Cognition

Unfortunately, both hospitals and community settings sometimes give inadequate pain advice and pain may be undertreated. Therefore it is important that patients understand that they have an important role in ensuring that their pain is alleviated. For example, patients who are undergoing surgery should be taught what to expect following surgery and how to properly communicate with their medical and nursing staff. Patients with pain should be encouraged to voice concerns about their pain management.

Acute pain

There are several critical distinguishing characteristics of acute pain.
- It is associated with a well-defined cause.
- It normally subsides as healing takes place, i.e. it has a predictable end.
- It is of brief duration—<12 weeks (which is often closely related to the severity of the injury and the time course for healing).
- It may become chronic if not treated effectively.
- It is usually of sudden onset.
- It can range from mild to severe.
- It can usually be relieved by treatment.

Acute pain can cause suffering, anxiety, and negative physiological effects for the patient. Changing the patient's position, performing a physical examination, toileting, and performing activities associated with daily living and comfort measures may exacerbate acute pain. Therefore, patients should be handled carefully, should be informed of what is happening, and should be involved in measures to relieve their pain. As a general principle, no one should be left waiting for acute pain control in a hospital setting.

Causes
- Trauma
- Burns
- Myocardial infarction
- Inflammation
- Infection
- Exacerbation of chronic medical disorders, e.g. chronic obstructive pulmonary disease (COPD)
- Surgery
- Migraine
- Diagnostic procedures
- Invasive procedures (e.g. blood draws, cannula insertion)
- Intramuscular injections

Possible physiological responses
- Stimulation of the autonomic nervous system and stress-related hormones
- Metabolic changes leading to protein breakdown and poor healing repair
- Cardiovascular effects (hypertension, tachycardia, myocardial ischaemia)
- Hypercoagulability (increased risk of blood clots)
- Poor respiratory function (increased risk of chest infection)
- Disturbance in the gastrointestinal tract
- Increased risk of chronic pain due to sensitization of the nervous system

Possible psychological responses
- Anxiety
- Fear
- Insomnia

Possible behavioural responses

Behavioural responses to pain are very individual.

- Guarding and protecting the affected area to reduce additional damage
- Holding oneself, rocking, or rubbing the affected area
- Moodiness
- Social withdrawal
- Short temper
- 'Out-of-character' verbalizations
- Severe restlessness
- Discomfort
- Crying, moaning, frowning, grimacing, and facial distortions

Chronic pain

There are several critical distinguishing characteristics of chronic pain.
- Its natural history is unclear.
- It does not subside even though healing has apparently taken place.
- It is of extended duration (beyond the expected time of healing or when associated with a long-term condition).
- It is a more complex problem than acute pain.
- It affects the complete lifestyle of the patient.
- It is described as ongoing or persistent pain, and can be severe in nature.
- It can be difficult to control.

Chronic pain can arise from stimulation of pain receptors or nociceptors (nociceptive pain) or from damage to the nerves themselves (neuropathic pain). It differs from acute pain in that the common physiological responses to acute pain such as tachycardia and hypertension do not continue. Chronic pain can be divided into malignant pain (associated with cancer) or non-malignant pain.

Chronic pain can have a significant effect on the sufferer's physical, psychological, and social well-being. Patients may experience a range of emotional responses including fear, anxiety, and depression. Treatment of chronic pain may involve a combination of pharmacological, physical (e.g. heat/cold, massage, TENS), behavioural (e.g. cognitive behavioral therapy) and complimentary therapies (e.g. acupuncture, hypnosis). The approach to treatment must consider the need to promote the patient's ability to remain active or to provide a comfortable end of life.

Causes
- Musculoskeletal pain, e.g. rheumatoid or osteoarthritis, back pain, ankylosing spondylitis
- Headache
- Peripheral neuropathy (e.g. diabetic neuropathy, hepatic neuralgia)
- Phantom limb pain
- Diseases of the central nervous system, e.g. multiple sclerosis
- Peripheral vascular disease
- Angina
- Leg ulcer
- Abdominal pain
- Fibromyalgia
- Cancer (classed as malignant pain)

Possible physiological responses
- Changes in body weight
- Fatigue
- Sleeplessness
- Muscular wasting, loss of strength
- Painful joints and stiffness

Possible behavioural responses
- Frustration and anger not only with the pain but with health professionals, family, and friends
- Decreased social contact, isolation, and depression
- Disrupted libido and relationship with partner; patient may become over-dependent and demanding
- Moodiness, hopelessness, despair, and suicidal thoughts
- Feelings of loss and poor self-esteem
- Anger with cultural norms and beliefs, questioning the concept of religious support and spirituality

Pain assessment

Pain is whatever the person experiencing it says it is, and it occurs whenever the patient says it does.' Because the pain experience varies from person to person and from situation to situation, the pain assessment must involve the patient. Each patient must be respected as an individual with unique needs.

Reactions to pain vary among individuals and may depend on past experiences, state of health and level of fitness, age, personality, culture, and beliefs. The amount of tissue damage is not an accurate predictor of pain intensity; therefore, the type of medical condition and the type of surgery is not a reliable guide of the reaction a patient will have to pain. Patients who have similar medical conditions or who are undergoing the same surgical procedure may have very different reactions to pain.

The pain assessment must be systematic, and holistic, and involve as many factors as possible, including biological, psychological, cultural, and social factors. Pain can be measured using a variety of different measurement tools and scales. An initial assessment should be performed on first encounter with the patient to establish a baseline. Subsequent assessments should be more involved and investigate more complex issues as well as monitor the effectiveness of nursing and medical interventions.

Effective pain control is dependent upon good assessment. The formal assessment of the patient's pain conveys three essential meanings to the patient:

1. That their report of pain is believed.
2. That their pain is being taken seriously.
3. That you want to know what it is like to experience the pain.

Nursing assessment

A thorough assessment should be performed to characterize the pain complaint. To this end, several pain assessment tools are available. The pain assessment should include:

- Full past medical history
- Verbal description of the pain
- Location, duration, frequency, and intensity of the pain
- Associated features, such as sweating, diarrhoea, or vomiting
- Aggravating and relieving factors
- Patient's thoughts and feelings about the pain experience
- Effects of the pain on the patient's lifestyle and ability to concentrate and work
- Usual ways of coping with pain
- How long the patient has had the pain
- Whether the pain affects the patient's rest and sleep

Physical assessment
- Head-to-toe review of the patient which includes looking for erythema, swelling, atypical body temperatures, tenderness, sweating, and deformities
- Vital signs (blood pressure, pulse, temperature, respiration, oxygen saturation)
- Observation of the patient's posture (Is the patient guarding or protecting an area of the body?)
- Observation of the patient's body language (Does the patient appear anxious or restless?)

Pain assessment tools

Patient self-report is the gold standard for measuring pain and a wide variety of pain assessment tools are available. Intensity rating scales measure the intensity of pain, but other more multidimensional pain assessment tools are also available. Most tools use the patient's self-report and therefore can only be used when the patient is able to report pain. Behavioural observation tools are available for patients who cannot self-report.

Visual analogue scale

A visual analogue scale is a horizontal or vertical line drawn on paper, anchored by 'no pain' at one end and 'unbearable pain' at the other end. Patients place a mark on the line to indicate the severity of their pain. Visual analogue scales are frequently used in research but many patients find them difficult to use. One limitation of this type of scale is that it can be difficult to quantify a meaningful change. This type of scale cannot be used to compare one patient with another, but may be useful for assessing whether an intervention is helpful for an individual.

Visual analogue scale

no pain --------------------------------------unbearable pain

Descriptive scale

A descriptive scale consists of a range of words on a continuum ranging from 'no pain' to 'severe pain'. Patients select the description that best describes their pain.

Verbal rating scale

no pain---------mild pain------moderate pain------ severe pain

Numerical rating scale

A numerical rating scale consists of numbers that patients use to rate the intensity of their pain. Typically the scale ranges from 0 = no pain through 10 = unbearable pain, but other numbers can be used. The tool can be administered verbally or on paper where a 10-cm line is drawn and a mark is placed along the line indicating pain intensity.

Numerical scale

0-----1-----2------3------4------5------6-----7-----8-----9-----10

Face rating scale (Fig. 23.1)

For the face rating scale, various pain intensities are represented by faces on a continuum ranging from smiling to grimacing and crying. This scale is frequently used with children and may be useful with adults who have difficulty conceptualizing their pain as words or numbers.

The above scales are quick and easy but may limit the patient's choice. In some cases, a combination of the above scales can be used. For example, a descriptive scale can be combined with a numerical rating scale:

No pain 0-------mild pain 1-------moderate pain 2--------severe pain 3

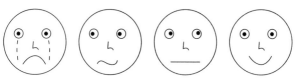

Fig. 23.1 Face rating.

McGill pain questionnaire (Fig. 23.2)

The McGill pain questionnaire developed in 1971 is an example of a multidimensional pain assessment tool. The questionnaire uses a complex range of scoring categories to assess a patient's pain. This type of scale is most often used in chronic pain clinics because it encompasses a wider range of factors affecting the pain experience.

3 Not Done

A. PLEASE DESCRIBE YOUR PAIN DURING THE LAST WEEK. (*Check off one box per line.*)

	None	Mild	Moderate	Severe
1. Throbbing	0 ☐	1 ☐	2 ☐	3 ☐
2. Shooting	0 ☐	1 ☐	2 ☐	3 ☐
3. Stabbing	0 ☐	1 ☐	2 ☐	3 ☐
4. Sharp	0 ☐	1 ☐	2 ☐	3 ☐
5. Cramping	0 ☐	1 ☐	2 ☐	3 ☐
6. Gnawing	0 ☐	1 ☐	2 ☐	3 ☐
7. Hot-burning	0 ☐	1 ☐	2 ☐	3 ☐
8. Aching	0 ☐	1 ☐	2 ☐	3 ☐
9. Heavy (like a weight)	0 ☐	1 ☐	2 ☐	3 ☐
10. Tender	0 ☐	1 ☐	2 ☐	3 ☐
11. Splitting	0 ☐	1 ☐	2 ☐	3 ☐
12. Tiring-Exhausting	0 ☐	1 ☐	2 ☐	3 ☐
13. Sickening	0 ☐	1 ☐	2 ☐	3 ☐
14. Fear-causing	0 ☐	1 ☐	2 ☐	3 ☐
15. Punishing-Cruel	0 ☐	1 ☐	2 ☐	3 ☐

B. PLEASE RATE YOUR PAIN DURING THE LAST WEEK.

The following line repesents pain of increasing intensity from 'no pain' to 'worst possible pain'.
Place a vertical mark (I) across the line in the position that best describes your during the last week.

No
Pain

Worst
Possible
Pain

Score in mm
(*Investigator's use only*)

C. CURRENT PAIN INTENSITY

0 ☐ No pain
1 ☐ Mild
2 ☐ Discomforting
3 ☐ Distressing
4 ☐ Horrible
5 ☐ Excruciating

Questionnaire Developed by: Ronald Melzack

Copyright R. Melzack, 1970, 1987

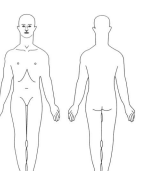

Fig. 23.2. © Copyright 1970, 1987 Ronald Melzack. Reprinted with permission from Dr R. Melzack.

Methods of relieving pain

Effective pain relief is dependent on continuous accurate assessment and evaluation of the patient's pain, and generally requires a multimodal approach using pharmacological and non-pharmacological interventions. The goals of pain management include:
- reducing pain to a level that is acceptable to the patient
- providing optimal comfort so that the patient expresses satisfaction and feels a sense of control
- enabling the patient to carry on with their normal or adjusted lifestyle
- eliminating or reducing side effects from the interventions used.

Pharmacological interventions
- *Non-opioid drugs* (e.g. paracetamol and NSAIDs such as ibuprofen, indometacin, and diclofenac) exert their analgesic effects on pain associated with inflammation. Non-opioid drugs are used for mild-to-moderate pain. Paracetamol is primarily metabolized by the liver and should be avoided by patients with moderate-to-severe liver problems. NSAIDs can damage the lining of the gut and may lead to ulcers, and are contraindicated for patients with some conditions.
- *Opioid drugs* (e.g. morphine, pethidine, codeine) inhibit the transmission of pain through receptors in the brain and spinal cord. Opioid drugs are used for severe pain and have demonstrated efficacy in a variety of visceral pain conditions. There may be concerns about dependency with opioids, and they are covered under the Misuse of Drugs Act 1971. Tramadol is classified as an opioid drug because it appears to have both opioid and non-opioid properties
- *Adjuvant agents* comprise a variety of classes of drugs with a primary purpose other than pain (e.g. antidepressants, anti-epileptics, muscle relaxants, corticosteroids, and local anaesthetics). For example anti-epileptics have demonstrated efficacy for neuropathic pain.
- *Regional analgesia* interrupts pain transmission over a localized area (e.g. Emla® cream to skin, local anaesthetics for nerve blocks, and steroids for reducing inflammation when given as an injection).

Issues relating to drug use in pain control

- Analgesic drugs may be used alone or in combination.
- The intensity and nature of the pain should determine the type of drugs used.
- Non-opioid drugs have a ceiling (i.e. beyond a certain dose there will be no further effect), and in opioid use the ceiling may be affected by the patient's pain response and by other treatments.
- Long-term use of opioids leads to tolerance and dependence and therefore increased doses may be required to manage chronic pain.
- For terminally ill patients both the dose and the frequency should be adjusted.
- Pain relief should be constantly monitored and updated.
- Analgesic ladders are frequently used in the control of chronic pain (See Fig. 23.3), particularly when the patient requires more than one analgesic for the control of their pain. Of note, the WHO analgesic ladder was designed for and validated in cancer pain only but is extrapolated often inappropriately elsewhere.
- Analgesic drugs can be administered through a variety of routes including oral, transdermal, subcutaneous, intramuscular, and intravenous (via a pump) routes.
- The patient and their relatives should be kept up-to-date and informed regularly of the pain control and drugs used.
- Some patients may be able to control their own administration of drugs for pain control.

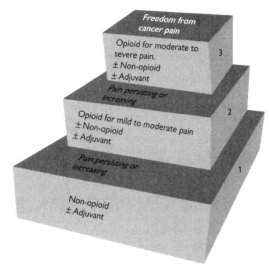

Fig. 23.3 WHO pain relief ladder. Reproduced with permission from WHO. World Health Organization (2003). *Palliative care: symptom management and end-of-life care*, p12, WHO, Geneva.

Non-pharmacological interventions to manage pain

Non-pharmacological interventions should not be used in place of pharmacological interventions but are useful adjuncts in relieving pain and discomfort. This should be discussed with the patient.

Cognitive behavioural therapy is based on the idea that an individual's thoughts and behaviour patterns affect the experience of pain. This type of therapy uses a range of techniques such as education, distraction, guided imagery, deep breathing, and relaxation. Patients are taught about the meaning of pain and how to deal with negative thoughts and feelings. These techniques are often combined with exercise and other elements of a multidisciplinary pain management programme that have been shown to be effective in a range of chronic pain states. These techniques can also be used independently. When using distraction, patients should be encouraged to recall an interesting or pleasant experience or focus their attention on an enjoyable activity. Music may be helpful. The patient may be encouraged to close their eyes and listen. This type of therapy may be particularly helpful with short episodes of pain.

Guided imagery aims to help the patient concentrate on a peaceful pleasant image. The patient is asked to give details of the image, what it is like, how it sounds, smells, tastes, and feels. The patient is asked to concentrate on an object and breathe deeply, slowly inhaling and exhaling. Patients are asked to note the rise and fall of their abdomen and the weightlessness of their breathing.

Muscle relaxation involves the patient focusing on a particular muscle group in the body. Patients are asked to start with the hands and gradually work their way around the body ending with the feet. Patients are asked to tense the muscles for 5–7 seconds and then to relax and concentrate on the sensations that relaxation brings.

Meditation is another method used to counteract the stress associated with pain and anxiety by producing a relaxation response.

Other interventions

Several other non-pharmacological interventions are available but have limited evidence to support their efficacy.

- *Transcutaneous electrical nerve stimulation (TENS)*. Electrodes placed around peripheral nerves transmit electrical impulses which block pain pathways.
- *Thermotherapy*. Heat is applied to decrease pain, relieve stiff joints, and ease muscle aches and spasms. A hot water bottle or heat pads can be used.
- *Hydrotherapy*. Depending on the patient's problem, warm or cold water can be used. When the body is in water, the weightlessness experienced reduces stress on joints, muscles, and other connective tissue.

- *Vibration*. A vibrating device is used to ease pain by inducing numbness in the treated area. The device can be a vibrating cushion, chair, or bed. It can also be a handheld device that a nurse, carer, or patient applies to the affected area.
- *Exercise*. Increased exercise can be a valuable therapy for both acute and chronic pain. During exercise, endorphins (the body's natural painkillers) are released which may promote a sense of comfort and alter the perception of pain. Patients can be shown a range of motion exercises permitted by the involved joint.

Complementary therapies for pain relief

These approaches require careful and considered handling and nurses should be appropriately trained in their use. The NMC recommends that nurses ensure that the introduction of these therapies is safe, that the therapies are in the best interest of the patient, and that the patient has consented to their use. Often these therapies form part of a wider multidisciplinary team approach to pain control and care.

Aromatherapy involves the use of essential oils to treat a medical condition or to induce relaxation. Aromatherapy may or may not include massage. It is important to determine whether there are particular odours that patients do not like, that upset them, or that they have allergies to.

Massage involves a therapeutic manipulation of the soft tissues of the body. It is usually carried out over and around the site of the pain. It is contraindicated in areas that are actively inflamed or where there are open wounds, damaged skin, or lumps/tumours. There are now a variety of massages including Indian head massage, hand massage, full body massage, and foot massage.

Acupuncture originates from China where it has been practised for thousands of years. It involves the placement of fine needles in the skin at specific points on the body. Some evidence is available to support this approach.

Acupressure is similar to acupuncture but uses finger pressure on the acupuncture points rather than needles.

Reflexology is based on the belief that the body's natural healing mechanisms can be enhanced by the application of pressure to certain areas of the feet and hands. There is no firm evidence basis for this mode of treatment.

Homeopathy is a treatment based on the belief that a substance that produces the symptoms of a health problem may also cure it (i.e. treating like with like). Extracts of plants, animals, or minerals are diluted repeatedly to provide a water-based solution used to provide a treatment. There is no firm evidence basis for this mode of treatment.

Hypnotherapy is the use of hypnotic techniques in the treatment of certain conditions. The patient is hypnotized into a trance-like state which allows them to become more compliant, relaxed, and open to suggestion. Special discs or tapes can be used to aid this process for patients at home. Hypnotherapy is contraindicated in patients with severe psychological health problems such as depression or psychosis.

Nursing care and interventions

- When nursing the patient with pain always demonstrate empathy by spending time listening to their account of the pain.
- Continue to monitor the patient's pain and the efforts to control it.
- Document the subjective information elicited from the patient, using their own words.
- Note the location, quality, and duration of the pain and any precipitating factors.
- Choose pharmacological interventions that are appropriate for the patient's level of pain.
- Administer drugs on time as prescribed; never keep a patient waiting for pain relief.
- Anticipate adverse effects from drug use, especially with an older patient, and treat them appropriately. The most common adverse effects are respiratory depression, sedation, constipation, nausea, and vomiting.
- Use a multidisciplinary approach to manage pain.
- Include non-pharmacological approaches.
- Ensure good nursing comfort measures to help the patient in pain.
- Reposition the patient 2-hourly to reduce muscle spasms and tension.
- Relieve pressure on bony prominences.
- Use pillows and special aids to support the patient when in bed or sitting in a chair.
- If appropriate, elevate limbs to reduce swelling, inflammation, and pain.
- Give massage if trained to do so and appropriate.
- Perform passive range-of-motion exercises to prevent stiffness and further loss of mobility.
- Provide oral hygiene and keep the patient's mouth fresh and clean.
- Provide any other necessary nursing care based on an assessment of the patient's need.
- Contact the pain nurse specialist or chronic pain care team if further help is needed.

Patient teaching

Patients and their families often times have misconceptions about pain and its treatment. Effective pain management is dependent on an adequate understanding of the concept of pain-controlled analgesia and the value of other forms of pain control.

- Educate patients and their carers about their prescribed drugs, including their adverse effects.
- Teach coping methods appropriate to the needs of the individual and their family.

Discharging patients home with pain problems

- Patients and their family or carers should understand that they have an important role to play in the control of pain when the patient is cared for in the community.
- Patients and their carers should understand the importance of taking drugs at the times they have been prescribed. The need to establish a new routine when at home should be stressed.
- Patients and their carers should understand that drugs should be taken exactly as they have been prescribed. Drugs should not be overdosed or abused.
- Patients and their carers should be taught that mild over-the-counter analgesics have side effects and should not be overused.
- Physiotherapy and/or complementary therapy should be arranged, if appropriate.
- People with learning disabilities or mental health problems, the elderly, and children are at risk of poor pain care and control in the community. Relatives and carers of such people are critical to the success of pain management and should be taught to establish good communication with the patient to ensure that their needs are being met.
- With the increasing number of special pain clinics and outreach teams from hospitals visiting the community, confusion may arise over the roles of various health care professionals. Community nurses should be informed on what is happening and what their role is with respect to the patient.
- Cultural issues affect the pain experience and nurses should be sensitive to various ethnic needs.
- Patients with pain may feel isolated and become depressed. Patients who may be vulnerable to isolation should be referred to appropriate resources, such as volunteer organizations, local churches, and religious groups.
- Patients with pain need encouragement and support. Local support groups and pain clinics can be a valuable resource for patients.
- It may be helpful for patients to maintain a special pain diary.

Lifestyle changes/adaptations

Workplace changes

Some patients may need to alter their work situation or may be unable to work altogether. Advice about income support or disability benefit should be provided. In such cases, referral to a social worker and an occupational therapist may be warranted.

Adaptations/equipment in the home

Occupational therapists can assess the patient, conduct a home visit, and advise on equipment and adaptations to maximize a patient's independence.

Common drugs used for pain management

Common drugs used for pain management are listed in Table 23.1. **All drug doses listed in this table are adult doses and not children's doses**. This table is only to be used as a guide and the current BNF should be consulted for further advice. Nurses should involve themselves only in the administration of medications which fall within their sphere of competence.

Table 23.1 Common drugs used for pain management

Non-opioid analgesics	Dose	Common side effects
Paracetamol	500–1000 mg every 4–6 hours to a maximum of 4 g daily	Rare but rashes and blood disorders reported. *Important –* liver damage (and less frequently renal damage) following overdose

NSAIDS
(💷 Table 17.1 Common drugs used for orthopaedic and musculoskeletal disorders: Anti-inflammatory drugs, p.635)

Compound analgesic preparations	Dose	Common side effects
Co-codamol 30/500	1–2 capsules/tablets every 4 hours; maximum 8 capsules/tablets daily	As above for paracetamol plus constipation, drowsiness
Co-dydramol 10/500	1–2 tablets every 4–6 hours; maximum 8 tablets daily	As above

Opioid analgesics	Dose	Common side effects
Dihydrocodeine	30–60 mg every 4–6 hours when necessary	Nausea and vomiting, constipation, drowsiness; side effects as for morphine (see below) may be seen with larger doses

Table 23.1 Common drugs used for pain management *(continued)*

Non-opioid analgesics	Dose	Common side effects
Morphine (including diamorphine)	Dose and frequency dependent on condition being treated and formulation used (See BNF for details)	As above; larger doses may cause respiratory depression, hypotension, and muscle rigidity; other side effects include difficulty with micturition, ureteric or biliary spasm, dry mouth, sweating, headache, facial flushing, vertigo, bradycardia, tachycardia, palpitation, postural hypotension, hypothermia, hallucinations, dysphoria, mood changes, dependence, miosis, decreased libido or potency, rashes, urticaria, and pruritis
Tramadol	50–100 mg up to a maximum of every 4 hours; total of more than 400 mg not usually required	As for morphine above; also abdominal discomfort, diarrhoea, hypotension and occasionally hypertension; parathesia, anaphylaxis, and confusion reported

Neuropathic and functional pain	Dose	Common side effects
Amitriptyline (for post-herpetic neuralgia) NB unlicensed indication	Initially 10–25 mg at night, increased gradually to 75 mg at night; higher doses at night under specialist supervision	Dry mouth, blurred vision, constipation, nausea, difficulty with micturition; cardiovascular side effects (electrocardiograph changes, arrhythmias, postural hypotension, syncope, tachycardia); many more side effects (See BNF)

Trigeminal neuralgia: 📖 Table 13.3 Common drugs used for neurological disorders: Carbamazepine, p.484.

Nursing patients with body image problems

Body image

Body image is a complex and multifaceted construct. It was originally defined by Schilder (1935) as 'the picture of our own body that we form in our mind, that is to say, the way in which the body appears to ourselves.' It has since been defined in many different ways. A useful definition, which includes the key elements identified by Schilder as well as key elements included in more recent definitions, is provided by Grogan (1999) as 'a person's perceptions, thoughts and feelings about his or her body.'

Models

No one model currently provides a comprehensive understanding of body image, but a number of factors are likely to be important in its understanding. Fig. 24.1 shows a framework adapted from Rumsey and Harcourt (2005) that offers a basis for understanding how body image and appearance concerns might develop and persist, as well as offering a model for focusing treatment interventions.

Altered body image

The terms 'body image concern' or 'body image disturbance' emphasize the dimensional nature of the construct and its links to a universal concept. Their use facilitates application of Rumsey and Harcourt's framework to clinical interventions.

Body image problems

Body image problems arise when individuals differ in the ease and speed with which they adapt to changes in both visible and invisible appearance. Markers that suggest body image may be problematic (e.g. changes in appearance have not been well adjusted to) include:
- Anxiety
- Avoidance
- Negative emotions, such as hostility and anger
- Poor psychological wellbeing

Assessing body image

Several tools have been developed to assess body image, but to date no one comprehensive measure exists. Each measure assesses a very specific aspect of body image, tied to the researcher's interests and to different aspects of what is understood as body image. Dolan and Birtchnell (1997) provide a summary of the most common measures, grouped into four methods of assessment:
- Body silhouettes – require judgements or responses to pictures or stimuli related to different shapes/weights.
- Objective measures – typically involve estimation of actual body size, yielding a measure of body image 'distortion.'
- Projective tests – ask patients to provide their own idiosyncratic view of their body image.
- Questionnaires – require a response to a set of predetermined questions.

Predisposing factors ⟹	Intervening processes ⟺	Consequences
• Demographic • Sociocultural (influences from parents, peers, society and culture, including religious beliefs, beliefs about how the body works) • Hereditary • Anatomical and biological, genetic factors	• Salient features and most noticeable body image changes to self and others • Ideals for self and cultural ideals and values for appearance • Beliefs about the importance and significance of physical appearance • Comparison of appearance with that of others • Attributional style (e.g. tendency to believe problems are caused by oneself) • Coping style (e.g. tendency to avoid discussing concerns, tendency to cope with problems with humour) • Social support • Physiological and biological changes due to normal ageing and development, trauma, injury, surgery, and abnormal growths such as cancer	• Social anxiety • Social avoidance • Isolation • Decreased psychological wellbeing (e.g. lower quality of life, depression) • Specific emotional reactions, including shame, hostility, anger, embarrassment • Request for support/ treatment

Fig. 24.1 A framework for understanding body image concerns.

Source: Rumsey, N and Harcourt, D, *The Psychology of Appearance*, ©, 2005 Reproduced with kind permission of Open University Press. All rights reserved.

Further information

Schilder PM (1935). *The image and appearance of the human body*. International Universities Press, New York, NY.

Grogan S (1999). *Body image*. Routledge, London.

Rumsey N and Harcourt D (2005). *The psychology of appearance*. Open University Press, Berkshire

Dolan B and Birtchnell S (1997). 'Measuring body image', in Salter M (ed) *Altered body image: the nurse's role*, 2nd edn. Balliere Tindall, London.

Factors associated with body image problems

A range of factors are associated with increased body image distress including demographic, sociocultural, hereditary, anatomical and biological, and genetic factors (See Fig. 24.1). In relation to demographic and sociocultural factors there is some, albeit limited, support for the suggestion that adolescent and young women are more distressed. Increased vulnerability to body image concerns may also be related to several psychological, particularly cognitive, factors:

- Low general self-esteem
- High investment in appearance (for example, as an important contributor to overall self-esteem)
- Unfavourable comparisons with other people
- Low general optimism
- Poor coping strategies
- Poor interpersonal skills

Some factors appear to reduce or ameliorate distress. Level and extent of social support is a commonly identified protective factor for body image. Physical characteristics and treatment related factors (e.g. nature, extent, severity of the objective difference in appearance, and nature and type of treatment undergone) do not generally predict distress or adjustment.

Medical conditions that alter body image

Cancer

Many patients with cancer undergo one or more treatments that alter body image.

- Surgery is commonly performed to diagnose and remove malignant tumours. Reconstructive surgery is also common in patients with cancer. Surgery can result in scarring, potential loss of function, lymphoedema, and reliance on prostheses or appliances.
- Chemotherapy can result in hair loss, weight changes, and feelings of nausea and vomiting. Some patients find the means of administration intrusive and threatening to body image.
- Radiotherapy can result in fatigue and skin reactions that may lead to permanent scarring.
- Steroids and hormonal therapy can also have an unwelcome impact on body image. These therapies can cause menopausal-like symptoms and can cause patients to experience emotional distance from others.

Breast removal/reconstruction

This normally results from breast cancer and affects women more often than men. Many of the consequences on body image will be as noted above.

Breast removal itself, whether partial or whole, can alter body image in ways that have implications for sexuality and sexual relationships. This is a highly sensitive topic for most women. Although not all women wish to discuss this topic, others are relieved if someone else broaches the subject.

There is often a range of choices to be made about what type of surgery the patient should undergo (e.g. whether to have reconstructive surgery or breast reduction). Involving the woman in those discussions enables her to gain some sense of control over what is happening to her and has been associated with better outcome.

It is important for the nurse to recognize that the meaning of breast surgery may differ significantly according to cultural and religious background.

Gynaecological issues

Both hidden and visible changes can affect a woman's body image, including surgery such as hysterectomy, as well as infertility and sterility, miscarriage, sexual violence, and abortion. Each may affect a woman's body image and perception of her identity as a woman.

In many women bodily changes will have significant and individual meaning to the woman. Her sense of femininity and personal identity is likely to be affected. As with breast surgery, the impact on sexuality (sexual confidence in one's bodily appearance; fears concerning sexual intercourse, etc.) may be important and will need careful exploration. However, some women may prefer not to discuss this.

Stoma

Patients with a stoma face changes in their body image, including some related to other's reactions.

- Patients may have false information or false expectations about the experience of having a stoma, which must be identified and corrected.
- A stoma can serve as a constant reminder of illness, and can be a source of extreme embarrassment and social avoidance, which in turn can affect self confidence and availability of social support.
- Intimate relationships are often avoided or considered impossible. Patients involved in intimate relationships may benefit from their partner's involvement in the decision, surgery, personal care routine, and any discussions of body image implications, particularly for sexuality and sexual relationships.

Burns

Burn injuries cause sudden and often widespread damage, and the events and circumstances surrounding the injury can be emotionally charged.

- Patients may have a difficult time reconciling the extent of the damage with a seemingly small accident. They may watch others closely for their reactions to their wounds.
- Scar management appliances may not be used due to dislike of their appearance and reactions from others.
- Appropriate management (e.g. protection from sunlight) may make the patient feel conspicuous, especially during warm weather.
- The ultimate outcome is typically uncertain, which can result in unrealistic expectations and delayed adjustment.
- The scars may serve as a permanent reminder of a traumatic event.

Skin conditions

Contrary to popular belief, disfiguring skin conditions increase in prevalence with age and are not confined to adolescence. Most conditions are not life-threatening, but their impact on body image is often overlooked.

- Stress appears to play a role in onset and maintenance of a skin condition.
- Some patients may find it difficult to camouflage or conceal their condition using make-up.
- In a holistic care plan, it may be important for the nurse to address the impact of such a condition on the patient's body image.

Other medical conditions

A wide range of other medical conditions may affect body image and these concerns may need to be addressed.

- Stroke may result in hemiplegia, a profound disturbance in which patients may deny that parts of their body belong to them.
- Endocrine disorders that cause myxoedema (e.g. diabetes and hypothyroidism) may result in body image changes.
- Changes may also result from neurological disorders such as Parkinson's disease, motor neuron disease, myasthenia gravis, and multiple sclerosis.

- Medical devices such as indwelling catheter, peg feeding tube, intravenous cannula, and pacemaker can alter body image.
- Medications including hormones, tranquillisers, and psychotropic medications can cause changes in the patient's experience of their body. Although most of these changes may not be visible, they may feel frightening for the patient.
- Paralysis, injuries due to trauma, and amputation can also alter body image.

Nursing care in helping patients adjust to changes in body image

Establish a good relationship

Establishing a trusting relationship is a prerequisite for any intervention with a patient who has body image concerns. The nurse needs to make time to listen, to be sensitive to what may be very personal concerns, and, if appropriate, to give reassurance.

It is important to recognize that a patient's reaction to changes in the body cannot be predicted objectively. For example, the extent of scarring cannot predict the effect it will have on a patient's body image. Any changes to the body can cause distress and concern, and individuals differ greatly in their response to the same event or damage. Listening, reassuring, and providing general support is likely to be particularly important in the early stages.

While recognizing individual variation, it is important that the nurse monitors the patient's reaction and is aware when this deviates greatly from the typical changes that might be expected over time. Some patients will require time, gentle prompting, and specific questioning in order to express any worries or concerns.

Encourage expression of feelings about their body

At all stages of treatment, including preoperatively, patients should be encouraged to express how they feel about any changes in their body. The nurse should be alert to any signs of extreme distress and concern and to any significant difficulties in adjustment the patient is experiencing. While realizing that adjustment takes time, some patients may require referral for psychological help.

Preparation

Before surgery or in any situation where change is likely to impact on body image, carefully prepare the patient for what is going to happen. Explain what the likely effects might be, including impact on body image.
- Written information that includes pictures (e.g. photographs of scars) can be particularly helpful.
- Generally, any information that might help alleviate the patient's anxieties should be given.

Advice on appliances and reconstructive surgery

Discuss with the patient any opportunities for appliances, reconstructive surgery, or methods of disguising appearance, e.g. using make up. Inform the patient about the advantages and disadvantages of each.

Prior to discharge

As discharge approaches patients' concerns may change as they contemplate facing other people, including strangers. Identify any concerns, and help prepare patients for practical and social problems that are likely to occur. For example, offer guidance about how to deal with stigma and curious behaviour and questions from other people.

Throughout hospitalization encourage patients, who often feel less acceptable and lacking in confidence at first, to socialize and integrate with others including other patients, if appropriate. Also encourage them to have visitors.

Provide patients with adequate information and education. Be aware of relevant support groups, both statutory and voluntary, and inform patients how to contact these groups. If necessary, facilitate this contact for the patient. Also be aware of available written and internet information that might be helpful to patients.

Partners and family

Provide partners, relatives, and friends with information about likely changes to the patient's body image, and likely patient concerns.

Culture

It is important to be sensitive to the different cultural, social, and religious issues that may be relevant. This involves putting aside one's own values and priorities to avoid influencing any nursing interventions, advice, or support offered to patients from different backgrounds. Areas of particular concern and significance to some cultures include:

- hair loss
- breast removal
- decreased fertility and stoma (e.g. a stoma can create problems with religious observance for Muslims).

Developmental/lifespan issues

It is important to take the patient's age and life-stage into account when considering the likely impact. The concerns and reactions of adolescents, for example, may differ from those who are elderly, as both groups will be facing different developmental and lifespan challenges.

Psychological referral

Despite good nursing care some patients will require more specialist psychological help. A range of psychological interventions are offered by specialists in psychiatry and psychology, and the nurse should be aware of local services, their referral criteria, and how to make such a referral, if it seems appropriate. The decision to refer is influenced not only by body image concerns, but in the case of trauma or life-threatening illness, also influenced by anticipated difficulties that the patient may have in adjusting to the trauma or illness itself. Such patients may display symptoms of clinical depression or post traumatic stress disorder.

Further information

Grogan S (1999). *Body image*. Routledge, London.
Rumsey N and Harcourt D (2005). *The psychology of appearance*. Open University Press, Berkshire
Price B (1990). 'A model for body image care'. *J Adv Nurs*, **15**, 585–93.

Nursing patients with cancer

The cancer problem

- Each year 10.9 million people worldwide are diagnosed with cancer and 6.7 million die from it, equating to around 12% of annual deaths worldwide.
- The most common cancers worldwide are lung, breast, bowel, and stomach.
- The proportion of all deaths caused by cancer varies, from 4% in Africa to 23% in North America. (Cancer is mainly a disease of older age and much of this difference is explained by differences in the age of the population in regions of the world.)
- In 2005 just under 290,000 people were diagnosed with cancer in the UK.
- Although there are more than 200 different types of cancer, four types (breast, lung, bowel, and prostate) account for more than 50% of cancer diagnosed each year in the UK. (See Fig. 25.1.)
- Cancer causes 28% of all deaths in the UK. In the UK in 2007, there were more than 155,000 deaths from cancer.

Further information

Cancer Research UK Website: http://info.cancerresearchuk.org/cancerstats/
Excellent resource for UK cancer statistical information.

Characteristics and causes

Normally, when cells wear out or are damaged, cells within the same tissue divide to form identical new cells. This process of cell division is highly controlled by several genes and usually ensures that cells only divide when necessary. Damage to these genes (causing genetic mutation) can cause uncontrolled growth in a cell. As the cell continues to divide in an uncontrolled manner it can lead to the development of a cancerous growth or tumour (primary cancer). Tumours are swellings or masses of tissue that may be benign or malignant.

Characteristics of cancer cells

Cancer cells differ from normal cells in many ways. Cancer is a mono-clonal disease, i.e. all the cells in a tumour come from only one ancestral cell. The transformation of a normal cell into its malignant counterpart is an accumulative, multistage process of gene mutation. As each mutation occurs, the cell's DNA becomes less stable. Many cancers exhibit loss of control of the cell cycle. This is the sequence of stages through which a cell passes between one division and another.

Infiltration of neighbouring tissues. The most important difference between cancer and normal cells is cancer cells' ability to spread and invade other tissue space and grow at other sites. This is the most dangerous aspect of cancer, and it is the reason for most cancer deaths.

Proliferation and angiogenesis. Cancer cells can invade local blood and lymphatic vessels and proliferate throughout the body. One of the key reasons cancer can spread in this way is because a tumour is able to establish its own blood supply (or blood vessels). The new blood vessels not only provide oxygen and nutrients for the tumour but also create a route for metastatic colonization.

Metastasis. Most cancers do not spread completely haphazardly; they have favoured sites, e.g. breast cancer commonly spreads to lymph nodes, liver, bones, and lungs. The four most common sites of metastases from cancer are lung, liver, bone, and brain.

Note: A breast cancer that spreads to the liver is not a liver cancer, but a metastatic (secondary) breast cancer. The cell histology will be more akin to a breast cell and treatment may well be very different from a primary liver cancer.

Tumour classification

Benign tumours
- Cannot spread by invasion or metastasis; only grow locally.
- Less likely to be life-threatening; an exception is benign brain tumours.
- Some may transform into malignant tumours, e.g. adenomatous polyps in the colon.

Malignant tumours
- Able to spread by invasion and metastasis.
- Often known as cancers; some diseases are classified as 'cancers' but may not make swellings which is the true meaning of 'tumour'.

Main cancer types

Cancer is classified by tissue type and point of origin within the human body. Cancer is loosely classified into five main types.

- Carcinoma (epithelial tissue origin)
- Sarcoma (supportive and connective tissue origin)
- Myeloma (myeloid blood cells)
- Leukaemia (leukocytes)
- Lymphoma (all haematological in origin)

Tumour of unknown origin: In about 5–6% of cancer diagnoses the tumour is of 'unknown origin'. The overall prognosis of such tumours is generally poor, with median survival less than 4 months.

Note: Some cancers are discussed in more detail in the relevant sections of the handbook. 📖 Chapter 8, Oesophageal and stomach cancer, p.218; 📖 Chapter 8, Colorectal cancer, p.230; 📖 Chapter 11, Urological cancers, p.382 📖 Chapter 12, Skin cancer, p.420; 📖 Chapter 13, Brain tumour, p.476; 📖 Chapter 16, Leukaemia, p.588; 📖 Chapter 16, Lymphomas, p.590; 📖 Chapter 19, Gynaecological cancers, p.664; 📖 Chapter 19, Testicular cancer, p.679, 📖 Chapter 19, Breast cancer, p.684.

Causes of cancer

Many tumours are swellings or masses of tissue that may be benign or malignant.

- Cancers occur due to exposure to carcinogens (cancer-causing substances) that cause mutations to genes that control cell division, plus the random damage to DNA that occurs during one's lifetime.
- Approximately 5% of cancers are caused by inherited cancer-related genetic mutations, e.g. *BRCA-1*, which increases the risk of breast and ovarian cancer.
- Hereditary cancers tend to occur at an earlier age and individuals have a higher risk of multiple tumours.
- The most common risk factors for cancer causation are tobacco use, dietary factors, infective causes, and UV light.

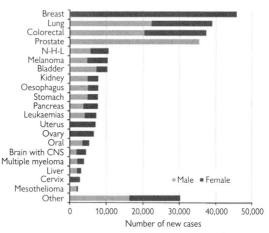

Fig. 25.1 The 20 most common cancers in the UK—incidence 2005*. Statistics used courtesy of Cancer Research UK. Reproduced with permission of Cancer Research UK 2006, http://info.cancerresearch.org/cancerstats/incidence/commoncancers/

* Non-melanoma skin cancer (NMSC) is omitted from the CRUK statistics shown here. It is a very common condition but is virtually always curable. Registration is known to be incomplete and up to 100,000 cases might be diagnosed each year in the UK.

Cancer prevention

Though the actual cause of an individual's specific cancer is often not known, many common forms of cancer have causative factors related to lifestyle, such as smoking, sunbathing, and poor diet. They are therefore potentially preventable, so prevention rather than attempts at cure may have a greater impact on rates of death from cancer.

Primary prevention

Strategies that reduce individuals' exposure to carcinogens include:
- **Medical** interventions such as immunization against human papilloma virus and hepatitis B, which reduces risk of cervical and liver cancer, respectively.
- Most strategies are **behavioural**, involving health education, lifestyle and environmental modification (e.g. dietary changes that reduce risk of stomach, bowel, and bladder cancers; smoking cessation programmes; and limiting exposure to the sun to reduce risk of skin cancer).

Secondary prevention

Cancer screening
- This involves testing a population of asymptomatic individuals and applying a specific screening process to detect either a cancer or a pre-cancerous condition that might benefit from early treatment.
- Early detection is believed to increase the outcomes of treatments.
- Common screening strategies include:
  - Breast cancer screening: mammography
  - Cervical cancer screening: pap smear and liquid based cytology
  - Colon cancer: faecal occult blood (FOB) test, sigmoidoscopy
  - Prostate cancer: prostate specific antigen (PSA) test
- In the future there may well be more targeted programmes of screening such as genetic screening.

Screening may intuitively seem the right approach to take with many cancers. This is reflected in pressure from the public and the media in many countries to increase screening uptake. However, screening can be potentially harmful for some individuals. It often produces a false-positive or a false-negative result. At best, screening benefits only a few people. For example, in breast cancer, approximately 500 people are screened to reduce mortality by one. The risks and benefits of population screening are highlighted in Table 25.1.

Early detection measures
Include individual and public education about common warning signs of cancer (See Table 25.2 for European code against cancer).

Effective prevention approaches

Evidence on cancer prevention suggests that it is most effective when political interventions are combined with individual interventions, e.g. banning of smoking in public places combined with well-resourced smoking cessation services. A combination of different approaches is required including:
- properly resourced health promotion and screening services
- skilled professionals who receive training
- using the media
- targeting services in schools and the community
- financial support for those living in poverty.

Table 25.1 Risks and benefits of screening for cancer

Costs involved (cons)	Benefits (pros)
Morbidity of screening test	Life years gained for those with curable cancers
Longer morbidity for those with unaltered prognosis	Avoidance of morbidity from radical treatment
Overtreatment of questionable abnormalities	Reassurance with negative results
False positives, giving unnecessary treatment	
False negatives, giving false reassurance	Reassurance that the disease is at an early stage
Screening expenses	Avoid cost of expensive treatment for advanced cancers
Cost of additional cases treated	
Cost of early treatment and extra follow up	
Diversion of resources from primary prevention and treatment.	Extra years of productivity

Adapted from Chamberlain J (1988) 'Screening for early detection of cancer', in Tiffany R and Pritchard AP (eds) *Oncology for nurses and health care professionals*, vol 1, pp. 155–73. Harper Row, New York.

Table 25.2 European code against cancer

Adopting a healthier lifestyle

Do not smoke; if you smoke, stop doing so. If you fail to stop, do not smoke in the presence of non-smokers.

Avoid obesity.

Undertake some brisk, physical activity every day.

Increase your daily intake and variety of vegetables and fruits to at least five servings daily. Limit your intake of foods containing fats from animal sources.

If you drink alcohol, moderate your consumption to two drinks per day if you are a man and one drink per day if you are a woman.

Avoid excessive sun exposure, particularly in children and adolescents.

Apply all regulations and follow all health and safety instructions that restrict exposure to substances that may cause cancer. Follow advice of national radiation protection offices.

Accessing public health programmes

Women over 25 years should participate in cervical screening programmes.

Women over 50 years of age should participate in breast screening.

Men and women from 50 years of age should participate in colorectal screening.

Men and women should participate in vaccination programmes against Hepatitis B virus infection.

Adapted from the *European code against cancer and scientific justification*, version 3 (2003). http://www.cancercode.org/code.htm

Diagnosis

Early diagnosis offers the best opportunity for cure or extended survival for many types of cancer. Therefore, fast and accurate diagnosis is essential to ensure the most effective and appropriate approach to managing cancer. Unfortunately no single test is specific and sensitive enough to determine the exact diagnosis of an individual cancer. Therefore a range of tests, both invasive and noninvasive, must be carried out before an individual patient can have an accurate diagnosis. It is essential to find out:

- **type** of cancer and histology
- extent of spread (**stage**)
- cellular structure and behaviour of cancer cells (**grade**).

This allows for prognostic information and planning of appropriate treatment.

Signs and symptoms

Obtaining a detailed patient history and identifying signs and symptoms assists in narrowing down possible diagnosis and guides appropriate use of more invasive tests. 🔲 Cancer signs— 'Caution' p.835. Patients with these signs and symptoms should be referred urgently to cancer specialists. Nurses should help patients articulate and interpret their problems and concerns relating to these symptoms.

Laboratory studies

- FBC and ESR
- Biochemical profile: U&E, LFTs, and bone profile (calcium, phosphate, and ALP)
- FOB, if gastrointestinal cancer is suspected

🔲 Chapter 39, Common laboratory tests and their interpretation, p.1168.

Tumour markers

Certain tumours (e.g. ovarian, breast, colorectal, and prostate) produce hormones, enzymes, or antigens (**tumour markers**). They can be useful in assessing response to treatment. 🔲 Chapter 39, Tumour markers, p.1183.

Surgical/specialist viewing

Obtaining an accurate tissue sample (a biopsy) is essential in establishing cancer diagnosis.

- Core or fine needle aspirate (breast/thyroid)
- Laparoscopy (ovarian, gastrointestinal)
- Endoscopy (lung, gastrointestinal)
- Bone marrow aspirate (haematological cancers)

Radiological imaging

Radiological imaging is used to provide a detailed understanding of primary tumours, their likely routes of spread, and their response to treatment. X-rays, CT scans, and MRI scans are commonly used for many cancers. Positron Emission Tomography (PET) is being introduced into UK practice. It offers improved accuracy in staging several cancers, including non-small cell lung, upper GI, lymphomas, and recurrent bowel cancer.

Staging

The TNM (Tumour, Node, Metastases) system is the most commonly used method of determining the extent of cancer spread. It involves the following staging categories:

- T: size of primary tumour (T_{1-4})
- N: absence or presence of regional lymph nodes (N_{0-3})
- M: absence or presence of distant metastases (M_0 or M_1)

Information from each part is combined to determine the stage of the cancer. Most cancers are then staged from Stage 1–4. (Staging is not useful in some cancers, including primary CNS and haematological cancers.)

Grading

Determined by a pathologist and can be:

- Low-grade or grade 1 (similar to local tissue)
  - Well differentiated
  - Slow growth
  - Less likely to spread
  - Generally good outlook
- High-grade or grade 4 tumours
  - Contain many abnormal cells
  - Poorly differentiated
  - Often spread early and grow rapidly
  - May respond well to chemotherapy
  - Aggressive nature tends towards a poor overall prognosis

Cancer signs—'Caution'

The American Cancer Society advises the use of the following mnemonic to assess cancer signs:

Change in bowel or bladder habits
A sore that doesn't heal
Unusual bleeding or discharge
Thickening or lump in the breast or elsewhere
Indigestion or difficulty in swallowing
Obvious change in a wart or mole
Nagging cough or hoarseness

NB: Any progressive symptom that does not disappear after 2–4 weeks should be investigated.

Supporting the patient through diagnosis

For many people, a cancer diagnosis initiates a series of confusing events that unfold in an unfamiliar hospital environment and in unfamiliar medical language. Many people do not fully comprehend the implications of a life-threatening illness at the time of diagnosis. Initial reactions may include shock, numbness, and disbelief. It is normal for people to have difficulty absorbing bad news and information associated with diagnosis. Diagnosis can cause high levels of anxiety.

Diagnosis can be a point for potential delays, which can impact on overall survival. Therefore, the role of the nurse is to help individuals begin making sense of the seriousness of the situation so that the most effective treatments can be initiated. Nurses should also help the individual understand the implications for their hopes and aspirations.

Many members of the health care team will be involved. Effective coordination of the multidisciplinary team is essential to ensure an efficient and well-supported patient journey through this difficult time. Patient pathways have been designed for many cancers to reduce diagnostic and treatment delay. Nurses are heavily involved in this process, supporting the patient with information, explaining tests, and offering emotional support. Clinical nurse specialists may coordinate the multidisciplinary team and evaluate the patient pathway. Some specialist nurses may also be involved in actual diagnostic tests such as digital rectal examination and cystoscopy, or in telling patients their actual diagnosis.

Nursing assessment

Routine health assessment may reveal key signs and symptoms that lead to a diagnosis of cancer (📖 Cancer prevention, p.832 and 📖 Chapter 5, Factors that determine health promotion, p.88). The nurse should be alert to this and also to the possible effects of a diagnosis of cancer on the patient.

Assessment in cancer care

Assessment can be particularly complex in cancer care due to a patient's varied needs stemming from the disease itself, side effects of treatments, and reactions to the illness by relatives and others. Effective assessment focuses on the patient and family's needs. The assessment should be interactive and provide an information exchange between the nurse and patient. It is an opportunity for both to get to know each other and identify personal and health care priorities. A holistic assessment covers several aspects.

- Disease and symptoms
- Physical functioning
- Psychological well-being
- Cognitive function
- Spiritual well-being
- Social, occupational, and financial concerns

Assessment is an ongoing process and should occur regularly throughout the patient's journey. There are several key time points for conducting assessment:

- At diagnosis
- Prior to and during treatment
- At the end of treatment
- Upon recurrence of the illness
- As the patient enters the terminal phase of illness

Assessment tools

Many wards have a proforma for assessment that guides the questioning. A holistic assessment will cover the different dimensions of a patient's experience of illness, treatment, and life. Assessment tools are a means of ensuring consistency across assessments or across different team members. They also serve as a guide so that the nurse inquires about specific problems or symptoms. Examples of assessment tools used in cancer care include *Cancer Care Monitor* (screening and assessment tool for symptoms and quality of life, QOL, in cancer patients) and *Concerns Checklist* (aid to elicit primary concerns of people with cancer).

Impact of cancer

Cancer precipitates strong emotional reactions, such as fear, sorrow, shock, or secrecy. Many patients and their families find it difficult to use the word. Euphemisms such as 'growth', 'tumour', 'mass', or 'malignancy' are often used as substitutes.

It is essential that the nurse establishes good communication, sensitivity, and rapport with the patient and their family. The nurse should evaluate the patient and family's level of understanding of the cancer and find out how they normally cope with stressful or demanding situations. This gives the best indication of how they will cope with the demands of the cancer.

Nursing advice for patients with cancer

- Recognize that fear of having and facing a diagnosis or re-diagnosis of cancer is very understandable.
- Get the support you need—the multidisciplinary health care cancer team are there to help you. Engage and work with them.
- It is useful to have someone with you for support and help during the vulnerable times (e.g. confirmation of diagnosis, treatment options, and prognosis). You may find comparing what you and your 'supporter' pick up from the consultation may help you better understand the information.
- Tell someone if you are not satisfied with the service you are getting. If you find this difficult there are advocates available in many hospitals and services such as PALS (Patient Advisory Liaison Service) to support you.
- Let everyone know what your individual needs are and what you want. Keep everyone up to date with your progress, from your point of view. You should have access to a site-specific clinical nurse specialist who will act as your key worker and can support you from diagnosis onwards.
- Take charge of your situation and do not be persuaded into decisions that are against your will. Before you commit to a particular treatment, be sure you understand both its potential benefits and side effects.
- Take time to absorb and clarify information, and to make decisions.
- Try to prepare yourself, physically and psychologically, for treatments and care. Many hospitals offer a range of services that can assist with this, e.g. dietitians, counsellors, complementary therapists, and benefits officers.

Nursing care and communication

- Help prepare the patient and their family for the physical and psychological outcomes of diagnosis, treatment, and nursing care. Some patients will need counselling or group support to help them accept the shock and disruption caused by the diagnosis. Skilled psychological assessment may help identify patients most in need of this support. Choose the appropriate environment to elicit good interaction.

- Encourage the patient to talk, express their feelings, ask questions, and enter into a constructive dialogue with all members of the health care team. This takes time and involves complex communication and therapeutic skills. Find out how much the person wants to know. Share information on diagnosis, treatment. 📖 Chapter 3, Individualizing nursing care practice, pp.56–58.

- Demonstrate to the patient that you are interested in them as an individual and are willing to support them on their cancer journey. Patients should have access to a site-specific clinical nurse specialist who will act as a key worker from the point of diagnosis onwards.

- Effective information and support is key to empowerment for cancer patients. Provide information or advice in a supportive manner and make sure patients and their families understand the information they are given. Tell them where they or their family can get further details that they might need. There are some excellent national websites, such as Cancer Backup and Cancer Help. 📖 Further reading, p.853.

- Encourage the patient and their family to be involved in decision-making about their care and treatment. Decisions can be particularly difficult when curative treatment is no longer an option. It can be very important at these times to provide further support and to talk options through.

- Help the patient reflect on how they are responding to what is happening to them. Listen to their stories and encourage an optimal frame of mind.

- Encourage the use of complementary or alternative medicine to promote optimal health throughout their experience. These therapies encourage a mind–body approach and can help reduce anxiety, depression, stress, and grieving. Many hospitals now offer access to a range of complementary therapies. Ensure that patients are aware of the availability of such services and encourage them to discuss the use of any complementary and alternative therapies with their consultant or clinical nurse specialist.

- There is evidence for the use of counselling, cognitive therapy, problem-focused therapy, and psychoeducational programmes in patients with cancer. Other therapies that may be potentially useful include group work, listening to an 'expert' patient, art, music, drama, keeping a journal, dream therapy, relaxation methods, meditation, and visualization. Inform patients about the various therapies or services that are available and how to access them.

- Encourage the patient to be assertive which will help them make their own decisions and feel involved in their care.

Treatment

Surgery, radiotherapy, chemotherapy, and hormone therapy constitute the main forms of cancer treatment, though a range of other biological therapies are also increasingly being used. The goal may be to provide radical treatment and attempt to cure (i.e. *curative* treatment), or to make patients more comfortable by alleviating symptoms caused by the tumour (i.e. *palliative* treatment).

Nurses should encourage patients to take a careful and measured approach to their choice of treatment. Consulting a variety of sources and not rushing into decisions can be time well spent. However, patients may also be extremely anxious to get started on treatment as soon as possible, either because of fear about cancer continuing to grow or because of particular symptoms from the disease.

Combination therapy

Though the following treatments are described separately it is more common for several different treatment modalities to be used together, either sequentially (one after the other) or concurrently, as in the use of combined chemo-irradiation. This more 'aggressive' approach to treatment has improved survival rates for some cancers, but increases overall toxicity. 📖 Side effects of treatment, p.846.

Case example

A woman with breast cancer may have initial surgery to the breast and axilla; chemotherapy, to reduce the risk of distant relapse; radiotherapy to the breast to reduce local relapse; trastuzumab (an anti-cancer drug); and then several years of hormone therapy.

Surgery

- Aim is to remove the tumour and a margin of surrounding normal tissue to reduce the likelihood of any malignant cells remaining.
- Removal of all possible cancer from the body is vital, as some tumours secrete proteins that can cause further growth in other organs.
- Following surgery the patient may need further treatment such as radiotherapy, chemotherapy, hormone therapy, or a combination of these.

Radiotherapy

- Aim is to damage or destroy cancerous cells so they cannot mature and divide.
- Involves the use of high-energy ionizing radiation directed at cancerous cells.
- Many different types of radiation are available ranging from high energy external beam x-rays produced by a linear accelerator to internal radiation by radioactive needles or seeds.

Chemotherapy

- 'Systemic' cancer treatments that reach all parts of the body (i.e. not localized as with surgery or radiotherapy).

- A variety of anticancer drugs are available that work by disrupting cell division and replication.
- Rapidly dividing cancer tends to respond more effectively to chemotherapy due to its mechanism of action.
- Different chemotherapy drugs may be combined to increase the chance of killing as many cancer cells as possible within acceptable limits of toxicity.
- Most drugs are given by specialist nurses via IV drip. There is increasing use of oral chemotherapy.

Hormone therapy

- Some cancers are stimulated to grow by endogenous hormones, e.g. testosterone or oestrogen.
- Specific therapy is used to inhibit the growth of hormone-dependent cancers.
- Most commonly used in breast and prostate cancer treatment.

Biotherapies

Recent advances in understanding cancer biology have enabled the development of more effectively targeted cancer therapies. New targets include cell signaling pathways, metastatic spread, and cancer blood vessel development (angiogenesis). These drugs can be used alone or, more commonly, in conjunction with conventional therapies. The most common of these are:

- Monoclonal antibodies – These drugs recognize particular protein markers on the surface of some cancer cells and use a variety of mechanisms of action to prevent replication or destroy them. Several of these are now standard treatments in specific cancers, e.g. trastuzumab in breast cancer and rituximab in non-Hodgkin's lymphoma.
- Immunotherapy – Interferons and interleukins are used to stimulate antibody production and cell-mediated immunity to attack and destroy cancer cells. Bone marrow transplantation and stem cell transplantation can restore haematological and immunological function in some cancer patients.

Other biotherapies include cancer vaccines, gene therapy, and anti-angiogenesis drugs.

Other treatments

A range of other modalities are less commonly used to treat cancer including laser therapy, cryotherapy/cryosurgery, and ultrasound.

Cancer breakthroughs

Mention of new miracle cures and breakthroughs are rife in the media and patients will often search the internet for new and experimental treatment. This can lead to confusion, false hope, and anxiety for some patients and their families. Patients should be warned about this likelihood and should be encouraged to discuss any findings with their oncologist. Patients should also be made aware of current clinical trials that are open, where relevant. Several websites list the various open clinical trials both in the UK and elsewhere. 📖 Further reading, p.853.

Preparing the patient for treatment

It is essential that patients are fully informed about their proposed treatments and that they understand what is going to happen, the rationale for each treatment, the duration of treatment, and possible side effects and their management.

Surgery

Cancer surgery can be physically and psychologically mutilating. Patient's nutrition may also be poor and many cancer patients have major co-morbidities (e.g. cardiorespiratory limitation) that can increase the number of perioperative complications and reduce effective recovery and wound healing. This can delay other treatments, such as chemotherapy, therefore increasing anxieties. A good preoperative assessment determines whether an individual will be able to tolerate surgery and its side effects, both physically and psychosocially. Any treatment plan must be discussed with the patient and family prior to consent being sought for the surgery.

- Refer to dietitian preoperatively for full nutritional assessment. Try to maximize calorie intake preoperatively.
- Assess cardiac and pulmonary function; administer oxygen as required.
- Promote preoperative comfort measures such as pain control and relief of nausea. Provide detailed preoperative pain assessment and education.
- Prepare patient for any complications, such as stomas.

Preparing patients for radiotherapy

Undertaking a course of radiotherapy can be an emotionally and physically demanding time for patients and their families. Radiotherapy may last several weeks plus the initial planning time, and it may require daily travel, often over a long distance.

- Recognize that radiotherapy may occur after or alongside other treatments, adding to the potential for debilitating side effects. Potential side effects will vary depending on the site of treatment, stage of disease, and general health of the patient (See Table 25.3).
- Clarify the individual's beliefs and concerns about radiotherapy treatment during the initial assessment. Many patients have misunderstandings about the nature of the treatment with concerns of getting other cancers or being a danger to others, e.g. 'Will I be radioactive?'

Preparing patients for chemotherapy

The impact of chemotherapy treatment varies greatly from regimen to regimen.

- Anticipate common side effects including nausea, hair loss, fatigue, and risk of infection. The severity and frequency of these varies greatly from regimen to regimen.
- Provide accurate and supportive information to prepare patients and to dispel any myths or inaccurate preconceptions.
- Most chemotherapy is given intravenously, therefore careful assessment of venous access is required. Some patients (*in fact a minority*) require central venous access such as Hickman lines or peripheral inserted central catheters.

Side effects of treatment

Undergoing cancer treatment can be an emotionally and physically demanding time for patients and their families. Treatments may last several months, may require regular travel to and from hospital, and may cause multiple debilitating side effects. After treatment is completed patients may continue to experience acute and long-term side effects.

Side effects of surgery

Any surgery can be debilitating. Cancer surgery is often mutilating, causing long-term body image alteration such as the loss of a breast, formation of a stoma, or facial disfigurement (Chapter 24, Nursing patients with body image problems, p.813). This can lead to a range of psychosocial difficulties from sexual problems to social withdrawal. The greater the postoperative changes the greater the difficulties are likely to be.

Side effects of radiotherapy

- Common side effects of radiotherapy are summarized in Table 25.3.
- Side effects are generally localized to the area being treated.
- Moist desquamation may occur, particularly in skin folds.
- Most patients do not have skin soreness when an internal tumour site is treated, but may have skin soreness when a surface site such as the breast, neck, or axilla is treated.
- The main systemic side effect of radiotherapy is fatigue.
- There are two phases of radiation reaction.
  - **Acute reactions** occur during treatment, last for a few weeks afterwards, and resolve completely.
  - **Late reactions** arise no sooner than 6–9 months after treatment and there is an ongoing risk year by year e.g. radiation enteritis, dry mouth, vaginal fibrosis.
  - The two phases of radiation reaction are distinct. Only rarely do consequential reactions occur when a severe acute reaction fails to heal (e.g. a radionecrotic ulcer).
- Management of radiotherapy side effects often involves many health care professionals including an oncologist and their medical team, oncology nurses, therapeutic radiographers, dietitians, speech and language therapists, physiotherapists, psychologists, and community health care professionals.

Side effects of chemotherapy

- Common side effects of chemotherapy are summarized in Table 25.4.
- Many side effects are related to the impact chemotherapy has on rapidly dividing cells, e.g. gut, skin, bone marrow, and reproductive system.
- Some side effects are specific to the particular chemical make up of the drug and vary from regimen to regimen.

Side effects of hormonal therapy

- Menopausal symptoms, e.g. hot flushes, night sweats, fatigue, depression, vaginal dryness, body image problems, osteoporosis
- Impotence and decreased libido
- Nausea and vomiting

Table 25.3 Side effects of radiotherapy

Area being treated	Acute side effects	Long-term side effects
Brain/CNS (including spinal cord)	Raised ICP, headache, nausea, blurred vision, tiredness	Neurological defects including CNS necrosis, cognitive dysfunction, neuroendocrine abnormalities, spinal cord myelopathy if excess dose given (in practice great care is taken to avoid this)
Head and neck	Dysphagia, mucositis, skin reaction, xerostomia, fungal infection, weight loss	Dysphagia, xerostomia, in high doses mandibular bone necrosis
Breast	Skin reaction, tiredness	Skin pigment changes (rare with modern linear accelerators), lymphoedema, bone necrosis (ribs), lung fibrosis, psychosocial problems. If high doses are given to the axilla then brachial plexopathy may be seen
Thorax	Breathlessness, cough, haemoptysia, dysphagia, weight loss, tiredness	Pericardial constriction, lung fibrosis, pneumonitis
GI tract (including oesophagus, small and large bowel)	Nausea, vomiting, colicky pain, diarrhoea, weight loss, tiredness	Oesophagus: dysphagia, Small bowel: malabsorption syndromes, hypermotility, diarrhoea, fistulas, perforation, ischaemia, bleeding Large bowel: colitis, stricture, bowel obstruction, ulceration, fistulas, perforation, ischaemia, tenesmus, bleeding
Pelvis (including bladder/prostate, gynaecological)	Dysuria, difficulty in micturition, frequency, nocturia and urgency, diarrhoea, tiredness	Bleeding, vaginal stenosis and vaginal dryness, fibrosis, chronic cystitis, urinary incontinence, erectile dysfunction, urethral stricture, large bowel complications (see above)

Table 25.4 Short to medium side effects and complications of chemotherapy

Short to medium side effects

Gastro-intestinal	**Skin and nail**
Nausea & vomiting (can be delayed with some drugs e.g. cisplatin)	Alopecia
Mucositis	Plantar-palmar erythrodysaesthesis (hand/foot syndrome)
Constipation	Rash, Erythema
Diarrhoea	Hyperpigmentation
Anorexia	Extravasation
Taste changes	Ridging of nails
Metallic taste (e.g. cyclophosphamide)	Nail loss, e.g.docetaxel
Bone marrow	**General side effects**
Myelosuppression, neutropenia, thrombocytopenia and anaemia.	Fatigue
	Flu-like symptoms
Is prolonged and delayed with some drugs e.g. carmustine, lomustine, melphalan, mitomycin C.	Fluid retention & oedema, e.g. docetaxel
Reproductive system	**Cardiac**
Amenorrhea/early menopause	Tachycardia and other rhythm disturbances, hypertension, cardiomyopathy (mainly anthracyclines, trastuzumab)
Infertility (particularly alkylating agents)	
Neurological	**Renal and bladder**
Peripheral neuropathy	Hyperuricaemia
Autonomic neuropathy	Coloured urine (doxorubicin, epirubicin, mitoxantrone)
Cranial nerve neuropathy	
Ocular nerve toxicities	Haemorrhagic cystitis (cyclophosphamide, ifosfamide)
Pulmonary	**Neurological**
Pulmonary toxicity (e.g. pulmonary fibrosis with bleomycin)	Neurotoxicity, e.g. oxaliplatin, vinca alkaloids
	Ototoxicity (tinnitus and hearing loss with cisplatin)
	Cognitive dysfunction, e.g. lack of concentration, memory lapses

📖 Management of common side-effects see page 850. For a more detailed exploration of side-effect management see: Tadman M and Roberts D (2007) *Oxford Handbook of Cancer Nursing*, Oxford, OUP

Management of common side effects

(Table 25.5)

Table 25.5 Management of common treatment side effects

Common side effects	Narrative
Oral mucositis	Sore mouth is a common complication of cancer chemotherapy and head and neck radiotherapy. Good dental assessment is important pretreatment. Scrupulous mouth care may help to prevent this complication (mouth rinses, teeth brushed with soft brush). Poor oral hygiene can be a focus of blood-borne infection.
Bone marrow suppression/risk of infection	Nearly all cytotoxic drugs cause bone marrow suppression. Use of steroids, poor nutrition, and damage to mucosa all increase the risk of infection. The danger is rapidly developing infection leading to life-threatening sepsis/septic shock. Patients and family require education about this danger and the signs and symptoms of infection. They also need 24/7 emergency contact numbers. If fever occurs, immediate treatment with IV antibiotics may be required.
Alopecia	Reversible hair loss varies between individual drugs and patients. There is no pharmacological method to prevent this. However, in some regimens scalp hypothermia (cooling) can be effective.
Nausea and vomiting	About 70% of patients having cancer chemotherapy will have some level of nausea or vomiting. This may be anticipatory (prior to treatment), acute (first 24 hours post-treatment) and/or delayed (longer than 24 hours post-treatment). Susceptibility to nausea and vomiting can increase with increased exposure to chemotherapy. Prevention is the key. Accurate assessment of the regimen (classified as mildly, moderately or highly emetogenic), the patient (history of motion sickness, pregnancy sickness, anxiety, young age can all increase risk), and other causes of sickness (tumour site, other drugs).
a) Anti-emetic use	Combined use of 5HT3 antagonists, domperidone/metoclopramide, and dexamethasone is the gold standard. Anti-anxiolytics can help with anticipatory nausea.
b) Non-pharmacological management	Some suggest 'patients find' that muscle relaxation techniques, guided imagery, or acupressure bands can help prevent nausea and vomiting.
Reproductive function	Most cytotoxic drugs are teratogenic. Alkylating agents carry the risk of causing male sterility. Discussion is required about infertility, early menopause and possible solutions such as sperm banking.

Table 25.5 Management of common treatment side effects *(continued)*

Common side effects	Narrative
Radiotherapy skin damage	Radiotherapy prevents cell division within the basal layer, delaying re-population. Reactions can range from erythema (reddening in treated area) to moist desquamation (skin peeling, weeping with exudate). Common areas for acute skin reactions are breast, head and neck and groin.
	General advice: Gentle washing (no perfumed products), avoid friction, avoid exposure to sun, application of aqueous cream.
	Hydrogel, hydrocolloid or alginate dressings can be used for moist desquamation.
Fatigue	One of the most common side effects of cancer treatment and can be the most distressing. Can severely restrict activities, lead to isolation and depression, and impact relationships. Causes include all major treatments, the disease process, and impact of diagnosis.
	There is no easy solution. Detailed assessment can identify treatable causes, such as anaemia or depression. Non-pharmacological management includes advice on exercise, energy conservation, and psychosocial interventions. Useful drugs include low dose steroids.
Altered bowel function	Many cytotoxic drugs and abdominal/pelvic radiotherapy can cause altered bowel function. Diarrhoea: Management includes prevention with anti-motility drugs (loperamide, codeine), antispasmodics and antibacterials if infective cause. Advise patients about diet, importance of fluid replacement, skin care, use of barrier creams.
	Constipation: many drugs (cytotoxics, opioids, anti-emetics), abdominal disease, fatigue, and lack of mobility can all cause constipation.
	Management requires effective assessment, dietary advice, use of appropriate laxatives, management of pain, mobility and other exacerbating causes.
Nutritional disorders	Cancer and its treatments can have a major nutritional impact. Nausea, sore mouth, dysphagia, diarrhoea, intestinal malabsorption, pain, and fatigue can all contribute to causing malnutrition.
	Management includes nutritional screening, management of preventable causes, dietary advice and use of supplements—oral, enteral and parenteral.

Nursing advice and help for carers

One of the most important ways to help patients with cancer is to provide good support and advice for those who care for them. Caring for a person with cancer is a stressful and harrowing experience. Reactions to the diagnosis are similar to those of the patient: shock, grief, and a feeling of disbelief. A carer could be a spouse, lifelong partner, another family member, close friend, or neighbour.

Although the patient may receive enough support, the carer may not. They can become isolated and ignored as attention is directed to helping the patient. The carer may experience feelings of frustration in not knowing what is going on. They may feel that their world and lifestyle is about to change dramatically in some way. This may lead to anxiety and fear of the unknown.

The intensity of the feelings of the carer will depend on the nature and closeness of the relationship with the patient, the prognosis, and their own hopes and aspirations for the future. Partners, family members, and friends may have to take on significant amounts of caring work.

Roles within the family may have to be re-allocated, either because the person with cancer can no longer continue in their role as parent or carer or they need additional care from others. This will happen whether or not family members are prepared, willing, or able to do this.

In certain circumstances a carer may be plunged into grief and feel too emotionally involved to keep up the previous relationship. This may lead to withdrawal from the patient or 'distancing'. Carers may feel trapped or overwhelmed by the sense of responsibility that the diagnosis of cancer brings.

The nurse may perceive a variety of emotional and psychological reactions in the carer. It is important not to be judgemental, but to support the carer in trying to adjust to the changes caused by the diagnosis.

- Encourage the carer to talk about their feelings and anxieties. Offer them the opportunity of a trained counsellor or support group if available.
- Advise and support carers in adjusting to the changes in their role. Explain that they can still remain in a close relationship with the patient, even if they withdraw from some elements of care. Many carers will feel guilty 'handing over' some aspects of care to professionals.
- Help the carer find other ways in which they can support patients and continue to involve them in decisions as much as they wish. A good carer can still be part of the overall support team, even if the nature of their relationship with the patient has changed.

Further information

Carers' National Association: Tel. 0345 573369 (Mon.–Fri.); 029 20880176 (Cardiff)
Crossroads—Caring for Carers: Tel. 08454500350; www.crossroads.org.uk

Nursing tips for patient's carers

- Be there for the patient during the vulnerable times, e.g. while waiting for test results, critical decisions about treatment, information relating to prognosis, and outcomes.
- Try to give emotional support, such as love, encouragement, hope, and ideas, and provide a sense of humour.
- Listen to the patient. Encourage them to express their feelings and emotions.
- Be part of and share their cancer journey.
- Help them with everyday tasks and activities, such as writing letters, arranging finances, making wills, and managing their home and personal affairs.
- Help the patient clarify and understand medical information and knowledge about their illness.
- Act as a link and information provider to others concerned about the well-being of the patient.
- Be willing, if necessary, to help with simple or more complex nursing care for the patient if appropriate.
- Accompany the patient on visits, holidays, and social events.
- Acknowledge own needs and seek appropriate support and guidance.

Further information

Grundy M (2006). *Nursing in haematological oncology*, 2nd edn. Baillière Tindall, Edinburgh.

Kearney N and Richardson A (2005). *Nursing patients with cancer: principles and practice*. Elsevier Churchill Livingstone, Edinburgh.

Souhami, RL and Tobias JS (2005). *Cancer and its management*, 5th edn. Blackwell, Oxford.

Tadman M and Roberts R (2007). *Oxford handbook of cancer nursing*. Oxford University Press, Oxford.

Weinberg R (1998). *One renegade cell: quests for the origin of cancer*. Weidenfield & Nicholson, London.

Cancer Backup: www.cancerbackup.org.uk

Cancer Help: www.cancerhelp.org.uk/

Cancer research UK: http://www.cancerresearchuk.org/

Macmillan Cancer Relief: www.macmillan.org.uk; information@macmillan.org.uk

Tel. 0845 6016161; concern line 0808 808 2020

Marie Curie Cancer Care: www.mariecurie.org.uk

National cancer Institute: www.cancer.gov/

Common drugs used in cancer care

Common drugs used in cancer care are listed in Table 25.6. **All drug doses listed in this table are adult doses and not children's doses**. This table is only to be used as a guide and the current BNF should be consulted for further advice. Nurses should involve themselves only in the administration of medications which fall within their sphere of competence.

Table 25.6 Common drugs used in cancer care and common side effects

All cytotoxic drugs may cause life-threatening toxicity and most are teratogenic. Because of the complexity of dose regimens in cancer treatment, many of which vary in combination with other cytotoxic agents, dose statements have been omitted from this section. Many doses are based on body surface area together with haematological and renal function reports. In all cases refer to specialist literature.

Common side effects for virtually all cytotoxics	Narrative
Extravasation of IV drugs	This follows leakage of drugs or IV fluids from veins or inadvertent administration into the subcutaneous or subdermal tissue. Cytotoxic drugs commonly cause extravasation injury which must be dealt with **promptly**. See BNF for prevention and treatment of extravasation.
Oral mucositis	Sore mouth is a common complication of cancer chemotherapy and is most often associated with fluorouracil, methotrexate, and anthracyclines. Good mouth care helps prevent this complication (mouth rinse, teeth brushed with soft brush) and sometimes sucking on ice cubes for short duration infusions is helpful. Poor oral hygiene can be a focus of blood-borne infection.
Hyperuricaemia	Treatment of non-Hodgkin's lymphoma and leukaemia can lead to this condition which may result in uric acid crystal formation in the urinary tract and possible renal dysfunction. To minimize this, allopurinol should be started 24 hours before treatment begins and patients should be adequately hydrated.
Bone marrow suppression	All cytotoxics cause this except vincristine and bleomycin; it commonly occurs 7–10 days after treatment (may be delayed in certain drugs, e.g. carmustine, lomustine and melphalan). Fever can occur in neutropenic patients and treatment with antibiotics (often quinolones 📖 Table 20.1 Common drugs used for infectious diseases: Quinolones, p.730) or bone marrow growth factors is required.
Alopecia	Reversible hair loss varies between individual drugs and patients. There is no pharmacological method to prevent this.

Table 25.6 Common drugs used for cancer care *(continued)*

Common side effects for virtually all cytotoxics	Narrative	
Reproductive function	Most cytotoxic drugs are teratogenic. Alkylating agents carry the risk of causing male sterility.	
Thromboembolism	Chemotherapy increases a patient's risk of thromboembolism.	
Nausea and vomiting	This is fairly common in cancer chemotherapy (see local hospital anti-emetic protocol) and may be acute (use deleted since granisetron is a serotonin antagonist and this class is referred to already to be given +/− dexamethasone, domperidone or metoclopramide, or a serotonin antagonist (see below) +/− other agents, e.g. dexamethasone, lorazepam); delayed (dexamethasone +/− metoclopramide or prochlorperazine); or anticipatory (add lorazepam to anti-emetic treatment). Susceptibility to nausea/vomiting can increase with increased exposure to chemotherapy. See *Oxford Handbook of Palliative Care*, Chapter 6B for more details.	
	Mildly emetogenic drugs	Fluorouracil, etoposide, methotrexate (less than 100 mg/m²), the vinca alkaloids
	Moderately emetogenic drugs	Doxorubicin, immediate and low dose of cyclophosphamide, mitoxantrone, and high doses of methotrexate (0.1–1.2 g/m²)
	Highly emetogenic drugs	Cisplatin, dacarbazine, and high doses of cyclophosphamide

Cytotoxics	Dose	Common side effects
Anastrozole	1 mg daily	Hot flushes, vaginal dryness, vaginal bleeding, hair thinning, anorexia, nausea, vomiting, diarrhoea, headache, arthralgia, bone fractures, rash (including Stevens-Johnson syndrome), asthenia, drowsiness, slight increases in total cholesterol
Tamoxifen	Breast cancer – 20 mg daily	Hot flushes, vaginal bleeding, vaginal discharge, suppression of menstruation in some premenopausal women, pruritus vulvae; increased risk of thromboembolism; many more side effects (See BNF)

Table 25.6 Common drugs used for cancer care *(continued)*

	Dose	Common side effects
Goserelin	Subcutaneously into anterior abdominal wall; 3.6 mg every 28 days or 10.8 mg every 12 weeks	Hot flushes, sweating, sexual dysfunction, gynaecomastia, transient changes in blood pressure, signs and symptoms of prostate cancer may worsen initially, paraesthesia
Bicalutamide	50 mg daily (in gonadorelin therapy start 3 days beforehand)	Gastrointestinal disturbances, asthenia, gynaecomastia, breast tenderness, hot flushes, pruritus, dry skin, alopecia, hirsutism, decreased libido, impotence, weight gain
Alkylating agents	**Common side effects (many of the above are in addition to those below)**	
Cyclophosphamide	Haemorrhagic cystitis is rare (more likely with high doses) but potentially very serious. (Ifosfamide is related to cyclophosphamide and may be given instead to reduce urothelial toxicity. Alternatively, increase fluid intake if appropriate for 24–48 hours before cyclophosphamide. In high-risk patients, consider mesna as a prophylactic measure.)	
Chlorambucil	Side effects apart from bone marrow suppression (as above) are rare but rash may occur and if so treatment should be stopped and substituted with cyclophosphamide.	
Melphalan	Interstitial pneumonitis and life-threatening pulmonary fibrosis	
Cytotoxic antibiotics	**Common side effects (many of the above are in addition to those below)**	
Doxorubicin	Cumulative dose should be limited to 450 mg/m^2 to minimize the likelihood of symptomatic (and potentially fatal) heart failure. (Epirubicin is a related drug and cumulative dose should be limited to 0.9–1 g/m^2 for the same reasons)	
Bleomycin	Progressive pulmonary fibrosis at doses greater than 300,000 units or in the elderly is the main problem with this drug. Little bone marrow toxicity is caused but dermatological toxicity is common. Hypersensitivity reactions (fever, chills) commonly occur a few hours after the drug has been given and may be prevented by simultaneous administration of a corticosteroid, e.g. hydrocortisone. Anaesthetists should be warned if a patient requiring general anaesthesia has received a cumulative dose over 100,000 units.	

Table 25.6 Common drugs used for cancer care *(continued)*

	Dose	Common side effects
Mitoxantrone		Myelosupression and dose related cardiotoxicity can occur.
Antimetabolites		**Common side effects (many of the above are in addition to those below)**
Methotrexate		Folinic acid can be given to prevent methotrexate induced mucositis or myelosuppression (📖 Common drugs used for haematological disorders, p.600).
Fludarabine		Generally well tolerated but does cause myelosuppression which may be cumulative and immunosuppression. Increased risk of Pneumocystis infection for which prophylactic co-trimoxazole may be given.
Fluorouracil		Toxicity is unusual but may include myelosuppression and mucositis.
Vinca alkaloids and etoposide		**Common side effects (many of the above are in addition to those below)**
Vincristine		Neurotoxicity and myelosuppression are dose limiting side effects of all vinca alkaloids. Neurotoxocity occurs less often with vinblastine, vindesine, and vinorelbine and symptoms include paraesthesia, loss of deep tendon reflexes, constipation, and abdominal pain.
Etoposide		Alopecia, myelosuppression, nausea, and vomiting
Platinum compounds		**Common side effects (many of the above are in addition to those below)**
Cisplatin		Requires intensive IV hydration to reduce toxicity which includes nephrotoxicity, ototoxicity, peripheral neuropathy, and hypomagnesaemia. Also causes myelosuppression, severe nausea, and vomiting.
Carboplatin		Better tolerated than cisplatin in all side effects above other than myelosuppression where cisplatin is less myelosuppressive.
Oxaliplatin		Neurotoxic effects for this drug are dose limiting. Other side effects are myelosuppression, gastrointestinal disturbances, and ototoxicity. Monitor renal function.
Taxanes		**Common side effects (many of the above are in addition to those below)**
Paclitaxel		Bradycardia and asymptomatic hypotension are more common. Hypersensitivity reactions may occur. Other side effects include myelosuppression, peripheral neuropathy, cardiac conductive defects, alopecia, muscle pain, nausea, and vomiting.

Table 25.6 Common drugs used for cancer care *(continued)*

Taxanes	Common side effects (many of the above are in addition to those below)
Docetaxel	Side effects are similar to paclitaxel but include persistent fluid retention (commonly as leg oedema which worsens during treatment). Hypersensitivity reactions may also occur and dexamethasone by mouth is recommended to reduce this and fluid retention.

Other agents commonly used include hormone antagonists and anti-emetics (see below) plus antifungals (📖 Table 20.1 Common drugs used for infectious diseases, p.730).

Hormone antagonists	Dose	Common side effects
Anastrozole	1 mg daily	Hot flushes, vaginal dryness, vaginal bleeding, hair thinning, anorexia, nausea, vomiting, diarrhoea, headache, arthralgia, bone fractures, rash (including Stevens-Johnson syndrome), asthenia, drowsiness, slight increases in total cholesterol
Tamoxifen	Breast cancer – 20 mg daily	Hot flushes, vaginal bleeding, vaginal discharge, suppression of menstruation in some premenopausal women, pruritus vulvae; increased risk of thromboembolism; many more side effects (See BNF)
Goserelin	Subcutaneously into anterior abdominal wall; 3.6 mg every 28 days or 10.8 mg every 12 weeks	Hot flushes, sweating, sexual dysfunction, gynaecomastia, transient changes in blood pressure, signs and symptoms of prostate cancer may worsen initially, paraesthesia
Bicalutamide	50 mg daily (in gonadorelin therapy start 3 days beforehand)	Gastrointestinal disturbances, asthenia, gynaecomastia, breast tenderness, hot flushes, pruritus, dry skin, alopecia, hirsutism, decreased libido, impotence, weight gain

Table 25.6 Common drugs used for cancer care *(continued)*

Anti-emetics	Dose	Common side effects
📖 Table 8.4 Common drugs used for gastrointestinal disorders, p.262.		
Serotonin (5HT3) antagonists	e.g. ondansetron – moderately emetogenic chemotherapy or radiotherapy: orally 8 mg 1–2 hours before treatment, then 8 mg every 12 hours for up to 5 days (for rectal administration give 16 mg and follow same schedule) For severely emetogenic chemotherapy see BNF	Constipation, headache, sensation of warmth or flushing, hiccups, and other side effects (See BNF)

Nursing patients with palliative care needs

Principles of palliative care

Palliative care, as defined by the World Health Organization, is an approach that improves the quality of life of patients and their families facing problems associated with life-threatening illness. The aim of palliative care is to prevent and relieve suffering by controlling the patient's symptoms. This is done through means of early identification of the patient's needs, impeccable assessment, and treatment of pain and other problems (e.g. physical, psychosocial, and spiritual). The focus of palliative care is on symptom management, and acute medical interventions are used only where appropriate. Palliative care also aims to support the patient and the family throughout the illness and the family after death.

Palliative care is a system of intensive care that requires careful assessment and detailed monitoring of the patient's condition. Care of the whole patient is important, and many holistic and complementary therapies and treatments may be used.

Characteristic principles of palliative care[1]

- Provides relief from pain and other distressing symptoms.
- Affirms life and regards dying as a normal process.
- Intends neither to hasten nor postpone death.
- Integrates the psychological and spiritual aspects of patient care.
- Provides a support system to help patients live as actively as possible until death.
- Provides a support system to help the family cope during the patient's illness and in their own bereavement.
- Uses a team approach to address the needs of patients and their families, including bereavement counselling.
- Enhances quality of life and may also positively influence the course of illness.
- Is applicable early in the course of illness in conjunction with other therapies that are intended to prolong life (e.g. chemotherapy or radiation therapy) and includes those investigations needed to better understand and manage distressing clinical outcomes.

Palliative care is intended neither to hasten nor postpone death. However, it involves ethical decision making such as withdrawing or withholding treatments, resuscitation, and truth telling.

Further information

1 World Health Organization (2006). *Definition of palliative care*. www.who.int/cancer/palliative/definition.

Hospice care

The hospice movement dates back to the 4th century and relates to institutions that cared for Christian pilgrims, the destitute, the sick, and the dying. More recently, Dame Cicely Saunders (a nurse who later became a physician) pioneered the hospice movement by founding St Christopher's Hospice outside London in 1967. Although hospice care started in the setting of a dedicated building, it now has developed day-care centres and home-care as an integral part of its service. Dame Cicely always viewed hospice care more as a philosophy of symptom control that could be incorporated into different settings and with diseases other than cancer.

Hospice care is well recognized as best practice for end-of-life care. Indeed, the hospice-care philosophy is now being transferred out of the traditional hospice environment into other areas of care. Palliative care, which is based on the hospice model, is carried out in other care settings such as nursing homes and patient's homes.

Palliative care nurses work with hospital and community nurses, forming a multidisciplinary team comprising physicians, therapists, chaplains, social workers, and volunteers. These nurses often have more time to give support and care to patients and their families and provide specialist advice on all aspects of health and social care. Individualized patient centred nursing care is the key. The patient and their family are involved and participate where appropriate. Support and care are provided 24 hours a day, 7 days a week, if necessary and where possible.

Commissioning of palliative care services remains inadequate and controversial in the UK, with about two-thirds of the cost nationally borne by the charitable sector. Much of that fundraising has been directed at end-stage cancer care. Other diseases, especially chronic neurological and cardiac conditions, are at present inadequately supported and, although some frameworks have been put in place governmentally, there are still many areas of chronic disease management that would benefit from more attention by the NHS and also specifically by palliative care services.

Patients often wish to die at home. In Britain two-thirds of those dying wish to end their days at home, but less than a quarter achieve this. The Charity 'Help the Aged' report that the needs of older people who are dying are often ignored. They are more likely than younger people to experience multiple medical conditions, repeated hospital admissions, lack of preventative planning, under-recognition of symptoms, and physical or mental impairment. Old people are often described as 'the disadvantaged dying'.

All patients who are dying at home should have access to their primary care team, i.e. GP and district nurse (DN), with support from specialist services such as palliative care and allied health care professionals. Those patients who prefer to have hospice care rather than home care will require the hospice physicians/team to liaise with the patient's GP in order to take over the patient's primary care from the GP, if the patient consents.

Palliative care interventions

Dying is the end stage of life and some key decisions must be made. Palliative care aims to help and provide:

- The opportunity to discuss and plan end-of-life care.
- The opportunity for the patient to 'put their house in order' or to organize their will, business, and family matters.
- Assurance that physical and mental suffering will be attended to.
- Assurance that comfort measures and nursing care will be individualized, linked to cultural needs, and will be of the highest possible quality.
- Assurance that preferences for withholding or withdrawing life-sustaining interventions will be honored, within acceptable ethical standards (e.g. an advanced directive and the Mental Capacity Act).
- Assurance that the professional palliative care team will not abandon the patient or their partner and will continue to support the family or carers.
- Assurance that peace and dignity will be a priority.
- The opportunity for the patient to pursue a variety of measures, both medical and complementary, to relax and explore meaning and spirituality at this stage in their lives.
- Assurance that the potential difficulties of their dying with all the associated physical and emotional factors will be minimized.
- Interventions to meet the patient's own specific wishes and goals.
- Information relating to cardiopulmonary resuscitation and to ensure that the patient has been consulted on, 'DNR' (Do Not Resuscitate) notices, and that this has been recorded in the patient's notes.
- Assurance that family and friends will be supported with accepting the patient's condition and any bereavement problems when the patient dies.
- Clear and consistent information for the patient and their family in order that they are given the opportunity to discuss end-of-life care, outstanding issues, and the place of death in a supported and sensitive way.

A key factor in providing palliative care is involving the dying person in the decision-making process. It requires that the patient has consented to their family being involved in their care and that the physician has discussed issues with the family. Ultimately the physician has the final say in treatment options and will act in the patient's best interest.

The Liverpool Care Pathway (LCP) for the dying patient

The LCP aims to translate best practice, i.e. hospice-based care, into a template of care to guide health care professionals with limited or infrequent experience of caring for dying patients. The three sections of the LCP include:

- initial assessment and care of the dying patient
- ongoing care of the dying patient
- care of the family and carers after death of the patient.

The multidisciplinary team must agree that the patient is in the dying phase. In this phase, the patient is no longer responding to their treatment and their condition is deteriorating at a rate that significantly means they are entering the final stages of their disease. The DNR order should be reviewed and signed accordingly. All members of the team should be aware of the outcome of this discussion, with the form filed clearly in the notes.

The LCP promotes discussion, integrates local and national guidelines into practice, is an educational tool, ensures patients die a dignified death, and ensures carers receive appropriate support (See Fig. 26.1).

COMFORT MEASURES	**Goal 1: Current medication assessed and non essentials discontinued** Yes ❑ No ❑ Appropriate oral drugs converted to subcutaneous route and syringe driver commenced if appropriate Inappropriate medication discontinued
	Goal 2: PRN subcutaneous medication written up for list below as per protocol (see blue sheets at back of ICP for guidance) Pain — Analgesia — Yes ❑ No ❑ Nausea and vomiting — Antiemetic — Yes ❑ No ❑ Agitation — Sedative — Yes ❑ No ❑ Respiratory tract secretions — Anticholinergic — Yes ❑ No ❑
	Goal 3: Discontinue inappropriate interventions Blood test — Yes ❑ No ❑ N/A ❑ Antibiotics — Yes ❑ No ❑ N/A ❑ IVs (fluids/medications) — Yes ❑ No ❑ N/A ❑ Not for cardiopulmonary resuscitation — Yes ❑ No ❑ (Please record below & complete appropriate associated documentation–policy/procedure)
	Goal 3a: Decisions to discontinue inappropriate nursing interventions taken Yes ❑ No ❑ Routine turning regime – reposition for comfort only – consider pressure relieving mattress–and appropriate assessments re skin integrity– Taking Vital Signs
	Goal 3b: Syringe driver set up within 4 h of Doctor's order Yes ❑ No ❑ N/A ❑
PSYCHOLOGICAL/ INSIGHT	**Goal 4: Ability to communicate in English assessed as adequate** a) Patient — Yes ❑ No ❑ Comatosed ❑ b) Family/other — Yes ❑ No ❑
	Goal 5: Insight into condition assessed Aware of diagnosis a) Patient — Yes ❑ No ❑ Comatosed ❑ b) Family/other — Yes ❑ No ❑ Recognition of dying c) Patient — Yes ❑ No ❑ Comatosed ❑ d) Family/other — Yes ❑ No ❑
RELIGIOUS/ SPIRITUAL SUPPORT	**Goal 6: a) Religious/spiritual needs assessed with patient** Yes ❑ No ❑ Comatosed ❑ **b) Religious/spiritual needs assessed with family/other** Yes ❑ No ❑ Patient/other may be anxious for self/others Consider support of chaplaincy team Religious tradition identified, if yes specify:............... Yes ❑ No ❑ N/A❑ Support of chaplaincy-team offered — Yes ❑ No ❑ In-house support Tel/Bleep No: .... Name .... Date/Time .... External support Tel/Bleep No: .... Name .... Date/Time .... Special needs now, at time of impending death, at death and after death identified:-
COMMUNICATION WITH FAMILY/OTHER	**Goal 7: Identify how family/other are to be informed of patient's impending death** — Yes ❑ No ❑ At any time ❑ Not at night-time ❑ Stay overnight at hospital ❑ Primary contact name .... Relationship to patient .... Tel no: .... Secondary contact .... Tel no:.........
	Goal 8: Family/other given hospital information on:- Yes ❑ No ❑ Concession car parking; accommodation; dining room facilities: payphones; washrooms and toilet facilities on the ward; visiting times. Any other relevant information
COMMUNICATION WITH PRIMARY HEALTHCARE TEAM	**Goal 9: GP Practice is aware of patient's condition** Yes ❑ No ❑ GP Practice to be contacted if unaware patient is dying
SUMMARY	**Goal 10: Plan of care explained & discussed with:-** a) Patient — Yes ❑ No ❑ Comatosed ❑ b) Family/other — Yes ❑ No ❑
	Goal 11: Family/other express understanding of care plan Yes ❑ No ❑ Family/other aware that LCP commenced and their concerns identified and documented

Fig. 26.1 Initial assessment and care of the dying patient. From: Ellershaw JE and Wilkinson S (2003). *Care of the dying: the Liverpool pathway to excellence.* Oxford University Press, Oxford. With kind permission of Dr Susie Wilkinson.

The importance of the family in palliative care

Working with the patient's family or equivalent group of close friends is an integral part of palliative care. Family members can be an invaluable support for the patient, bringing with them physical and psychological resources that the nurse can use to the advantage of the patient.

Family members may experience problems such as depression, sleep disorders, difficulty concentrating, hypertension, severe stress, and anxiety. Attention must be paid to the health needs of family members and the possible effects on the family's ability to function as a unit.

The nurse should be aware of the changing dynamics within the family group. Certain members of the family will play more dependent and more supportive lead roles. Such role changes may help others to cope with the difficulties they are having and enable them to adapt to the stresses and strains of the situation.

Family conflicts and arguments may increase with some members finding it difficult to communicate easily.

Family care interventions

Palliative care involves helping the family as well as helping the patient. Apart from the physical aspects of caring for someone, this is particularly relevant to a family's emotional and psychosocial needs. Where possible, ensure that the patient is involved in these discussions and that their permission has been sought to discuss medical and nursing care with family members.

- Arrange family conferences which may assist them in accepting what is happening.
- Teach family members various nursing techniques that they can use to care for the patient.
- Keep the family informed about the patient's journey, changes they are going through, treatments, symptom control, and up-to-date care plans.
- Give family members with an opportunity to talk about their needs.
- Give emotional support and encourage individuals to express their feelings. Listen carefully to what they are saying.
- Be alert to family members who are suppressing their feelings and who may have many unmet needs.
- Encourage family members to acknowledge that their health is important both as individuals and as a family unit.
- Determine whether those who have been caring for the patient at home are suffering from carer fatigue. If so, respite care might be appropriate in a long-term situation.

Symptom control: overview

Nurses support patients and family in maintaining control over their individual lives as much as is possible to ensure dignity and self-esteem. Control of symptoms is an essential element of this process.

Symptom interactions

Management of the dying patient may be complicated by the interaction of the symptoms of the disease. For example, treatments that produce relief from one symptom may introduce new problems, e.g. analgesics cause troubling constipation and nausea. Therefore it is important to be aware of the possibilities and complications that may occur.

Treatment of distress caused by fear of potential uncontrolled physical symptoms will significantly improve quality of life. Psychological, social, and existential or spiritual distress may increase the intensity of physical symptoms (e.g. depression and anxiety may increase the experience of pain; anxiety may increase dyspnoea). Pain, fatigue, nausea and vomiting, diarrhoea, constipation, and dyspnoea are among the most frequently occurring symptoms at the end of life. Delirium, depression, and anxiety are extremely common at the end of life and can be under-recognized, undiagnosed, and under-treated, leading to unnecessary distress for patients and families. Maintenance of comfort, both physical and emotional, is of the essence. 📖 Chapter 21, Nursing patients with intimate and sensitive care needs, p.736.

Terminal restlessness

This is a state of uneasiness, agitation, and fidgeting where the patient appears to be irritated by something. It is important to exclude any possible cause for this, such as pain or inadequate positioning, problems in the environment, or other physical factors affecting the patient's comfort.

Interventions
- Constantly review the nursing care and care plan to ascertain whether there are any identifiable causes that can be treated.
- Observe the patient's behaviour and try different techniques when handling, moving, or positioning the patient, if the methods in use appear to cause discomfort.
- Involve the patient's close family and friends to identify possible causes and factors that calm the patient.
- In some cases medications such as midazolam can help, which can be combined with morphine or diamorphine.

Symptom control: pain

Pain is an unpleasant sensory and emotional experience associated with actual or potential damage or described in terms of such damage. (For other definitions of pain terms see Table 26.1.) 📖 Chapter 23, Nursing patients with pain, p.788.

Pain is a source of great fear for many patients with advanced incurable disease and is one of the most prevalent symptoms across terminal illnesses. It may impair psychosocial functioning, cause enormous psychological distress (anxiety and depression), and limit the patient's capacity for relaxation, enjoyment, and spiritual thinking.

Unfortunately, misconceptions about dependency and addiction to opioids, the risks of oversedation, and regulatory problems associated with opioids have contributed to poor pain interventions and control for patients.

Assessment

Assessing the patient's pain accurately is the key to good pain control. Several tools are available for assessing pain. 📖 Chapter 23, Pain assessment tools, pp.796–98.

Causes

All causes of pain should be investigated.
- Pathological disturbances, e.g. due to cancer, tumors or related problems
  - Bone
  - Nerve compression/infiltration
  - Soft tissue infiltration
  - Visceral muscle spasm
  - Lymphoedema
  - Raised intracranial pressure
- Treatment-related conditions
  - Surgery
  - Postoperative scars/adhesions
  - Radiotherapy
  - Fibrosis
  - Chemotherapy

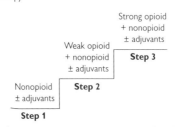

Fig. 26.2 The analgesic ladder. Reproduced with permission from *Cancer pain relief: with a guide to opioid availability*, 2nd edition, World Health Organization, 1996.

- Conditions such as low back pain, arthritis, heart disease, angina, and trauma
- Other associated factors
  - Constipation
  - Pressure ulcers
  - Bladder spasm
  - Stiff joints
  - Post hepatic neuralgia

Table 26.1 Definition of pain terms[1]

Allodynia	Pain caused by a stimulus which does not normally provoke pain
Analgesia	Absence of pain in response to stimulation which would normally be painful
Causalgia	A syndrome of sustained burning pain, allodynia and hyperpathia after a traumatic nerve lesion, often combined with vasomotor dysfunction and later trophic changes
Central pain	Pain associated with a lesion in the central nervous system (brain and spinal cord)
Dysaesthesia	An unpleasant abnormal sensation which can be either spontaneous or provoked
Hyperaesthesia	An increased sensitivity to stimulation
Hyperalgesia	An increased response to a stimulus that is normally painful
Hyperpathia	A painful syndrome characterized by increased reaction to a stimulus, especially a repetitive stimulus, as well as an increased threshold
Neuralgia	Pain in the distribution of a nerve
Neuropathy	A disturbance of function or pathological change in a nerve
Neuropathic pain	Pain which is transmitted by a damaged nervous system and is usually only partially opioid sensitive
Nociceptor	A receptor preferentially sensitive to a noxious stimulus or to a stimulus which would become noxious if prolonged
Nociceptive pain	Pain which is transmitted by an undamaged nervous system and is usually opioid responsive
Pain	An unpleasant sensory and emotional experience associated with actual or potential tissue damage or described in terms of such damage
Pain threshold	The least experience of pain which a subject can recognize
Pain tolerance level	The greatest level of pain which a subject is prepared to tolerate

1 Mersky H and Bogduk N (1994). *Classification of chronic pain*, 2nd edn. IASP Press, Seattle. Reproduced with permission.

Treatment

Analgesic ladders are frequently used in the control of chronic pain (See Fig. 26.2), particularly when the patient requires more than one analgesic for the control of their pain. Adjuvant drugs are commonly used in addition to a nonopioid or opioid drug (See Table 26.2).

Morphine

- Strong opioid of first choice for moderate-to-severe cancer pain.
- Patient is usually started on immediate release (i/r) morphine liquid or tablets. Later modified release (m/r) morphine.
- Morphine is titrated (i.e. slowly increased) according to the patient's needs, e.g. 5 to 10 to 15 to 20 to 30 to 40 to 60 to 80 to 100 mg.
- Very few patients will require more than 600 mg morphine daily.
- Morphine can be given via the rectal route (i.e. suppositories).
- Laxatives should be prescribed concurrently with morphine.
- An anti-emetic may be needed for nausea and vomiting, e.g. haloperidol.
- Diamorphine is commonly used as the injectable strong opioid in a syringe driver for subcutaneous infusion because of its high solubility.
- If needing to convert oral morphine to SC diamorphine, divide the total daily dose of oral morphine by 3 (e.g. 10 mg oral morphine every 4 hours = 60 mg oral morphine as a total daily dose is equivalent to 20 mg diamorphine SC given over 24 hours). See also the 'Palliative Care' section of the BNF for other examples of equivalence for doses of morphine (oral and IV) and diamorphine (IM and SC).

Alternatives to morphine are fentanyl and methadone.

Table 26.2 Examples of use of adjuvant drugs[2]

Corticosteroid	Pain caused by oedema	Night sedative:	when lack of sleep is decreasing pain threshold
Antidepressant	Neuropathic pain		
Anticonvulsant	Neuropathic pain		
Muscle relaxant	Muscle cramp pain	Anxiolytic:	when anxiety is contributing to pain
Antispasmodic	Bowel colic		
NSAID	Inflammatory pain	Antidepressant:	when depressed mood is contributing to pain
Antibiotic	Infection pain		

Taken from Watson M, Lucas C, Hoy I, and Back A (2005). *Oxford Handbook of Palliative Care.* Oxford University Press, Oxford. Reproduced with permission from Oxford University Press.

2 World Health Organization (1996). *Cancer pain relief: with a guide to opioid availability,* 2nd edn. WHO, Geneva.

Symptom control: appetite loss

Appetite is the desire for food and is a pleasant sensation felt in anticipation of eating. Appetite is learned through enjoying a variety of foods that smell, taste, and look good.

- Loss of appetite may be temporary or persistent.
- Loss of appetite will affect the patient's nutritional status.
- Possible causes include sore mouth, nausea and vomiting, taste changes, diarrhoea, side effects of medical treatments and drugs, and the illness itself.

Assessment

- Observe the physical appearance of the patient's mouth and tongue.
- Talk to the patient and find out what their food preferences are.
- Carefully monitor and record food and fluid intake of the patient, including the times of the day the patient feels their appetite is not so badly affected.
- Assess the patient's nutritional status and food and fluid intake; involve a dietitian.

Treatment

- Encourage fluids and liquid nutritional diet, with the aid of a special feeding cup or straw.
- Encourage the patient to eat small frequent meals or snacks and to eat slowly and relax when eating. Identify foods that the patient likes.
- Try, if allowed, a small amount of alcohol such as sherry.
- If sore mouth, choose foods with plenty of sauce or gravy.
- Moisten food with milk or butter.
- Encourage soft foods such as pasta dishes and creamy soups.
- Keep mouth clean, brush teeth, and encourage use of mouthwashes.
- Avoid foods that may irritate the situation.
- Nutritional supplements may assist food intake.
- Appetite stimulants have not proven effective.

When patients are no longer able to take oral fluids, hydration *may* be provided by SC fluid administration (500–1500 mL/24 hours of normal saline or 5% dextrose and normal saline). Enteral feeding and PEG feeding may be used to strengthen the patient in the initial stages of palliative care.

Symptom control: nausea and vomiting

There are often many causes of nausea and vomiting in patients receiving palliative care. The symptoms are very distressing and often leave the patient weak and restless. It is particularly common in patients with advanced cancer.

Assessment

The key to assessing the patient suffering from nausea and vomiting is to set up a good communication system between the nurse and the patient.

- Determine whether there are particular times of the day that are worse than others.
- Identify any factors that may precipitate an attack.
- Record food and fluid intake or maintain a diary of the type and quantity of fluids being swallowed.
- Encourage the involvement of a dietitian and cook to advise on appropriate food and meals.

Causes

Oral causes

- Examine the mouth for oral thrush and stomatitis.
- Determine whether the patient has pain on swallowing.
- Hiccups may indicate uraemic cause.

Gastric causes

- Epigastric pain—may indicate gastritis or ulcer
- Nausea—may indicate constipation
- Heartburn—may be gastro-oesophagal reflux
- Examine abdomen—may be enlarged and tender due to a large liver, tumours, or ascites
- Digital rectal examination—constipation or faecal impaction
- Hypercalcaemia—dehydration, confusion
- Intestinal obstruction
- Inflammation—peritonitis
- Gastric stasis—drugs, anticholinergics
- Gastric irritation—blood alcohol, drugs, e.g. aspirin

Neurological causes

- Vomiting without nausea may indicate raised intracranial pressure.
- Vomiting exacerbated by movement may be due to a brain tumour.

Urinary causes

- Assess elimination—dysuria may indicate a urinary tract infection.

Psychological causes

- Nausea without vomiting may result from fear and anxiety or may be a reaction to offensive smells.

Chemical causes

- Drugs—morphine, digoxin
- Toxic states
- Chemotherapy
- Hypercalcaemia
- Uraemia
- Radiation exposure

Treatment and nursing interventions for nausea and vomiting

Non-drug measures

- Assess possible causes; ask patient what may help.
- Make food presentable and appealing.
- Reduce cooking smells or other unpleasant odours.
- Maintain good oral hygiene.
- Give stimulating small drinks, ice chips, or sips of clear cool fluid, or what the patient fancies.
- Monitor bowel movements.
- Monitor urine output and keep strict fluid balance.
- Review the patient's medications.
- Use complementary therapies such as relaxation technique.
- Provide good mouth care. Mouthwashes are an essential aspect of nursing care after a patient has vomited.

Drug measures

Anti-emetics should be chosen for the most likely cause of the nausea and vomiting.

- Metoclopramide for vomiting due to gastric stasis, irritation, and opioid-related vomiting.
- Haloperidol for uraemia.
- Cyclizine for motion sickness, raised intracranial pressure, radiotherapy, chemotherapy, and cerebral metastasis.
- Lorazepam for chemotherapy and anxiety states.

Symptom control: psychological symptoms

Anxiety

This is an unpleasant emotional state ranging from uneasiness to intense fear. The patient may complain of a variety of physical symptoms such as palpations, chest pains, and breathing problems. It is the most common symptom of distress in patients suffering from terminal illnesses and may stem from fears of shortness of breath, fear of pain, unremitting symptoms, and uncertainty about the future. The nurse must carefully assess the causes as they may be multifactorial, e.g. include the physical condition and medications. Supportive psychotherapy with drug treatment may be used (📖 Chapter 31, Anxiety and depression p.986). Patients nearing the end of life may have problems controlling emotions and underlying personality problems may emerge such as anger and hostility (📖 Chapter 31, Nursing patients with mental health needs, p.984).

Depression and depressive symptoms

These symptoms are characterized by emotional feelings of sadness, hopelessness, and lack of interest in social activities. There may be associated physical feelings of appetite loss, difficulty sleeping, tiredness, and poor concentration. Patients with severe depression may have suicidal thoughts, feelings of worthlessness, hallucinations and/or delusions (📖 Chapter 31, Anxiety and depression p.986). These symptoms are common when a patient has been diagnosed with a terminal illness and they are considered part of a normal stage of the grieving process. A prior history of bipolar disorder or dysthymia suggests a long-standing problem that may be exacerbated during end-of-life care. Patients require careful assessment, especially as the role of depression is common in requests for physician-assisted suicide. Treatment includes psychological support, psychotherapy, and medication. Antidepressants and psychostimulants are of proven value, but can take 4–6 weeks to work. Also, their possible interactions with other medications must be considered. 📖 Chapter 31, Nursing patients with mental health needs, p.983.

Fatigue, cachexia, and feelings of weakness

Fatigue is a term closely associated with weakness, weariness, and reduction in effort and energy. It affects most patients especially those treated for cancer. Cancer-related fatigue is defined by the National Comprehensive Cancer Network as 'a persistent subjective sense of tiredness related to cancer or cancer treatment that interferes with usual functioning.' (Mock et al. 2000) It is often caused by a disease advancing through the body and has both subjective dimensions and objective properties. It may result in lack of sleep and rest, anxiety, depression, and a general feeling of lethargy.

Cachexia involves involuntary loss of weight that is not caused simply by anorexia in patients with cancer (i.e. cancer cachexia). It also includes the presence of anaemia and immunosuppression along with other biological changes. It affects more than 80% of patients with advanced cancer. It may have a negative psychological impact due to body image change and may affect social mobility and interaction. It leads to feelings of frustration and intolerance to treatment and condition. It is not improved by increasing nutritional input, which can cause frustration and distress in families.

Weakness involves lack of strength or power. It can cause patients to feel fragile and vulnerable to not being able to cope with their daily living activities.

Care and management

- Assess the degree of fatigue.
- Explore with the patient and their family any other possible causes and effects, e.g. emotional concerns, pain, sleep disturbance, and drugs.
- Help the patient establish priorities for maximum energy needed to achieve their goals.
- Review drugs and treat other possible causes.
- Treat any physical causes such as anaemia and hypothyroidism.
- Suggest an individualized exercise programme which may help to improve mood and movement.
- Seek nutritional advice from a dietitian and encourage fluids.
- Encourage rest, sleep, and an individualized care plan of activities and emotional support.
- Involve the family and significant friends of the patient.
- Consider use of drugs such as corticosteroids, which may help.

Further information

Mock V et al. (2000). 'NCCN Practice Guidelines for cancer-related fatigue'. *Oncology (Huntington)* **14**(11A), 151–61.

Symptom control: respiratory symptoms

Dyspnoea

This is defined as difficult, uncomfortable, or laboured breathing (the individual feels the need for more air). It is the most frequent symptom in patients with end-stage respiratory disease. There are many causes and it is important to exclude physiological causes such as fluid overload and respiratory tract infection. It is commonly linked to anxiety and fears of choking or suffocation. By definition, dyspnoea is subjective and its severity can be gauged only by the patient. Because dyspnoea can be so frightening to the patient, adequate management must be a high priority for the nurse.

Care and management

- Measure oxygen saturation and give oxygen as required.
- Ask patient whether they are producing any sputum, and, if so, check its colour. Send a specimen for microbiology.
- Encourage the patient to express their feelings and work with them to help alleviate the difficulties.
- Position patient in a sitting or semi-sitting position as that will probably be the most comfortable. Teach relaxation techniques.
- Ensure the patient's immediate area is well ventilated. Open a window or place a fan near the neck/face of the patient so that the receptors around the lower face and neck respond to the cool air and have an effect on the alveoli in the lungs. For a breathless patient the air must blow across the face. Blowing a fan somewhere in the room is of little benefit.
- Continue drugs, nebulizer treatments, and oxygen therapy as prescribed.

Cough

Cough is a physiological mechanism to clear the airways of foreign substances or excessive secretions. If present, determine the source and establish the time of day the cough presents, any exacerbating and relieving factors, and any contact with other people with a cough. It is commonly caused by a chest cancer or metastatic involvement of the lungs or pleura, chronic airways disease, respiratory infections, heart failure, sinusitis, and certain medications.

Treatment

For a dry hacking irritation use simple linctus, codeine, or current medications via nebulizer. For wet cough with sputum, encourage steam inhalations or nebulizer, with chest physiotherapy. If the patient is too weak to expectorate the sputum, then give appropriate drugs such as atropine, morphine, or dexamethasone. Suction may be necessary, especially if there is bleeding into the throat, if secretions become trapped, or if the patient has a tracheostomy. Continuing oral antibiotics can often help stop further production of purulent sputum but will not alter the course of the dying process.

Other symptoms and factors relating to palliative care nursing

Numerous symptoms and nursing problems can occur at this stage of life. 📖 Chapter 24, Nursing patients with body image problems, p.814. Many of these are specific to certain medical conditions and are covered in many other sections of this book. Patient education is an essential component of care to ensure a collaborative approach to symptom management.

Loss of control of independence in living

Irrespective of the patient's age, loss of independence in self-care is extremely distressing for the individual and the family. Therefore the nurse should be particularly sensitive when assisting the patient with these activities. The nurse should encourage involvement and do things in the way the patient wishes, or when this is difficult, in a way that has been negotiated and agreed with them. Involvement of the occupational therapist and physiotherapist may help maintain the patient's independence.

Loss of control of bodily function and other fundamentals of nursing care

These are most distressing for the patient, especially urinary and faecal incontinence. Sometimes it is necessary for the patient to be catheterized and this may cause severe embarrassment. It is important to explain the need for this and that it may be a long-term solution. Ensure dignity is preserved by discreetly hiding the catheter bag and tubing, maintaining patency and flow. Explore ways of controlling faecal incontinence, especially if the patient wants to remain at home with their partner and sleep together.

Emotional considerations in palliative care

Working with the patient and their carer is crucial, and requires very careful and empathetic nursing. 📖 Chapter 2, Models for delivering nursing care, p.14.

- Be compassionate.
- Make yourself available and present for the patient and their family.
- Maintain the patient's dignity and encourage choice and control of their situation.
- Encourage hope and strategies to support or restore hope in some way.
- Get to know the patient and their family by listening and discussing their feelings as psychological and emotional feelings are severely tested during this stage of the patient's life.
- Facilitate exploration, self awareness, and discovery for the patient.
- Let the patient make decisions and find meanings.
- Use therapeutic touch, where and when appropriate.
- Help close family members cope with the patient's situation, particularly as they are going through their own grief and loss issues. If necessary, encourage the involvement of grief counsellors.

- Work with the patient to express their feelings and share their journey through their illness. Involving their family and friends takes time and patience.
- Keep a written account of key conversations and/or a log or diary which may help both the patient and carers, including the palliative care team.

Ethical and spiritual considerations

Many ethical questions about treatment and care may be raised e.g. 'Why bother with me?' 'Let me die,' 'I don't want to be a burden,' 'Please stop this treatment and care,' 'Help me to end my life,' 'Life has lost all meaning.' Some may be linked to their condition, others to their treatment and meaning of life. 📖 Chapter 35, Ethical issues, p.1125.

- Encourage patients to express their views and concerns.
- Find ways of helping patients and encourage previous coping and spiritual methods that they have used in the past.
- Consider the patient's religious and spiritual needs and involve the appropriate people, e.g. priests and clergy. Faith practices can be very helpful, particularly in times of stress, e.g. prayer, meditation, rituals, and sacraments. Independent non-religious counsellors may be helpful.
- Aromatherapy, painting, music therapy, and other non-religious practices can also help.

The concept of spirituality, which may seem abstract and unreal to some nurses, is ignored at the peril of providing substandard holistic nursing care (📖 Chapter 21, Nursing patients with intimate and sensitive care needs, p.735). The hospice and palliative care movement is one solution to what is a very emotive and challenging problem for society today.

Euthanasia ('the action of inducing a gentle and easy death'; Oxford English Dictionary) is controversially seen by some as a way of helping the minority of patients for whom symptom control is impossible. It is not a legalized option in the UK, but is in some countries elsewhere in Europe.

Nursing the dying patient

Principles of care of the dying

As each person is unique, so too is his or her death. Whether patients are resigned to their death or struggling desperately until the bitter end, the nurse's role remains to make them as comfortable as possible. To ensure that patients die with dignity, a holistic approach to care is needed.

Unfortunately, death-bed experiences may not always be ideal. Fear of pain is among the most commonly reported sources of anxiety about dying. Therefore, pain assessment and control is a priority. Fear of abandonment is the second most commonly reported anxiety. Therefore, relatives and friends should be involved. Dying people may ask for someone to be with them when they die. Sometimes the very presence of the nurse is needed to bring this comfort. 📖 Chapter 2, Models for delivering nursing care, p.14. The death-bed scene depicted by film and television, of a family gathered around the bed of the dying patient to witness the moment of death, is not one commonly encountered, although family and friends should be encouraged to visit. Death may not occur when the family is conveniently present, however.

While the final hours of life can be a profound shared experience, such moments rarely allow for profound differences between the dying patient and their family, if present, to be completely resolved.

The nurse should make sure that all involved in the patient's care are aware that they are 'not for resuscitation', including checking with the physician that a DNR form has been formally logged in the notes. The nurse should check that any agreement over organ donation has been discussed with a physician and appropriate permission received.

Terminal care, final hours

Caring for patients in the final hours of their life can be very distressing for the patient's partner, closest family members, and friends. It can also be very stressful and emotional for nurses and the caring team. A template of care to guide health care professionals with limited or infrequent experience of caring for dying patients, the Liverpool Care Pathway (LCP), has been developed (📖 Chapter 26, The Liverpool Care Pathway for the dying patient, pp.865–6). Involve the chaplain or appropriate religious representative, as applicable (📖 Chapter 21, Nursing, religion, and spiritual needs, pp.754–9).

Preparing everybody for the final stage is important, particularly for the changes they may see and experience. Some of the most common changes are:

- Patient becomes restless and agitated—may pull or throw off bed linens (known as terminal restlessness).
- Level of consciousness may lessen but the patient may still respond or be aware of the presence of others.
- Hearing is one of the last senses to disappear according to studies carried out in intensive care units.
- Face may become grey and very drawn.
- Eyes may become sunken and glazed.
- Lips may become cyanosed.
- Mouth may become very dry; swallowing is very difficult.
- Skin may become cold, mottled, and bluish in colour, especially the extremities.
- Small uric acid crystals may appear on skin.
- Breathing becomes noisy (death rattle) and irregular (known as Cheyne–Stokes breathing).
- Urine becomes concentrated.
- Patient may become incontinent of urine and faeces.
- Blood pressure falls and pulse rate becomes thready and weak.
- Muscle twitching/grimacing of the face may occur.

The nurse's role

The nurse's role is to make the dying patient as comfortable as possible.

- Keep lips and mouth moist and clean.
- Change patient's position regularly, for comfort measures only.
- Keep skin clean and dry.
- Review medications—oral preparations may no longer be possible.
- Discontinue enteral feeding only after multidisciplinary team discussion with family.
- Review any intravenous therapies, such as fluid, and stop if no direct benefits.
- Ensure a suitable environment for care of the dying. Consider privacy, lighting, noise, and situation.
- Encourage those present to speak quietly to the patient and hold their hand or touch the patient in a manner that is soothing and relaxing.

The nurse also has a role to comfort and support the relatives throughout the dying process.

- Make sure the patient is pain free. 📖 Chapter 23, Nursing patients with pain, p.788 and 📖 Chapter 26, Nursing patients with palliative care needs, p.862.
- Inform relatives that the physical changes associated with death do not mean that the patient is in distress.
- When death occurs, be prepared to deal with grief experienced by the family and friends. Reactions to grief may vary from sadness and weeping to shouting and running away, fainting, and hyperventilation syndrome.
- Allow the family time alone with the body.

Caring for the patient's body after death

In cases of expected death the nurse has responsibility to inform the relatives and the patient's physician. A medical certificate stating the cause of death will be provided for the relatives.

'Last offices' is a nursing tradition that involves washing the body and laying it out in an appropriate manner for transfer to the mortuary. It is the last thing the nurse will do for the patient and is a way of ending the nurse–patient relationship. It involves:

- respecting and collaborating with any relevant wishes or cultural and religious beliefs. 📖 Chapter 2, Nursing religious and spiritual needs, pp.754–9.
- caring for, respecting, and protecting the body until it is removed
- leaving the body for relatives to sit with for a while
- appropriate care of bereaved relatives
- appropriate support for other patients, informing them of what has happened
- appropriate support of staff
- preparing the body in a careful and systematic way for the mortuary staff and undertakers
- providing care and safe custody of patient's property.

Offer relatives further opportunity to view the body. Involve the chaplain or appropriate religious representative. Discuss the death with the relatives and give time for questions. Explain relevant administrative and legal procedures. Carry out 'last offices' systematically and respectfully or leave to others if requested by relatives.

Nurse's role following the death of a patient on the ward (general guidelines—check your own organization's policy)

- Ensure the patient's privacy to prevent the distress of other persons.
- Ask the physician to certify the death.
- Inquire whether the next of kin wish to view the body.
- Document in the nursing notes details of the death and action you have taken.

Once death has been certified (📖 Chapter 21, Nursing, religion, and spiritual needs, pp.754–9 provides details on how to deal with the body of people of different religions).

- Wear gloves and lay the patient flat, face up with their limbs in a natural position and their arms by their side. Rigor mortis occurs 2–4 hours following death; after this time positioning of the body will be difficult.
- Remove all tubes and drains, unless otherwise instructed, to reduce health hazard.
- Wash the body as for bed bath for general hygiene purposes.
- Redress all wounds with waterproof dressing, thereby reducing the potential problems of leakage of body fluids. When drains or tubes are left in position, these should be covered with a waterproof dressing.
- Remove any jewellery except the wedding ring (which should be secured with tape if loose and documented) and sacramental/religious jewellery. 📖 Chapter 37, Patients' property, p.1143.
- In some situations the patient or relatives may have requested some jewellery to be left on the body. In this case, make sure you record where on the body this has been left and any detail to describe the item.
- If the patient has false teeth, clean them and replace in mouth to enhance the aesthetic appearance of the deceased.
- Change bed linen as appropriate and place an incontinence pad under the body.
- Gently close the eyes to improve the facial appearance.
- If relatives want to view the body, consider the patient area and the possible use of a flower arrangement.
- Dress the body in a shroud (adhering to your trust policy).
- Complete body identification slips and secure to the wrapped body (adhering to your trust policy).
- Secure patient's property noting all items in patient property book (including money and such jewellery as it has been appropriate to remove) with a witness present. Place property in a secure place.
- When appropriate, contact porters to take the body to the mortuary and screen off the other beds in the bay.

Breaking bad news

Overview

'Bad news' can be defined as any information that drastically alters the recipient's view of their future for the worse. The breaking of bad news is commonly encountered in the care setting and is not necessarily related to the news of a prognosis of death or the news of a death to relatives.

Patients respect physicians and nurses who give them the information they need and the opportunity to discuss their situation. Bad news is easier to hear from someone who is trusted. Trust depends on a good nurse–patient relationship, competence, reputation, communication, and respect.

The sharing of bad news with the patient can often best be achieved by the physician and the nurse working together. Particular sensitivity should be observed when communicating bad news to certain sensitive people such as those with a learning disability or a mental health problem.

Delivering news of poor prognosis

Usually it is the physician's role to tell the patient the prognosis and prospects regarding their medical diagnosis. Often it is the nurse who is left to support and care for the patient once this information has been given.

Bad news may come as a shock to the patient and may cause severe emotional distress. A patient has a right to hear bad news and it should be delivered in a sensitive way, taking into consideration the patient's background, personality, and ability to understand the information necessary at this stage in their illness. Patients not only want to be given information, they want the opportunity to talk things through and reflect on the information they have been given. It is often helpful for the nurse to be present when the patient is given this information.

It is the nurse's role to encourage this reflection and check the patient's level of understanding. If the patient has misunderstood something, then nurses should correct information that they feel able and competent to correct. The nurse should also refer the patient back to the physician if there are problems.

It is important to ask the patient's permission to speak with their relatives. Do not assume the patient wants every relative involved. It may be appropriate to have the patient's family present when discussing bad news and prognosis.

Delivering bad news to families

Where patients have died without family members being present, the nurse will often be the first member of the medical team encountered. In these circumstances the nurse should check carefully who the relatives (or close friends) are, and their relationship with the patient. The nurse may be called upon to deliver the bad news, and, if so, the considerations given to the breaking of bad news (📖 Key factors in breaking bad news, p.893) should be followed.

Key factors in breaking bad news

- Identify a telephone-free room.
- Find a comfortable environment and a box of tissues.
- Take precautions to avoid interruptions.
- Know all the facts before the meeting.
- Find out who the patient wants to be present.
- Find out what the patient and relatives want to know.
- Outline any boundaries (there may be areas that only the consultant or a member of the medical team can cover).
- Check the patient and relative's level of understanding (ask the patient and relatives to recall the information they know). Listen to words and phrases used.
- Identify the patient and relative's concerns.
- Give a warning shot—'I'm afraid it looks rather serious' (if appropriate at this stage).
- Allow denial.
- Explain by narrowing the gap step by step. The details will not be remembered, but the way you explain will be.
- Listen to concerns.
- Answer any questions using terms that are understandable to the patient and relatives.
- Allow the patient time for reflection alone or with relatives.
- Encourage the expression of feelings and concerns.
- Summarize the patient and relative's concerns; plan further options, treatment, support, aspects of nursing care; and foster hope.
- Be available to offer further support.
- Offer guidance and information with regard to any further counselling needed (such as bereavement counselling).

Breaking bad news concerning death to family and close friends takes into consideration all of the salient features of this protocol.

Bereavement, loss, and grief

Bereavement is the loss of a close relation or friend through their death, or the loss of function of a body part through illness, injury, or amputation. Grief is the intense sorrow that results from this loss. There can be profound physical and mental effects on individual sufferers.

It is suggested that grieving people go through stages or follow an overall pattern in coming to terms with their loss (📖 Tasks of bereavement, p.895). However, there is much debate about this and many bereavement counsellors believe that the 'stages' theory is often too rigidly applied. Elizabeth Kübler-Ross proposed a 'stage' model of what may happen in grief. This consists of shock, denial (not disbelief), anger, guilt, fear, anxiety, despair/depression, and acceptance/resignation. Some people may go through these stages in some type of order or may experience just a few of these proposed feelings. Others may get stuck at a certain stage. Whatever happens, the nurse should be aware of these stages and assess and counsel patients appropriately, bearing in mind that there is often a time factor related to each of these stages and each can take days, weeks or years to be resolved.

There is no 'right' way to grieve. Each person reacts in their own individual way. Adjustment and healing come slowly. Some people find it easier to show their emotions, while others do not. The bereaved may suffer a variety of physical symptoms including breathlessness, tiredness, insomnia, and loss of appetite. Existing conditions may be exacerbated by the pain and distress of grief. If the bereaved do not experience any feelings intensely or if feelings persist and worsen, then grief is often labelled as 'abnormal' and psychiatric help may be needed.

Dying and death often bring into sharp focus philosophical and spiritual questions about self and existence. The nurse's role is to listen and encourage the bereaved to talk. Referral may be needed to specialist counselling organizations such as Cruse Bereavement Care or a local group.

Further information

Cruse Bereavement Care: Cruse House, 126 Sheen Road, Richmond, Surrey, TW9 1VR. Tel: 0208 940 4818) www.crusebereavementcare.org.uk

Kübler-Ross E (1969). *On death and dying*. Tavistock Publications, London.

Worden JW (1991). *Grief counselling and grief therapy*, 2nd edn. Routledge, London.

Tasks of bereavement

Worden (1991) suggests bereavement can be conceptualized as four tasks:
- to accept the reality of the loss
- to experience or work through the pain of grief
- to adjust to an environment in which the deceased is missing
- to emotionally relocate the deceased and move on with life.

Supporting the bereaved

- Being there, even though you feel helpless, is of utmost importance.
  📖 See Chapter 2, Models for delivering nursing care, p.14.
- If you are familiar with the person and if intimacy and closeness have pre-existed in your relationship, then touching may be beneficial and reassuring.
- Do not just touch because you do not know what else to do.
- Provide gentle reassurance and listen to the person.
- Allow the bereaved to talk and cry if they want. (In sudden death some feelings may be more intense and emotional.)
- Take the bereaved to a quiet area away from the situation.
- Remain passive, giving the person non-verbal permission to express their grief in their own way.
- Anger may lead to destructive behaviour; therefore say such things as, 'I can't let you do this' or 'It distresses me to see you doing this'. (In this way the nurse takes the responsibility for the inhibition and does not lay another negative on the bereaved.)
- Encourage the person to tell or re-tell their story.
- If the intensity of the sadness and situation distresses you, ask others to relieve you.
- Be aware of cultural variations in response to bereavement.

Anticipated grief

Anticipated grief occurs when the person who will be bereaved begins the grieving process while the patient is still alive. This often happens in cases where the patient's death is long and expected. The partner, relative, or friend comes to expect the inevitable and, following the death of the patient, adjusts to the bereavement more quickly. When someone dies suddenly, there is no opportunity for anticipated grieving.

Further information

Asian Family Counselling Service. Tel: 020 8571 3933
Cancer BACUP Counselling. Tel: 020 7833 2451. www.cancer.bacup.
  org.uk
Compassionate Friends. www.compassionatefriends.org
Cruse Bereavement. Tel: 0870 167 1677. www.crusebereavementcare.org.uk
Samaritans/Age Concern/Citizen's Advice Bureaux: See local telephone directory

What information should nurses give to relatives following a death?

Firstly remember that the death of a loved one is often a shattering and bewildering experience. Express your deepest sympathy and be supportive.

Be aware that relatives often want to know what happened, why their loved one died, and whether they experienced any pain. Even when death has occurred suddenly, relatives need answers to these questions and reassurance about the nature of the death. Sometimes it is appropriate for relatives to speak to the nurse and the physician together.

Following the death of a patient, nurses should give relatives the following information:
- What happened and what caused the death (be factual).
- When and where they can obtain the death certificate.
- When and where they can view the body. Explain that the body is taken to the hospital mortuary and arrangements can be made through the bereavement officer in the hospital to see the body in the chapel of rest. (Check with local policy.)
- How to register the death (your ward should have written information).
- Inform the relatives if the death is to be reported to the coroner and tell them why. (Deaths are usually reported following a sudden or unexpected death or when certain questionable circumstances surround the condition of the patient.)

Give relatives the following leaflets:
- Registering a death.
- Letter from the bereavement officer.
- Letter from the hospital chaplain.
- How to make funeral arrangements.

Nursing the older person

Principles of nursing older people

Care of the sick and frail older person has always been entrusted to the family and those individuals who occupy a nursing role in society. Today older people depend on nurses not only for help, but also for advocacy and specific care when they are in general and specialist medical facilities.

Gerontology is the study of the ageing process and of problems encountered by older people. It focuses on the processes and effects of normal ageing. Geriatrics is the study and practice of the medical problems and care of older people with diseases. The term 'geriatric' has also, however, acquired negative connotations and today the term is not as widely used as it was.

Modern gerontological nursing draws from a large body of knowledge and research and seeks new evidence-based practices to promote healthy ageing, prevent illness, treat disease, and provide rehabilitation for older people. It is a nursing speciality that is essential practice for all nurses working in areas where older people receive health care. Statistically, older people make up the majority of patients seen in many adult clinical hospital units and certainly they form one of the largest numbers of clients seen by community nurses.

Conclusions drawn from early studies of ageing were based on cross-sectional studies of ill and institutionalized old people. These tended to portray the elderly and the ageing process in a very negative manner. Today new directions in research have shown how positive and fulfilling life can be for older people, and many are now living longer and are more active than ever before.

Nursing older people is aimed at helping the individual come to terms with their illness, get better, or improve their health care situation and to achieve and maintain the highest level of physical and social functioning that the older person feels is appropriate to their lifestyle and needs.

The multidisciplinary team (which includes doctors, nurses, physiotherapists, occupational therapists, social workers, and care managers) is now recognized as being the key to successful rehabilitation, adaptation, and recovery from acute illness for the older person.

National Service Framework for Older People (March 2001)

Key recommendations and standards

- *Standard 1:* abolish age discrimination, making sure all services are provided for older people regardless of age.
- *Standard 2:* person-centred care.
  Treat older people as individuals and enable them to be involved in their own care and make choices. A single assessment process and integrated provision of services should be provided.
- *Standard 3:* intermediate care.
  Access for older people to a range of services designed to promote independence, unnecessary hospital admission, rehabilitation, and appropriate discharge from hospital.
- *Standard 4:* general hospital care.
  Provision of specialist multidisciplinary care in hospitals.
- *Standard 5:* stroke.
  Action to provide appropriate stroke prevention, treatment, and care.
- *Standard 6:* falls.
  Action to prevent falls and reduce injuries.
- *Standard 7:* mental health in older people.
  Provision and access to appropriate mental health services for older people.
- *Standard 8:* the promotion of health and active life in older age.
  An emphasis on health promotion and local social and voluntary support services.

Recent updates relevant to the above:

- NMC (2008). *Standards for medicines management.* Available at: www.nmc-uk.org. 📖 Chapter 4, Medicines management, p.74 addresses the importance of this subject.
- Department of Health OPD (2006). *A new ambition for old age: next steps in implementing the National Service Framework for Older People,* Department of Health, London

Assessing older people

An illness can have far reaching psychosocial implications for an older person, such as loneliness and lack of mobility. These implications must be actively sought during assessment and addressed in order to maximize the return to health and adaptation to disability, if present. Often certain generations of older people are culturally reluctant to express or talk about health issues that affect their lifestyle.

All nursing models can be used in addition to the typical medical and social model to assess older people's health problems. Orem's self-care model and Roper's activities of living model are examples. Whichever model is chosen, the following are key points to look for when assessing and examining the older patient.

- Observe the patient's general appearance and non-verbal communication.
- Include questions on psychological and social details when exploring physical aspects of assessment.
- Encourage mutual interaction and collaboration with the patient, fostering the expectation that they will participate in decision making and care.
- Review the patient's life history, culture, and experience of ageing to help identify unresolved issues that may be affecting their current health and lifestyle.
- Explore concerns about possible adaptations in lifestyle to chronic or acute illness, altered social and family networks, changes in health status, and expectations for the future.
- Involve the family and other key carers in discussions to learn how the patient usually behaves or has changed over the past few days, months, and years. This will be particularly relevant if the patient has difficulties communicating and giving a history.
- Remember that illness in older people presents atypically and non-specifically; causes greater morbidity and mortality; progresses more rapidly; and has health, social, and financial consequences for the patient. Comorbidity is common and patients have a low physiological reserve. Identifying and correcting several minor disorders may help to improve the overall health of the older person.
- An elderly person with multiple problems may give a history that is hard to unravel; therefore follow things up during your nursing care.
- Be aware of labels that are applied to older people and terms that may be misleading by non-experts in the speciality of care for older people.
- Some older patients suffer from acute or chronic cognitive impairments which may affect the assessment process.
- Some older patients have very complex social situations.
- Make sure to give older patients adequate time to respond and come back to you about their health and social problems. Don't rush them.
- Develop an atmosphere of trust, respect, and mutual interest in their life history, which may increase their willingness to participate and accept nursing care.

Key areas of assessment

During the assessment, focus on understanding the usual (pre-morbid) function and the current functional level of the patient. Key areas to be explored with patient/relatives/friends include:

- General health status, personal cleanliness and hygiene in the past and recently.
- Physical functioning, i.e. independent, supervision, limited assistance, extensive assistance, or total dependence.
- Ability to perform activities of daily living.
- Bed mobility, transfer, walking, dressing, eating, toileting, personal hygiene, bathing, use of mobility appliances, stick, frame, wheelchair. (Standardized assessment tools such as Barthel scale may be helpful.)
- Use of prosthesis and aids such as false teeth, hearing aid, spectacles, writing pad for communication.
- Continence levels: bladder, bowels, frequency, soiling.
- Nutritional and oral status: nutritional problems, dietary needs, feeding support, weight, hydration.
- Skin condition: problems with circulation and ulcer status. Pressure areas and pressure sores or skin breakdown, bruises. (Use of Waterlow assessment tool may be helpful.)
- Rest and sleep: insomnia, wakefulness, and sleep habits.
- Cognitive function: memory, daily decision making, confusion, mini-mental status. (📖 Assessment of confusion, p.918).
- Pain assessment.
- Communication and hearing patterns: speech, non-verbal expression, making self understood.
- Emotional and psychological well-being: signs of sadness, grieving, bereavement, loss, depression, anxiety, self-perception and concept, fatigue, mood.
- Values: beliefs and spirituality.
- Falls assessment.
- Social issues: responsible legal guardian, next of kin, friends and community support, social workers and voluntary support services received.
- Any advanced directives: living will, do not resuscitate, organ donation.
- Medication methods and restrictions, use of special containers and memory aids, self medicating, use of others and special precautions and allergies.
- Types of disease and medical problems related to activities of daily living status, mental and behavioural functioning, and provision of nursing care, i.e. heart/circulation, neurological, pulmonary, sensory, endocrine, and other.

Further information

Orem D (1980). *Nursing: concepts of practice* (2nd edn). McGraw-Hill, New York.
Roper N, Logan W, Tierney A (1980). *The elements of nursing*. Churchill Livingstone, Edinburgh.

The ageing person

- Ageing changes appear in most organs in the body, but there is wide variability between individuals.
- Cellular changes occur which make more cells vulnerable and susceptible to damage.
- Connective tissue loses elasticity.
- Bone structure changes throughout life and by old age there is gradual loss of bone. Trabecular bone is affected more than cortical bone. Women lose more bone mass than men.
- The shape of long bones changes with increasing age; the internal cavity increases in diameter while the outer cortical layer becomes thinner. These changes result in weaker bones.
- Gait changes with age as a result of the interaction between ageing and disease processes. The person may become slower and take less regular steps, with shuffling.
- Older individuals have consequent increases in bone fractures, increased wound healing time, and increased need to mobilize using walking aids.
- Muscle wasting may occur in the proximal muscles due to disuse. This may lead to difficulty in rising from a chair or sitting position.
- Pupils are often small and react sluggishly to light. Eyes appear sunken and vision and accommodation to variable light is impaired as the lens becomes inelastic.
- Loss of high-frequency hearing occurs and there is particular difficulty when background noise is present.
- Ear wax becomes more viscous and may need removal.
- Changes in the mouth, particularly related to the teeth and gums, results in dental problems and ill-fitting dentures.
- Cellular changes occur in the cardiovascular system with decline in stroke volume, cardiac output, and oxygen consumption. All these can be improved by regular aerobic exercise.
- Although many physiological changes occur to the respiratory system with age, because of the lungs' large reserve capacity, significant clinical issues only occur when an elderly person becomes sick.
- Age changes affecting the gastrointestinal system are loss of sense of smell and taste, impaired swallowing, reduced gastric acid and pancreatic function, and reduced small and large bowel motility.
- In old age renal function is reduced and urinary output is affected with the failure of the kidney to concentrate urine. This may cause nocturia. Prostatic size increases with age leading to difficulties in passing urine in men. Renal function may suffer as a result of certain disease processes such as hypertension and diabetes.
- Women often complain of incontinence due to changes in their pelvic floor. Men most often complain of erectile dysfunction or prostate gland problems.
- Both men and women may feel that their sexual drive and ability to have intercourse is changing due to increasing time to arousal and orgasm. Women additionally may suffer a loss of vaginal lubrication.

- There is a reduction in lean body mass and body water and usually a relative increase in fat. Various hormonal changes occur resulting in susceptibility to fluid and electrolyte problems, and endocrine problems such as diabetes mellitus.
- Skin changes are mostly confined to the dermis which becomes thinner, more transparent, more fragile, and less elastic. There is also a change in sweating and sebaceous excretion, and a reduction in damage repair to the skin.
- Pressure sores and leg ulcers are the most common serious skin problems in old age.

Common nursing problems

Alteration in bowel elimination

Diarrhoea

- *Causes:* viral or bacterial gastroenteritis, misuse of laxatives, food intolerance, improper hyperosmolar tube feedings, side effects of medicines (especially antibiotics), inflammatory colitis, malignancy, and faecal impaction.
- *Nursing interventions:* keep stool chart, observe stool, perform digital rectal examination for faecal impaction. Obtain medical, drug, and diet history. Take care when handling, use barrier nursing technique, and maintain strict handwashing. Obtain stool samples for culture and sensitivity, look for ova cysts of parasities, and check for *Clostridium difficile* (culture and toxin). See How to deal with the problem, a DH and HPA publication, Jan 2009, www.hpa.org.uk.

Constipation

Constipation is a decrease in the frequency of bowel movements accompanied by difficulty in evacuation of stool, straining, and a feeling of incomplete evacuation.

- *Causes:* decreased mobility and exercise, malignancy, obstruction, poor nutrition, lack of fluids, depression, certain medical conditions, medications, misuse of laxatives, and sedentary lifestyle.
- *Signs and symptoms:* abdominal pain, cramping, and bloating; straining during defecation; small hard faeces (🕮 Appendices, Bristol stool form scale, p.1205); acute confusion; nausea; and loss of appetite.
- *Nursing interventions:* use the Sussex/UCE constipation care pathway (🕮 Appendices, Management of constipation, p.1206). Confirm the problem with a digital rectal examination. Monitor bowel movements. In the short term use laxatives, suppositories, or enemas to empty entire bowel. Try to prevent recurrence by encouraging high-fibre diet, adequate fluid intake, and reduced or regular use of laxatives. Check for environmental causes when using the toilet or bedpan/commode, mechanical problems such as appropriate position when toileting, and time for evacuation. It may be necessary to manually remove the stools, but this is a very specialized procedure and must only be done following RCN guidelines, by a qualified person.

Loss of hearing due to cerumen (wax) impaction

This is easily treatable; however, many older people do not realize they have the problem. Cerumen impaction results in hearing loss, itching, and feeling of fullness in the ear. Blockage can sometimes be seen on inspection of the ear canal. Confirm using an auroscope. (Deafness may be caused by presbycusis.) Insert warm olive oil drops or appropriate medication, instruct patient to lie on their side for a few minutes. Perform ear irrigation or suction, if necessary. This should be confirmed by a nurse specialist or physician. Encourage patient to express any emotions over hearing loss and introduce regular ear examination. 🕮 Chapter 14, Nursing assessment of patients with ear problems, p.504.

Falls and fall prevention

Falls are a leading predictor of morbidity and mortality among older people and their incidence increases with age. Falls are one of the most common reasons for hospital admission in older people. In general hospitals, most inpatient incident forms relate to falls. About 40% of patients who fall experience more than one fall and for those over 85 years of age, a fall may prove fatal.

The use of bed rails only prevents falls in the unconscious patient. For confused and agitated patients, they can be a source of danger and an added obstacle. Many clinical areas now have special instructions and directives relating to the use of bed rails.

Falls often occur during the busiest times of the day when there are many obstacles about or there is a lack of nursing supervision. In all settings, most falls take place in the bedroom or bathroom and are related to going to or from the bathroom, transferring to and from bed, or getting out of chairs. Up to 15% of falls result in physical injury, usually fractures and/or soft tissue damage. Psychological problems from falls include anxiety and worry about future independence, loss of self-esteem, and fear of performing ADLs.

Risk factors

Among older people, falls usually result as a combination of factors and not just one cause.

Physiological factors
- Age
- Gender (more women than men)
- Sensory impairment (e.g. vision and hearing)
- Medical conditions that affect certain body systems (i.e. neurological, cerebrovascular, cardiovascular, musculoskeletal)
- Other conditions (e.g. cancer or other chronic progressive diseases, gain and balance changes, and polypharmacy)

Social factors
- Disorientation, wandering, and acute confusion
- Getting up too quickly from a bed at night for toilet purposes
- Environmental traps (e.g. objects, wet surfaces, poor lighting, clothing and footwear)
- Bed rails. 📖 Falls and fall prevention, above
- Walking devices
- Alcohol abuse
- Medications or medical devices (e.g. tubes)

Nursing interventions

- Assess older person for risk of falls.
- Consider age, mental status, continence, activity and mobility, gait and balance, medications, environment, and history of falling.
- Monitor and document falls and always assess patient following falls for any injuries.
- Record actions taken on incident forms and in patient records.

Foot care

Often neglected, foot care is particularly important for bedridden patients, diabetics, and those especially susceptible to foot infections and poor circulation.

- Ensure meticulous cleanliness and regular observation for signs of skin breakdown.
- Protect from injury and avoidance of extremes of heat and cold.
- Trim toenails carefully and encourage patient to see a podiatrist especially when there is any problem with nails, calluses, or injuries.
- When washing, soak the feet well; carefully remove debris on skin and between toes and toe nails.
- Apply appropriate skin lotions and lightly dust water-absorbent powder between toes to absorb moisture.

Preventing dehydration and encouraging good nutrition

- Assess the patient's nutritional and fluid needs, checking carefully if help is needed in assisting patients with their meals and preparation of food.
- Review patient's diet, especially for calcium and fibre intake.
- Monitor fluid intake and output. To maintain adequate hydration older people need 1–3 litres of fluid a day.
- Provide 'tasty' beverages and fluids.
- Provide appropriate feeding cups.
- Assess skin turgor and mucous membranes.
- Monitor laboratory tests such as U&E, albumin and FBC. Assess urine osmolality if urine output is low.
- Weigh regularly.

Urinary continence and incontinence

Disturbances in urine elimination are common among older people and usually follow any loss or impairment of urinary sphincter control. Contrary to popular opinion, urinary incontinence is not a disease and is not part of normal ageing. It is a common consequence of urinary tract infections and may occur after catheter removal. It should not be accepted as part of ageing, rather a cause should be sought. It may be caused by confusion, dehydration, faecal impaction, or restricted mobility.

Consequences of incontinence include restricted social activity, altered self-concept, decreased self-esteem, and skin problems such as rawness and breakdown. There are various types of incontinence and it is important to identify the type and its main causes.

Nursing interventions
- Assess patient's intake and voiding patterns.
- Encourage a regular voiding schedule, i.e. initially 2-hourly and increasing to 4-hourly.
- Teach relaxation techniques such as deep breathing which helps reduce the sense of urgency.
- Position bed near bathroom or portable toilet.
- Limit fluid intake after 6 p.m.
- Answer patient's call for toileting promptly.
- Be positive and encourage positive attitude in patient.

- Evaluate related problems such as urinary hesitancy, frequency, and urgency.
- Note that nocturia is very common in older people because of their decreased ability to concentrate urine, increased use of diuretics, better perfusion of kidneys in a supine position, and altered sleep patterns that result in easier arousal during sleep.
- Keep patient dry and clean. Use special pads where necessary and appropriate.
- Assess the patient's mental and general physical state and maintain the patient's dignity and privacy at all times.
- Avoid the use of catheters.
- Carry out laboratory tests or use a dipstick test for signs for urinary infections.
- Manage stress incontinence with pelvic floor exercises, i.e. *teach* the patient how to locate the muscles of the pelvic floor. Instruct them to tense the muscles around the anus, as if to retain stool or intestinal gas. Then teach the patient to tighten the muscles of the pelvic floor to stop the flow of urine while urinating and then to release the muscles to restart the flow.
- Keep in mind that intervention depends on cause. Sometimes bladder training as mentioned above does not work for sphincter incompetence; therefore a bladder stabilizing medication may be used for urge incontinence.

Psychological factors

Three key areas of psychology are relevant to nursing the ageing patient.

1. *Cognition* is the mental process by which knowledge is transformed, reduced, elaborated, stored, and retrieved in the body by thought, experience, and the senses. Memory, hearing, and attention may be affected by disease processes. Short- and long-term memory especially can be affected with age.

2. *Self-concept* is a key component of personality and can be viewed as an attitude towards the self. Personality type influences self-concept and adaptation to role transitions and adaptation to old age. Problems related to self-concept include depression, isolation, rigidity, and stubbornness.

3. *Morale* represents the confidence, enthusiasm, and discipline of a person. Morale may be affected in older patients due to losses and changes in their lives. However, many older people remain happy despite the difficulties and changes they face. It is therefore important to explore why older people are happy, e.g. could be due to surviving a war, personal ambition, family success, or longevity.

Emotions

All behaviours are associated with underlying emotions and these are personal experiences. Observe and understand emotions in older people by putting oneself in their place, i.e. empathize, ask questions, and pick up clues.

Examples

- You look worried. Are you worried?
- You don't seem happy today. Is there something on your mind?
- You seem to be feeling angry about something. What is it?

Key signs of emotions

- *Anger:* frowning, tearfulness, clenched teeth, intensive staring, flushed or pale face.
- *Anxiety:* trembling, shaking, flushed face, sweating, dry mouth, wrinkled brow, lip biting or lip quivering.
- *Depression:* no eye contact, self-neglect, not speaking, withdrawing from social contact, listlessness, crying, sad expression.

Behaviour

Identify and describe behaviours in older people carefully using descriptive terms, e.g. cooperative, uncooperative, sociable, suspicious, unpredictable, isolated, in character, out of character, agitated, wandering, shouting, calling.

Common mental health problems in old age

Depression

This is the most common psychiatric disorder in later life. It is characterized by sadness, low mood, pessimism about the future, self-neglect, self-criticism, self-blame, retardation, agitation, slow thinking, difficulty in concentrating, and disturbances in appetite and sleep.

Possible predisposing factors
- Biological changes
- Genetic predisposition
- Specific diseases
- Chronic medical conditions
- Drugs
- Sensory deprivation
- Loss of physical functioning

Psychological causes
- Difficulty adapting to old age
- Loss of social contacts and work
- Poor support mechanisms
- Chronic stress, life events, and daily hassles

Signs
Most characteristic of depression are a sad expression, withdrawal from social interaction, agitation, frequent crying, clinging, and other expressions of dependency and helplessness. Older people differ from younger people in that they may deny changes in mood or feelings of depression and instead may complain of bodily changes and problems. Cognitive impairment, i.e. pseudo-dementia, may be an important sign of depression.

Categories of depressive disorders in later life
Major depression or *unipolar depression* – lasts >2 weeks and consists of some of the following symptoms: depressed mood; loss of interest or pleasure; significant weight loss or gain; insomnia, agitation, and fatigue; guilt; and suicidal thoughts. Treatment includes hospitalization if there are signs of suicidal intent, psychotic features, or resistance to drug treatment; appropriate drug therapy, which includes antidepressants; and possibly psychotherapy.

Minor depression – less severe than major depression and occurs more frequently. There is marked loss of interest or pleasure in most activities and depressed mood. Treatment includes drug therapy and some psychosocial interventions.

Bipolar disorder – exhibits a manic episode after having had at least one depressive episode. Treatment includes antipsychotic medications for acute agitated behaviours and lithium carbonate for prevention of recurrent symptoms of mania.

Other types of depressive conditions are bereavement and reactive depression or adjustment disorder with depressed mood. Both are related to severe losses in later life and problems of coping. Both are treated with social and psychological supportive measures, and with individual and group psychotherapy.

The use of the Geriatric Depression Scale may be helpful. (See Fig. 28.1)

Instructions

Undertake the test orally. Ask the patient to reply indicating how they have felt over the past week. Obtain a clear yes or no reply. If necessary, repeat the question. Each depressive answer (bold) scores one.

1	Are you basically satisfied with your life?	YES / **NO**
2	Have you dropped many of your activities and interests?	**YES** / NO
3	Do you feel that your life is empty?	**YES** / NO
4	Do you often get bored?	**YES** / NO
5	Are you in good spirits most of the time?	YES / **NO**
6	Are you afraid that something bad is going to happen to you?	**YES** / NO
7	Do you feel happy most of the time?	YES / **NO**
8	Do you often feel helpless?	**YES** / NO
9	Do you prefer to stay at home, rather than going out and doing new things?	**YES** / NO
10	Do you feel you have more problems with memory than most?	**YES** / NO
11	Do you think it is wonderful to be alive now?	YES / **NO**
12	Do you feel pretty worthless the way you are now?	**YES** / NO
13	Do you feel full of energy?	YES / **NO**
14	Do you feel that your situation is hopeless?	**YES** / NO
15	Do you think that most people are better off than you are?	**YES** / NO

Scoring

0–4	No depression
5–10	Mild depression
11+	Severe depression

Fig. 28.1 The Geriatric Depression Scale. Taken from Bowker LK, Price JD, and Smith SC (2006). *Oxford Handbook of Geriatric Medicine.* Oxford University Press, Oxford. Reproduced with permission from Oxford University Press.

Social factors and ageing

Social factors that may be particularly impacted at this time of life include: change in financial situation, housing, lifestyle, social support networks, work, and recreational activities. Issues that older people previously may have grappled with or ignored often tend to have more impact or may become important issues to them such as ability to keep fit and independently mobile.

Because of chronic illness and changes in social contacts and support from family and friends, older people are more vulnerable. Many changes occur at this stage in life and unfortunately there are many losses.

- Loss of health
- Loss of status and independence resulting from retirement
- Loss of spouse and other loved ones
- Sensory losses
- Death of a pet
- Sale of a home
- Wealth may be affected depending on pension and savings or investments
- Driving may need to be given up at some stage
- Mobility and fitness difficulties may reduce trips and social visits

It is important for the nurse to remind patients that there are also advantages associated with ageing. It is important to emphasize and build on these.

- Opportunity to redesign lifestyle and to promote health (e.g. more time to exercise)
- Opportunity to do things that they were unable to do or did not have time for earlier in life
- New interests bring new contacts and relationships
- Opportunity to help other people and charities
- Time to travel, visit, and explore

Most people do not develop psychiatric disorders in old age, but social problems can make older people more vulnerable to mental health and emotional problems. Some social problems require interventions from social workers, from the local community, and from church groups. Nurses should be aware of the extent social problems influence the health status of older people.

Organic brain disorders (confusion)

Organic brain disorders are impairments in the functioning of the brain that cause disturbances of behaviour and awareness. The most common conditions of organic brain disorder that lead to confusion are delirium and dementia.

Confusion

An impairment of memory, thought processes, and awareness of surroundings. The emotions and coordinating functions of the brain are also disturbed.

Delirium or acute confusional state

Can occur at any age but frail older people are more susceptible to it, especially when they suffer from ill health and cognitive impairment. Usually it disappears when the underlying illness or cause is resolved (i.e. it is reversible).

Many people, irrespective of their age, exhibit delirium or confusion on admission to hospital. In some patients these conditions may develop as a reaction to hospitalization itself. For older people these conditions may be more common, especially in patients with less cognitive reserve. The level of consciousness may fluctuate from drowsiness to stupor or coma or the individual may be restless or hyperactive.

Perceptual disturbances may precipitate misinterpretation of factors in the environment leading to illusions or hallucinations (usually visual). Other symptoms include disorganized thinking, incoherent speech, depression, irritability, anger, apathy, euphoria, mood changes, fear, and sleep disturbances.

Causes

- Infections
- High fever
- Chest and urinary sepsis
- Cerebral hypoxia or hypoperfusion
- Toxic substances and drugs
- Withdrawal of alcohol
- Injury to the brain
- Constipation
- Fluid and electrolyte imbalances
- Hypothermia
- Sensory overload or deprivation

Nursing interventions and care

- Recognize and identify the cause.
- Protect patient from harm.
- Provide a calming environment, consistent carer/nurse, soft lights, music, and familiar objects.
- Simplify patient's world; keep informed of time, day, and surroundings; explain all routines and procedures.
- Use simple direct language—do not lie or play fantasy games.
- Give constant reassurance.

- Restrict visitors to close friends and relatives at appropriate times.
- Where restlessness is a problem, care for patient in a low bed. Do not use restraints; take them for walks.
- Reduce light and noise at night.
- Explain the nature of delirium and nursing actions to relatives.
- Regularly assess mental and emotional status.
- Report and record behaviour in nursing records.
- Slowly introduce more active and complex routines when patient is improving.
- Minimize medications and review those needed for patients being treated for acute confusion.

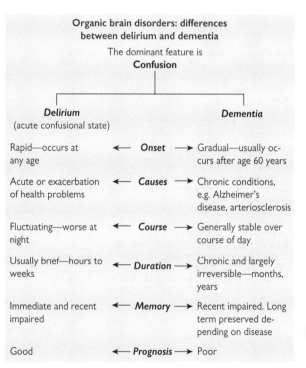

Organic brain disorders: differences between delirium and dementia

The dominant feature is
Confusion

Delirium (acute confusional state)		**Dementia**
Rapid—occurs at any age	← **Onset** →	Gradual—usually occurs after age 60 years
Acute or exacerbation of health problems	← **Causes** →	Chronic conditions, e.g. Alzheimer's disease, arteriosclerosis
Fluctuating—worse at night	← **Course** →	Generally stable over course of day
Usually brief—hours to weeks	← **Duration** →	Chronic and largely irreversible—months, years
Immediate and recent impaired	← **Memory** →	Recent impaired. Long term preserved depending on disease
Good	← **Prognosis** →	Poor

Assessment of confusion

JOMAC method
- J: *Judgement* – Ask patient how they make judgements in certain situations and for certain tasks, e.g. how they decide which social activities to become involved in, or, when feeling ill, at what point they decide to call or visit the doctor.
- O: *Orientation* – Ask patient time, place, person.
- M: *Memory* – Ask questions relating to recent events and to events in the distant past.
- A: *Affect* – Ask about feelings and moods and observe behaviour for appropriateness.
- C: *Cognition* – Ask questions relating to new material and ability to comprehend its meaning.

Other signs of confusion
- Decreased ability to perform daily living activities
- Signs of wandering or intrusive behaviour
- Verbal disruption or noise
- Physical aggression
- Emotional dependence
- Danger to self and others
- Attention-seeking or difficult behaviour

Key to successful nursing care
- Protect the patient.
- Work with family and friends.
- Encourage orientation and honesty with what is going on in the patient's environment.
- Do not rush the patient.
- Understand the patient's world.
- Use reminiscence therapy.
- Reduce stress and encourage a calm environment.
- Provide appropriate positive stimulation suited to the individual patient, e.g. music therapy.
- Aim to create a calm, cheerful, and confident atmosphere.

Dementia

Dementia most commonly occurs in patients >60 years, but may occur earlier (referred to as early-onset dementia). It is an irreversible chronic condition that leads to decline in mental and physical abilities. The progress of the disease is slow and patients have an unpredictable life expectancy.

Causes
- Alzheimer's disease (60–70%)
- Multi-infarct or vascular disease (10–20%)
- Mixed pathology (especially Alzheimer's and vascular)
- Trauma and infections
- Rare conditions—severe alcoholism, AIDS, brain tumours, Lewy body dementia, and Parkinson's disease with dementia
- Treatable causes of dementia (<5%) include thyroid disease, drugs, subdural haematoma, normal pressure hydrocephalus, and pseudodementia due to disease.

Diagnosis
No single test is available to diagnose dementia. A detailed medical and psychiatric history is required. Special mental tests are done in a series over time (See Fig. 28.2). Other diagnostic tests include FBC biochemical profile, MSU, ESR, thyroid function tests, serum B_{12} and folate, chest x-ray, ECG, and imaging such as MRI or CT scans.

Clinical features
- Insidious gradual process with functional loss and permanent impairment of intellectual ability and memory
- Loss of interest and initiative – inability to perform up to usual standard
- Minor episodes of muddled thinking and confusion
- Increasing episodes of bizarre inappropriate behaviour
- Difficulty making decisions
- Inability to learn new tasks
- Increasing forgetfulness
- Inability to remember recent events
- Eventually capacity to remember past disappears
- Lack of concern and callousness to loved ones
- Inappropriate sexual and social behaviour
- Restlessness, wandering, and hoarding of useless objects and rubbish

Nursing interventions and care
- Observe and assess the patient carefully.
- Involve close family members and friends who know the patient. Ask them to describe the patient's past and present behaviour.
- Note onset, speed, and progression of symptoms. Usually there is a progressive decline in cognitive function over several years leading to complete dependency. Deterioration may be stepwise, abrupt, or rapid depending on causes.
- Be aware that some patients may have been labelled incorrectly as having dementia, e.g. patients who are deaf, dysphasic, delirious, depressed, or under the influence of drugs.

The Abbreviated Mental Test Score

The Abbreviated Mental Test Score (AMTS) is a widely applicable, well validated, brief screening test of cognitive function (See Fig. 28.2). It was derived by Hodkinson from a 26-item test, by dispensing with those questions which were poor discriminators of the cognitive sound and unsound.

Age	Must be correct (years)
Time	Without looking at timepiece; correct to nearest hour
Short-term memory	Give the address '42 West Street' Check registration Check memory at end of test
Recognition of two persons	For example doctor, nurse, carer
Year	Exact, except in January when previous year is satisfactory. Replies '206', '207', etc. in place of 2006, 2007 should be considered correct, as they confirm orientation
Name of place	If not in hospital ask type of place or area of town
Date of birth	Exact
Start of World War I	Exact
Name of present monarch	Exact
Count from 20 to 1 (backwards)	Can prompt with 20–19–18, but no further prompts. Patient can hesitate and self-correct but no other errors are permitted

Scoring

8–10	Normal
7	Probably abnormal
<6	Abnormal

Fig. 28.2 A dementia test. Adapted with permission from *Classification of Chronic Pain*, 2nd edition, Merskey, H and Bogduk, N (editors), IASP Press, Seattle, 1994.

General guidelines for carrying out intimate procedures such as bathing on people with dementia

- Focus more on the person than the task.
- Observe the person's feelings and reactions. (Is there fear or pain?)
- Always protect privacy and dignity.
- Be flexible—modify approach to meet the needs of the patient.
- Use persuasion not coercion.
- Give choices, negotiate.
- Use distractions such as conversation.
- Praise the person often.
- Be prepared for the task and collect all equipment and prepare environment.
- Stop if person becomes distressed. Look for underlying reasons of the distress.
- Seek help if appropriate.
- Many dementia patients dislike being bathed

Types of disease and patterns of health

There are three major categories of disease in older people.
1. Diseases that occur to varying degrees in a large proportion of aged persons, e.g. arteriosclerosis or cataracts.
2. Diseases that have an increased incidence in aged persons but that do not occur universally, e.g. neoplastic disease, diabetes mellitus, and some dementing disorders.
3. Diseases that have more serious consequences in the elderly because of their reduced ability to maintain homeostasis compared with the young, e.g. pneumonia, influenza, and trauma.

The incidence of acute and chronic conditions can increase with age. More than 80% of older people suffer from a chronic disease, and many suffer from more than one. Older people also suffer disproportionately from functional disabilities related to the normal activities of daily living. Their problems are frequently multiple and complex and require careful assessment, diagnosis, care, and treatment.

Hospital admission

Older people are the greatest users of hospital beds (65% of inpatients are >65 years of age in some acute hospitals). Occupancy rates have never been so high and may become even higher due to people living longer. There are several common reasons for hospital admissions in older people.
- Type of disease process, acute and chronic conditions
- Exacerbations or deterioration in chronic illness
- Frailty and decreased reserve due to chronic disease processes
- Impaired homeostasis leading to problems with coping with an acute illness
- Polypharmacy and the effects of age on pharmacokinetics and pharmacodynamics
- Living alone and social disadvantage, resulting in lack of social care support and nursing care at home
- High incidence of falls

Common reasons for admission of older people to hospital

Note, some of the reasons given below cut across the three areas given.

Physical

- Various infections, including urinary tract infection, pneumonia, and influenza
- Fractures of neck of femur, wrist/arm and pelvis
- COPD
- CCF
- Stroke/TIA/syncope
- MI
- Osteoporosis
- Rheumatoid arthritis
- Parkinson's disease
- Constipation/diarrhoea
- GI Bleed
- Diabetes
- Continence problems
- Cataract
- Glaucoma
- Hernias
- Leg wounds, ulcers and cellulites
- Delirium due to physical causes
- Nutritional problems and dehydration
- Poor appetite and weight loss
- Cancer
- Immobility
- Collapse/generally unwell
- Acute myeloid leukaemia
- Anaemia
- Accidents

Social

- Falls
- Isolation
- Loneliness
- Self neglect
- Environmental problems at home
- Nutritional problems and dehydration
- Decreased mobility
- Medication errors

Mental health

- Loss
- Bereavement issues and not coping
- Depression
- Dementia
- Anxiety
- Psychosis
- Attempted suicide
- Alcoholism

Management of medicines

- Drugs are very powerful therapeutic agents with the potential to cause great harm in older people as well as alleviate symptoms and cure disease.
- Individuals >65 years are the greatest consumers of prescription drugs.
- 75% of older patients have one or more medicines discontinued and new ones started during a hospital stay.
- Some health care professionals fail to properly distinguish between normal biological effects of ageing and disease processes that the elderly patient is suffering. Therefore, prescribers should be very alert to possible drug–disease interactions. Some drug reactions are more common with age because of altered drug dispensing, e.g. digoxin.
- More information is needed on the interactions between severity of illness, age, and altered response to drug therapy.
- The UK National Service Framework for Older People has prioritized the need for appropriate and rational prescribing for older patients.
- Nurses often seek sedation for patients rather than taking the time to understand the underlying cause of the agitation or behavioural problem.
- Drugs can cause adverse reactions and trigger exacerbation of common syndromes (e.g. cognitive impairment, falls, mobility problems, incontinence, and bowel problems such as constipation and diarrhoea).
- Risk factors that predispose to adverse drug reactions include multiple disease, poor health status, and polypharmacy. Inappropriate prescribing can lead to improper use, inadequate dosage, potential drug interaction, therapeutic duplication, no indication for use, or allergy present.
- Start patients on low doses of drugs; make sure the patient has the ability to comply (e.g. rheumatoid arthritis may make it difficult to take pills physically); review treatment and the response regularly; and watch for drug related symptoms.
- The possibility of medication errors should be considered when prescribing many medications, as this may lead to errors in dosage and compliance difficulties. Practice varies from location to location; however, more than five concurrent medications is often held to be 'too many' and the patient's medications may consequently be reviewed in line with their condition.
- Adverse drug reactions may occur as a result of poor concordance.

Common side effects of drugs

Alterations in thought processes and confusion are a common adverse side effect of medication use in the elderly. Because of this baseline mental status testing should be performed in older patients before new regimens are started. When mental alterations due to drug side effects are suspected, nurses should specify the domains of function that are impaired and communicate these to the prescriber. The risk of falls rises with the number of drugs the person is taking. Drugs that interfere with postural control by acting on the autonomic nervous system include beta-blockers, antidepressants, and antipsychotics.

Dizziness is an adverse effect of phenytoin, lithium, and the benzo-diazepines. Syncope is associated with anti-arrhythmics and with hypotension caused by vasodilators, antihypertensives, antidepressants, and diuretics.

Nurses should focus particular attention on teaching older persons and their carers about drugs. Evaluate and monitor drug therapy. Most medications can be discontinued abruptly without adverse complications. However, certain medications cannot. Slow careful withdrawal from a medication can decrease or eliminate the risk of side effects.

Factors to consider when assessing an older patient for medications
- Amount, type, frequency, and purpose
- The individual's ability to take the drug
- Potential for drug interactions and adverse drug reactions
- A baseline from which to evaluate effectiveness of the therapeutic regimen
- Whether any drugs can be discontinued or decreased in dose

Key points for drug taking in older patients
- Limit the number of medications to as few as is necessary.
- Review regularly.
- Increase doses slowly.
- Monitor for drug interactions and side effects.
- Involve patients and carers in their drugs.
- Recognize that older people commonly forget to take medications.
- Teach patients and their carers about the drugs and side effects.
- Regularly reinforce patient and carer teaching, evaluating concordance and progress.

Good nurse–doctor communications over medication management in older people is crucial to good prescribing.

Effects of hospitalization

- Admission to hospital often leads to acute disorientation and confusion. This is exacerbated by moving the older patient from ward to ward or from bed space to bed space.
- Pressure sores result from lengthy waits on hospital trolleys and failure to change the patient's position frequently enough.
- There is concern that many deaths of elderly patients in hospital are precipitated by poor prescribing.
- Many older patients are not given adequate and appropriate nursing time to care for and identify their problems. 📖 Assessing older people, p.902.
- More than 10% of all hospital inpatients suffer from cross-infection, especially MRSA and *Clostridium difficile*, which is now in UK hospitals becoming the biggest nosocomial killer. See 'How to deal with the problem' DH and HPA publication, Jan 2009, www.hpa.org.uk.
- Failure to communicate appropriately with older people leads to misunderstandings about their needs and about their responses to medical and nursing care.
- Broad-spectrum antibiotics may precipitate growth of *Clostridium difficile* and lead to death from severe diarrhoea. See 'How to deal with the problem' DH and HPA Pub., Jan 2009, www.hpa.org.uk.
- Loss of contact with friends and relatives may lead to social isolation and loneliness. (Older people tend to have older relatives who find it difficult to visit, especially in evenings.)
- Dependency and unwillingness to be involved in self-care may develop due to poor staff attitudes and practices that fail to encourage rehabilitation and patient involvement.
- Falls are common because of lack of supervision; agitated and restless behaviour; unsteadiness, poor mobility, or functional problems; and inappropriate use of bed rails and physical and pharmacological restraints.
- Poor nutritional status and dehydration is exacerbated by staff not encouraging and assisting patients with their meals.
- The loss of loved ones and other patients may lead to grief, bereavement, and depression.
- Elder abuse may occur because of lack of knowledge, understanding, and skills essential for nursing older people. 📖 Elder abuse and neglect, p.931.
- Demands on hospital beds may lead to older patients being discharged too soon. This may be precipitated by lack of community services and support.

Ten essentials of nursing care for older people

1. Perform an assessment to determine their level of functioning and nursing need.
2. Develop an individualized nursing care plan specific to their needs.
3. Be involved whenever and wherever possible in their care.
4. Ensure their position is changed regularly, at least 2 hourly, and assess pressures areas, if necessary.
5. Maintain a position that does not compromise their safety, comfort, breathing, feeding, and ability to communicate.
6. Encourage good nutritional and fluid intake.
7. Ensure their mouth is moist and clean.
8. Attend to their personal hygiene and comfort needs.
9. Maintain regular interpersonal communication and pay attention not only to physical needs but also to psychosocial and spiritual needs.
10. Encourage health promotion and rehabilitation where possible.

Ageing is not a disease, but rather a unique life stage with its own rewards and issues.

Ageism

Ageism refers to prejudice or discrimination towards people based on their chronological age or on symbols of old age such as grey hair, physical appearance, or slow shuffling gait. Three elements that cause ageism are stereotyping, biased attitudes, and discriminatory behaviour.

Unfortunately, health care professionals are often guilty of stereotyping of older people. Ageist beliefs and attitudes often cause older people to receive inappropriate treatment or to be excluded from opportunities. Through awareness of the widespread beliefs associated with ageism and through more astute and accurate assessment of older people's needs, nurses can help their elderly patients combat ageism.

Although there is no place for ageism in providing health care to older patients, there are important considerations that must be made when caring for older patients. There needs to be an evidence base for carrying out medical treatments on older people. Some interventions may carry a higher risk of harm or injury than others. Therefore consent from the patient or their relatives is essential and should be obtained carefully and considerately. Chapter 30, Consent to treatment, principles of the Mental Capacity Act, pp.976–7.

Elder abuse and neglect

Elder abuse and neglect refers to the wilful infliction of physical pain, injury, debilitating mental anguish, unreasonable confinement or the wilful deprivation of services that are necessary to maintain physical and mental health of older people.

Physical abuse includes rough handling, forcing patients to sit down or stay in one position, force feeding, smacking, punching, withholding, or inappropriately forcing medical and nursing tasks/procedures on patients.

Psychological abuse includes shouting and verbal assaults, demands to perform demeaning tasks, making threats, isolating an older person, calling them names, and making fun of them.

Financial and possession abuse includes theft, mismanagement of money and personal belongings, and persuading or ignoring the old person's opinion regarding their home and its contents.

Common indicators
- Abrasions
- Cuts and lacerations
- Bruises
- Burns from various sources
- Sprains
- Fractures
- Dislocations
- Pressure sores
- Injuries inconsistent with history
- History of falls
- Untreated medical problems
- Inappropriate clothing
- Poor hygiene
- Excessive drowsiness
- Over-medication
- Malnutrition/dehydration
- Unusual behaviour—signs of anger, fear, or nervousness especially when a certain person is present or has visited the patient

Social abuse

- Includes restricting movement, forcing the person out of their own home, and not allowing social contacts and family and friends to visit.
- Neglect refers to a lack of services that are necessary for the physical and mental health of the older person who is living alone or who is not able to provide self-care. Neglect may be by self or another. It is more difficult to define than abuse because it is a more subtle form of mistreatment.
- Passive neglect occurs when the carer is incompetent to help and active neglect occurs when the carer intentionally withholds help and services.
- Self-neglect occurs when the older person themselves refuses help and chooses an unhealthy and unsafe lifestyle. This right to self-determination is a closely guarded value in Britain, and raises many ethical and legal issues.
- Abuse may occur in residential and nursing homes. The NMC and professional misconduct statistics in the UK provide evidence that elderly people are most likely to be abused by carers and nurses, irrespective of where the patient is nursed.
- Risk factors for elder abuse include social isolation, female gender, advancing age, past history of family conflict or abuse, alcohol abuse, and stressed carer.
- Educational programmes and physical help aimed at families who are caring for older people may help reduce abuse occurring.

How to manage suspected abuse

1. Document your suspicions carefully based on accurate observations and by recording what precisely the patient has said and what you have seen.
2. Support the patient and explore ways of dealing with the abuser and their behaviour.
3. Reduce the likelihood of it occurring by removing the patient from the situation.
4. Keep a close observation on the situation and involve other members of the multidisciplinary team.
5. You may need to approach the carer as the cause of the abuse can be due to carer strain and help with caring may be a solution.
6. Inform your senior manager, specialist nurse, and the medical staff/GP.
7. Involve other agencies such as social services, local authorities, and (rarely at first) the police.

Further information

Action on Elder Abuse www.elderabuse.org.uk

Health promotion and education

- Recognize that ageing is not a disease, but rather a unique life-stage with its own rewards and issues. Older people can slow the ageing process and enhance the quality of their life by engaging in healthy habits such as exercise, nutrition, and modifying their risk factors to disease.
- An important nursing intervention in the case of older adults is to encourage greater personal responsibility for health through health promotion.
- Be aware of how culture affects beliefs and values as it can have a profound effect on a patient's health behaviour. Ageing is viewed differently by different cultures.
- Encourage older adults to perform as many activities of daily living as possible, taking extra time if needed.
- Encourage physical activities and exercise.
- Set progressive physical activity goals with the patient, suitable to the patient's health condition to maintain patient autonomy and involvement with their care.
- Identify and eliminate hazards in the environment.
- Identify educational needs and learning methods suitable for teaching health promotion to older people.
- Carefully assess an older adult's risk factors for experiencing a fall and plan interventions to reduce the risk.
- Encourage older people to have regular check-ups, especially blood pressure, serum cholesterol, pap smear, eye and ear examinations, prostate checks, and bone density scans for osteoporosis. Not all these are easily available through the GP, but there are now other services developing such as pharmacy, drop in centres, and private assessment clinics.
- Encourage annual influenza and pneumonia vaccination.
- Recognize that patient education and teaching is one of the most important components of caring for an older person with a chronic illness. Provide written materials/handouts to augment topics and eliminate distractions, and frequently summarize information. Keep teaching/learning sessions relatively short and schedule frequent breaks. Evaluate and audit effects of teaching and education.

Methods to promote mental activity

- Solving crossword puzzles
- Reading
- Completing jigsaw puzzles
- Cooking with new recipes
- Sewing and needlepoint
- Dancing
- Exercising
- Debating
- Writing

Methods to promote physical activity

- Exercise regularly.
- Maintain a healthy body weight.
- Decrease alcohol consumption.
- Eat a healthy diet, low in sodium and fat.
- Avoid smoking.
- Dance.
- Keep a pet.

Community and home care

- The goal of community-based services is to promote the independence of older people and to provide an alternative to traditional hospital care. It can consist of special nurses and members of the hospital or community multidisciplinary health care team following up patients immediately they are discharged home. In some situations some acute hospitals have arrangements with nursing homes for intermediate care. These are known as 'step down' beds. Community hospitals also commonly provide step down care.
- Transferring patients out of hospital back home requires the implementation of home assessment and risk reduction strategies. These will be assessed by the multidisciplinary team in conjunction with the patient and their home carers.
- The multidisciplinary team consists of occupational therapists, physiotherapists, dietitians, speech therapists, social workers, care managers, physicians, and nurses.
- Home assessment involves determining whether the older patient and, where available, their carer can cope with their health problem at home and what help and possible devices or home adaptations they may need.
- For many frail older people, home care is often preferable to having to give up their independent life style. It may therefore be possible to provide nursing and social care support at home. Meals on wheels, shopping, laundry, and cleaning services may also be provided for older people at home.
- Community nurses provide essential nursing care for patients in their own homes and also attend those in care homes as well. Such nursing care includes wound care, palliative care, attention to certain long-term care treatments and the fundamentals of nursing, such as mouth care and bed bathing.
- Special day centres have also been developed to provide care for older people, e.g. there are special centres for people with dementia. Other day centres provide luncheon clubs and a variety of other services such as exercise classes, social activities, and educational opportunities.
- Day hospitals provide special health facilities and rehabilitation services for older people who require more physical and mental health care while living at home.
- A wide variety of voluntary and social support agencies provide services for older people in their own homes, e.g. good neighbours and special home visiting services and transport for isolated individuals.
- Nursing or 'care' homes, as they are now referred to, provide institutional alternatives for older people with chronic nursing and social care needs. They provide a vast variety of services geared to individual needs. These homes are monitored much more stringently now than they were in the past.
- Sheltered housing and warden-controlled flats provide social independent living.

Discharging older patients home

Key considerations

- Type of community/home support
- Availability of spouse, family member, or carers
- Any pre-hospital problems
- Home environment layout and design
- Need for adaptation or assistive devices
- Need for specialized medical equipment, e.g. oxygen, pain relief devices
- Supplies for needs such as wound care, diabetes, and ostomy care
- Amount of professional intervention and back up services needed, type of package of care, e.g. GP follow up, community nurse care
- Ability to care for self and functional activities of daily living
- Risk of falls and self-neglect
- Medication concordance
- Adequate health care teaching and information to cope at home
- Any relevant care plans and information for future carers
- Mental health status
- Sensory deficits
- Pressure care equipment, e.g. pressure-relieving mattress
- Referral to district nurse for 'over 70s visit'
- Transport needs

Skin care for older people

Major skin care changes are one of the many features occurring with ageing. It is estimated that >70% of older people suffer from skin problems. The Associate Parliamentary Group on Skin (APGS, 2000) conducted a report into skin problems in the elderly and highlighted, among other things, the importance of basic skin care including the regular and correct use of emollients to prevent common skin problems such as dryness, itching, and asteatotic eczema in older people. Unfortunately, the skin care needs of older people are often neglected.

Changes in the skin due to ageing

- The epidermis gradually becomes thinner and thus more susceptible to mechanical injury, due to moisture, friction, and trauma.
- The dermis changes and results in fewer sweat glands and reduced production of sebum.
- Changes to the epidermis and dermis make the skin more vulnerable especially when the skin is cleansed with soaps which increase the skin's pH to an alkaline level.
- The skin's surface is further put at risk by the effects of dehydration, alteration in the normal bacterial flora, and colonization with more pathogenic species.
- A reduction in elastin fibres results in the skin becoming easily stretched and at the risk of tearing and trauma.
- The thickness of the dermis is reduced by 20%, giving the skin its 'paper thin' appearance.
- There is a reduction in the blood vessels, nerve endings, and collagen which may lead to decrease in sensation, temperature control, rigidity, and moisture retention.

Nursing history and assessment of the older person with skin problems

Ask the patient

- How long has the condition been present?
- What have they noticed or experienced with their skin problem?
- How often does it occur or recur?
- Are there any seasonal variations?
- Are there any known allergies?
- Is there a family history?
- What previous treatments have they had and how effective were they?
- What factors do they think influence their condition?

The nurse should also review the patient's medications and any other source of drugs or applications to the skin. Discuss possible emotional and stressful situations in the patient's life. Assess:

- The presence of any medical condition which may affect the skin.
- The overall general health of the patient and their medical history.

Examine the patient

- Perform a careful assessment of the whole area of the patient's skin – head to toe. 📖 Chapter 12, Nursing assessment of patients with dermatology and skin needs, p.396.
- Assess skin characteristics, e.g. changes, breaks, colour, texture.
- Note signs of infestation, scratching, rashes, and condition of the nails.
- Note where the skin problem exists and how widespread the condition is.
- Record carefully in the patient's nursing notes the condition of the skin and any areas of concern.
- May need to draw a diagram of the patient's body and problem site(s). Record dimentions of any lesions and consider photographing areas such as pressure sores for reference (obtain patient's permission).

Common skin conditions affecting the older person

Skin disease categories are shown in Table 28.1.

Table 28.1 Skin disease categories (Norman, 2003)

Eczematous

Eczematous conditions are very common in this age group and include

Asteatotic eczema (eczema cragueie)

Gravitational eczema (stasis or varicose)

Allergic contact eczema

Irritant contact eczema

Discoid (nummular) eczema

Infections

Bacterial – impetigo

Viral – herpes zoster

Fungal – Candidiasis, tinea pedis, tinea cruris and onychomycosis

Infestations

Pediculosis (lice) – head, body and pubic scabies

Lesions

Benign – seborrhoeic keratosis, actinic keratosis

Malignant – basal cell carcinoma, squamous cell carcinoma, melanoma

Others

Nutrient deficiency disorders – chronic diseases and poor diet may contribute to vitamin deficiencies. Iron deficiency may also cause pruritis (itch)

Vascular – chronic venous insufficiency and peripheral vascular disease, purpura, caused by thrombocytopenia, platelet abnormalities, vascular defects, trauma and drug reactions.

Bullous pemphigoid

Eight key areas of skin care for older persons
- Effects of pruritus
- Dry, vulnerable tissue
- Damage to the skin due to pressure (pressure ulcers)
- Effects on the skin due to incontinence
- Effects on the skin due to maceration
- Skin tears
- Environmental factors
- Changes in normal skin lesions

Pruritus
Pruritus (itchy skin) induces scratching and is often linked to an underlying skin condition such as eczema or systemic disease such as iron deficiency but is often idiopathic. Apart from scratch marks, the skin itself may look normal. Occasionally it may be due to a psychogenic cause. Pruritus may lead to sleeplessness, and exhaustion and disrupt daily living activities.
- Keep the environment cool and dust free and instruct patients to wear loose cotton clothing.
- Ensure emollients are used to wash and moisturize the skin.
- Avoid products that may irritate the skin such as perfumes, bubble baths, soap based products, and talcum powder.
- May use sedating antihistamines, emollients and topical antipruritics such as menthol in aqueous cream.

Dry, vulnerable tissue
This can be dangerous because as skin becomes dry it splits and cracks which can lead to exposure to bacterial contamination and infection.
- Use a soap substitute emollient and moisturizer.
- Gently rub soap substitute into the skin and wash off, then apply an emollient or moisturizer immediately after.
- Apply lightly when the skin has a high water content.
- Use twice a day or more according to the condition of the skin.

Pressure ulcers
📖 Chapter 12, Pressure ulcers: assessment and prevention, p.424 and 📖 Chapter 12, Pressure ulcers: management, p.426.

Older people are vulnerable to pressure ulcers which are caused by direct pressure, shearing, and friction. They usually occur over a bony prominence such as the sacrum, ischial tuberosity, and heels (See Fig. 28.3 and Fig. 28.4). Other factors which exacerbate the situation include moisture; poor mobility and movement; poor nutrition; and underlying medical conditions, medications and poor physical state of the person.
- Assess carefully using special risk assessment aids.
- Treat and avoid by altering the patient's position regularly.
- Nurse on special pressure relieving support surface.
- Treat according to expert advice and evidence-based guidelines.
- Involve specialist nurses.

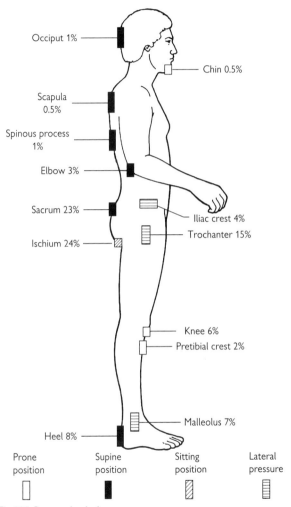

Fig. 28.3 Pressure ulcer body map.

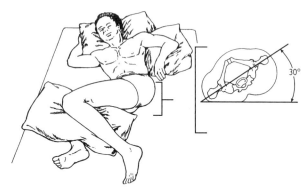

Fig. 28.4 Thirty-degree lateral position at which pressure points are avoided.

Effects on the skin due to incontinence

Older people have a higher incidence of both faecal and urinary incontinence which can quickly affect the skin. Skin pH levels are changed from a mean of 5.5 (slightly acidic) to alkaline, and ammonia is produced when micro-organisms digest urea. The perianal area is most at risk. Incontinence may lead to skin reaction, excoriation, and breakdown.

- Clean the skin and dry it carefully.
- Use a protective barrier cream or spray.
- Check the patient regularly, keep dry, and encourage regular toileting.
- Refer to a specialist continence adviser. 📖 Urinary continence and incontinence, p.908.

Effects on the skin due to maceration

Maceration refers to the process of softening due to soaking. Maceration causes skin to become soft and wrinkled leading to skin breakdown. It may be due to incontinence, excess moisture from sweating, wound exudates, or peristomal exudates. Treatment involves protecting the skin from maceration and as above for incontinence.

Skin tears

These are common in the older person as the dermis becomes thinner, dryer, and less elastic. They commonly occur on the arm and shin and are caused by trauma, shearing, and friction. The three categories of skin loss are: 1 = no loss, 2 – partial loss 3 = full thickness.

- Treat immediately as an open wound.
- Keep clean.
- Seek specialist advice if necessary.

Environmental factors

Premature ageing of the skin occurs due to overexposure to sun (photoageing), repeated ultraviolet (UV) exposure, environmental pollutants, and smoking. Protect and teach older people about effects and avoidance of exposure.

Changes in normal skin lesions

Skin lesions, moles, and warts may change as the skin ages. These changes may be a signal of malignancy. Look for some aspect of the lesion to have changed in size or shape, irregular edge of lesion, colour (blacks, browns, reds, greys, etc. in the same lesion). Note that symptoms usually develop over time. Symptoms that develop rapidly (e.g. overnight) may be due to trauma. If in doubt refer to specialist nurse or doctor. Excision biopsy and removal may be necessary.

Nail care for older people

- Older people's nails are affected as any other person's nails would be by congenital anomalies, trauma, and disease or ill health.
- Longitudinal ridging is very common as is ischaemic dystrophy of the toenails which results in thickened, brittle, and hard nails.
- Crumbly nails occur with fungal infections.
- Check the older patient's nails regularly and skin condition of the feet.
- Keep nails short and clean.
- Refer to a chiropodist for expert help and advice.

Further information

www.dh.gov.uk
www.statistics.gov.uk/focuson/olderpeople
www.scotland.gov.uk/topics/people/olderpeople
www.wales.gov.uk/topics/olderpeople
www.olderpeoplewales.com
www.patient.co.uk/showdoc137/seniorshealthinfo
www.ageconcern.org.uk
www.opin.org.uk (older people's information network)
www.rcpsych.ac.uk/mentalhealthinfoforall/olderpeople

Mouth care for older people

- Nursing assessment and help with older people's dental/mouth care is essential, especially if they are unable to care for their own needs
  - Check patient's mouth care regularly especially if they are showing signs of a dry mouth and lips.
  - Observe and examine the patient's mouth with a good source of light.
  - Look for any soreness of the tongue (which might be due to the effects of drugs, fungal infections of the mouth, or oral candidiasis), acute bacterial parotitis (especially in frail older people), mouth ulcers (sometimes due to ill-fitting dentures or inflammatory bowel disease), and the condition of any teeth.
- Poor oral and dental health contributes to poor appetite and malnutrition.
- Refer the patient to a dentist if they are complaining of any pain and discomfort and have not had a recent dental check.
- In some older people dentures may not fit very well and a reassessment is needed.
- Consider helping patients use their toothbrush if they are having any difficulties conducting their own oral hygiene or if care is poor.
- Consider chlorhexidine mouthwashes regularly following meals.

Sleep and rest needs in older people

- With increasing age less sleep is needed, but sleep pattern changes with more daytime 'catnapping' and less sleep at night.
- Around 25% of older people suffer from chronic insomnia and this figure is higher in older people with psychiatric and medical conditions.
- Assess the possible causes such as noisy wards, pain at night, breathing difficulties, depression, and the effects of medications.
- Treat by reducing or stopping daytime catnapping, and avoid stimulants such as caffeine, heavy meals, and too much alcohol.
- Check environment is conducive to sleeping.
- Use relaxing techniques and warm drinks.
- Finally consider short courses of sedative drugs.

Nursing the child and adolescent

Standards of children's care

The health and well-being of children depends on socioeconomic and environmental factors as well as health factors. Therefore, health, social, and education agencies must work closely together to ensure the well-being of children. The Children's National Service Framework (NSF) set out 11 standards for improving child health.

- *Standard 1: promoting health and well-being, identifying needs, and intervening early.* This requires putting a joint agency programme in place to promote the standards set out in *Every Child Matters: Change for Children* including promoting a healthy lifestyle, reducing health inequalities, and ensuring children and young people have access to relevant services and support.
- *Standard 2: supporting parents.* Parents should have information, services, and support to ensure they can provide their children with optimum life chances and to ensure their children are healthy and safe.
- *Standard 3: child, young person, and family-centred services.* This aims to ensure that children and their families receive information, that they are listened to and respected (i.e. their views are considered when planning and commissioning services), and that staff who work with children are appropriately trained and ensure safe practice.
- *Standard 4: growing up to adulthood.* This aims to ensure that age-appropriate services are provided for children as they grow and mature as adolescents and that a planned and coordinated transition to adult services occurs.
- *Standard 5: safeguarding and promoting the welfare of children and young people.* This aims to ensure agencies work together to safeguard children and prevent them from being harmed.
- *Standard 6: children and young people who are ill.* This requires children to have access to comprehensive and integrated local services, support and advice to provide self-care, and access to trained and competent professionals and high quality treatment.
- *Standard 7: children and young people in hospital.* This aims to ensure children have access to evidence-based safe practices in appropriate settings to meet their needs.
- *Standard 8: disabled children and young people and those with complex health needs.* This aims to ensure early diagnosis and interventions for health problems, easy access to well-planned services, palliative care, and the promotion of social inclusion for children with complex needs.
- *Standard 9: the mental health and psychological well-being of children and young people.* This requires that children receive specialist support from early years. Staff working with children should be able to offer mental health promotion and early interventions.
- *Standard 10: medicines for children and young people.* This aims to ensure that safe medicine practices for children are followed. It includes providing clear information for patients and their parents about risks and benefits. It aims to ensure that safeguards are in place for all children, but especially for those in special circumstances, e.g. with mental ill health.

- *Standard 11: maternity services.* This aims to ensure that women have supportive high-quality maternity services which provides the right start for health and development of children.

Further information

Glasper EA and Lowson S (2006). 'Contemporary child health policy: the implications for children's nurses', in Glasper EA and Richardson J (eds) *A textbook of children's and young people's nursing*, pp. 33–53. Churchill Livingstone, Elsevier, Edinburgh.

Department of Health (2004). *National Service Framework for children, young people and maternity services.* Department of Health, London.

Principles of nursing

- The child's and family's needs are the focus of care and the nurse must consider the central role of the family in the child's life. Parents should be given information, service, support, and teaching to enable them to be involved in decision making about their child's care.
- Children and young people should be cared for in specific wards that:
  - have restricted access
  - are bright and cheerful
  - are safe and secure with play areas
  - have separate treatment rooms
  - have separate areas for adolescents which reflect their specific needs.
- Specially trained children's nurses should provide care. All general hospitals should have a senior nurse to oversee the provision of care for children and young people. General nurses caring for children should have appropriate supervision or special training, for example in areas such as emergency departments where sick children receive care.
- Specially trained play staff are a key part of the team.
- Distraction techniques should be used during invasive procedures to reduce stress and pain.
- Wards should have a school teacher or links to the local Education Authority to ensure that children with long-term conditions continue their education and retain links with their school.
- Parents should be encouraged to have a presence on the ward and participate in care. Residential facilities with appropriate amenities (e.g. toilets, showers, and rest rooms) should be available.
- Children should be prepared in advance for hospital.
  - Use videos, leaflets, books, stories, and visits, if possible.
  - Provide simple and accurate explanations to the patient, parents, and siblings.
  - Describe different staff roles, ward routine, facilities available, and procedures.
  - Answer questions honestly.
  - Give specific instructions about what to bring, what is allowed, and what is not allowed. Most hospitals have a pre-admission service for this.
- Children admitted to an emergency department have special needs and should not be exposed to hostile sights and sounds. Separate areas for assessment and treatment of children in emergency departments and specially trained children's nurses as part of the skill mix are components of best practice.
- Administration of medications for children is important. Two nurses should carefully calculate the correct dosage, promote concordance, and be familiar with how to administer the medication by different routes. Simple explanations for the purpose of the medications should be given.
- The nurse should ensure that the child receives adequate nutrition. Alternatives should be chosen if the child is unwilling or unable to eat.

- Maintaining fluid balance is important in caring for a sick child. Periods of fasting should be kept to a minimum and the child should be carefully monitored to prevent dehydration. IV therapy should be given if necessary.
- Assessment of a child's pain is essential and specially tailored tools can be used. Medication and physical and psychological interventions should be used to help reduce the pain and the child's fears.

Further information

Smith L, Coleman V, and Bradshaw M (2006). 'Family central care', in Glasper A and Richardson J (eds), *A textbook of children's and young people's nursing*, pp. 77–88. Churchill Livingstone, Elsevier, Edinburgh.

Nursing assessment

Assessment is the basis for making decisions about how to nurse a sick child. Both subjective and objective data should be gathered within a conceptual nursing framework. The assessment and planning of care should be undertaken in partnership with the family.

The environment should be reassuring, specially created for children, and should create an opportunity for the nurse to develop a relationship with the child and parents.

Observe the patient
- General appearance: lethargy, unresponsive, clean, or dirty
- Airway and breathing: signs of respiratory distress (e.g. grunting, apnoea, recession, nasal flaring), body position and posture, rate and depth of breathing, blocked nostrils, sweating, cough, wheeze, stridor
- Colour: pallor (shock, anaemia), cyanotic (cardiac or respiratory problems), flushed (pyrexia), jaundice (hepatic problems), dehydrated (dry mouth, lips, mucous membranes; sunken fontanelle in babies)
- Temperature: pyrexia or hypothermia
- Vital signs: pulse rate and pattern (tachycardia, bradycardia), blood pressure (ensure the cuff is the correct size for the child)
- Irritability, agitation, changed level of consciousness (decreased level may be due to shock, sepsis, ingestion of depressants, metabolic abnormalities, hypothermia, or head injury); bulging fontanelle suggests raised intracranial pressure
- Head-to-toe physical assessment
  - Weight, height, and head circumference to check if in normal range
  - Chest and abdomen for asymmetrical movement, abdominal distension, bowel sounds
  - Skin for turgor, rashes (purpura, petechiae, macules, papules), bruises (clotting disorders, injuries), injuries (e.g. fractures, lacerations, non accidental or incidental)
  - Body fluids—urine, faeces, vomit, sputum characteristics and amount
  - Signs of pain, including body position and crying

Ask the patient and parents about
- Their views of the patient's needs and concerns
- The patient's normal temperament and behaviour and what any changes might indicate (e.g. relationships with other children, siblings, problems at school)
- Developmental history and delay
- Normal activities of living; normal diet history, food likes and dislikes; rest and activity patterns; special routines at bedtime; hobbies
- The patient's usual home routine—to help create a familiar environment in hospital
- Previous experiences of illness or hospitals; immunization history; previous illnesses, conditions, and accidents; long-term conditions; care arrangements; resources; coping strategies and support required; and impact on family
- Current problems, onset and duration, medication history, duration, concordance, reactions

Creating a positive environment for assessment

- If possible, spend time talking to the child and parents before the assessment to gain their confidence and establish a positive relationship. Observe the child and the parents and their interactions.
- Depending on the age of the child, consider using toys or books to comfort the child or to help them understand what is going to happen to them, e.g. take a doll's temperature to demonstrate what will happen to the child.
- Explain things to the child and parents in a way that they understand so that they can provide informed consent. Select words carefully as they can be interpreted differently by a child.
- Be sensitive while questioning the child to prevent any embarrassment and to reduce anxiety. Some older children and young people may be more willing to answer questions or confide in the nurse if the parents are not present.
- Carefully plan observations, assessments, and interventions to ensure the minimum amount of time is spent disturbing the child, especially if they are very sick.
- Where possible, encourage the child to participate, e.g. let them handle a stethoscope but ensure they understand which equipment they must not touch.
- Some children may find some aspects of the assessment and examination embarrassing, e.g. undressing. Take care to ensure privacy and dignity as would be done for an adult.

Further information

Casey A (2006). 'Assessing and planning care in partnership', in Glasper A and Richardson J (eds). *A textbook of children's and very young people's nursing*, pp 89–103. Churchill Livingstone, Elsevier, Edinburgh.

Common medical problems

Febrile convulsions

A febrile convulsion or febrile seizure (FS) is an event precipitated by fever in children. It is relatively common in children between 6 months and 5 years of age. Pyrexia is usually over 38.8°C and the FS usually occurs as the temperature rises. Risk factors include:

- Family history
- Temperature <40°C for the first FS
- Age <15 months for first FS

Nursing care

- Prepare to manage an unconscious child, in extreme cases.
- Position the patient so that they come to no harm.
- Give antipyretics as prescribed.
- Administer rectal diazepam or buccal midazolam for repeated convulsions.
- Provide explanations to parents to reduce fear and advise what to do if an FS recurs.

Diarrhoea and vomiting

Proper diagnosis and treatment depends on an assessment. Is the vomiting projectile? (may indicate pyloric stenosis) Is it bile stained or faecal? (may indicate obstruction) Is it due to regurgitation or haematemesis? Is it accompanied by abdominal pain or distension, pyrexia, or signs of dehydration? Treatment depends on the cause. Determine whether anyone in the family is suffering from the same symptoms.

Nursing care

- Focus on rehydration (oral, NG, or IV fluids).
- Ensure hygiene, mouth care, and prevention of skin excoriation.
- Provide adequate relief of pain.
- Monitor vital signs and symptoms.
- Reduce pyrexia.
- Note the characteristic of the stool (loose, watery, offensive smell).
- Obtain specimens for microscopy, culture, and sensitivity to detect infection.
- Give support and education to the parents and child.
- Implement infection control measures to prevent cross-infection when gastroenteritis is suspected.

Anaemia

The oxygen-carrying capacity of the blood is reduced. Tiredness, lethargy and listlessness, anorexia, and pallor are early signs of anaemia in children followed by weakness, tachycardia, and palpitations at a later stage. Types of anaemia include iron deficiency, megaloblastic (folic acid and B_{12} deficiency), aplastic (depression of blood production), haemolytic (rapid destruction of red blood cells), and sickle cell (abnormal Hb). Thalassaemia (deficiency in synthesis of α or β globulin in Hb) and haemophilia (lack of factor VIII for clotting) are also types of anaemia. Treatment depends on the type of anaemia. 📖 Chapter 16, Anaemia, p.576.

Nursing care

- Give dietary advice and support (foods rich in iron or that facilitate iron absorption) and suggest suitable meals; refer to dietitian.
- Administer blood transfusions, if required, and take safety precautions to minimize risks.
- Give advice on prevention of sickle cell crisis (importance of maintaining hydration and how to recognize fluid loss and prevent infection).
- Teach how to recognize signs of bleeding in haemophiliacs and stress the importance of seeking prompt medical help if signs of sickle crisis occur.
- Provide education, support, and advice for parents of children/young people with long-term anaemias and give details of support agencies to enable them to cope at home.
- Stress the importance of wearing alert bracelets.
- Educate the family regarding the prescribed medication and importantly its safe storage.
- Remember iron supplements can be extremely toxic when taken in excess.

Further information

Harrison M (2006). 'Care of a child with febrile convulsions', in Glasper EA, McEwing G, and Richardson J. (eds), pp. 260–61. *Oxford handbook of children's and young people's nursing.* Oxford University Press, Oxford

Pengelly T (2006). 'Gastroenteritis', in Glasper EA, McEwing G, and Richardson, J (eds), pp. 348. *Oxford handbook of children's and young people's nursing.* Oxford University Press, Oxford

Price J (2006). 'Anaemia', in Glasper EA, McEwing G, and Richardson J (eds), pp. 868–9, *Oxford handbook of children's and young people's nursing.* Oxford University Press, Oxford

Common respiratory conditions

Upper respiratory tract infection

This type of infection usually includes acute rhinitis and inflammation of pharynx, but also otitis media, epiglottitis, croup, and sinusitis. Most are caused by viruses, and a small percentage by bacteria such as *H. influenzae*. Therefore, antibiotics are usually of little value. Extreme care should be taken if taking a throat swab from any unvaccinated child as rarely the illness can be caused by epiglottitis. 📖 Chapter 14, conditions of the throat, p.534.

Nursing care
- Explain to the child and parents that antibiotics are not effective.
- Advise on symptomatic relief, e.g. offer small amounts of clear fluids and milk often to prevent dehydration; give paracetamol to reduce fever.
- Although there is not a strong evidence base for the use of increased humidity, its use as a placebo is still advocated. Instruct parents on how to increase humidity in the home environment.
- Stress the importance of good handwashing and proper disposal of tissues to prevent the spread of infection and the importance of a smoke-free environment to prevent complications.

Bronchiolitis

Inflammation of the bronchioles usually occurs in the first 6 months of life, but can occur up to a year. It can affect all infants but may be more serious in premature infants, in those with respiratory or cardiac diseases, and in those who are immunosuppressed. It presents with acute coryza, irritable cough, tachypnoea, and feeding difficulty, and may progress to breathlessness, wheeze, cyanosis, pyrexia, and life-threatening apnoea. The causative organism is often the respiratory syncitial virus (RSV) and is one of the commonest causes of hospital admission in young children. Oxygen saturation of <92% in air requires hospitalization and treatment. Continuous monitoring of oxygen saturation with pulse oximetry is mandatory.

Nursing care
- Nurse patients in an isolation cubicle.
- Give humidified oxygen and monitor for bradycardia and apnoea (ventilation may be required).
- Give paracetamol for pyrexia.
- Administer antibiotics if there is evidence of secondary bacterial infection.
- Provide NG feeds or IV fluids as necessary.
- Give support and explanations to parents during this stressful period.

Asthma in children

Approximately 20–25% of children experience asthma to some extent during childhood with 5% having significant problems. Bronchoconstriction, oedema, and hypersecretion of mucus occur in response to many triggers. It occurs primarily with viral (upper) respiratory infections. Wheeze may also be precipitated or exacerbated by atmospheric pollution, house dust mites, or rarely food, drink, and medicines (e.g. NSAIDs). In many children, asthma resolves with time. Children may be asymptomatic between attacks but then develop airway obstruction resulting in wheeze, breathlessness, and occasional cough. Symptoms are worse at night. Chest tightness, vomiting, and loss of appetite may occur. Symptoms are more severe in an acute episode and may be life threatening.

Nursing care
- Support the child in a position that eases respiratory effort.
- Give humidified oxygen therapy.
- Administer drugs (bronchodilators and anti-inflammatory agents, e.g. steroids) and ensure the patient and parents can use the relevant dispenser (e.g. nebulizer, spacer devices).
- Educate the parent and child to improve their understanding of the condition, including how to manage acute episodes, how to avoid triggers and how to use inhalers.

Further information

Slee B (2006). 'Bronchiolitis', in Glasper EA, McEwing G, Richardson J (eds) *Oxford handbook of children's and young people's nursing*, pp. 284, Oxford University Press, Oxford

Parker AN (2006). 'Health problems in early childhood', in Glasper A and Richardson J (eds) *A textbook of children's and young people's nursing*, pp. 665–85, Churchill Livingstone, Elsevier, Edinburgh

Kelsey J and McEwing G (2006). 'Respiratory illness in children', in Glasper A and Richardson J (eds) *A textbook of children's and young people's nursing*, pp. 423–43, Churchill Livingstone, Elsevier, Edinburgh

Surgical care

In addition to general surgical care (📖 Chapter 22, Nursing patients requiring perioperative care, p.761), the following special considerations for children and parents should be made.

- Tailor preparation to the child's developmental level.
- Refer patients and their parents to pre-admission clinics or talks to groups of children (e.g. Saturday clubs), which can help prepare patients and their parents for planned surgery.
- Consider using colouring books to help children understand what will be happening to them or consider asking them to draw, which may reveal concerns or anxieties about the effect of surgery on body image.
- In an emergency situation, give as much information as possible to the child and parents.
- Ensure preoperative weight is measured accurately to calculate anaesthetic and postoperative drugs.
- Ensure both the child and parents are fully informed and give consent.
- Check for loose teeth.
- Encourage parents to accompany child to the anaesthetic room and ensure a favourite toy or comfort blanket accompanies the child.
- Encourage parents to stay with the child when they come round from the anaesthetic.
- Use pain assessment tools specifically for children.

Common surgical procedures

Elective

- Circumcision—surgical removal of the foreskin due to phimosis or for religious or personal reasons
- Correction of orthopaedic deformities, e.g. talipes equinovarus (club foot) or calcaneovalgus (foot is dorsiflexed and everted)
- Orchidopexy—for undescended or partly descended testes
- Dental extractions—may be done for caries
- Correction of squint—to correct abnormal alignment of the eyes
- Tonsillectomy—removal of the tonsils for children with recurrent tonsillitis or airway obstruction

Emergency

- Appendectomy—commonest surgical emergency; appendicitis presents with low-grade fever, abdominal pain, tenderness, and guarding; initially centrally then localizing in the right iliac fossa
- Hernias—usually inguinal or rarely umbilical (often relieved without surgery) or congenital diaphragmatic hernia (present as neonate); risk of strangulation if repair is not carried out
- Pyloric stenosis—presents with projectile vomiting in a hungry, usually well fed baby; there is hypertrophy and hyperplasia of the pylorus muscles in the stomach; pyloromyotomy (Ramstedt's procedure) is done
- Trauma—e.g. stabilization of fractures, head injury, wounds, etc.

Further information

Shields L and Tanner A (2006). 'Children and surgery', in Glasper A and Richardson J (eds) *A textbook of children's and young people's nursing*, pp. 278–308, Churchill Livingstone, Elsevier, Edinburgh

Mental health problems

Mental health and emotional problems occur in 15–20% of children. As a result, non-specialist nurses may be involved in the care of these children. The role of the non-specialist nurse is as follows.

Identify mental health problems early

These are manifested by abnormalities of behaviour, including conduct problems (e.g. alcohol intoxication, overactivity, tantrums, truancy, stealing, delinquency, sleep problems), delays in development, eating disorders (e.g. anorexia nervosa), elimination problems (e.g. encopresis, enuresis), emotional disorders (e.g. unhappiness, misery, anxiety, phobias, or depression) that may lead to suicide attempts (e.g. drug overdose), or complaints of physical symptoms without cause (e.g. abdominal pain).

Be aware of the risk factors

Recognizing risk factors will help with identifying problems. These include genetic factors; pre- and perinatal injuries; physical disease, especially chronic or neurological disorders (brain injury, infections, tumours); low IQ or learning disabilities; family problems (death, family breakdown and disharmony, hostile relationships); child abuse; parental problems (psychiatric illness, substance abuse); drug and other substance abuse; and socioeconomic disadvantage.

Manage specific events

Eating disorders include anorexia nervosa (obsession with being thin) or bulimia (binge eating followed by weight-controlling activities, e.g. self-induced vomiting, taking diuretics and laxatives, or rigorous exercise; it is usually accompanied by depression). Management includes developing a positive rapport with patient and family; using a firm non-punitive approach where non-eating is not negotiable and privileges depend on eating and gaining weight; and supporting all the family. Family therapy is required.

Self-harm and suicide attempts have an increased incidence in the late teens. Following the management of an acute episode, provide careful and close observation of the child to identify continuing signs of risk, e.g. withdrawn behaviour, expression of ideas about how to kill themselves, feelings of isolation, failure, and hopelessness, and focusing on their problems. It is necessary to provide support for child, parents, and siblings.

Refer to relevant multidisciplinary team members

This may include psychiatrists, members of the Child and Adolescent Mental Health Services (CAMHS) team, social workers, community psychiatric nurses, child and educational psychologists, music or art therapists, and occupational therapists. Continuing liaison with the GP, school, and paediatrician is also important.

Promote emotional and mental health

📕 Promoting emotional and mental health in children and young people, p.959.

Promoting emotional and mental health in children and young people

- Ensure close interaction among health care professionals, social workers, education agencies, the child, and parents.
- Provide good antenatal care to minimize the risk of birth injury. Parentcraft sessions are essential in preparing parents to cope with the child's early development and behaviour.
- Suggest life skills sessions for children in schools to develop problem-solving and coping skills, effective communication skills, self-esteem, and confidence (e.g. coping with bullies and stressful situations) and to develop respectful partnerships with parents and others.
- Educate about the effects of alcohol and drugs and minimizing access to such substances.
- Educate about sexual health and strategies to prevent the risk of teenage pregnancies and sexually transmitted infections.
- Encourage young people to talk through feelings and worries.
- Ensure easy access to school counselling services and particularly school nurses who can identify problems early.
- Find out and address the cause of problems (e.g. bullying or abuse), otherwise treatment is unlikely to be effective.
- Encourage parental guidance and restricting access to violent and aggressive films, programmes, and games.
- Provide explanations about expected behaviour, clear boundaries, and high levels of supervision and training for children with behavioural problems.
- Suggest interventions to help children cope with crises and stressful life events (e.g. bereavement, child abuse, bullying) and to help them and their families develop coping skills and supportive strategies.
- Ensure access to peer support and to help lines, e.g. Samaritans or Childline.
- Advise parents on how to manage their child's behaviour, how to create time to spend with the child, and how to develop effective relationships.
- Advise parents on support services and self-help groups available during periods of crisis such as divorce or when there are specific parent–child relationship problems.
- Guide parents to financial and social support when there are socioeconomic problems.

These can be achieved by all agencies working collaboratively to promote the outcomes framework for children recommended in *Every Child Matters: Change for Children*.

Further information

DH (2004). *Every child matters: change for children*, DH, London.

Cooper M (2006). 'Child and adolescent mental health. The nursing response', In Glasper A and Richardson J (eds), *A textbook of children's and young people's nursing*, pp. 700–19, Churchill Livingstone, Elsevier, Edinburgh

Children/adolescents with long-term conditions

Long-term conditions (LTCs) in children are varied and include physical, sensory, or learning disabilities. Common chronic conditions include cystic fibrosis, coeliac disease, and diabetes. LTCs have an impact not only on the child or adolescent, but also on parents, siblings, grandparents, and other members of the extended family.

Effects of LTC

The diagnosis of LTC has a devastating effect on the family, especially if the condition is potentially fatal. Feelings of shock, denial, anger, guilt, worry, sadness, helplessness, confusion, and depression are common.

For the child/young person there may be disruption of schooling leading to difficulty in learning; problems with relationships, meeting people, making friends, and having a social life; difficulty coping with the physical consequences of the illness (pain, restricted diet, drugs, side effects of treatment); or feelings of dependency. This may lead to poor concordance with treatment plans.

For the parents there may be financial worries if a parent needs to give up work to care for the child; unwillingness to discuss the condition with others and share the burden; inability to spend sufficient time with other family members who feel neglected; difficulty coping with the anxieties, questions, and fears of the child; overprotection of the child; and social isolation if no one can provide respite care for the child.

For siblings there may be jealousy of the attention given to the ill child or feelings that they are being neglected and unloved. There may be feelings of guilt if they are healthy or feelings of worry about being affected themselves.

The role of the nurse

- Recognize the intense grief reaction and help the child, parents, and family express their feelings. Take time to listen.
- Help the family understand the condition and treatment, and what it will mean to them now and in the future. This requires simple straightforward explanations, access to information materials, several opportunities for discussion, further information from support groups and other families in similar circumstances, and possibly counselling.
- Treat each patient as an individual and encourage them to make decisions about their care.
- Recognize the parents' expertise and ensure they have high levels of participation in the child's care; allow them to make choices.
- Help the family establish a support system to share the burden and involve all family members in decision making.

- Identify the family's resources for caring for the child and the support they need including financial and respite care.
- Do not judge the parents if their behaviour is poor; they are likely to be concerned and acting as the child's advocate.
- Ensure continuity of care.

Further information

Elliot B, Callery P, Mould J (2006). 'Chronic Illness and the family', in Glasper A and Richardson J (eds) *A textbook of children's and young people's nursing*, pp. 723–738, Churchill Livingstone, Elsevier, Edinburgh

Childhood infectious diseases

Infections are likely to occur when children first mix with others at nursery, play group, or school. The child can normally be cared for at home, but if symptoms are potentially damaging or life threatening, admission to hospital may be necessary. The benefits of immunization are great in preventing serious infectious diseases.

- *Measles* is a very infectious viral disease. The incubation period is 8–15 days. It presents with fever, coryza, conjunctivitis, and cough followed by Koplik's spots on mucosa of the cheeks and a blotchy pink rash spreading downwards from the head over the whole body. Respiratory complications (e.g. bronchopneumonia and otitis media or encephalitis) may occur. Immunization programmes have reduced morbidity and mortality.

- *Rubella* is usually a mild, but highly infectious, viral condition that may go undetected. The incubation period is 2–3 weeks followed by little or no fever, malaise, a pink rash, and enlargement of the lymph nodes. Rare complications include purpura (with normal or low platelets), encephalitis, and arthritis. Congenital defects and severe disability can occur in the developing fetus if a pregnant mother contracts the infection during the first trimester of pregnancy.

- *Mumps* is a viral infection with fever, malaise, and enlargement of the parotid glands. The incubation period is 2–3 weeks. Symptoms include difficulty swallowing because of pain, tenderness, and swelling, and subside after 7–10 days. Meningitis or epididymo-orchitis, which can reduce fertility in males, may develop as a complication. Immunization reduces the incidence.

- *Chickenpox (varicella)* is highly infectious and is caused by the same virus that produces herpes zoster (shingles). The incubation period is 11–18 days and is followed by mild fever and itchy rash with spots developing from macule to papule to vesicle which dry and leave scabs that usually separate without scarring. Complications are uncommon in immunocompetent children but include shingles, pneumonia, encephalitis, and hepatitis.

- *Pertussis (whooping cough)* is caused by *Bordetella pertussis* and results in a prolonged respiratory illness. After 7 days incubation there is a catarrhal cough and the child is unwell with an upper respiratory tract infection. This is followed by an increasingly severe paroxysmal cough that may be followed by an inspiratory 'whoop' with cyanosis, apnoea, and exhaustion. The cough may last up to 3 months, and may be complicated by pneumonia. Immunization is available.

- *Glandular fever (infectious mononucleosis)* occurs most commonly in adolescents and young adults but also in children. It is caused by the Epstein–Barr virus. Following an incubation period of 4–14 days there is malaise, fever, sore throat, anorexia, swelling, and tenderness of lymph nodes. A macular rash may occur, especially if antibiotics (e.g. amoxicillin) are given. Hepatitis is a complication.

- *Meningitis:* 📖 Chapter 13, Meningitis, p.452.

Nursing care

- Ensure adequate pain relief.
- Keep the child clean and comfortable.
- Encourage fluid intake and light nutritious diet.
- Encourage proper mouth care.
- Teach measures to prevent spread of infection.
- Reassure the child and family.
- Observe for signs of complications.

Further information

Scanlon K and Sorrentino AL (2006). 'Health problems during infancy', in Glasper A and Richardson J (eds) *A textbook of children's and young people's nursing*, pp. 637–664. Churchill Livingston, Elsevier, Edinburgh, www.immunisation.nhs.uk/

Safeguarding children and young people (child protection)

Abuse of a child or adolescent may be physical, psychological, emotional, or sexual. Harm is inflicted either temporarily or over a period of time, intentionally or unintentionally, or harm may be caused by neglect. The perpetrator may be a family member, a non-family member, or another child. All health care professionals must be aware of the special needs and vulnerability of children and have a duty and responsibility to act when there are issues of concern. Abuse can take place anywhere: at home, in nurseries, at school, and in hospitals.

- *Physical abuse* may be physical hurt or injury or even death. Bruising, (frequent, old, and new pinch marks), bites, scratches, knife and razor wounds, burns (e.g. cigarette burns), or fractures (old, healed and new) may be seen.
- *Emotional or psychological abuse* is due to maltreatment, rejection, constant ridicule, and intimidation. It affects the child's behavioural and emotional development. The child may be withdrawn, may display attention-seeking behaviours such as truancy and running away, and may have difficulty with relationships.
- *Sexual abuse* may be incest or other unlawful sexual activities. It results in bleeding and soreness in genital and anal areas, sexually transmitted infections, and emotional trauma.
- *Neglect* is the failure to meet basic essential needs. It results in failure to thrive, hunger, tiredness, destructive behaviours, stealing, low self-esteem, truancy, general poor health, and unclean and unkempt appearance.
- *Fabricated and induced illness* (FII) is where a parent or guardian claims their child has developed an illness when in fact they themselves have made up the symptoms. FII is not diagnosed in the mother or guardian but is identified for the child where there has been
  a) False reporting of symptoms
  b) and/or falsification of specimens, chart changes, etc.
  c) and/or actual induced harm.

The term Munchausen's Syndrome by Proxy is no longer used by health care professionals.

Policies for safeguarding children and young people

- These policies require interagency working and the involvement of hospital physicians, nurses, play leaders, therapists, midwives, health visitors, social workers, GPs, police, school teachers, and others.
- Each local authority has a Local Safeguarding Children's Board (LSCB) with child protection procedures.
- Health care professionals have the autonomy and duty to report concerns to social services in relation to children. All nurses should be aware of their local procedures including reporting out of hours. Anyone can make a referral if they suspect child abuse. Nurses should report suspected child abuse to their line manager, if in accordance with local policy.

- Child Protection Register—contains details of children who are considered at risk or where concerns have previously been raised and should be checked by staff who have concerns, e.g. in the emergency department.
- Each hospital should have a designated physician and nurse for child protection and a lead across the local authority who can provide advice.

Further information

Powell C and Ireland L (2006). 'Protecting children: the role of the children's nurse', in Glasper A and Richardson J (eds) *A textbook of children's and young people's nursing*, pp. 297–308, Churchill Livingstone, Elsevier, Edinburgh

http//www.rcpch.ac.uk/publications/recent/recent_publications/FII.pdf

Child health

Immunization programmes

These have a significant benefit to child health. Table 29.1 summarizes the full immunization programme for children.

Table 29.1 The full immunization programme for children (2006)

When to immunize	What is given	How it is given
2 months old	Diphtheria, tetanus, pertussis (whooping cough), polio and *Haemophilus influenzae* type b (Hib) (DTaP/IPV/Hib)	One injection
	Pneumococcal infection (Pneumococcal conjugate vaccine, PCV)	One injection
3 months old	Diphtheria, tetanus, pertussis, polio and *Haemophilus influenzae* type b (Hib) (DTaP/IPV/Hib)	One injection
	Meningitis C (meningococcal group C) (MenC)	One injection
4 months old	Diphtheria, tetanus, pertussis, polio and *Haemophilus influenzae* type b (Hib) (DTaP/IPV/Hib)	One injection
	Meningitis C (meningococcal group C) (MenC)	One injection
	Pneumococcal infection (Pneumococcal conjugate vaccine, PCV)	One injection
Around 12 months old	*Haemophilus influenza* type b (Hib) and meningitis C (Hib/MenC)	One injection
Around 13 months old	Measles, mumps and rubella (German measles) (MMR)	One injection
	Pneumococcal infection (PCV)	One injection
3 years and 4 months to 5 years old	Diphtheria, tetanus, pertussis (whooping cough) and polio (dTaP/IPV or DTaP/IPV)	One injection
	Measles, mumps and rubella (MMR)	One injection
13 to 18 years old	Diphtheria, tetanus, polio (Td/IPV)	One injection

Role of the nurse
- Provide advice about immunization and risks, listen to fears, and answer questions.
- Encourage parents to keep calm, which will help keep their child calm.
- Reassure the child.
- Distract the child at the time of injection.
- Praise the child and give a special treat such as a bravery sticker if old enough.
- Encourage parents to keep a record of the immunization (parent-held record) in a safe place and to record details of each vaccine.
- Advise parents to take a record when travelling.
- Ensure vaccines are stored and administered safely and according to agreed policies.

Child surveillance

This consists of a series of checks and reviews at regular intervals to assess a child's growth and development (physical, mental, and emotional) against 'norms' or expected levels (See Table 29.2). Health visitors are required to understand normal growth and development and the influences of social, family, environmental factors, communication, and teaching. Records should be kept in the parent-held record.

Health education

This is undertaken to minimize hazards and provide optimum physical and mental health. 📖 Health promotion, p.970.

Further information

www.immunisation.nhs.uk

Table 29.2 Key developmental milestones

Age	Activity
General motor skills	
4–6 weeks	Hold head up momentarily
18–30 weeks	Sits alone
6–10 months	Pulls self up to stand
7–13 months	Walks holding furniture
11–18 months	Walks unaided
Language and hearing	
0–1 months	Makes soft noises when talked to
1–3 months	Turns toward sounds at ear level
14–30 weeks	Turns to voice
10–12 months	Says 'dada', 'mama'
14–24 months	Puts two words together
Fine motor skills	
8–12 weeks	Loses primitive grasp reflex
6–12 weeks	Follows moving person with eye
10–20 weeks	Reaches out for object
12–24 months	Scribbles round and round
Personal and social	
1–2 months	Smiles back at parents
1.5–3 months	Smiles spontaneously
4–8 months	Smiles at self in mirror
6–16 months	Drinks from cup
18–38 months	Dry during day

Health promotion

- Taking account of the developmental stage of the child is essential.
  - From birth to 2 years—focus on teaching the parents.
  - From 2–7 years—recognize that children interpret explanations literally; simple drawings and stories can help explanations; comparisons with other children are not helpful as they cannot generalize; reassure the child that no one is to blame for his pain or condition; use popular heroes to help explain treatment, e.g. Dr Who (antibiotics) destroying the Daleks (infections).
  - From 7–12 years—use drawings and models to explain; begin to relate care to others' experiences; use child's particular interests (e.g. science) to explain.
  - Young people are developing the ability to think in abstract and can reason deductively and should be taught in a similar way to an adult; however, motivation and readiness to learn will differ.
- The environment needs to encourage the child's participation and jargon needs to be replaced so that children can understand.
- Health promotion should be focused on the needs of the child and may be targeted at the parents and/or the child.
  - Nutrition: breast or bottle feeding, weaning, healthy eating, weight control
  - Baby and child care: importance of play, managing behaviour and importance of relationships, e.g. with siblings and other children
  - Exercise: short- and long-term benefits
  - Toilet training
  - Dental hygiene: low-sugar diet, effective teeth cleaning, use of fluoride, regular dental check-ups
  - Participating in surveillance programmes: importance of attending child health clinics for developmental and growth checks
  - Immunization programmes: effects of infectious diseases
  - Sex education: HIV, AIDS, STIs and long-term effects, family planning, and unplanned teenage pregnancy
  - Substance misuse: effects of smoking, alcohol, and illicit drugs
  - Accident prevention: road safety, wearing cycle helmets, using infant and child car restraints and seat belts, protective clothing for sports (e.g. joint protectors for skate-boarding), fire safety, home safety (e.g. gates on stairs, and guards on fires and heated areas)
  - Safe storage of medicines, chemicals, equipment, plastic bags, and general belongings
  - Importance of hand hygiene before and after eating and after using toilet

Further information

Rhodes C and Wilbourn V (2006). 'Promoting child health and health promotion models', in Glasper EA, McEwing G, Richardson J (eds) *Oxford handbook of children's and young people's nursing*, pp. 18–20, Oxford University Press, Oxford

Discharge and continuing care

- Involve the family and plan from the time of admission. Give an estimated date of discharge as soon as possible.
- Follow the local discharge policy and work with the multidisciplinary team.
- Inform the child and parents of which nurse will be coordinating the discharge arrangements for the child.
- Assess the parents' and child's perceptions of their condition and ability to cope; talk through coping strategies. Ensure support is available from social services, counsellors, and community children's nursing team and health visitor, if necessary.
- Hold frequent discussions to give and reinforce information about the discharge together with a written discharge plan that identifies what care needs to be carried out, the services to be provided, and the frequency.
- Ensure any equipment (e.g. wheelchair or dressings) is ordered well in advance.
- Ensure the child and/or family have been taught, have practised, and feel confident in aspects of self-care (e.g. injections of insulin, tube feeds, nebulizers) and understand how to care for and maintain equipment. Provide telephone numbers and instructions about what to do if equipment breaks down.
- Ensure community services, GP, and specialist practitioners are notified of the discharge early and information about the child's needs is communicated with them. Confirm transport arrangements.
- Undertake an assessment of the family home environment if necessary, e.g. space for equipment, home renovations, availability of peer/parent support and transport.
- Ensure that discharge times are convenient for the family and for community and social services.
- Provide telephone numbers or contact details of relevant members of health care team and what to do in an emergency.
- Provide information about self-help groups for both child and parents.

Further information

Walmsley J (2006). 'Preparing for discharge', in Glasper EA, McEwing G, and Richardson J (eds) *Oxford handbook of children and young people's nursing*, pp. 74, Oxford University Press, Oxford

BNF for Children

For all issues relating to the use of medicines for managing childhood conditions use the special BNF for Children. See www.bnfc.org.

The BNF for Children is revised yearly and all copies should be replaced when the new edition is published.

Doses are expressed for specific age ranges, for example:
- Neonates 0–28 days
- Child 1 month–4 years
- Child 4–10 years
- Adolescents 12–18 years

A pragmatic approach is urged in prescribing depending on the child's physiological development and condition, and if weight is appropriate for the child's age.

The difference between the BNF for Children and the standard BNF for adults

Whereas the standard BNF is used for medications for individuals of all ages, the BNF for Children focuses specifically on the use of medicines in children.

The BNF for Children is for use by all professionals in all sectors of health care who are involved in prescribing, administering, or managing medicines used for children.

Warning

All nurses working in the field of adult nursing care should be very careful when handling and administering medicines for children and adolescents.

Nursing patients with learning disability

Principles of care

Definition of learning disability

A learning disability is a lifelong condition where the person has a reduced ability to understand new and complex information or to learn new skills, and has a reduced ability to cope independently. This has a lasting effect on the individual's development.

People with learning disability

- Are unique individuals with different abilities, needs, likes, and dislikes.
- Are susceptible to the same general medical conditions as the rest of the population but are more likely to have epilepsy, thyroid disease, hearing and visual impairments, obesity, osteoporosis, mental health problems, gastric disease, respiratory problems, and dental disease. They may have chromosomal abnormalities.
- Have difficulty accessing services and health screening. Health needs are poorly met because of:
  - lack of staff expertise in communicating and understanding the individual
  - difficulty in diagnosing illnesses
  - lower expectations by health professionals for acceptable standards for people with learning disabilities.
- Are less likely to receive health education and health promotion, and to learn about healthy lifestyles.
- Are sometimes unable to recognize dangers and causes of illness or accidents. Therefore, they fail to take preventive action and as a result may need to access health care more frequently.
- Often feel vulnerable and frightened when admitted to hospital.
- Have reduced ability to understand information presented in a complex way.

Nursing care

- Work with experienced learning disability nurses to develop policies, guidelines, and practices to meet needs.
- Implement systems to highlight special needs, e.g. longer appointments to enable more time for communication, specific communication aids.
- Provide pre-admission visits if possible.
- Develop effective relationships with each individual and their carer.
- Use specially formulated assessments to establish the abilities and needs of the individual. Seek out and use any personal profile or care plan that the person carries with them or that their carer uses for communicating their needs and characteristics.
- Maintain continuity of existing skills to promote independence.
- Have communication aids readily available to promote choice and involvement in decision making, e.g. picture cards.
- Recognize that people with learning disability have equal rights with other citizens and ensure that no inequity exists in standards of response, equipment, nursing care, or resuscitation.
- Ensure access to an effective advocate, key worker, or similar.
- Ensure there is a list of organizations and key people who can offer support in the care of people with learning disability.

Communication

Difficulties in communication

These arise when professionals fail to provide appropriate levels of explanation, communicate exclusively with the carer and ignore the patient, fail to work with carers who know the patient well, or misunderstand nonverbal communication and behaviours.

People with learning disability often use behaviours to communicate. They may have difficulty expressing pain and discomfort, or appear threatening or over-friendly because of limited communication skills. Examples may include shouting, crying, changing posture, silence, and gesticulation. They may have an acute awareness of other people's nonverbal communication.

Improving communication

- Work with carers to identify behavioural patterns that indicate specific meanings, needs, and wants and to identify patient's communication system.
- Spend time on a one-to one basis with the individual to develop a relationship. Observing behaviours will help in understanding what the individual is trying to communicate.
- Focus on the communication skills that the individual possesses.
- Use nonverbal gestures to reinforce verbal communication, e.g. nodding to demonstrate understanding, gestures to show empathy.
- Use clear and simple language, even-paced conversation in a calm tone, and summarize what is said.
- Keep conversations short but frequent. Allow extra time to allow patients to process the information.
- Ensure body posture and stance is non-threatening.
- Present information in an accessible format, e.g. use pictures, drawings, flash cards, and symbols, or use other augmentative communication systems such as Makaton if the patient is familiar with them.
- Use an advocate, key worker, or family member who knows the individual well to assist with communication.
- Consult with local user forums on how best to communicate.
- Seek guidance from a speech and language therapist.

Consent to treatment

People with a learning disability have the same rights as other people, including the right to make informed decisions and choices about their care and treatment. Sometimes people with learning disability are not able to give or withhold informed consent because they lack the mental capacity or because they are unable to communicate their decision. The Mental Capacity Act 2007 is specifically designed to cover situations where someone is unable to make a decision because their mind or brain is affected. It covers day-to-day occasions (e.g. what to wear) as well as more serious decisions (e.g. having an operation).

Criteria for assessing capacity to give informed consent

Having mental capacity means that a person is able to make their own decisions. The law says that a person is unable to make a particular decision if they cannot do one or more of the following:
• understand information given to them
• retain the information long enough to be able to make the decision
• weigh up the information available to make the decision
• communicate the decision, e.g. by talking, using sign language, blinking an eye, or squeezing a hand.

Assessing the capacity to give informed consent may be difficult for patients with learning disability who may have deficits in verbal and memory ability, difficulties in problem solving, problems with processing complex information, difficulties with comprehension and reasoning, and difficulties in articulating a decision.

Principles of the Mental Capacity Act

• Every adult has the right to make his or her own decisions and must be assumed to have capacity to do so unless it is proved otherwise.
• People must be supported as much as possible to make their own decisions before anyone concludes that they cannot make their own decisions.
• People have the right to make what others might regard as unwise or eccentric decisions.
• Anything done for or on behalf of a person who lacks mental capacity must be done in their best interests.
• Anything done for or on behalf of people without capacity should be the least restrictive of their basic rights and freedoms.

Assessment of capacity

• Assessment of capacity is decision specific, i.e. it must be made about the particular decision and not about a range of decisions.
• If someone cannot make complex decisions it does not mean they cannot make simple decisions.
• Normally friends, family, carers, or an Independent Mental Capacity Advocate will participate in assessing capacity.

Helping people make decisions for themselves

- Does the person have all the relevant information needed to make the decision? Has information on the alternatives been given?
- Could the information be explained or presented in a way that is easier for the person to understand, e.g. pictures, videos, sign language?
- Are there particular times of the day when a person's understanding is better or is there a place where they feel more at ease?
- Can anyone else help or support the person to understand the information, e.g. friend or advocate?
- If there is reason to believe a person lacks capacity, check the following:
  - Has everything been done to help and support the person to make a decision?
  - Does this decision need to be made without delay?
  - If not, is it possible to wait until the person does have the capacity to make the decision for themselves?
- It is the responsibility of the health care professional proposing the treatment to determine whether the patient has the capacity to give valid consent.
- A record of the assessment of the patient's capacity, why the health professional believes treatment is in the best interest of the patient, and the involvement of people close to the patient should be recorded on the standardized NHS forms.
- If there is lack of consensus on what is 'in the best interests' of the patient, involve an advocate who is independent of all parties; get a second opinion; hold a case conference; go to mediation; and, if necessary, apply to the Court of Protection for a ruling.

Maintaining patient safety

Some patients with learning disability are not always able to communicate their needs and have difficulty evaluating dangers and risks, especially in a strange environment. Nurses should be proactive and reduce the risks as follows.

Reducing risks

- Discuss with relatives and carers where best to place the patient. Do not assume that a side room is best to prevent upsetting others. Having company may reduce boredom or being near the nurses' station may allow better supervision.
- Keep the patient occupied if well enough. Do not assume that relatives will be able to stay every day. Find out what the patient is able and likes to do.
- Active curiosity in the surroundings may result in the person removing dressings, tampering with equipment, and wandering. Consider whether additional staff are required to support and supervise the patient.
- Failure to identify changes in condition and recognize levels of pain and discomfort may arise because of lack of knowledge of staff of the needs of people with learning disability. Ask relatives and carers to identify usual ways of communication. Allocate the same nurses to ensure an effective relationship is built with the patients.
- Failure to diagnose underlying medical conditions may also arise because of lack of knowledge of staff of working with people with learning disability. Nurses should recognize physical disabilities and medical conditions associated with learning disabilities, e.g. Down syndrome, hypothyroidism, leukaemia, epilepsy, osteoporosis, mental ill health, and increased risk of myocardial infarction, stroke, cancer, and fractures.
- Improved awareness of the needs of people with learning disability and how to address these will help to prevent problems. A designated nurse who preferably is supported and advised by a learning disability nurse to act as lead for all in patients with learning disability will be helpful in addition to policies covering admission, exchange of information, and involvement of relatives and carers.
- Some people with learning disability inflict injuries on themselves, e.g. head banging, biting, scratching, pinching, and hair pulling. This may arise if there is insufficient stimulation in the environment. Discuss with carers and relatives any triggers and usual forms of management.
  📖 Challenging behaviour, p.979.

Challenging behaviour

About 16% of people with learning disability have challenging behaviour. It increases with age during childhood and reaches a peak between 15 and 34 years. It may include aggression, property destruction, and self-injurious behaviour, and is more commonly identified in males than females. It may be associated with psychiatric disorders, e.g. anxiety disorders and compulsive behaviours are more common in people with self-injurious behaviour.

The degree of challenging behaviour is variable and may occur rarely or several times a day, may prevent an individual taking part in normal activities, may require intervention by one or more staff members, or may result in major injury to the individual, another person, or a member of staff, e.g. broken bone, cuts, or stab wounds.

Managing a patient with challenging behaviour

- Each person is different. It is important to be aware of what triggers the behaviour and be able to recognize the type of behaviour and how it starts in order to diffuse it. Therefore a detailed discussion with the individual's carers to elicit this information is essential. Work with the usual carers to develop a suitable management plan in the new environment.
- Determine whether the patient is on any medication and ensure this is maintained.
- Prepare the environment. A calm quiet environment with subdued colours is helpful. This can be difficult to achieve in an acute general hospital which is often busy and noisy, and where it is difficult to get away from people. A balance of company and peace and quiet should be sought. Certain areas may need to be made out of bounds, e.g. lock kitchens, treatment rooms, and offices. Ensure equipment that may be used for self-injury is locked away (e.g. scissors); supervise mealtimes, if necessary; ensure knives are removed.
- Ensure personal safety. Staff should understand the risks of wearing jewellery (face and body piercing which may be pulled or ripped out) and long hair not being tied up.
- Use breakaway techniques and strategies. Staff must be trained in the techniques that will enable them to break away from holds and escape from dangerous situations.
- Policies and procedures should be available locally which indicate the legal and ethical implications of violence arising from challenging behaviours and additional support that can be called upon in emergency situations.

Networks of support

Nurses in hospital must work together with specialist services to improve the care provided for patients with learning disability. It is helpful to have a list of resources with names and contact numbers that are available in your local workplace, including the following:

- The individual's lead practitioner or key worker who takes responsibility for assessment, planning, and review in partnership with the client and their carers and/or the community learning disability team
- The individual's family and carers who will provide support in many circumstances but may also need the advice and support of professional carers, for example when the individual experiences care in a new environment such as a hospital
- The individual's Health Facilitator (HF) and/or Community Learning Disability Nurse
- The individual's GP
- Social worker and relevant social services department contacts
- Members of the multidisciplinary team in the hospital including physiotherapist, occupational therapist, speech and language therapist, and dietitian
- The hospital's Patient Advice Liaison Service (PALS) or similar information service that will often have links to local support groups and networks
- Voluntary and charitable organizations. Further information, p.981.
- Local Authority Learning Disability Partnership Boards or similar bodies which aim to bring together public, private, community, and voluntary sectors and oversee interagency planning and commissioning of services
- Social Care Institute of Excellence—source of expertise on learning disability
- Ideally, the same team members will manage the same patients, to build up a relationship and familiarity and put the patient at ease

Further information

Association for Real Change ARC—Membership organization which supports providers of services www.arcuk.org.uk

British Institute of Learning Disabilities (BILD)—a charity to improve the quality of life of all people with learning disability www.bild.org.uk

Challenging Behaviour Foundation—a charity to improve the lives and conditions of people with learning disability and challenging behaviour and their carers www.thecbf.org.uk

Department of Health www.dh.gov.uk

Learning Disability website www.learningdisability.co.uk

MENCAP www.mencap.org.uk

Social Care Institute of Excellence www.scie.org.uk

Nursing patients with mental health needs

Recognition and assessment of mental health problems

It is important for general nurses to be aware of patients with physical illness who may also experience mental health problems. For example patients admitted with surgical or medical conditions may develop a new mental health problem or may have a pre-existing mental health condition. It is therefore important that nurses:

- Develop an effective relationship with the patient and their family (if patient agrees) and encourage the patient and family to express and verbalize their feelings and concerns.
- Recognize that it is common for a patient to experience psychological reactions, e.g. anger, tearfulness, frustration, anxiety during a physical illness.
- Include a mental health assessment in the holistic assessment of the patient. 📖 Chapter 3, Mental status examination, p.36.

Observe the patient

- Degree of activity and agitation—restlessness, trembling, irritability
- Rapidly changing behaviours, e.g. euphoria, depression, aggression. (This may not be obvious in the timeframe of the interview.)
- Physical appearance—signs of self-neglect or weight loss or gain
- Level of alertness and orientation to time, place, person, people, and environment
- Ability to concentrate and respond to questions appropriately, remember what was said, and cooperate with simple requests
- Changing thought processes—flight from one subject to another
- Check temperature, pulse and blood pressure, and blood glucose for hypoglycaemia
- Skin lesions, e.g. self-cutting, needle tracks, bruising

Ask the patient about

- *Recent changes in behaviour or mood:* feelings of restlessness, being wound up, or poor concentration; any ritualistic behaviours, panic attacks, phobias, suicidal thoughts, or self-harm potential; social withdrawal; hallucinations or delusions.
- *Recent emotional difficulties:* e.g. divorce, bereavement, survival or guilt, feelings of worthlessness, loneliness, family problems and relationships, and emotional support available.
- *Previous history of mental health issues:* when, duration, how they felt, and coping strategies they used including family support, treatment, and medication, whether admitted to hospital or under GP, and any follow-up offered and accepted.
- *Physical problems:* poor sleep pattern, loss of appetite, changes in weight, fatigue, long-term conditions, e.g. arthritis, pain, recent surgery, head injury, infections, GI, or cardiovascular problems.
- *Sexual history* may be relevant.
- *Drug, solvent, or alcohol use:* type, duration, amount, effects and route together with any risk behaviours.
- *Prescribed medication:* type, dose, frequency, and whether concordant.

- *Family history of mental illness:* relationship with patient, difficulty coping, or emotional problems.
- *Ongoing support* from other agencies, family, or links with support groups.

Common symptoms of mental disorder

Anxiety – this is a normal response to an unusual or stressful event. It is abnormal when severe or prolonged, it occurs in the absence of a stressful event, or impairs the individual's ability to function.

Panic attack – is a discrete period of severe anxiety that is associated with unpleasant symptoms which may be spontaneous or related to a situation.

Depression – is a mood disorder with predominant feelings of sadness with possible changes in appetite, weight, sleep patterns, and poor concentration.

Insomnia – is the inability to sleep or abnormal wakefulness.

Confusion – is a form of disorientation. 📖 Chapter 28, Nursing the older person, pp.916–17.

Memory loss – is the inability to remember or recall events, people, words, names, etc.; it may affect short-term or long-term memory; it may be transient or permanent. 📖 Chapter 28, Cognition, p.910.

Delusions – usually a false belief that is unshakeable and held on unsatisfactory grounds, is not amenable to rational argument, and is not explicable in terms of the individual's background.

Elevated mood – the mood is greater than excitement and is coupled with impatience and irritation.

Hallucination – is a false perception without an external stimulus that may be simple phenomena (e.g. noises, lights) or more complex (e.g. hearing voices).

Anxiety and depression

Anxiety disorders

It is often difficult to distinguish the different anxiety and mood disorders. In anxiety disorder, patients tend to be apprehensive, have panic attacks, irritability, poor sleeping, and poor concentration.

- *Generalized anxiety disorder* is defined as worry and tension on most days for at least 6 months and possibly fatigue, trembling, irritability, restlessness, breathlessness, tachycardia, dry mouth, feeling wound up, and poor concentration.
- *Panic disorder* is the presence of unexpected panic attacks or displays of concerns. Phobias such as agoraphobia (anxiety about being in places from which escape is difficult) or fears about life-threatening illnesses (heart attack) are associated with panic disorder. Avoiding action may be taken to prevent having these feelings.
- *Obsessive-compulsive disorder* is the presence of obsessions (unwanted intrusive thoughts, images, and urges) and compulsions (repetitive unwanted behaviours, e.g. repeated hand washing, ritualistic behaviours that the individual feels driven to perform). These disorders occur at all ages and often start in childhood.
- *Specific phobias*, e.g. spiders, mice, or social situations.
- *Post-traumatic stress* may follow a stressful event or threatening or catastrophic situation. Symptoms may develop immediately or may be delayed. These include:
  - Re-experiencing the event – flashbacks, nightmares, intrusive images
  - Avoidance – of people, situations, or circumstances
  - Hyperarousal – sleep problems, irritability, and poor concentration
  - Emotional numbing – feeling detached
  - Depression, drug or alcohol misuse, anger, or unexplained physical symptoms

Depression

This is a common psychiatric problem affecting all ages, sometimes related to people with physical illness especially chronic conditions, e.g. arthritis, respiratory disease, stroke, and cancer. It is also linked to heart disease. Women and the unemployed are more commonly affected as are those experiencing life changes, e.g. fears about future, loss of role, identity, or partner. Patients with depression present with low mood, loss of interest and enjoyment, reduced energy and appetite, weight changes, sleep problems, feelings of worthlessness, lack of concentration, and obsessive thoughts of death. Alcohol and substance misuse and suicide are problems associated with depression.

- *Mild to moderate depression* is characterized by depressive symptoms and some functional impairment and it may recur.
- *Severe depression* also includes agitation and functional impairment.
- *Psychotic depression* may also present with hallucinations and delusions.
- *Postnatal depression* affects 10–15% of women after childbirth. It may lead to hospital admission or even suicide.

Further information

CEMACH (2007). *Saving mothers' lives. The 7th report on confidential enquiries into maternal deaths in the UK.* www.cemach.org.uk

Callaghan P and Waldock H (2007). *Oxford handbook of mental health nursing.* Oxford University Press, Oxford

General principles of treatment for anxiety and depression

- Give patient all options for treatment where possible and consider patient preference in deciding treatment.
- Give appropriate level of information on treatment and side effects in simple language.
- Give information on self-help and support groups.
- Take account of the patient's psychological, social and physical characteristics; health; living conditions; and social situation.
- Assess the risk of self-harm or harm to others and consider whether referral to a specialist mental health team is required.

Treatment and management of anxiety

Non-pharmacological measures
These include breathing exercises, yoga, hypnosis, relaxation CDs, tensing/relaxing muscles.

Cognitive behavioural therapy
This is a form of therapy which combines cognitive and behavioural therapy and aims to weaken the connections between troublesome situations and negative reactions to them. It aims to help people identify negative thoughts and behaviour patterns that reduce their mood level, changing these, and enabling them to return to health. This can be helpful for both depression and anxiety disorders and should be a first-line therapy for children and young people with mild to moderate disorders.

Pharmacological treatments
Psychopharmacology is the use of drugs that act on the central nervous system and modify mood, thought perception, and behaviour.
- Benzodiazepines are effective for general anxiety disorder; are not usually used beyond 2–4 weeks; and should not be used for panic disorder.
- Selective serotonin reuptake inhibitors (SSRIs).

Self-help
'Self-help' as a term concerns an activity whereby an individual or group engages in bettering themselves. Typically, this involves the use of written material to help people understand their problems and change behaviour to overcome them.

Treatment and management of depression
Guided self-help and cognitive behavioural therapy should be considered. Antidepressants may be used in moderate depression.

Counselling
Types of talking therapies that aim to offer help in changing attitudes and behaviour. It may take place on a one-to-one or group basis.

Exercise
Alone or combined with other treatments improves mild to moderate depression.

Mental health specialist teams
May be required to care for patients with moderate and severe depression or where depression is resistant to treatment, recurrent, or atypical. This may be in the community or in hospital. Medications or electroconvulsive therapies may be used.

Other common mental health disorders

Schizophrenia

This is a disorder characterized by auditory hallucinations, delusions, and disordered thought processes with changes in behaviour. It usually develops in early adulthood (earlier in men than women). Risk factors include family history, cannabis use, developmental difficulties, and acute life events. Assessment by the psychiatric team is essential.

Symptoms

- *Hallucinations* – These are false perceptions of a sensory experience with no external stimulus. They may be auditory (hearing voices), visual (seeing faces, insects, or anything unpleasant), olfactory and gustatory (smelling and tasting), or tactile (feeling sensations).
- *Delusions* –These are unshakeable beliefs that are held even when cast iron evidence to the contrary is presented. Delusions are not affected by rational argument.
- There may also be thought blocking, mood changes (e.g. depression, anxiety, irritability, euphoria), demotivation, reduced emotion, and functional deterioration (e.g. self neglect).

Treatment

(See NICE guideline CG1)

- The choice of drug and drug dosage is guided by individual responsiveness and may be limited by side effects.
- Drugs may be given by mouth or depot injection.
- Follow-up must be provided by the community mental health team to:
  - Check medication concordance and side effects.
  - Check for deterioration in condition.
  - Promote lifestyle changes, e.g. avoid illicit drugs and alcohol.
  - Support return to employment.
  - Ensure support is available with finances and housing.
  - Encourage to develop social networks.
- Family members should be encouraged to support the patient to prevent relapses.

Bipolar disorder

This is also called manic depression, and is a mood disorder that affects 1–2% of the population and is more common in women. Patients with bipolar disorder experience extreme fluctuation in mood and activity, from euphoria with hyperactivity (i.e. mania) to severe depression with decreased energy. Normal mood may also be present. In severe mania psychotic symptoms may develop such as grandiose ideas, suspiciousness, irritability and aggression, loss of insight into the real world, and self neglect. Patients may be cared for in primary or secondary care and should see health care professionals regularly. Drug treatment such as lithium or olanzapine may be used for long-term treatment (See NICE Guideline 38).

Further information

National Collaborating Centre for Mental Health (2002). *Schizophrenia: core interventions in the treatment and management of schizophrenia in primary and secondary care*. National Institute for Clinical Excellence, London, www.nice.org.uk

National Collaborating Centre for Mental Health (2006). *Bipolar disorder: the management of bipolar disorder in adults, children and adolescents, in primary and secondary care.* National Institute for Clinical Excellence, London, www.nice.org.uk

Nursing patients with mental health problems on an acute general ward

Patients with a mental illness may be admitted from the community to a general hospital for surgery, from medical care on a planned or emergency basis, or they may be transferred from a mental health unit for treatment. Patients may also develop a new mental health problem in the context of a physical illness. General nurses should be able to identify and meet their basic needs, whether physical, psychological, or social, and not label or marginalize patients because of their mental health disorders or overlook their physical needs because of concerns about possible behavioural problems.

- Spending time with the individual is important to develop an effective relationship. The patient may initially be suspicious and unwilling to communicate. Effective communication skills, especially listening, appearing patient, unhurried, and non-judgemental will be helpful.
- Inexperienced nurses may be anxious about approaching patients when they are unsure of how they will respond, and the support of a more experienced nurse will be welcomed.
- Information from the patient's family and carers (including a key worker if the patient has one) will be helpful, but this should not replace discussion and assessment directly with the patient.
- Encouragement and support for patients in carrying out self-care may be helpful, including a daily routine for some patients who lack concentration, motivation, or self-worth.
- Information about their medication, its effects, and the consequences of not taking it should be provided. Patients should be observed to ensure they are taking their medicines as prescribed, though it must be remembered that patients can refuse treatment. Patients detained under the MHA can still refuse treatment; the issue is that their refusal can be over-ridden. Section 58 also allows for an assessment of mental capacity including seeking a SOAD (Second Opinion Appointed Doctor).
- Observation of the patient's behaviour, mood, appetite, sleep patterns, and activities should be made and carefully recorded along with expressions about their feelings. These should be discussed with the multidisciplinary team. In certain circumstances, e.g. when there is a risk of self-harm, the patient should be observed continuously. A specific risk assessment should be undertaken and advice from a psychiatrist or mental health liaison nurse obtained. The environment should also be checked to restrict access to dangerous equipment or substances. 📖 Suicide and deliberate self harm, p.995.
- If there are concerns about aggressive or disruptive behaviour look for triggers or reasons. Seek advice from the mental health team. 📖 Violent and agressive patients, p.1118 and 📖 The mental health team, p.1000.
- If in doubt about the patient's nursing care related to their mental health needs, advice should be sought from colleagues from the local mental health team or from colleagues with more experience.

Alcohol and substance misuse

Definitions

Substance misuse is the harmful use of any substance, such as alcohol, pre-scribed medications (e.g. diazepam), illicit drugs (e.g. heroin, methadone, cannabis, cocaine, and amphetamines), and other substances (e.g. glue and lighter fluid). Drug misuse commonly coexists with alcohol misuse.

Harmful use is the continuing misuse of substances despite the evidence of damage to the person's mental health and social, occupational, or family well being.

Dependence includes physical and psychological dependence. If consump-tion of the substance stops, the individual experiences withdrawal.

Withdrawal includes physical dependence where abstinence leads to features of withdrawal. Clinically significant withdrawals may be seen in alcohol, opioids, benzodiazepines, amphetamines, and cocaine.

Complicated withdrawal is development of seizures, delirium, or psy-chotic features.

Dual diagnosis, or comorbidity, is the coexistence of a mental illness and substance use (e.g. psychosis, schizophrenia, and substance misuse). From 8–15% of clients have dual diagnosis and prisons have a high preva-lence. It is more common in homeless people. There is an increased burden on the family and carers, and there is often poor concordance with medication.

Alcohol misuse

This is the most common form of substance misuse, and there is a high prevalence in general hospitals and emergency admission. It often coexists with a medical problem, e.g. GI problems, hypertension, peripheral neuritis, and pancreatitis, and may be related to recurrent accidents, poor sleep patterns, and weight changes. Denial is common.

Assessment

- Observe for smell of alcohol, tremor, sweating, agitation.
- There are a number of assessment tools that can be used to assess alcohol dependence. One such tool is the CAGE questionnaire.
  - Have you ever felt you should **C**ut down on drinking?
  - Have people **A**nnoyed you by criticizing your drinking?
  - Have you ever felt **G**uilty about drinking?
  - Have you ever had a drink first thing to steady nerves or get over a hangover (**E**ye-opener)?

Alcohol dependence is likely if patient gives 2 or more positive answers.

- Observe for signs of withdrawal—tachycardia, hypotension, tremor, sweating, fits, hallucinations, and delirium tremens.

Alcohol withdrawal

Alcohol withdrawal may be a presenting feature or may occur as an unex-plained development in a patient who has been admitted for other reasons and is deprived of alcohol. Features of alcohol withdrawal can appear 6–72 hours after the last drink. The range and severity of symptoms depends on such factors as degree of alcohol dependence and current level of consumption. Nursing management should include the following:

- Recognize and assess alcohol withdrawal – signs and symptoms include:
  - Mild withdrawal – mild anxiety, slight sweating, insomnia, slight tremor, tachycardia, fever, GI symptoms
  - Moderate withdrawal – malaise, marked anxiety, depression, irritability, profuse sweating, noticeable tremor, fever,↑ blood pressure, tachycardia
  - Severe withdrawal – as above plus increasing confusion, disorientation, hallucinations, restlessness, ataxia, vestibular disturbances, possible convulsions, seizures, and blackouts
- Follow local policy on alcohol withdrawal management.
- Provide patients with reassurance and general support.
- Optimize nutrition and fluid levels; manage seizures and changes in conscious level; and provide safe environment to ensure patient safety when confused, agitated and disorientated.
- Administer prescribed medication with the aim of preventing features of withdrawal without over-sedation, e.g. chlordiazepoxide or lorazepam if there is liver impairment. Parenteral thiamine is prescribed to prevent thiamine deficiency that can cause Wernicke's encephalopathy (WE). Patients at high risk of WE should have IV Pabrinex.
- Recognize delirium tremens (DTs) – usually develops up to 5 days after alcohol cessation and causes increased confusion and disorientation, sever tremors, visual and auditory hallucinations, and delusional beliefs. Prompt recognition and treatment with benzodiazepines usually prevents this.
- Liaise with Drug and Alcohol Liaison Team or equivalent, if available.

Drug misuse

The symptoms produced depend on the type of drug or substance used, the quantity, and route of administration. Frequent requests for prescriptions, lack of self-care, unusual behaviour, and mood lability are common.

Assessment

- Elicit current and past use of drugs and alcohol.
- Check for complications, e.g. signs of poor nutrition, infected injection sites indicating HIV, hepatitis, DVT.
- Conduct physical, emotional, and psychosocial assessment.

Treatment

- NICE Guidelines 51 and 52 recommend offering motivational sessions to encourage behaviour change and provide non-judgemental feedback.
- Give information on self-help groups; management programmes to reduce illicit drug use; detoxification for people who are opioid dependent and have made choice to stop.
- Explain risks and benefits of treatment.

Further information

National Collaborating Centre for Mental Health (2007). *Drug misuse: psychosocial interventions.* National Institute for Clinical Excellence, London, www.nice.org.uk
National Collaborating Centre for Mental Health (2007). *Drug misuse: opioid detoxification.* National Institute for Clinical Excellence, London, www.nice.org.uk

Nursing alcohol and substance misuse problems

- Develop an understanding of the patient and their view of drugs and alcohol. This will vary with age, culture, gender, and religious beliefs.
- Develop a trusting and non-judgemental relationship by communicating respect, empathy, and genuineness; using effective verbal and nonverbal skills; and protecting confidential information.
- Work with other agencies and, where possible, the patient's family.
- Ensure the patient has the information they want to help them make decisions about their lifestyle. This may include the following information for alcohol:
  - The recommended safe levels of alcohol consumption (females <14 units per week; males <21 units per week)
  - Examples of 1 unit: a small glass (125 mL) of ordinary strength wine (12% alcohol per volume) or half a pint of ordinary strength beer or lager (3–4% alcohol per volume)
  - The health impacts of alcohol – impact on behaviour; risk of GI cancer and other GI conditions; risk of liver damage, renal damage, infections, pancreatitis; risk of cardiovascular problems; impact on reproduction and the fetus; risk of harm and crime
  - Information about support groups, e.g. Alcoholics Anonymous to support patients, Al-Anon to support relatives, and Al-Ateen to support teenagers
  - Managing problem drinking including how to reduce intake, availability of alcohol-free wine and beers, need to build up interests and hobbies and new activities, avoiding situations where there is peer pressure to consume large quantities of alcohol
  - Effects of withdrawal and how this can be managed with pharmacological treatment; support from community psychiatric nurses; support from family; group therapy and counselling; and how underlying problems can be managed, e.g. developing self-esteem, marriage guidance, financial problems
- Information that may be helpful for patients with substance misuse include:
  - The potential risks of substance misuse – violent behaviour; links with mental illness; risk of infections, e.g. HIV, hepatitis from needle sharing, thrombophlebitis from injections; accidents; crime; and overdose
  - Keeping healthy by using needle exchanges and practising safe sex
  - Information on what support is available – support groups (e.g. Narcotics Anonymous), local mental health services, and group therapy
  - Information on treatment, e.g. counselling; support for underlying problems, e.g. housing, financial; referral to specialized drug units for detoxification; residential rehabilitation, in order to live away from drugs and situations where there is peer pressure to continue the habit; and complementary therapies
  - Seeking support from family and friends

Suicide and deliberate self-harm

Definitions

- *Suicide* is the act of deliberately killing oneself. 📖 Chapter 33, The patient threatening or attempting suicide, p.1088.
- *Deliberate self-harm* (DSH) includes attempted suicide (a deliberate self-inflicted act by an individual with a non-fatal outcome) and parasuicide (a deliberate act that mimics the act of suicide but does not result in death). 11% of medical admissions to general hospitals are for DSH and the rate is rising. These acts may be impulsive or planned. The underlying suicidal intent varies considerably from being clearly intended to be nonfatal and manipulative to essentially leaving survival to chance. Intent is often later unclear even to the patient.
- *Self-cutting* may be superficial laceration of hands, wrists, and forearms or other parts of the body, or deep self-cutting and mutilation, and may be associated with feelings of tension or self-loathing.

Risk factors

- People who have committed non-fatal acts of DSH are at an increased risk of committing suicide at a later date.
- Suicide is more common in men and the mentally ill. It increases with age and being single, divorced, widowed, or unemployed. Individuals with chronic, debilitating, and painful physical conditions are also at greater risk. It is also more common in farmers, physicians, veterinarians, pharmacists, and dentists.
- DSH is more common in younger people and women. It is likely to be impulsive and involve self-poisoning, e.g. overdose with over-the-counter medicines (paracetamol is the most common form seen).
- People who commit suicide have often had contact with a health care professional in the preceding month.

Nursing role

- Use a sensitive non-judgemental approach and effective communication with the patient to develop trust and an effective relationship and to prevent them from feeling isolated.
- Work with patient, family, and multidisciplinary team to obtain the history relating to the present illness and identify problems (e.g. whether expressed suicidal ideas or behaviour, or if difficulties in family relationships exist) and assess the level of risk.
- Ensure the level of observation and location of the patient is appropriate for the severity of the patient's condition and assessed risk, and that this is maintained.
- Restrict the patient's access to dangerous equipment and materials.
- Ensure rapid referral to mental health nurses and psychiatrist for assessment of mental state, suicidal intent, and psychosocial history.
- Refer to 'suicide prevention' or 'deliberate self harm service' if available for problem solving and counselling, including family members; ensure follow-up and referral to other agencies.
- Seek advice from specialist mental health nurses in developing the patient's care plan while still in general hospital care.

Mental Health Act

The Mental Health Act (England and Wales) 1983 covers the detention of patients in mental health services. Most people who have mental health problems are treated on a voluntary basis either in the community or in hospitals and are often called 'informal patients'. A small proportion of patients are compulsorily detained under a specific section of the Mental Health Act and are often called 'formal patients'. The Mental Health Act is complex and covers such things as compulsory admission to hospital, consent to treatment, the right of appeal, guardianship, and patient's involvement with the legal system. There is a Code of Practice that gives best practice on the use of the Mental Health Act.

Role of the nurse in general hospitals

Patients are sometimes detained under a section of the Mental Health Act within a general hospital or are transferred for physical care while detained in a mental health unit. For most nurses this will be an infrequent experience but to be able to care for patients they should be aware of:

- Local policies and procedures for detaining and transferring patients detained under the Mental Health Act
- The key points of the sections commonly seen in general hospitals (Sections 2, 3, 4, 5 17, 58–61 and 132)
- Who is designated mental health administrator for the organization
- Who to contact urgently for help, support, and advice if a patient is admitted or transferred
- Local arrangements and contact details of specialist psychiatric nurses who can give advice on management and care
- Where to find relevant:
  - Statutory pink forms and where they should be kept
  - Information leaflets on patient's rights
- What to do if a patient is transferred
- Where to store the completed forms securely
- What to do if the time limits on the section are approaching
- Patient's rights and the code of practice
- What to do if a patient dies while detained on section
- What to do if a patient absconds while detained

Consent to treatment

There are a number of principles of law that guide consent to treatment of patients with mental health problems.

Informal patients – (over 16 years) have the right to refuse treatment except in the case of an emergency.

Common law – Patients may be treated under the common law doctrine of necessity in their own best interests. If the practitioner is acting in good faith and believes there is a serious risk to health and safety of the patient and others, the patient may be restrained to be given treatment. For example, if a person requires but refuses medical help but his life is immediately threatened (e.g. following overdose) then he may be treated.

Mental Capacity Act (England and Wales) 2005 – This provides a statutory framework to empower and protect vulnerable people who are not able to make their own decisions. It makes clear who can take decisions, in which situations, and how they should go about this. 📖 Consent to treatment, p.976.

Mental Health Act – Formal patients under Section 3 can be given certain treatments without their consent in certain circumstances for the first 3 months. After this time Section 58 consent is required or a SOAD (Second Opinion Appointed Doctor) may give consent. Special rules also apply to specific treatments such as electro-convulsive treatment (ECT).

Compulsory detention orders seen in general hospitals

Section 2
Allows compulsory detention for up to 28 days for assessment or assessment followed by treatment when:
- the individual has no history of admission and the diagnosis is unclear
- there is no treatment plan in place and assessment is required, *or*
- the effectiveness of compulsory treatment under the Act is not currently known.

The patient must be suffering from a mental disorder that warrants detention for a limited period and ought to be detained for their own health and safety or for the protection of others. The period of detention is not renewable. It may need to be followed by a Section 3 application.

Section 3
Allows compulsory detention for treatment for up to 6 months (but may not be needed for this length). This is renewable for a further 6 months and then for periods of 1 year. It is used when:
- the mental disorder is to a degree that makes it appropriate to receive treatment in hospital, *and*
- it is in the interests of the individual's health and safety or for the protection of others that the individual should receive such treatment and it cannot be provided unless they are detained. This should be signed by two doctors.

Section 4
Intended for genuine cases of emergency admission and requires a medical recommendation. It is used when obtaining a second medical recommendation causes undesirable delay. The grounds for the application are the same as Section 2 but the detention lasts only 72 hours.

Section 5(2)
This is for patients who are already voluntary patients in hospital. Section 5(2) prevents a patient from leaving hospital. Application is made by the doctor in charge of the patient's care. Also lasts 72 hours and cannot be extended. This time period should provide time to arrange Section 2 or 3.

Section 132
The managers have the duty to provide formal patients with information on the section they are detained under; their right to apply for a Mental Health Review Tribunal and/or appeal to the hospital managers; their right to be discharged; and consent to treatment rules, correspondence rules and the Mental Health Act Commission.

The mental health team

Many agencies, both statutory and voluntary, are involved in caring for people with mental health problems.

- *Primary care team:* most patients access the NHS through the primary care team, mainly the GP and practice nurses. Some patients will require referral to specialist services. 📖 Overview of primary care and public health, p.1004.
- *Accident and emergency services:* other patients access mental health care following contact with the emergency services, e.g. following accidents, injuries, or self-harm episodes.
- *Liaison psychiatry team:* works across traditional boundaries, e.g. between general hospital and psychiatric settings or between GP and community mental health team or with maternity services. Liaison with the prison service also occurs. This role involves mental health assessment and intervention for patients in non-psychiatric settings and may have a particular focus, e.g. self-harm or alcohol liaison.
- *Community mental health team:* this is a multidisciplinary team providing specialist assessment, treatment, and care to people in their own homes, including nursing, medical, social work, clinical psychology, occupational therapy, psychotherapy, art, music therapy, and pharmacy. Often provide assertive outreach (intensive case management) where the team provides practical support, care coordination, and advocacy as well as traditional therapeutic input.
- *Hospital mental health team:* the composition is similar to the above and may be provided in a:
  - local mental health unit
  - low secure unit—wards within local mental health units with locked doors, greater staff-to-patient ratios (high dependency/intensive care units)
  - medium secure unit—includes regional secure units that care for patients whose behaviour is too difficult or dangerous for local units
  - high secure unit provided by three special hospitals in England (Ashworth, Broadmoor, and Rampton) for dangerous and violent patients who require intensive supervision and observation.
- *A care coordinator* or key worker is responsible for coordinating the community programme approach reviews (written care plan). They usually have the most contact with the patient.
- *Social care:* social workers form part of the above teams but care is also provided in residential care homes by home helps and by other home care services.
- *Independent sector providers* may provide hospital and community care.
- *Carers:* family or friends who voluntarily look after mentally ill people.
- *Voluntary services* provide support, advice, and help to patients, family, and carers, e.g. Alcoholics Anonymous, drug lines, National Association for Mental Health (MIND).

Contacts for mental health

- Alcohol Concern — www.alcoholconcern.org
- Alzheimer's Society — www.alzheimers.org.uk
- Government drug guidance to professionals — www.drugs.gov.uk
- Manic Depression Fellowship — www.mdf.org.uk
- National Association for Mental Health (MIND) — www.mind.org.uk
- National Institute for Mental Health England — www.nimhe.org.uk
- Rethink — www.rethink.org
- National Treatment Agency for Substance Misuse (Special Health Authority) — www.nta.nhs.uk
- Obsessive Compulsive Disorder charity — www.ocduk.org
- SANE—meeting the challenge of mental illness — www.sane.org.uk
- SIGN (National Society for Mental Health and Deafness) — www.signcharity.org.uk
- Young Minds (promotes child and adolescent mental health) — www.youngminds.org.uk

Mental health promotion

Approximately 1 in 6 people of working age have mental ill health, often anxiety or depression or a psychotic illness such as schizophrenia (prevalence ~0.9%) or bipolar disorder (manic depression). It is often linked to vulnerable groups and those who experience social exclusion, e.g. unemployed, prison population, abuse, domestic violence, poverty, chronic physical conditions, refugees, some black and ethnic minority groups, and those with alcohol and drug problems.

Aims of mental health promotion
- Reduce psychiatric disease.
- Reduce mental distress and disability.
- Promote self-esteem, mental ability, and resilience.
- Reduce the need for inpatient care.

Actions to promote mental health
- Raising public and health care professionals' awareness about mental ill health to reduce the stigma attached to it and to prevent discrimination.
- Early assessment, identification, treatment, and ongoing support of pregnant and postpartum women with mental health problems by midwives and health visitors.
- Providing support for parents in child rearing, e.g. parenting classes, support groups, referrals to specialists for children with learning difficulties, follow-up by health visitors, access to preschool and nursery education.
- Developing programmes in schools aimed at raising understanding of what mental health is.
  - Improve life and coping skills.
  - Develop skills, self-esteem, and self-confidence.
  - Raise expectations.
  - Develop an anti-bullying culture.
- Implementing programmes in the workplace to help employees cope with work overload and develop health–work–life balance; training programmes to ensure they have the skills and knowledge to do the job; involving them in decision making and providing opportunities for exercise, relaxation, and stress management.
- Providing education to communities and individuals.
  - How to support others at times of stress.
  - Benefits of exercise and relaxation.
  - How to drink sensibly and avoid illegal drugs.
  - Where to get help and support when problems arise.
  - How to develop interpersonal awareness, coping mechanisms, self-confidence and self-esteem.
- Providing community support and access to specialist help for vulnerable groups, e.g. helping the unemployed find work, helping divorced people manage life changes, helping children whose parents are divorcing, providing bereavement support for the recently widowed, providing access to health services for the homeless, refugees, and asylum seekers, and supporting people released from prison.

Nursing in the community

Overview of primary care and public health

Primary care health services

Primary care is defined by the WHO as the first level of contact that individuals, the family, and community have with a national health system. It brings health care as close as possible to where people live and work. It is the first element of a continuing health care process that starts in the home, may progress to hospital, and then may return to home again. In the UK the core primary care services available in all areas include:

- 24-hour NHS helpline, e.g. NHS Direct, NHS 24
- General medical services (📖 General practice, below) and their 'out-of-hours' (OOH) GP services
- Midwifery
- Pharmacy
- Dentist
- Optician
- A variety of community health nursing services based in various community clinics, health centres, and GP surgeries:
  - Nursing in the home (e.g. district nursing)
  - Public health nursing (e.g. health visiting, school nursing)
  - Sexual health and contraceptive services

Other primary health care services available

- Chiropody, dentistry, optometry, speech and language therapy, occupational therapy, and physiotherapy for specific patient groups.
- A variety of specialist services that may be linked to hospitals, hospices, and other providers of health care such as:
  - Multidisciplinary specialist teams in palliative care, rehabilitation, chronic disease management, intermediate care, and rapid response.
  - Clinical nurse specialists, e.g. continence, diabetes, TB, and tissue viability.
  - 'Walk in' treatment and 'drop in' centres for assessment, prevention, identification, and treatment of minor injuries and health problems (usually staffed by specially prepared nurses).
  - Community hospitals whose admission and clinical management is usually through GPs and primary care nurses.

General practice

Most general practitioners (GPs) are not directly employed by the NHS. Their contract with the NHS specifies that they provide day-to-day medical care for the practice's registered patients. This care includes the management of:

- Minor and self-limiting illness
- Referral to secondary services and other services as appropriate
- Non-specialist care of those who are terminally ill
- Chronic disease management

In addition they may choose to provide:
- Cervical cancer screening
- Contraceptive services
- Vaccinations and immunizations
- Child health surveillance
- Maternity services
- Minor surgery procedures, e.g. curettage and cautery

Registration with a practice In the UK, people apply to register with a GP by handing in their NHS medical card to the GP practice reception or completing an application form. Temporary registration can be obtained if the person is a resident for longer than 24 hours but less than 3 months. People may change their GP without giving an explanation, giving a period of notice, or informing the GP.

Morbidity and mortality

Health is influenced by a multiplicity of factors as summarized in Fig. 32.1.

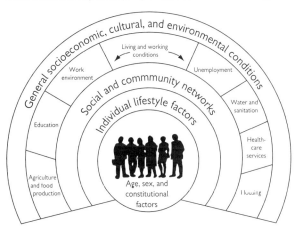

Fig. 32.1 Influences on health. Reproduced with kind permission of the authors Margaret Whitehead and Goran Dahlgren. Dahlgren G and Whitehead M (1993). *Tackling inequalities in health: what can we learn from what has been tried?* Working paper prepared for the King's Fund International Seminar on Tackling Inequalities in Health, Ditchley Park, Oxfordshire. London. Reproduced with permission of King's Fund. © 1993.

The major causes of death in the UK are:
- Cardiovascular disease, which has a male-to-female ratio of almost 2:1
- Cancer, with the commonest types being breast, lung, colorectal, and prostate
- Respiratory disease

Mortality rates vary with age and sex, e.g. for those aged 45–64 cancer is the leading cause of death (National Statistics Office, 📖 Further reading, p.1006).

Health inequalities

People are likely to experience worse health if they experience one or more of the following than if they do not:

- Economic disadvantage
- Lower educational attainment
- Insecure employment

There is also evidence that living in a materially deprived neighbourhood contributes to worse health for individuals. 📖 Chapter 5, Factors that determine health, p.88.

Public health

A definition of public health and public health nurses is '… the science and the art of preventing disease, prolonging life, and promoting physical and mental health through the organized efforts of society' (Independent Inquiry into Inequalities in Health, 1997). It takes a collective view rather than an individual view of the health needs and health care of a population.

Every primary care organization has a public health department. Its role is to:

- Provide advice to service commissioners.
- Monitor the health of the local population and the impact of services.
- Implement measures to prevent communicable infectious diseases.
- Address outbreaks of communicable diseases.
- Develop health promotion campaigns and may provide materials such as leaflets, etc.

The public health department's annual reports provide valuable information about the health needs of local populations for nursing in the community.

Further information

Association of Public Health Observatories: www.apho.org.uk/apho/
Health Protection Agency: www.hpa.org.uk
The National Health Service: www.nhs.uk/thenhsexplained
National Statistics Office: www.statistics.gov.uk/default.asp
World Health Organization (1978). Declaration of Alma Ata.
Acheson D, chairman (1997). Independent inquiry into inequalities in health. The Stationery Office, London.

Overview of primary care and community nursing

Nurses and health visitors working in primary care settings deliver services that range from providing public health services to providing preventative, curative, and chronic disease care to providing end-of-life care. Sometimes their main work roles are categorized by the type of care they provide:

- First contact services (e.g. in walk-in centres and nurse practitioners)
- Chronic disease (or long-term conditions) management services, including palliative care (e.g. adult community nursing services, practice nursing)
- Public health services (e.g. practice nursing, health visiting, school nursing)

Nurses in primary care can be generalists or specialists. Generalists are practice nurses who work with patients who are registered in the GP practice. Specialist nurses work with only one type of condition (e.g. people with sickle cell disorders), work with only one part of the population (e.g. travellers), or provide only one type of service (e.g. sexual health or contraceptive services).

In the UK more than 68,000 nurses and health visitors are employed by primary care organizations and more than 26,000 practice nurses are employed by general practices. The numbers are increasing as more health care is delivered in primary health care settings. The largest groups of nurses are within:

- District nursing services (adult community nursing services)
- Practice nursing (general practice nursing)
- Health visiting and school nursing services (children and family nursing services)

Most nurses work as small teams comprising registered nurses, health care assistants, and sometimes other staff such as nursery nurses (mostly health visiting). Practice nurses work only with patients registered to their practice. Adult community nursing teams may be affiliated with only one GP practice or may be affiliated with a cluster of practices. Specialist nurses working in the community in such areas as tissue viability, diabetes, and heart disease may also be linked to GP practices.

Smaller numbers of nurses work in community specialist services such as family planning services, sexual health services, walk-in centres, out-of-hours centres, and occupational health services. Some specialist nurses work in primary care as outreach from the hospital consultant led team, e.g. diabetes specialist nurses. Many services are evolving and changing constantly, sometimes introducing new roles (e.g. community matrons in England and nurse practitioners with advanced practice skills). Primary care offers a very dynamic environment for career development. Local as well as national advice should always be sought on educational pathways and the competencies required of different roles.

Working in primary care and domiciliary settings

Working in primary care and domiciliary (home) settings is very different than working in the hospital setting. The main differences (Drennan et al. 2005) are:

- Patients and their carers undertake most of their own health care and the overall nursing contribution is small.
- The patient is in control of all decisions. When providing services in the patient's home, the nurse is a guest who has no right of entry or action other than by invitation.
- Many systems and infrastructures support the delivery of health and social care; these are locally specific and variable. It takes time to familiarize oneself with the full range of local available services.
- Clinical decision making and care delivery are often done independently and at a physical distance from other colleagues.
- Nurses in primary care work with uncertainty. Changing situations and services require flexibility in the approach and assertiveness to work on the patient's behalf.

Even the most experienced hospital nurse may at first find the transition to a primary care setting difficult as the resources at hand are sometimes less immediately available. Additionally, the patient's role changes, in that they are now in their own home and are inviting the nurse in to care for them. All nurses and nurse learners new to working in primary care should ensure that they have:

- An orientation and induction process to their work and the setting
- A mentor who will review and discuss the nurse's clinical work
- An opportunity to work with other nurse role models and to shadow other professionals, e.g. social workers
- Access to information about the local service environment (e.g. directories, public health reports), the range of local services, referral mechanisms, key contacts, eligibility criteria, and funding mechanisms for different services
- Knowledge of risk assessment processes for both patient and personal safety, especially if working alone or providing services in a patient's home
- Information on how to navigate the area in which the service is delivered

Many community nursing teams produce and share community profiles of their areas, which include public health information, information on local services, local voluntary organizations, and detailed contact information.

Further information

NHS Nursing Careers: www.nhscareers.nhs.uk/careers/nursing/
The NHS Security Management Serivce—lone workers: www.nhsbsa.nhs.uk/

Nursing assessment and care management

Systematic assessment of need and care planning for adults with long-term conditions is one of the core skills of community nurses, and has the potential to substantially affect a person's quality of life. In primary care, assessment often involves other professionals and services (e.g. social services) and a recognition that most of the care will be done by the patient and/or their carers. High quality comprehensive assessment can be the means by which individuals can access care and services tailored to their needs. Assessment strategies are influenced by:

- The problem-solving framework of the nursing process, i.e. assessment, planning, implementation, evaluation
- Nursing models, theories, and values, e.g. focus on activities of daily living, partnership working, self-care, and health promotion
- Local policies, e.g. risk assessment and avoidance of unplanned hospital admissions, the use of local comprehensive assessment frameworks (CAF) shared across health and social care services
- Computerized records and databases, which can often dictate how assessment data are collected, recorded, and shared

Principles of assessment

Assessment should incorporate a sense of the patient's own rating of health status and focus on the needs of the patient and their carers. It should not be limited by what is available from the service. The assessment should include objective and quantifiable data as well as subjective, client focused data. The assessment leads to the development of an agreed care plan and provides the basis for selecting proper nursing interventions. Most individual health needs assessments will include obtaining a biographical profile and evaluating physiological, psychological, environmental, sociocultural, and spiritual domains.

At an individual level, theories of need have largely provided the basis for primary care nurses to understand how patients respond. For example, Maslow's hierarchy of needs suggest that an individual's lower level needs must be met before their higher level ones can be met, i.e. physiological → safety → belonging → esteem → self-actualization. Methods for directing assessments by nurses in primary care include:

- Nursing models (e.g. Roper)
- Biomedical (diagnostic) models, i.e. history taking, physical examination, requesting special investigations. (These are more commonly used in advanced and first-contact roles, e.g. nurse practitioners.)
- Health promotion models

Assessment and planning in primary care takes into account the environment, the housing, socioeconomic factors, family/social networks, and local health care facilities.

Older people

Standardized assessment tools should include the following domains: social, physical, mood, quality of life, and cognition. Integrated health and social care assessment processes for adults in need are being used in all

UK countries, e.g. Single Assessment Process (SAP). The scale and depth of the assessment is kept in proportion to older people's needs and avoids duplication of services.

Patients with long-term conditions and care management

Approximately 8.8 million people have a long-term condition (LTC) in the UK. Some have multiple conditions and complex care needs. Different levels of need among people with LTCs are described in the long-term conditions model of care, which is often represented as a triangle (See Fig. 32.2). The aim of this model is to treat patients sooner, in health care settings nearer to home, and earlier in the course of the disease. Care is focused on detecting conditions early, reducing effects of the disease, reducing complications, providing effective medicines management, reducing the number of crises, increasing independence, and prolonging and extending the quality of life.

Case (case management) is a particular approach to assessment and management of care of people with long-term conditions who have highly complex needs and are living in the community. The named case manager (akin to a key worker) has a responsibility to coordinate the care plan across services and coordinate regular review.

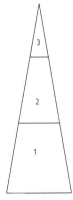

- **Level 3** Highly complex patients (5%) at risk, e.g. through numbers of hospital admissions, medical conditions, medicines, GP consultations, falls etc. Care coordinated by key worker/case manager with advanced clinical and prescribing skills, e.g. community matron.
- **Level 2** High-risk patients. Disease/care management needs met through primary care multidisciplinary teams, i.e. involving practice nursing or district nursing with specialist support and advice. The care delivery is informed by agreed standards and protocols, systems of identification, recall, and review.
- **Level 1** 70–80% of patients with LTC self-care with support from the primary care team, e.g. practice nurse may be involved in LTC monitoring and education. Patients and their carers are supported to develop knowledge, skills, and confidence to care for themselves and their condition effectively. Often referred to the expert patient programme (EPP).

Fig. 32.2 Levels of need among people with long-term conditions

Further information

Centre for Policy on Ageing. Materials for SAP: www.cpa.org.uk/sap/sap
Department of Health (2007). *The NHS and social care long term conditions model*: www.dh.gov.uk
Expert Patient Programme: www.expertpatients.co.uk

Delivering nursing care in the home

Nursing care is given in the home when the person is unable to leave their home and is unable to receive care at a general practice or at a clinic in the community health centre. Patients may also receive care in the home to prevent hospital admission or as a step down from hospital care. Types of nursing care delivered in the home are:

- Short-term intervention, e.g. post-surgery wound care
- Longer-term intervention, e.g. support, education and monitoring for someone newly diagnosed as diabetic who also has mobility problems
- Time-limited interventions, e.g. someone in a palliative care stage of their condition requiring, among other things, support with medication, bowel and bladder care, pressure sore prevention, and support to carers

Most adults receiving nursing services in the home have more than one condition. The most common conditions include cardiovascular disease, COPD, diabetes, peripheral vascular disease, neurological conditions (e.g. multiple sclerosis, Parkinson's disease), arthritis/musculoskeletal conditions, dementia, and cancer. A central tenet of community nursing is to support interdependence and the patient risk assessment is undertaken with that objective.

Community nursing team

This team operates just like a hospital nursing team except that its 'ward' patients are dispersed geographically. Likewise the health and social care team members belong to a number of different organizations. All the same principles of high quality nursing care apply in the home as in hospital, i.e. the delivery of appropriate, acceptable, timely, safe, and effective evidence-based care.

Good nursing practice for lone working and home visiting

- Schedule appointments and ensure the base office knows all intended visits, journey details, telephone numbers, and anticipated arrival and departure times.
- Do not visit alone if the patient, relative, or carer has a history of violence or if the location is considered unsafe.
- Carry key safety equipment including ID badge, mobile phone, map of the local area, personal attack alarm and torch, and emergency telephone numbers.
- Adhere to safe home visiting practices.
  - When the front door is opened, carry out a 10-second risk assessment and if the environment feels unsafe have an excuse ready.
  - Request any animals be secured prior to entry.
  - Shut the front door and be familiar with the door lock.
  - Maintain awareness of entrances and exits.
  - If uncomfortable, do not sit down and do not spread belongings out.
  - If feel unsafe, make an excuse and leave immediately.

Differences in the care delivery from hospital settings

There are differences between the home setting and hospital setting. These include the delivery of care (particularly in regard to nursing records), medicines and dressing (📖 Medicines and associated health care products, p.1014), aids to nursing, incontinence management (📖 Continence and incontinence management, p.1015), infection control, and clinical waste.

Record keeping

All record keeping follows NMC standards. Two sets of nursing records are kept to ensure effective communication.
- One is kept in the patient's home. This often has a section for joint record keeping with home care services, particularly if medication administration or medicine prompting is involved.
- One is kept in the nursing team base office. In addition, the nursing team may either enter data direct onto the GP patient record or provide the GP with regular written updates for the GP patient record.

Aids to nursing care

Community nurses can obtain aids to support nursing in the home through a joint equipment store (i.e. NHS with the local authority). The patient's permission must be obtained before any equipment is brought into their home. Types of equipment include:
- Pressure relief equipment, e.g. some types of beds, cushions, mattresses (alternating pressure, fluidized bead flotation, foam, low air loss, ripple, water)
- Varied height/position beds and raising aids (e.g. monkey poles, chair raisers) and transfer aids (e.g. hoists, slide sheets, turntables)
- Toilet aids, e.g. urinals, commodes, and incontinence aids

The public may buy aids for independent living at specialist centres or may obtain them following local authority assessment, provided they meet the eligibility criteria. 📖 Social care and support, p.1016.

Infection control and clinical waste

All the principles of infection control are applied in delivering care in the home. Many community nurses wear their own clothes, not uniforms. These should be washed at 65°C for the first part of wash cycle to minimize risks of cross-infection. Personal protective equipment (e.g. gloves and aprons) is provided by the employer and used as in hospital. Alcohol rubs, gels, foams, etc. are often used in home settings that have poor hand washing facilities. Local council authorities provide the patient and their household with sharps containers and clinical waste bags (for dressings, swabs, incontinence management products, stoma bags, etc.). These are collected by special waste disposal services. Each area will have agreed policies for the provision, transportation, and disposal of sharps containers units for care in the home.

Further information

Disabled Living Foundation provides a wide range of fact sheets and advice on aids to independent living: www.dlf.org.uk

The NHS Security Management Serivce—lone workers: www.nhsbsa.nhs.uk/

National Institute for Clinical Excellence (2003). *Prevention of healthcare-associated infection in primary and community care*. Clinical guideline 2. London: www.nice.org.uk

Medicines and associated health care products

All medicine administration in primary care, as in the hospital, is in accordance with legal requirements and NMC guidelines. There are a few differences to the hospital environment that impact on nursing practice.

Patient medicines

In primary care, medicines and associated health care products, such as dressing packs, bandages, wound care products, and catheters, are prescribed for individual patients by independent prescribers (e.g. GPs or nurses and pharmacists with additional qualifications) on NHS prescriptions (known as FP 10s or GP 10s in Scotland). These medicines are dispensed by local pharmacists and then become the property of the patient (not the NHS), mostly for self administration.

Primary and community nursing services do not have any stocks of medicines, dressings, lotions, catheters, stoma bags, and incontinence products. Everything is prescribed or obtained from central supplies (in the case of continence pads) on a named patient basis. Nurses with authority to prescribe on FP 10s do so either by using the GP practice computers/prescription pads or by specifying the GP practice code on the prescription (pads supplied on a named nurse basis by their employers).

Nurses are well placed to give advice on the safe storage and safe disposal of medicines in the home.

- Keep medicines in cool, dark place away from light, heat (including steam), or as directed on the instructions, e.g. fridge, and out of sight and reach of children.
- Keep medicines in their original containers as they have instructions, expiry date, etc.
- If a medicine reminder device is used, always label the contents.
- Return unused medicines to the supplying pharmacy for destruction rather than disposing of them at home as this may harm the environment.

Nursing staff administering home stored medicines

- Nursing staff must be aware of individual medicine storage requirements. If the drug potency is compromised by poor storage, new supplies need to be obtained for administration or prompting.
- Local guidelines are available on the involvement of nursing staff in filling and prompting from medicine reminder devices. Many guidelines are available but all focus on safety concerns, e.g. labelling, opportunities for mix-ups particularly if the person has cognitive problems, or multiple carers helping with medication. Many areas now have schemes for a pharmacist to dispense into sealed monitored dosage systems, e.g. blister packs.
- Community nursing services do not hold controlled drug registers as controlled drugs are prescribed for and held by individual patients.

Medicines following hospital discharge

When patients are discharged from hospital, they require a 5–7 day supply of any medicines and associated health care products (including dressings). This allows for enough time for the next prescription to be written by their GP, taken to the local pharmacist, and dispensed. People with poor mobility may rely on carers or on the local pharmacist's delivery services to obtain their medicines. Home carers that are funded through local social services will only pick up medicines if specified in the social workers care manager care plan.

Patient group directions

Nurses working in specialist clinics (e.g. sexual health or family planning) are often authorized under patient group directions to prescribe and dispense specific medicines for specific categories of patients in specific circumstances (e.g. antibiotics, immunizations, and oral contraceptives).

Continence and incontinence management

Urinary catheters and bags and stoma bags are prescribed and dispensed to the individual patient (□ Medicines and associated health care products, p.1014). Many continence products such as pads are provided through the local NHS, often a specialist community continence service. The range of products available and the mechanisms for delivery to the person are determined by local policy. Disposal of clinical waste will be in accordance with the local authority's policy. Laundry costs are usually the responsibility of the individual patient and carers. All clinical waste (e.g., soiled dressings) is disposed of in a similar fashion.

Further information

Continence Foundation: www.continence-foundation.org.uk

Promoncon: *Promoting continence and product awareness*: www.promocon.co.uk

Royal Pharmaceutical Society of Great Britain (RPSGB) (2005). *The safe and secure handling of medicines: a team approach*. RPSGB, London.

National Prescribing Centre (2007). *A guide to good practice in the management of controlled drugs in primary care in England*, 2nd edn. NPC, Liverpool.

Social care and support

Patients' health needs are often closely related to their social needs. Consequently, health and social care services aim to collaborate as partner organizations and as practitioners. Social care services also link with private health and voluntary and charitable social care providers. They provide:

- Statutory services
- Mobility aids
- Help with bathing, cleaning, shopping, and meals
- Day centres
- Sheltered housing
- Care homes
- Services that provide support to particular groups, e.g. people with learning disabilities, carers

NB. Every nurse in primary care must be familiar with local referral processes to social workers and to other local agencies offering social support.

Social services departments

These have legal responsibilities under the NHS and Community Care Act 1991 to use public funds to provide a range of care, support, and protection services for vulnerable adults who, by reason of age or disability, need assistance to live an independent life. Support is also provided to their carers. These departments work in partnership with health, education, housing, law enforcement, and the voluntary sector to meet the needs of vulnerable people. Social services take direct inquiries from the public as well as referrals by professionals. People are assessed by a social worker to determine needs. Social workers can provide:

- Information about available care and support services
- An assessment of need (sometimes known as a community care assessment)
- Practical (including financial) help and support for some people who meet eligibility criteria
- Information about other organizations that may help.

NB Most social care services are charged following an individual assessment of the person's ability to pay (📖 Care home fees, p.1017). Decisions are made according to local policies, priorities, criteria of eligibility, and waiting lists.

Social care and support services available for vulnerable adults and older people and their families

- Services for older people with physical and mental frailty and their carers, e.g. home care, personal care, meals on wheels, equipment and home adaptations, short-term breaks
- Support for people with physical and/or sensory disabilities, mental health needs, or learning disabilities, e.g. registration for disabled people, day centre, and group activities
- Support teams for people with substance misuse problems
- Support for carers. 📖 Working with carers, p.1018.

Care homes

Approximately 4% of people >65 years old and 20% of people >85 years old live in a care home. Most are women. Registered care homes either have onsite nursing care and registered nurses (previously known as nursing homes) or do not have onsite nursing care (previously known as residential homes). Care homes are run by not-for-profit voluntary organizations, by private companies or, less frequently, by local authorities and the NHS. Care homes can provide:

- Long-term care for adults who, through frailty or disability, need help with personal care and/or have nursing care needs
- Respite, intermediate, and palliative care
- Specialist elderly mentally infirm (EMI) homes

All care homes are inspected against nationally set standards and are registered by the Care Quality Commission (CQC), or in Scotland by the Care Commission. Complaints and concerns not addressed by a care home are referred to these inspection bodies (📖 Further information, below). Some care homes have specific registration for EMI patients. Local CQC offices and social service departments provide lists of registered care homes.

Care home residents are registered with GPs and should receive the full range of NHS services. Community and specialist nurses therefore provide nursing care when it is needed for residents in both kinds of care homes. Residence in a care home does not limit access to NHS nursing support, e.g. health assessments, advice, support, referral to specialist services, medication reviews, wound care, end-of-life care, etc. Unfortunately there is very little funding (if any) for dental, chiropractic and optical care in homes.

Care home fees

Rules for public financial assistance differ in the four UK countries. More than half of residents in care homes have fees paid by local authorities (LAs). The starting point in all countries is the assessment of need by (usually) a social worker care manager. Social services have a set ceiling for fees and a list of preferred providers. The proportion of fees that is to be paid by the individual is based on a financial assessment that includes income (e.g. pension), savings, shares, and property (including the individual's own home). A resident in a care home with nursing may have the nursing care element of their fees paid by the NHS. Primary care organizations will have agreed a system for assessing the need for a Registered Nursing Care Contribution (RNCC). Amounts differ in each country in the UK.

Further information

Age Concern: www.ageconcern.org.uk (linked sites for all countries)
Counsel and Care: www.counselandcare.org.uk
Care Quality Commission: www.cqc.org.uk
Scottish Social Care Services Council: www.sssc.uk.com

Working with carers

A voluntary carer is someone who provides care on an unpaid basis. They provide this care either in association with or instead of paid-for carers (e.g. care workers, nurses, and social workers). It is estimated that there are >6 million voluntary carers in the UK, and they are key to the support of dependent family members and friends in the community.

Most carers look after older people and may provide:
- Personal care
- Physical help with daily activities
- Practical support, e.g. help with medication and shopping

The experience of being a carer is affected by the quality of the relationship between the carer and the dependent person prior to the initiation of the caring role as well as by how both parties relate to each other. Many carers derive high levels of personal satisfaction in their role. This does not mean, however, that they do not need support and regular review. There is a significant financial consequence of being a carer, i.e. 70% of carers worry about finances. Moreover, caring can be very stressful and thus may be detrimental to health.

Meeting the needs of carers

Nurses are well placed to offer ongoing support, advice, and help to carers. All health professionals that are in contact with carers should ensure that the carer's needs are considered independently of the patient.
- Carers should have access to a proper assessment of their needs.
- Carers should be consulted on decisions that affect them.
- Carers should have access to information about benefits, services, respite care, and sources of peer and voluntary/charity based support.
- Services should NOT be withheld because a carer is present.
- The needs of carers from a variety of diverse cultures should not be overlooked. The Carers (Equal Opportunities) Act 2004 gives carers the right to an assessment by local authority social workers for help and support in their own right. The purpose of the assessment is to:
  - Discuss the help required to support the caring role, including housing and need for aids and adaptations.
  - Explore how an individual feels about being a carer.
  - Provide information about benefits.
  - Discuss how caring responsibilities can be balanced with other responsibilities, e.g. work and leisure interests.
  - Plan for the future, consider how responsibilities might change over time, and plan in case of emergencies.
  - If caring is likely to continue indefinitely, a review date should be set.

Young carers

These are defined as anyone <18 years old whose life is in some way restricted because of the need to take responsibility for someone else. Being a young carer can have several adverse effects:
- Schooling, e.g. learning and attendance
- Relationships with peers

- Relationships within the family
- Emotional and physical health and growth

Community nurses providing care to adults with long-term conditions are in a good position to offer support to young carers. Young carers should also have an assessment of their needs by a social worker under the terms of the Carers Act 1995 and the Children's Act 1989.

Help and support available to carers

Several programmes and services are available to provide help and support to carers, but there is considerable local variation. 📖 Social care and support, p.1016

- Help at home: means tested support from social services
- Voluntary organizations, e.g. local carer support groups; Crossroads offers sitting services
- Involvement of district nursing service and relevant specialist nursing support, e.g. admiral nurses for carers of people with dementia
- Day care, i.e. social services centres providing day care for older people
- Respite care, i.e. short-term residential care providing carer with planned breaks. (Social services may provide support with costs.)
- Aids and equipment either through social services or local voluntary sector
- Adapting the home environment, i.e. the carer may be eligible for a local authority home improvement grant
- Carer support offered by social services, e.g. help with taxi fares for hospital visits
- Financial support, e.g. Attendance Allowance, Carers Allowance, direct payments, vouchers to purchase care, Independent Living Fund
- Local pharmacy support, e.g. delivery of repeat prescriptions

Further information

Carers UK: www.carersuk.org.uk
Caring about Carers; Carers Strategy: www.carers.gov.uk
Princess Royal Trust for Carers: www.carers.org
Children's Society Young Carers Initiative: www.youngcarer.com

Emergencies

Nursing care of patient emergencies

This chapter is divided into two parts. The first part concerns basic first aid and emergency care principles which may be helpful outside the emergency department (ED), but still in a clinical setting/hospital. In some cases very basic advice is given so that the nurse can assist in situations outside the hospital and in the community setting when medical assistance is unavailable. The second part of the chapter focuses on some of the work carried out in an ED and gives the non-specialist or student a brief overview and introduction to emergency care in a specialist unit.

Medical emergencies

Key points

- A medical emergency is a critical life-threatening situation. It is often a sudden and unexpected event, happening anywhere, anytime.
- The nurse must be aware of the basic principles of first aid and how to deal with emergencies in their own clinical practice area.
- Trauma is the third largest cause of death in all regions of the world and is the leading cause of death in young people. A key influential factor affecting patterns of injury all over the world is the increasing abuse of alcohol and other drugs.
- The incidence of deaths from natural disasters and terrorist attacks appears to be rising.
- Emergency health care is increasingly provided by an integrated network and team made up of first responders, ambulance crews (paramedical staff), air ambulance, GPs, walk-in clinics, minor injury units, and trauma centres.
- Prevention of injury and the principles of how to deal with medical emergencies are important goals for nurses working in health promotion and patient/family health education.

Principles

The principles of managing patient emergencies are the same irrespective of the context in which the emergency occurs.

- Quickly assess the situation and the possible causes of the incident.
- Do not put yourself at risk—think before you act. Be aware of hazards in the environment and make the environment safe, if possible.

For all pre-hospital emergencies, start with:

- SAFE approach
  - **S** = Shout or call help.
  - **A** = Assess the scene for dangers to rescuer or patient.
  - **F** = Free from danger.
  - **E** = Evaluate the casualty
- Identify and correct any immediate life-threatening conditions. Use the ABCDE system and life support methods.
  - **A**—airway and cervical spine control
  - **B**—breathing
  - **C**—circulation with haemorrhage control
  - **D**—disabilities (detect and monitor other injuries; check level of consciousness)
  - **E**—exposure (protect the patient, prevent further injury and provide emergency/first aid care),
- Don't forget to send for help.

General principles of first aid for nurses

First aid is traditionally associated with the help given to someone who is injured or who is suffering from an acute medical problem and requires medical assistance. The British Red Cross Society defines first aid as 'the first assistance or treatment given to a casualty before the arrival of specially trained paramedical personnel/ambulance or medical team.' It is restricted to immediate or temporary care and is the first link in the chain of emergency medicine.

Various voluntary bodies such as the St John Ambulance brigade, the Red Cross, and St Andrew's First Aid in Scotland have traditionally dominated this area of care. In the UK, however, recent improvements in ambulance services have resulted in the development of the paramedic/ambulance crew who are now trained to a high level of expertise in emergency medicine. There are also specially trained 'first responders' in some areas of the country where ambulance access is difficult.

All nurses should be knowledgeable in first aid so that they can give immediate assistance to patients in any area of the hospital and community where they work. The incidence of accidents in the home and workplace is very high. Moreover, the increasing terrorist threat makes it essential that nurses be well prepared for an emergency wherever it may occur.

The Code of Professional Conduct expects nurses to act with a professional duty to provide care in an emergency, in or outside the work setting. The care provided by a nurse will be judged against what could reasonably be expected based on the nurse's knowledge, skills, and abilities when placed in those particular circumstances.

There is now a lot more advice emerging with regard to what to do if you are involved in out-of-hospital emergencies. For example what first aid care is appropriate, what equipment to carry and how to control and use bystanders. The NMC expects nurses to know the basics of first aid and to act in a sensible and reasonable manner if confronted with an emergency situation.

Good Samaritan acts

In the UK there has been great debate about what nurses should do if they encounter trauma situations as bystanders or passers-by. There is an ethical, moral, and professional duty to stop and render assistance. To encourage this help for accident victims, many states in North America have passed statutes that grant health care professionals immunity from liability for negligent acts.

It is assumed that in the UK a similar sensitivity would be shown to health care professionals acting in good faith. The exception to 'Good Samaritan acts' would be if a nurse acted wilfully with gross negligence towards a victim; then a judgement of liability may be possible.

Key legal points

- Nurses who intervene in any situation outside the course of their work will still be judged by the standards of the average professional skilled nurse.
- The situation and circumstances would probably be taken into consideration and the nurse's clinical judgment at the time.

- Any action undertaken for the benefit of another carries a risk if it goes wrong especially if the person delivering the first aid is a professional nurse.
- Although the NMC expects nurses to do their best and help if needed at an emergency, nurses can only be expected to work within their realm of experience and education.
- Nurses are accountable to patients, the public, their employers, and to the profession and have a duty to care for people.
- If first aid competence is considered to be an integral part of a registered practitioner's role, then the skills involved should clearly be part of nurse training at both pre- and post-registration levels.
- Continuous updating should be provided by employers who expect nurses to act in emergency situations.
- If a nurse is injured as a result of assisting a patient/casualty, then the nurse could take legal action against the person whose negligence led to the situation where help was needed.

Further information

British Association for Immediate Care (Basics): Tel: 01473 218 407; www.basics.org.uk/intropage.htm

Priorities when faced with an emergency situation

The principles of first aid as outlined in the first part of this chapter are very basic and are relevant to all areas of nursing and emergency medical care wherever they occur.

- Know what to do based on established guidelines for administering first aid care.
- Do not put yourself at risk.
- Assess a situation quickly and safely.
- Prioritize treatment and care.
- Know when additional help is needed.
- Stay as calm as possible.
- Know what measures to take to save a person's life.
- Know how to give immediate help and assistance.
- Determine what type of help is needed, e.g. physician, ambulance, fire service, police.
- Know how to protect casualties and prevent further injury.
- Give comfort and reassurance to victims.
- Be aware of one's limitations and be self-aware of what to do based on previous knowledge and experience.

After being faced with an emergency situation, it may be helpful to talk to a colleague about what happened and to be alert to any emotional reaction to the situation.

Calling for help

In the hospital, emergency medical assistance will be readily available and it is important to know the emergency number to call for help.

- When on duty in a hospital setting in the UK, the emergency number is 2222.
- There is also an emergency button or call system available in most UK hospitals, so check this out when you start working on a ward.
- In the UK, when working as a nurse in the community or when off duty, the nurse must dial 999 and use the emergency services. Dialing 112 can also be used to contact the emergency services on a mobile phone.

Administering first aid outside the hospital setting

- Quickly assess the scene (a major incident involves many people and multiple casualties).
- Ensure your own safety and that of other rescuers.
- If in a car, park it safely with hazard warning lights on.
- Be careful of fast oncoming traffic especially on a motorway.
- If available, wear a reflective protective jacket.
- Use protective gloves.
- If a mobile phone is available, dial 999 (or 112) and request emergency services. Remember to give the exact location and a brief description of the incident.
- If the incident is a road traffic accident, switch off all engines.
- Be aware of any fluid spillages such as petrol and chemicals.
- Apply hand brakes.

- Send bystanders to warn other drivers.
- Set up, if available, warning triangles and lights.
- Ensure that no one is smoking or displays a naked flame.
- Look for hidden casualties who may have been thrown some distance from the immediate scene.
- If electricity or chemicals are involved, be careful and seek expert help and advice.
- Talk to casualties to check if they are conscious and breathing.
- Examine the casualties and determine the priorities.
- Do not move the casualty unless it is absolutely necessary.
- Keep the casualty's head still in case of a neck injury if sitting in a vehicle.
- Seek information from any witnesses of what happened as this may help in determining the casualty's injuries.
- Use ABCDE system to assess the patient.
  - *Airway* – Protect cervical spine, if injury is possible. Assess airway for any signs of obstruction and keep patent.
  - *Breathing* – Check rate and chest movement. If casualty is not breathing, treat as an arrest (📖 Cardiopulmonary arrest, pp.1036–7). *Suspect cardiac arrest in any patient who is unconscious and who does not have signs of life.* May need to place the casualty in the recovery position if they are breathing and have not had a cardiac arrest but there is danger of them obstructing their airway (See Fig. 33.1).
  - *Circulation* – Check pulses at wrist (radial) and neck (carotid). If absent, treat as an arrest (📖 Cardiopulmonary arrest, pp.1036–7). Look for evidence of bleeding if casualty is in shock (📖 Shock, pp.1038–9).
  - *Disability* – Assess level of consciousness using AVPU score (**A**lert? Responds to **V**oice? To **P**ain? **U**nresponsive?). Check pupils for size, equality, and reactions. (Use principles of the Glasgow Coma Scale, See Table 33.1.)
  - *Exposure* – Check casualty's body carefully looking for signs of discomfort, immobility, and pain,
- *Ask them where they hurt and if they feel any internal pain and discomfort.*
- *Remove clothing very carefully and only if necessary to obtain a diagnosis.*
- *Leave protective helmets in place.*
- Prevent hypothermia. Use an emergency blanket if available.
- Keep talking to the casualty, reassuring them in a positive manner.
- Monitor their condition and look out for signs of deterioration and further signs of pain and discomfort.
- Carefully check pulse rate and enquire about any significant medical history.
- Unless medical equipment is available, it may be impossible to monitor vital signs such as blood pressure and oxygen saturation.
- The casualty should be transported to hospital and a written/verbal handover given to ED staff.
- For further help, see approved First Aid Manual which is regularly updated and published by Dorling Kindersley (www.dk.com/firstaidmanual).

Administering first aid inside a hospital but outside an ED

- Use the ABCDE system. 📖 Use of the ABCDE principles in the emergency department, p.1098.
- Check the patient's airway.
- Check the patient's breathing; if no response proceed to arrest situation. 📖 Cardiopulmonary arrest, p.1036.
- Check the patient's pulse. The wrist (radial) pulse is often unreliable in an emergency, therefore use the carotid or femoral.
- If no responses, proceed to arrest situation. 📖 Cardiopulmonary arrest, p.1036.
- Call for help by initiating the emergency call bell and dial for medical assistance (use 2222 if an arrest situation).
- Ask the patient or any witnesses what happened.
- Systematically scan the patient's body from head to toe looking for signs of injury or acute illness due to a medical emergency.
- Notice the patient's body position and their mobility and movement.
- If the patient has fallen or you suspect they have fallen, do not move them until you are confident they have not injured themselves.
- Get expert help to move the patient if serious injury is suspected.
- Look for signs of bleeding externally and control bleeding.
- Ask the patient if they have any particular pain and discomfort.
- Seek information about the patient from the members of staff and the medical/nursing records.
- Keep a record of any treatment given or drugs and IV fluids administered.
- Monitor the patient's vital signs and oxygen saturation.
- Continually reassure the patient, monitoring their condition.
- Reassure other patients who may have seen the incident.
- Inform close relatives of the incident, especially if the condition of the patient has changed.
- Record the event in the nursing records and fill in any relevant incident forms.
- Note the names of emergency medical staff who attended to the patient.
- Check and restock emergency trolley following the incident.
- Debrief the members of the ward team and evaluate their performance and procedures.

(a)

(b)

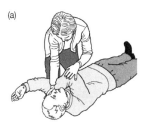
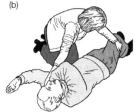

- Place the arm nearest to you out at right angles to his body, elbow bent with the palm uppermost.
- Bring the far arm across the chest and hold the back of the hand against the patient's nearest cheek.
- With your other hand, grasp the far leg just above the knee and pull it up, keeping the foot on the ground.

- Keeping the hand pressed against the cheek, pull on the leg to roll the patient towards you onto his side.
- Adjust the upper leg so that both the hip and knee are bent at right angles.
- Tilt the head back to make sure the airway remains open
- Adjust the hand under the cheek, if necessary, to keep the head tilted.
- Check breathing regularly.

(c)

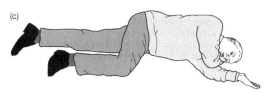

Fig. 33.1 The recovery position. Reproduced with kind permission of the Resuscitation Council UK. www.resus.org.uk.

Care of the unconscious patient (both within and outside the hospital environment)

There are several common causes of deteriorating consciousness or unconsciousness:

- Hypoglycaemia
- Drug overdose
- Head injury
- Stroke
- Subarachnoid haemorrhage
- Convulsions
- Alcohol intoxication
- Other causes include cardiac and respiratory failure, arrhythmias, hypovalaemic shock, anaphylaxis, hepatic and renal failure, hypothermia/hyperthermia, meningitis/encephalitis and malaria

Key priorities when caring for the unconscious patient (see Fig. 33.3)

- Assess and maintain the patient's airway and breathing. 📖 Maintaining a clear airway, p.1033.
- Check the pulse and circulation.
- Nurse in the recovery position to help maintain a clear airway.
  (If a spinal injury is suspected, three people will be required to help place in the recovery position: the first to steady the head, the second to turn the body, and the third to keep the back straight. This is known as the log-roll technique. (See First Aid Manual, DK, London.)
- Monitor the patient's vital signs, if the appropriate equipment is available.
  - Temperature
  - Pulse, blood pressure
  - Oxygen saturation
  - ECG
- Assess level of consciousness using the principles of the 'Glasgow Coma Scale' (See Table 33.1), and record if possible.
- Check the patient's colour and feel the skin temperature if no thermometer is available.
- Check blood glucose if in a hospital setting (initially by base medium plus glucose [BMG]).
- Obtain reliable venous access and replace IV fluids if indicated and prescribed. (Only for nursing personnel with appropriate training and experience.)
- Note whether the patient passes urine and check any signs of severe diarrhoea (recording fluid balance may be difficult but if it is possible it would be useful).
- Obtain any further information about how the patient was found and any relevant medical and health history; check patient's clothing and possessions for tablets and information relating to possible causes of condition.
- Interview close relatives and friends.

- Don't leave the patient alone.
- Make a note of or record on appropriate charts (if in hospital) any relevant progress, and any signs of recovery or deterioration.
- Further investigations may need to be carried out such as radiological investigations and CT scan.

Maintaining a clear airway

- Look and listen to check how the patient is breathing (breath sounds).
- Record breathing rate over one minute.
- Talk to the patient and listen to their reply.
- Observe for any paradoxical chest and abdominal movements, gurgling or snoring sounds.
- Look in mouth and pharynx.
- Clear any obstruction using Magill's forceps, if available. If forceps are not available, use a suitable rigid instrument.
- Suck out any liquid with a large rigid suction catheter if available.
- Check gag reflex; avoid precipitating coughing and vomiting.
- If neck injury is not suspected, then lift the chin and use the jaw thrust manoeuvre to open the airway.
- Do not tilt the neck.
- Look, listen, and feel to reassess the airway and breathing.
- If gag reflex is absent or poor, an oropharyngeal airway or in some situations a nasopharyngeal airway will be inserted.
- If airway is patent and the patient is breathing, then a high concentration of oxygen (15 l/min via a non-rebreathing reservoir mask) is given.

When a neck injury is suspected

- Avoid causing or exacerbating any neck injury.
- Someone should be instructed to hold the head and neck in a neutral position until the neck has been satisfactorily immobilized (See Fig. 33.2). See also Fig 33.3, How to move an unconscious patient.

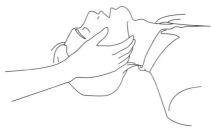

Fig. 33.2 Performing a jaw-thrust. Taken from Thomas J. and Monaghan T (2007). *Oxford Handbook of Clinical Examination and Practical Skills*. Reproduced with permission from Oxford University Press.

Table 33.1 Glasgow Coma Scale

Test	Score	Patient's response
Eye opening Spontaneously	4	Opens eyes spontaneously
To speech	3	Open eyes to verbal command
To pain	2	Opens eyes to painful stimulus
None	1	Does not open eyes in response to stimulus
Motor response Obeys	6	Reacts to verbal command
Localizes	5	Identifies localized pain
Withdraws	4	Flexes and withdraws from painful stimulus
Abnormal flexion	3	Assumes a decorticate position
Abnormal extension	2	Assumes a decerebrate position
None	1	No response, just lies flaccid
Verbal response Oriented	5	Is oriented and converses
Confused	4	Is disoriented and confused
Inappropriate words	3	Replies randomly with incorrect words
Incomprehensible	2	Moans or screams
None	1	No response
Total score		

AVPU system for a quick assessment of level of consciousness

A = alert
V = responds to voice
P = responds to pain
U = unresponsive

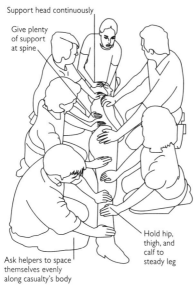

Support head continuously

Give plenty
of support
at spine

Hold hip,
thigh, and
calf to
steady leg

Ask helpers to space
themselves evenly
along casualty's body

Fig. 33.3 How to move an unconscious patient.

Cardiopulmonary arrest

This is the cessation of respiratory effort and cardiac activity (the heart and breathing stop). Basic cardiopulmonary resuscitation (CPR) and advanced life support (ALS) measures are required for successful resuscitation. 📖 Advanced life support, p.1103.

Basic life support

The three elements of basic life support include Airway, Breathing, and Circulation (i.e. ABC). See Fig. 33.4.

Adult sequence

- Ask, are you safe?
- Check patient's response—shake and ask.
- If no response:
  - Shout for help—call ambulance or arrest team.
  - Turn patient onto the back.
  - Open airway and lift chin.
  - Tilt head back.
  - Listen and check breathing for 10 seconds.
  - Look for chest movement.
- If not breathing:
  - Commence chest compressions.
  - Place heel of one hand in the centre of the patient's chest and other hand over it. Interlock fingers. (See Fig. 33.5.)
  - Give chest compressions at a rate of 100 per minute.
  - After 30 compressions open the airway and give 2 breaths.
  - Repeat until help arrives.
- Place patient in the recovery position if they have started breathing spontaneously and have a pulse.

Basic life support for children

Children sometimes do not receive resuscitation because potential rescuers fear causing harm. The Resuscitation Council recommends using the adult sequence with the following minor modifications:

- Give 5 initial rescue breaths before starting chest compressions. Note that the head is not tilted as far back in paediatric resuscitation as it is for adult resuscitation.
- If you are alone with the child, perform CPR for 1 minute before going for help.
- Compress the chest by approximately one-third of its depth. Use two fingers for an infant under 1 year; use one or two hands for a child over 1 year as needed to achieve an adequate depth of compression.

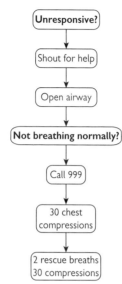

Fig. 33.4 Adult basic life support. Reproduced with kind permission of the Resuscitation Council UK. www.resus.org.uk. Don't forget to call 999 (or 112) or if in hospital 2222.
NB The rate should be 100 compressions per minute.

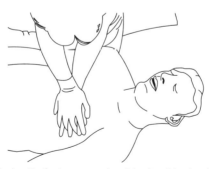

Fig. 33.5 Hand position for chest compressions. Taken from Wyatt J. et al. (2006) *Oxford Handbook of Emergency Medicine*. Reproduced with permission from Oxford University Press.

Further information

Resuscitation Council (UK): www.resus.org.uk

Shock

This is a life-threatening emergency. It occurs when the oxygen supply is inadequate to meet the demand at the cellular level. Usually this is due to failure of the circulatory system. In this hypoxic state, cellular metabolism is altered, metabolic acidosis develops, and organ damage and death may result.

Recognition of shock

- Hypotension—systolic blood pressure <90 mmHg in adults. Values may be higher in young, fit, or previously hypertensive patients.
- Changes in pulse rate—associated tachycardia (>100) is common but may not be present in patients with cardiac or neurological causes.
- Altered consciousness and/or fainting, especially on standing or sitting up.
- Poor peripheral perfusion—cool peripheries, clammy/sweaty skin, pallor. (In the early phase of endotoxic septic shock, vasodilation with warm peripheries may occur.)
- Low urinary output—oliguria (<50 mL/hour) in adults.
- A fast rate of breathing—tachypnoea.

Types of shock

- Fluid problems (hypovolaemia) caused by haemorrhage, dehydration, ruptured aortic aneurysm, ruptured ectopic pregnancy, severe fluid loss in burns, and gastrointestinal problems such as severe vomiting and diarrhoea.
- Cardiac pumping problems (cardiogenic) caused by myocardial infarction, contusion, tamponade, or cardiac disease. Also pulmonary embolus, and tension pneumothorax.
- Septic shock common in children and in older people. Associated with diabetes mellitus, renal/hepatic failure, and severe infections and those with immunocompromised problems.
- Anaphylactic shock—immunological condition caused by exposure to a foreign substance, e.g. drugs, vaccines, bee/wasp stings, foods such as nuts, and materials such as latex.
- Neurogenic shock.

Shock can be exacerbated by fear and pain; therefore it is important to give reassurance and comfort to the patient.

Physical signs and symptoms

- Pallor
- Sweating
- Distress
- Cold clammy skin
- Cyanosis
- Weakness and dizziness
- Nausea and vomiting
- Thirst
- Rapid shallow breathing
- Weak 'thready' pulse (vasodilation with a bounding pulse is suggestive of septic shock), or tachycardia
- Yawning and gasping
- Hypotension

Patients with anaphylactic shock may have swelling of the face, neck, and tongue, which may result in difficulty breathing. Also skin may become red and blotchy. Eyelids may be swollen and puffy.

Nursing care

- Stay with the patient as signs and symptoms may deteriorate.
- Remember priorities, i.e. airway, breathing, and circulation (ABC).
- Monitor the pulse for bradycardia or tachycardia.
- Monitor blood pressure, oxygen saturation, heart (ECG), level of consciousness, skin colour, respiratory rate, and urine output.
- Lay patient down and raise and support legs, loosen tight clothing, keep warm, and ensure nil by mouth.
- Provide reassurance and support as patient may be very anxious and stressed.
- Ensure patient is covered underneath and on top as body heat is lost to the ground, if outside.
- Remember that shock can be fatal. If the patient starts to slip into lethargy or silence rouse patients using a firm approach as doing so may keep them conscious and alive.
- Get expert medical care as soon as possible.

Hospital care involves securing an airway, high-flow oxygen, and fluid and blood replacement.

Management of shock in hospital setting

- Use the ABCDE principles. 📖 Use of the ABCDE principles in the emergency department, p.1098.
- Administer oxygen by high flow mask.
- Ensure venous access—use as large a cannula as possible.
- Perform laboratory tests (FBC, U&E, cross-match, blood glucose, blood cultures, clotting, and toxicology).
- Administer fluids (crystalloid fluids and blood) as prescribed
- Monitor fluid balance strictly.
- Insert a urinary catheter to monitor output, if indicated.
- Monitor vital signs, including pulse, blood pressure, oxygen saturation, and respiratory rate.
- Check arterial blood gas (ABG).
- Monitor ECG and obtain 12-lead ECG and chest x-ray.
- Treat causes, e.g. surgical intervention for aortic aneurysm.
- Administer antidotes for certain poisons.
- Administer antibiotics for certain sepsis.
- May need inotropic and vasoactive therapy, assisted ventilation and invasive monitoring via arterial and CVP lines.
- Maintain body temperature.
- Reassure patient and provide comfort.

Further information

Wyatt JP et al. (2008). *Oxford handbook of emergency medicine*. Oxford University Press, Oxford.

Breathing emergencies in the hospital/clinic setting I

Breathing problems result in lack of oxygen reaching the tissues (hypoxia). Always check the patency of the airway. Check the mouth for foreign matter. Clear with wide-bore Yankauer sucker, if available, or Magill's forceps for solids. Try jaw thrust or jaw lift if the patient is not fully conscious. Fig. 33.6 illustrates the treatment of choking in adults. Avoid head tilt if a cervical spine injury is suspected. When the patient is breathing spontaneously, reassure and monitor vital signs and oxygen levels.

Upper airway obstruction

- Foreign object (e.g. food, mucus, dentures)
- Croup
- Epiglottitis
- Anaphylaxis
- Angio-oedema
- Airway burns

Lower airway obstruction

- Asthma
- Chronic obstructive pulmonary disease (COPD)
- Aspiration of foreign body or vomit
- Trauma
- Seat belt bruising should raise concerns about possible internal injury (especially abdominal injury or ruptured thoracic aorta)
- Rib fracture/flail chest
- Pneumothorax/haemothorax
- Pulmonary contusion

Recognition—assessment

- Inspect and examine the patient's chest and neck.
- Assess level of consciousness.
- Follow ABC approach and resuscitate.
- Note nasal flaring, respiratory rate, and pattern.
- Recognize that severe bruising from seat belt mark on chest may arouse suspicion of fractured ribs.
- Recognize that a stab wound near nipple or scapula suggests possible damage to heart.
- Listen to patient and take past and present respiratory history. (If unable to talk, obtain from family or close partner.)
- Note possible exposure to inhaled toxins.
- Note any cough, sputum, or haemoptysis.
- Note raised temperature.
- Note skin colour and signs of dehydration.

Nursing care and treatment

- Maintain a clear airway.
- Position the patient to facilitate breathing—may be the recovery position or sitting upright, supported by pillows.
- Reassure and provide comfort.
- Administer oxygen by nasal cannula or facemask according to patient's problem and doctor's prescription. ▢ Chapter 6, Oxygen therapy, p.104.
- Monitor vital signs, oxygen saturation and respiratory rate.
- Refer to hospital.

Common breathing emergencies

Hyperventilation

This is breathing that occurs more deeply and/or more rapidly than normal. It may be primary (psychogenic) or secondary due to respiratory compensation for a metabolic acidosis.

Secondary hyperventilation is the most serious and requires hospital treatment. Patients are sometimes misdiagnosed as primary psychogenic hyperventilation when the problem is actually a physical cause such as pulmonary embolism. Other possible causes include:

- Metabolic acidosis due to ketoacidosis, uraemia, sepsis, or hepatic failure
- Poisoning due to drugs such as aspirin
- Pain/hypoxia
- Hypovolaemia
- Respiratory disorders such as asthma and pneumothorax

Primary hyperventilation (psychogenic or inappropriate) occurs commonly in females with a past history of panic attacks or episodes of hyperventilation, who are agitated and very distressed. Treatment includes reassurance and simple breathing exercises such as breathing in through the nose (count to 8), out through the mouth (count to 8), hold for count of 4, and repeat.

Haemoptysis

This is coughing up of blood and may be the patient's only complaint. It is a very important symptom and should be investigated as soon as possible.

- Possible causes
  - *Respiratory*—infections, carcinoma, bronchiectasis
  - *Cardiovascular*—pulmonary oedema, pulmonary embolism (PE)
  - *Coagulation disorder*—drugs such as warfarin and heparin, and rare inherited diseases
  - *Trauma*—penetrating or blunt injury
- Treatment and nursing care
  - Follow ABC, if necessary.
  - Observe amount and type of coughed up material.
  - Distinguish from possible vomited blood.
  - Observe vital signs.
  - Give reassurance.
  - Refer to medical care.

Treatment of choking in adults

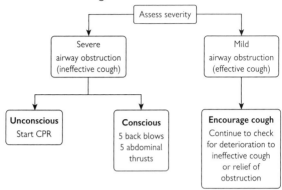

Fig. 33.6 The treatment of choking in adults. Reproduced with kind permission of the Resuscitation Council UK. www.resus.org.uk.

Back blow and abdominal thrusts

(a)

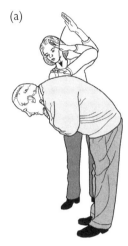

• If the back blows fail, carry out abdominal thrusts:

(b)

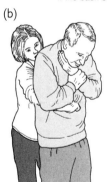

• Stand behind the patient and put both your arms around the upper part of the abdomen.

(c)

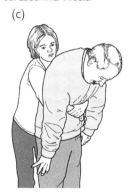

• Clench your fist and grasp it with your other hand.
• Pull sharply inwards and upwards with the aim of producing sudden expulsion of air, together with the foreign body, from the airway.

Fig. 33.7 Back blow and abdominal thrusts for choking. Reproduced with kind permission of the Resuscitation Council UK. www.resus.org.uk. *Advanced Life Support Manual*, Chapter 4.

Breathing emergencies in the hospital/clinic setting II

Table 33.2 Emergency response to acute breathing problems

Acute breathing problem	Emergency/first aid response
Choking adult	1. Administer 5 back slaps.
	2. Encourage coughing.
	3. Administer 5 abdominal thrusts (See Fig. 33.7).
Asthma attack	1. Check severity of attack based upon a combination of clinical features, peak flow measurements, pulse oximetry, and patient's ability to talk.
	2. Check pulse and respiratory rates.
	3. Make comfortable—sit patient upright, let them hold on to trolley sides or bed table.
	4. Administer inhaler or nebulizer plus high concentration oxygen.
	5. Encourage slow breathing.
	6. Get expert help urgently if patient remains breathless.
	7. Administer drugs, e.g. salbutamol or terbutaline and corticosteroids.
COPD	1. Make comfortable and reassure.
	2. Administer bronchodilator medications by aerosol treatment or IV.
	3. Oxygen via mask 24–28% plus nebulizer.
Pulmonary emboli	1. Make comfortable and reassure.
	2. Administer oxygen.
	3. Obtain ECG.
	4. Administer drugs, e.g. heparin, and analgesia.
	5. If breathless get expert help urgently.
Bronchitis	1. Administer bronchodilator.
	2. Collect sputum for culture and sensitivity.

Table 33.2 Emergency response to acute breathing problems
(*continued*)

Acute breathing problem	Emergency/first aid response
Pneumonia	1. Antibiotics, broad spectrum until sensitivity known.
	2. Sputum for culture and sensitivity if in hospital setting.
	3. Give oxygen as required.

See further care and treatment in Wyatt JP et al. (2006) *Oxford Handbook of Emergency Medicine*. Oxford University Press, Oxford.

Airway problems in trauma
- Soft tissue obstruction
- Oedema, haematoma, or swelling
- Foreign bodies
- Displaced facial bones
- Aspiration of gastric contents
- Burns—may cause severe oedema and airway obstruction
- Suspected cervical spine injuries (do not cause airway problems but make them more difficult to deal with)

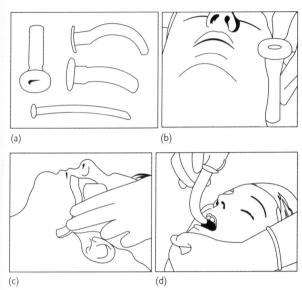

Fig. 33.8(a) Oropharyngeal and nasopharyngeal airways; (b,c) Sizing of an oropharyngeal airway; (d) Insertion of an oropharyngeal airway.

Haemorrhage and wounds: overview

Bleeding can occur both externally and internally in the body. External bleeding usually results from wounds caused by trauma or surgery. Internal bleeding occurs within body cavities and may be caused by injury. Internal bleeding may also occur spontaneously from such things as a stomach/peptic ulcer, oesophageal varices, aneurysms, and cancers.

Bleeding is usually classified into three types.
- *Arterial:* damage causes bright red oxygen-rich blood to spurt out of the body in time with the heart.
- *Venous:* damage causes dark red blood to gush out profusely, depending upon the extent of the damage.
- *Capillary:* red and brisk at times or oozing, depending on damage.

Control

Irrespective of its source, bleeding must be controlled. Direct pressure is initially the preferred way of managing external haemorrhage, but if an object is embedded in the wound then pressure is applied on each side of the embedded object or fragment. The limb should be elevated to reduce the bleeding.

(Tourniquets of any kind should not be used as they increase intraluminal pressure, distal ischaemia, and tissue necrosis.)

Internal bleeding should be suspected if a patient develops signs of shock without obvious blood loss. It is important to check for any bleeding from body orifices such as the ear, mouth, urethra, or anus.
- Observe the patient carefully and estimate how much blood is lost.
- Make patient comfortable.
- Call for assistance.
- Treat for shock (📖 Shock, p.1038) and be prepared to resuscitate.

Nursing, first aid, and treatment of wounds

Key objectives of wound care
- Stop any haemorrhage.
- Assess for blood loss (hypovolaemia).
- Obtain vascular access.
- Provide appropriate fluid resuscitation.
- Reduce infection risk.

Later key objectives
- Assess the extent of the wound.
- Observe for signs of complications (such as tendon, nerve or vascular injury, or damage to internal organs).
- Correct cleaning and closure of the wound.

Treatment of wounds
- Wear disposable gloves, if available, when dealing with wounds.
- Check the neurovascular status of the limb.
- Remove or cut clothing as necessary to expose the wound.
- Apply direct pressure with a sterile pad, if there is no object embedded in the wound.
- If an object is present, then apply indirect pressure either side of the object and apply a bandage and wound dressing carefully over the area.
- Raise and support injured limb.
- Lie patient down and protect from cold.
- Call for medical help or transfer to emergency department.

Wounds: types and treatment

Classification of wounds

Laceration occurs when blunt forces to the area cause the skin tissue to break open over a bony prominence. The extent of the laceration varies in length and depth and results in torn skin and irregular wound edges. Repair is usually achieved by surgical closure.

Incision results from a cut in the skin made by a sharp object such as a knife or broken glass. Stab and slash wounds are classified as incisions. The extent of the incision varies in length and depth and is characterized by clean-cut edges. Repair is usually achieved by surgical closure.

Contusions or bruises are a collection of blood under the tissue. No skin breakage occurs. Localized bleeding occurs and collects to form a haematoma. Discoloration may occur but it is not reliable to determine the exact age of a bruise. Contusions occur from blunt forces applied to the area. Usual treatments include applying cold packs to the area and administering mild analgesic medications.

Abrasions are 'grazes' which result from blunt injury and may contain dirt with the risk of infection. Treatment involves cleaning all dirt and debris that is imbedded in the skin to prevent a permanent skin tattooing effect. Abraded areas may be dressed with non-adherent material or left open to heal.

Avulsion refers to full-thickness tissue loss in which the wound edges cannot be approximated. Small avulsions heal by secondary intention. Larger avulsions may require skin grafting. A severe type of avulsion injury is a degloving injury in which the skin is peeled away from the underlying structures.

Puncture wounds are commonly caused by a sharp or, in some cases, a blunt object which has sufficient force to penetrate the skin. Underlying structures should be checked for further damage. Treatment involves cleansing the wound, removing any foreign objects, and careful surgical repair and closure.

Subungual haematomas or nail injuries result from a blunt force to the fingernail or toenail. Increasing pressure from blood accumulation under the nail causes a throbbing pain. Treatment involves relieving the pressure by making a small opening in the nail with a sterile needle or special pin.

Types of wounds and bleeding

Injuries to the head

Scalp wounds: These wounds often result in profuse bleeding due to the large number of small blood vessels close to the skin surface. This makes the situation appear worse than it is. Find the wound and cover it with a sterile dressing. If there is no possibility of foreign objects such as glass embedded in the wound, apply direct pressure over the dressing to control the bleeding. Do not apply pressure to 'boggy' swellings, as these are indicative of depressed skull fractures. Secure the dressing in place with a bandage. Lay the patient down. Monitor and record vital signs, level of response, pulse, and breathing. Assess all head injuries using the Glasgow Coma Scale (See Table 33.1) Be aware of the possibility of a neck injury with patients with head injury. Transfer to the hospital and get medical help.

Eye wounds: Cover with a sterile dressing and refer to the ED for assessment and treatment For specialist eye care see 📖 Chapter 14, Eye, p.485–503.

Ear injury: Help patient into a half-sitting position. Tilt head to the injured side to allow blood to drain away. Use a sterile dressing and refer to ED. For specialist ear care see 📖 Chapter 14, Ear, p.504–525.

Nose bleed: Sit patient down. Advise patient to breathe through their mouth; tilt head forward to allow blood to drain from nostrils. Pinch the soft part of the nose for 10 minutes. Use a clean cloth or tissues to clean any dribbling. After 10 minutes, release the pressure and reapply again for two further periods of 10 minutes. Once the bleeding has stopped, clean around the nose with lukewarm water. Refer to an ED or GP practice. If the patient has sustained a head injury and the blood appears thin and watery refer to an ED. 📖 Chapter 14, Nose and throat, p.526–548.

Bleeding from a tooth socket

Control bleeding by using a piece of gauze and telling the patient to bite down on it. With regard to any other bleeding from the mouth, try to determine the cause, use a sterile dressing, and refer for medical consultation. Be careful that the patient does not inhale the blood. Keep the tooth in milk for possible reinsertion later. Transfer to hospital for care of a dentist or advice from a maxilla-facial surgeon.

Penetrating chest wound

This type of wound usually involves a sharp object such as a railing spike, knife, or metal object. There may be damage to the pleura which can cause the lung to collapse (pneumothorax). Eventually the pressure may build up and affect the uninjured lung (tension pneumothorax). Lean the patient towards the injured side. Completely cover the wound with a sterile pad to stop air from entering and secure on three sides only to prevent accidentally causing a tension pneumothorax. Monitor vital signs, especially breathing. If the object is still *in situ* do not remove but transfer patient to hospital and seek senior medical and surgeon advice. Be aware of the possibility of heart or abdominal organ involvement—monitor the pulse as well as breathing.

Abdominal wound

Lie patient down, cover wound with dry dressing, apply pressure if needed, and monitor vital signs.

Internal bleeding

This type of bleeding may occur as a result of crush injuries or penetrating wounds, or may occur spontaneously from a peptic ulcer, ruptured aortic aneurysm, or ectopic pregnancy. Shock is the biggest risk and may occur without obvious blood loss. Check for any wounds and bleeding from orifices such as mouth, urethra, and anus. Patients become very pale, cold and clammy, thirsty, confused, and restless, with breathing problems and a rapid weak pulse. Treat as for shock (📖 Shock, p.1038). Lie the patient down, raise and support the legs, loosen clothing, and monitor vital signs. If the patient is in hospital an IV line should be inserted.

Vaginal bleeding

This type of bleeding is usually due to menstrual factors, miscarriage or abortion in pregnancy, internal disease, or trauma. Sit patient down, make comfortable, assess possible causes, be sensitive and supportive, and offer clean sanitary pads, and monitor blood loss and vital signs. Transfer to hospital for gynaecologist advice. 📖 Chapter 19, Menstrual problems and endometriosis, p.660.

Leg wounds

The most common types of leg wounds are cuts and grazes from falls, sport, and leisure activities and bleeding from varicose veins. Lay the patient down, raise the limb, and apply a clean dressing or pad. Apply pressure, if needed, or clean wound using surgical nursing technique. Bleeding from varicose veins may cause shock. 📖 Shock, p.1038. Therefore check and record the pulse. Check the neurovascular status of the limb.

Chest emergencies

Chest pain

📖 Chapter 7, Nursing patients with cardiovascular problems, p.135.

Chest pain is a non-specific symptom that must be carefully assessed. The following are some of the most common conditions associated with chest pain (See Fig. 33.9).

- **Myocardial infarction:** Vice-like central chest pain that often spreads to the jaw and down one or both arms. Pain lasts more than 15 minutes and does not ease with rest or glyceryl trinitrate (GTN) spray. It is caused by sudden obstruction of the blood supply to the heart.
- **Angina pectoris:** Vice-like central chest pain that often spreads to the jaw and down one or both arms, and eases with rest. Symptoms include shortness of breath, weakness, and anxiety. Caused by narrowing of coronary arteries.
- **Musculoskeletal:** Sharp localized pain that is worsened by movement, coughing, and deep breathing. Possible causes are muscle ligament strains, rib fracture, and pathological fractures due to tumours.
- **Pleuro-pulmonary:** Sharply localized 'stabbing' pain in the lateral aspect of the chest that has a sudden onset and is aggravated by movement, cough, and deep breathing. Pain may radiate to the shoulder or abdomen. Causes include pleurisy and pneumothorax.
- **Gastrointestinal disorders:** Lower substernal area pain in epigastric region spreading to chest or lower abdomen. Colic-like aching pain associated with meals.
- **Rarer conditions**
  - Pericarditis—sharp stabbing pain aggravated by deep breathing and chest rotation
  - Rib fracture
  - Gastro-oesophageal reflux disease
  - Dissecting aortic aneurysm—anterior chest pain radiating to back and abdomen, tearing pain
  - Skin factors such as herpes zoster
  - Sickle cell disease
  - Pancreatitis
  - Psychiatric factors such as anxiety disorders and substance abuse

Nursing and first aid care

- Observe patient carefully and establish a calm and quiet atmosphere.
- Assess characteristics of the pain. Using the word SOCRATES may help – S=site, O=onset, C=character, R=radiation, A=associated symptoms, T=timing, E=exacerbating and alleviating factors and S=severity of pain.
- Monitor airway and vital signs.
- Determine whether there is any history of cardiovascular or other medical condition that may be the cause.
- Make the patient comfortable (usually sitting up supported).
- Call for help especially if there is a possibility of myocardial infarction.

- When expert help is available, blood tests are performed, IV access is obtained, oxygen given and ECG performed, as appropriate.

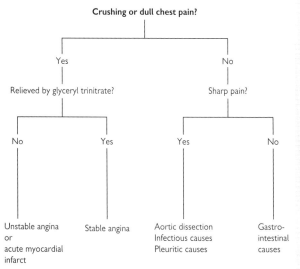

Fig. 33.9 Algorithmic approach to chest pain.

Heart and circulatory emergencies

📖 Chapter 7, Nursing patients with cardiovascular problems, p.135.

Heart problems – angina

Angina is defined as discomfort in the chest or adjacent areas due to myocardial ischaemia. It is usually brought on by exertion and associated with a disturbance of myocardial function without necrosis. It occurs when coronary artery blood flow fails to meet the oxygen demand of the heart muscle (myocardium). Where angina is suspected or the patient has a previous history of angina, the following first aid can be given.

First aid management
- Try to make the patient comfortable.
- Give reassurance and support.
- If the patient has medication for angina (e.g. tablets or a pump-action aerosol spray) let them, or help them, administer it.
- Keep the patient quiet and resting. If the pain persists, it may be a heart attack. Patient may prefer to sit up supported.
- Call medical assistance as soon as possible.
- Be prepared to use the ABCDE system.
- Constantly monitor and record vital signs.
- Observe airway and breathing. 📖 Use of the ABCDE principles in the emergency department, p.1098.
- Some patients with 'stable' angina may complain of angina when they exert themselves such as walking up a hill or climbing stairs. Such attacks may be predictable and may soon clear within 10 minutes of rest and their own treatment.

Unstable angina

This is more serious and may occur as worsening angina or as a single episode of 'crescendo' angina resulting in a myocardial infarction. It is important to monitor the patient closely and refer to hospital and medical assessment.

Acute myocardial infarction (MI)
- Ischaemic heart disease (IHD) is the leading cause of death in the Western world.
- It is caused by narrowing of the coronary arteries.
- It is a result of a sudden blockage or occlusion of a coronary artery or one of its branches by thrombosis.
- People with IHD are at risk of suffering an MI, particularly if they suffer additional stress that affects their heart.
- Emergency first aid consists of treating the patient's angina with their usual medications, placing them in a comfortable position, observing them closely, and calling for an ambulance as soon as possible (300 mg aspirin to chew slowly is recommended).
- Sometimes a patient's symptoms may be poorly localized and may appear to be seen as musculoskeletal or a gastrointestinal problem.
- ECG may be normal in a patient with myocardial infarction, and if symptoms suggest the possibility of an MI the patient should be admitted for observation, repeat ECGs, and blood tests such as troponin. Thrombolysis, if given quickly enough, can have

life-saving effects. PCI (percutaneous coronary intervention) may be more effective if available. 📖 Chapter 7, Myocardial infarction, p.152.

Transient ischaemic attack (TIA)

- A TIA is an episode of transient focal neurological deficit that lasts <24 hours.
- It can be a major warning for the development of a stroke.
- Causes include thrombo-embolic disease involving the heart or cranial blood vessels, hypertension, polycythaemia/anaemia, vasculitis, sickle cell disease, hypoglycaemia, any cause of hypoperfusion (e.g. arrhythmia, hypovolaemia).
- Signs and symptoms of a TIA are unilateral weakness, dysphasia/speech disturbance, visual disturbance, a sudden change in consciousness/ blackouts, bilateral motor or sensory changes, vertigo and ataxia.
- First aid care involves observing and reporting the effects of the attack, documenting if possible, and reassuring the patient while they are transferred to hospital for further assessment. If in hospital monitor and record patient's pulse, blood pressure, respirations, temperature, and oxygen saturations, and carry out neurological observations. Call for medical assistance.
- 📖 Chapter 13, Stroke and transient ischaemic attack: diagnosis and management, p.470.

Stroke

A stroke is an acute onset of focal neurological deficit of vascular origin that lasts >24 hours. It is caused by temporary or serious impairment of the blood supply to the brain.

Patients may become confused or disorientated and may lose consciousness. They may have problems with speech, swallowing, and movement, particularly on one side of the body. Patients may in some instances suffer from a headache, suggesting that the stroke may be haemorrhagic.

First aid care includes:

- Laying the patient down and placing in the recovery position (See Fig. 33.1).
- Calling for medical assistance and transferring to hospital as soon as possible.
- Loosening any tight clothing.
- Reassuring the patient and monitoring pulse manually at wrist or neck.
- Checking level of responsiveness.
- Clearing the airway and monitoring closely as patients may become unconscious.
- Keeping nil by mouth until a swallowing assessment has been made by speech therapist.
- Being prepared for CPR, especially respiratory arrest. 📖 Chapter 13, Stroke and transient ischaemic attack: diagnosis and management, p.470.
- Hypoglycaemia may cause signs typical of a stroke; therefore check blood glucose in any patient who appears to have had a stroke.
- Check pulse and blood pressure for possible hypertension.
- Thrombolysis is used in some stroke patients who have ischaemic rather than haemorrhagic strokes. Therefore time is critical and urgent assessment and CT scan is required.

Musculoskeletal injuries

📖 Chapter 17, Nursing patients with orthopaedic and musculoskeletal trauma problems, p.601.

This type of injury is usually caused by falls, collisions, and over-exertions that result in damage to bones, joints, muscles, tendons, ligaments, and surrounding soft tissues. Such injuries occur commonly in road traffic accidents (RTAs), sport and leisure activities, and falls in older people.

Classification

Musculoskeletal injuries are classified according to the structures damaged and the nature and extent of the damage.
- Fractures or breaks are injuries to the bones.
- Sprains are injuries to ligaments.
- Strains are injuries to muscles and tendons.
- Dislocations are injuries to joints.
- Subluxations are partial dislocations.
- Contusions or bruises are injuries to muscles and surrounding soft tissue.

Assessment of the injured patient
- Perform an initial assessment of the patient using the ABCDE system.
- Do not move the patient or their suspected damaged limbs until the extent of the injury has been assessed.
- Examine the patient carefully from head to toe.
- Ask the patient or a witness what happened and how the patient landed. For example, was there a trip, stumble, or fall, or was any type of force involved?
- Observe for deformity and discoloration.
- Check for wounds, e.g. open fracture with protruding bone, swelling, and shortening.
- Feel carefully for abnormal movement.
- Check pulses, temperature, and sensations.
- Palpate the suspected injury part very carefully. If pressure produces severe pain, assume possibility of fracture.

Blunt trauma is the term used to describe energy transfer to the patient over a large area. It can be further divided as follows:
- *Direct impact/compression* is the commonest type of force and causes injury by direct pressure. May result in haemorrhage, organ rupture, and fractures.
- *Shearing* causes organs to move and tear, damaging local structures and blood vessels, e.g. aortic rupture in a high-speed RTA.
- *Rotation* causes body part to twist and move, resulting in spiral and oblique fractures, ligament damage, and dislocations.

Fractures/traumatic injuries I

📖 Chapter 17, Specific musculoskeletal injuries: limb fractures, p.618.

A fracture is a partial or complete disruption in the continuity of a bone. Fractures are classified according to the nature of the break in the bone (See Fig. 33.10).

The following terms are used to describe fractures:
- Closed fracture: the skin surface is not broken over the fracture site.
- Compound or open facture: the bone punctures the surface of the skin leaving an open wound.
- 📖 Types of fractures, p.1061 and Fig. 33.10; Chapter 17, The femur showing sites of fractures, p.611.

Signs and symptoms
- Open wound may or may not be present
- Deformity
- Swelling and discoloration
- Pain
- Lack of movement or abnormal movement

General first aid
- Ask patient what happened, e.g. history of fall or impact.
- Immobilize before moving.
  - Use splints, making sure bandages do not interfere with circulation.
  - Pad splints, if possible, or use special types provided by the ambulance/paramedic crews.
- Control bleeding.
- Apply first aid dressings.
  - Basic support for wounds and injuries includes use of a triangular bandage or scarf.
  - Wound dressings can be applied underneath the triangular bandage or scarf to keep a wound clean and free from further harm (See Fig. 33.11)
- Treat for shock.
- Ensure nil by mouth.

Specific fractures

Skull fractures are caused by a blow to the head from an object or from a fall. Nurse in recovery position if no neck injury is suspected. If patient is conscious keep them lying or help to lie down. If fluid or blood is draining from an ear, cover the ear with a sterile dressing or pad. Control bleeding from scalp by pressing around the wound if no signs of a foreign body. Observe airway. Monitor vital signs and level of consciousness.

Clavicle (collar bone) fractures are caused by a fall or impact. Symptoms include a lump at site and pain. Apply an arm sling to injured site (See Fig. 33.11).

Arm fractures should be immobilized using a padded splint and sling (See Fig. 33.11).

Wrist and hand fractures should be immobilized with splint and sling (See Fig. 33.11).

Rib fractures are caused by impact. Do not bandage, but apply sling to arm of side affected.

Pelvic fractures are caused by RTAs and falls from horses and motorcycles. They are very serious and the patient should not be moved until expert help arrives. It is better to keep the legs together by fixing a scarf or triangular bandage around the feet and knees. Place padding between bony points. Monitor vital signs as fractures of the pelvis may result in severe bleeding from damage to pelvic veins, and internal organs such as the urethra and rectum.

Fractures of the lower limbs are treated by determining which bone is affected, applying splints, and bandaging legs together.

Neck injuries commonly occur due to sports injuries such as rugby, football, diving into the sea or a shallow pool, and motorcycle injury. Keep the patient flat and still. Immobilize with use of special spinal stretcher and head–neck brace. Observe for breathing and ask patient whether they have any feeling or movement in extremities. It is important not to move the patient without specialist help and appropriate apparatus. Chapter 17, Specific musculoskeletal injuries: spinal, muscular, and neurovascular, p.620.

Spine or vertebral column fractures are very dangerous. Do not move the patient unless they are in danger. Use the log-roll technique. Monitor their vital signs.

Types of fractures

- Transverse or simple – single transverse fracture of the bone with only two main fragments.
- Oblique – single oblique fracture with only two main fragments.
- Spiral – occurs in long bones as a result of twisting injuries, only two main fragments.
- Comminuted – complex fracture resulting in more than two fragments.
- Impacted – bone ends are driven into each other.
- Hairline – visible with no displacement.
- Greenstick – incomplete fracture of immature bone.
- Pathological – fracture due to underlying disease, e.g. osteoporosis, metastasis, Paget's disease.
- Stress – due to repetitive minor injury in certain bones that are prone to this type of fracture.
- Fracture-dislocation – fracture adjacent or in combination with a dislocated joint.
- Avulsion – bony attachment of ligament or muscle is pulled off.

Dislocations

Dislocations occur when a bone is displaced or separated from its normal place of articulation.

Signs and symptoms
- Pain located in and around the joint.
- Inability to move the part at the joint site.
- Deformity when compared with uninjured side (will appear abnormal with a possible lump, ridge, or disfigurement).
- Swelling may occur, especially if internal bleeding takes place.

Emergency first aid care
- Immobilize the joint with a sling so further movement does not contribute to pain.
- Apply ice or cold packs to assist in controlling bleeding.
- Care for shock. ⃞ Shock, p.1038.
- Transport for x-ray and expert medical treatment.
- Assess pain and give analgesics.

Sprains

This is stretching and/or tearing of the ligaments and soft tissue surrounding a joint. Depending upon the damage to the ligaments, sprains are classified as mild or severe.

Signs and symptoms
- Swelling, depending upon the extent of the damage.
- Discoloration eventually occurs, indicating internal bleeding.

Emergency nursing care
- Restrict movement and pressure on the joint.
- Apply ice or a cold pack.
- Observe circulation.
- Elevate the limb to keep gravity from pooling excess fluid into the injured joint.
- Transport for x-ray and expert medical advice.
- Assess pain and give analgesics.

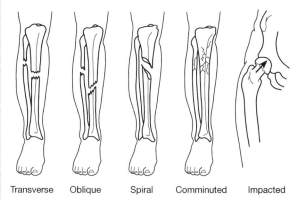

Transverse   Oblique   Spiral   Comminuted   Impacted

Fig. 33.10 Types of fracture.

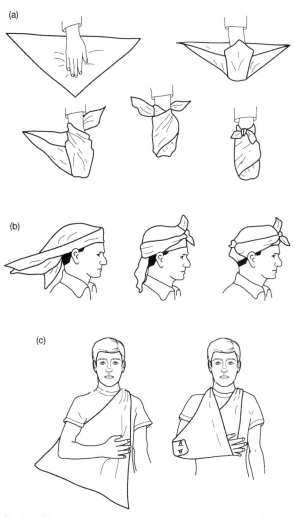

Fig. 33.11 Triangular bandages were once recommended as a good, overall, first aid cover for various types of injuries. Today they are only used in the hospital setting for the treatment of trauma to the wrist and forearm, to support the limb. The above diagram shows how they or a scarf or piece of material of similar size can be used in the out of hospital first aid setting. (a) Triangular bandage applied to hand. (b) Triangular bandage applied to head. (c) Triangular bandage used as a sling.

Fractures/traumatic injuries II

Strains

This is a stretching and/or tearing of muscle and tendon fibres. It is usually caused by overexertion, incorrect lifting, or sports injury. The muscles in the back and upper leg (hamstrings) are common sites of strains in athletes and in individuals participating in leisure activities involving running. Treatment for strains is the same as in sprains, i.e. ice or cold pack, compression, rest and elevation, and analgesia.

Contusions or bruises

These are caused by a direct blow to the body causing tissue damage. They result in localized pain, stiffness, and some disability. Discoloration appears after several hours. The treatment for contusions is often ineffective, but applying ice helps prior to full assessment by a GP or ED.

Care of patients with amputated parts

Initial care and treatment involves using the ABCDE approach (📖 Use of the ABCDE principles in the emergency department, p.1098). Good first aid and vascular spasm may reduce the bleeding, while compensatory mechanisms maintain the blood pressure. A careful assessment of the circulatory state of the patient must be made to avoid underestimating the degree of hypovolaemia. Control the bleeding with elevation and a pressure dressing. Tourniquets should only be used as a last resort in order to save life. Apply direct digital pressure and summon expert surgical help.

Care of the amputated part involves keeping it clean, covered in a single layer of damp (not dripping-wet) gauze or other clean material, depending on circumstances. Place the amputated part in a plastic bag, seal the bag, and then place the bag in a container of water–ice (See Fig. 33.12).

The amputated part should never be allowed to come into direct contact with ice as this will cause frostbite.

Crush injury

This may be caused by machinery, collapse of buildings, and RTAs and results in muscle, tissue, and bone damage. It is difficult to treat because of cellular destruction and damaged vascular and nerve structures. Compartment syndrome may develop due to pressure inside a limited body space. Observe for internal bleeding, severe pain, and, if lower body part is involved, urine output. Monitor vital signs and oxygen saturation. Crush injuries may lead to damage to internal organs such as kidney and cardiac complications.

Blast injury

This is caused by a blast wave of hot gas at the time of the detonation of an explosive charge. More severe injuries usually occur when a blast occurs in confined spaces. Patients suffer tympanic rupture and lung and bowel injuries. Secondary blast injuries are due to fragments from the device or surrounding area that penetrate the body. Tertiary blast injuries with amputation, burns, and crush injuries can also occur. Victims need ABCDE and psychological support because of the disfiguring nature of injuries.

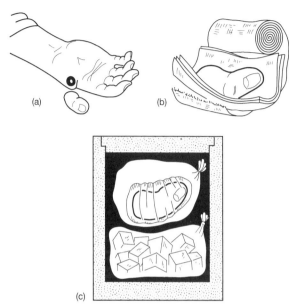

Fig. 33.12 (a) Rinse the wound with saline solution. (b) Rinse the amputated part in saline solution, wrap it in moist sterile gauze, and then place part in a plastic bag or container. (c) Place wrapped amputated part on plastic bags containing ice.

Temperature-related emergencies

Heat stroke

Heat stroke is very common in tropical or semitropical climates, during heat waves almost anywhere, in hot buildings and factories, and in hot gyms and on sports fields. The symptoms are caused by high body temperature, salt loss, and dehydration (See Table 33.3). Heat stroke is a medical emergency and should be treated as a life-threatening situation.

First aid/treatment

Because heat stroke is caused by the body's acute inability to lose heat rapidly enough, urgent treatment is required.
- Transport to hospital as soon as possible.
- Remove patient's clothing.
- Cool the patient's body using any means possible, e.g. ice bath or cold water sheet.
- Encourage cold drinks. Will need IV fluids, possibly in hospital.
- Monitor and record vital signs.
- Rest in a cool room.

Heat cramps

These usually occur when the environmental temperature is high, but there are exceptions to this. The condition often affects sportspeople, particularly when exercise levels are high, sweating is profuse, and salt replacement is inadequate. It is diagnosed by painful muscle spasm of the arms, legs, and abdomen in usually healthy people. Treatment includes drinking water that is diluted with a very small amount of salt (less than a teaspoonful) or drinking a special hypotonic sports drink. Ice can be applied to the cramped muscle.

Heat exhaustion

This is the most common of the heat-related emergencies and is most likely to occur during heat waves. It is caused by dehydration, salt depletion, or both. Thirst cannot be relied on as an indicator for water replacement as dehydration occurs before thirst occurs and is often quenched long before the water loss is replaced. See Table 33.3 for signs and symptoms of heat exhaustion. Treat by encouraging the patient to lie in the coolest place available and drink cold drinks. Cold hypotonic drinks help speed up hydration.

Table 33.3 Comparison of signs and symptoms for heat exhaustion and heat stroke

	Heat exhaustion	Heat stroke
Face	Pale	Red and flushed
Skin	Moist	Hot and dry
Sweating	Profuse	None
Temperature	Normal	Extremely high
Pulse	Weak and rapid	Strong and rapid
Unconsciousness	Not usually	Usually

Burns

A burn is damage to the skin by a source of heat or high energy, such as electricity or exposure to the sun. Burn injuries vary in severity depending on the amount of total body surface that is injured. They are also classified according to the depth of skin damage (See Fig. 33.13).

There are many possible causes of burns.
- Dry burn due to flames or friction
- Moist or scald due to steam or hot liquids
- Electricity from high-voltage currents and lightning strikes
- Cold injury due to frostbite, freezing materials, and vapours such as liquid oxygen
- Chemical burns from a variety of sources
- Radiation burns from the sun or ultraviolet rays and exposure to radioactive sources

Emergency treatment and nursing care
- SAFE approach:
  - **S** = Shout or call help.
  - **A** = Assess the scene for dangers to rescuer or patient.
  - **F** = Free from danger.
  - **E** = Evaluate the casualty.
- Stop the burning process. Remove the patient from the burning source. Remove all burnt clothing (unless it is stuck to the patient). Remove jewellery carefully.
- Cool the burn wound. Use running tap water for 10 minutes. If the burn area is small (<5%), a cold wet towel can be placed on the burnt area on top of Clingfilm. If the burn area is particularly extensive do not apply cold water for long periods, as this may intensify shock. Patients with chemical burns may need a longer period of irrigation under tap water. Maintain burn warmth.
- Apply dressings. Clean the burnt area and cover with a cellophane-type wrap. In chemical burns, after irrigation/cooling, Clingfilm may worsen the burn effect; therefore the affected area should be irrigated thoroughly until pain or burning has decreased and only wet dressings should be used. Care should be taken with the management of powder injuries, which may be worsened with water. If available, data regarding the likely chemical should be taken to hospital with the patient.
- Assess the patient for any other injuries. Administer high-flow oxygen via a non-rebreathe mask (15 l/min).
- Assess the burn severity. The Wallace rule of nines or the 'half burnt/ half not' approach should be used (See Fig. 33.14). The following should be noted:
  - Time of burn injury.
  - Mechanism of injury (flame, scald, etc.).
  - Any possible respiratory inhalation. Watch for upper airway obstruction if inhaled hot gases, suspect if singed nasal hairs/change in voice.
  - Pain assessment. Refer the patient to an ED.

- Cannulation and intravenous fluids. These are used for administration of titrated opioid analgesia. Fluid replacement with 0.9% normal saline or Hartmann's solution.
- IV fluids are usually needed if the burned area is > 15% in adults or 10% in children.
- Provide analgesia. This is best accomplished by cooling and covering the burned area.

Special considerations

For electrical burns, make sure that the contact with the electrical source is broken. For chemical burns to the eye, put on protective gloves and hold patient's affected eye under gently running cold water for at least 10 minutes. Monitor vital signs and assess pain. Do not use ointments and creams. Burns that do not require transfer to a burns unit are best treated by dressing with petroleum-jelly-based dressings. Significant hand burns, which cannot be dressed with paraffin gauze, can be placed in silver sulphadiazine bags.

Physiological reactions to severe burns

- Thirst
- Rapid breathing
- Increased heart rate
- Slowed gastric motility
- Increased blood glucose
- Increased metabolic rate and caloric needs
- Fluid retention
- Generalized oedema
- Weight gain
- Decreased urinary output
- Occult blood in stools

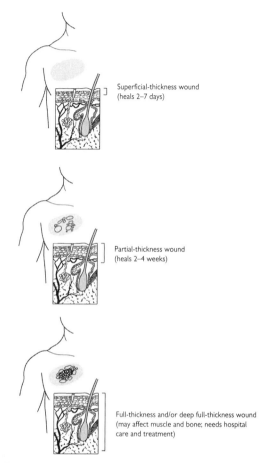

Superficial-thickness wound
(heals 2–7 days)

Partial-thickness wound
(heals 2–4 weeks)

Full-thickness and/or deep full-thickness wound
(may affect muscle and bone; needs hospital
care and treatment)

Fig. 33.13 Classification of burns by depth of tissue destruction

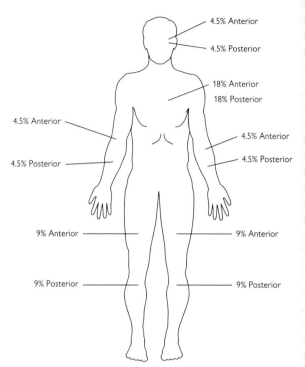

Fig. 33.14 The rule of nines for estimating burn percentages.

Hypothermia

This occurs when the body temperature falls below 35°C (95°F). It can occur inside as well as outside in cold environments. Moving air has a much greater cooling factor than still air. This is known as the 'wind chill factor'. When treating hypothermia outside:

• Prevent further heat loss by sheltering the patient.
• Remove wet clothing and apply dry clothing and blankets. If available, use a polythene survival bag.
• Protect the patient, especially from the cold surface they may be lying on.
• Transport as soon as possible to a warm environment.
• Give warm drinks and high-energy foods.
• Monitor vital signs, especially breathing.
• Do not give alcohol because it dilates superficial blood vessels and allows heat to escape.

Hypothermia is a particular risk not only for climbers and walkers in the winter, but also for infants, homeless people, the older person, and those who are inactive, thin, and frail. Prevention is the best cure but the key treatment in any situation is to:

• Prevent the patient from losing heat.
• Re-warm the patient. Care must be taken not to do this too quickly or it may lead to sudden vasodilation and shock.
• Give warm drinks and high-energy foods.
• Monitor vital signs.
• Transfer to a warm hospital ward for further assessment, especially if the person is elderly.

Frostbite

This is destruction of tissue by freezing, particularly at the extremities, i.e. fingers and toes. In many instances the person is unaware that the condition is occurring. Frostbite makes the skin white and numb. Eventually the tissue dies. Treatment for frostbite involves the usual treatment for hypothermia (📖 Hypothermia, above), plus specifically:

• Handle the frostbitten areas carefully.
• Clean and dress affected areas after re-warming in warm water at around 40°C (104°F).
• Raise or elevate frostbitten parts and protect from contact with bed clothes.
• Ensure affected part is not near direct heat such as a radiator.
• Monitor vital signs and observe dressings.

Poisoning

Types of poisoning

Accidental poisoning is common in inquisitive children (age 1–3 years) who swallow tablets, household chemicals and plants. Older children and adults may be poisoned by toxic fluids decanted into drinks bottles or by chemicals at work.

- Carbon monoxide poisoning may occur at any age, often in several family members at the same time due to a faulty heater or boiler.
- Poisoning by prescribed drugs may result from confusion about doses.
- Drug smugglers who swallow illegal drugs wrapped in condoms, or stuff them in their rectum or vagina may suffer poisoning if the packages leak.
- Bites from poisonous snakes are a hazard in many countries but are rare in the UK.

Deliberate self-poisoning is the commonest form of poisoning in adults and may occur in children as young as 6 years (usually with a family history of self-poisoning). Overdoses are often taken impulsively, as a cry for help or to manipulate relatives or friends. Suicidal intent is uncommon, but patients must be assessed for this. A few patients leave suicide notes and conceal the drugs or poison to evade detection.

Non-accidental poisoning occurs occasionally in children deliberately poisoned by a parent as a fabricated illness. Homicidal poisoning is rare and may involve acute or chronic poisoning with chemicals or drugs. Deliberate release of poisons by terrorists could affect many people simultaneously and cause widespread panic.

Information about poisons

The patient or relatives/friends may say what drugs or poison has been taken, but this information is not always accurate. Many patients take overdoses while under the influence of alcohol and may not know the drug or quantity involved. Check bottles or packets for the names and amounts of drugs or poisons that were available. If a patient is severely poisoned find out what drugs had been prescribed. Record the time of ingestion of the drug or poison.

- In the UK information about poisons is available at all times from the National Poisons Information Service (telephone 0844 892 0111) and their internet database TOXBASE (http://www.toxbase.org). TOXBASE is password protected and restricted to NHS clinical staff in the UK and to hospital staff in Ireland.
- In Ireland advice is available by telephone from the National Poisons Information Centre, Dublin (telephone 01 809 2566).
- Telephone enquiries to Poisons Information Centres are answered by an information officer using TOXBASE and other reference sources. Medical staff with specialist toxicology experience are available for advice about seriously poisoned patients.

Treatment of poisoning

Many children eat household products or tablets which are known to be non-toxic and so require no treatment. However, the circumstances of the poisoning must be considered in order to prevent another episode.

Poisoned patients should be assessed in hospital if there is any risk of toxicity. In severe poisoning intensive supportive treatment is needed with care of the airway, breathing, and circulation and appropriate nursing care while the poison is metabolized or excreted. Only a few poisons have specific antidotes, e.g. acetylcysteine for paracetamol (Paracetamol poisoning, p.1077), naloxone for opioids (Opioid poisoning, p.1077), and glucagon for beta blocker poisoning.

- Clear and maintain the **airway**. In an unconscious patient a cuffed endotracheal tube is needed if there is no gag reflex. If an oral or nasal airway is used, nurse the patient in the recovery position to reduce the risk of aspiration if vomiting or regurgitation occur.
- If **breathing** appears inadequate ventilate with oxygen using a bag and mask (not mouth-to-mouth in poisoned patients). Hypoxia and carbon dioxide retention are common in deep coma. Monitor respiratory rate and oxygen saturation. Check arterial blood gases if patient is deeply unconscious or breathing abnormally. Give naloxone for respiratory depression due to opioids (Opioid poisoning, p.1077).
- Record **pulse** and **blood pressure**. If blood pressure <90 mmHg elevate the foot of the trolley and give IV fluids, such as gelatin 500 mL. Record and monitor ECG if the patient is unconscious, has tachycardia or bradycardia or has taken drugs or poisons with a risk of arrhythmias.
- Assess and record **conscious level** frequently. Check blood glucose in all patients with altered mental status, coma, or fits.
- Check temperature. **Hypothermia** may occur in coma from drugs such as clomethiazole and phenothiazines: it usually responds to insulation and passive rewarming. **Hyperthermia** may be due to amphetamines, ecstasy, or other drugs: convulsions and rhabdomyolysis may occur. Active cooling, chlorpromazine, and possibly dantrolene may be needed.
- Urinary retention is common in coma, especially after tricyclic poisoning. Suprapubic pressure often stimulates bladder emptying but a catheter may be needed to empty the bladder or to measure urine output.
- Prolonged coma and immobility risks pressure areas and occasionally causes nerve palsies, compartment syndrome, or rhabdomyolysis.

Investigations in poisoned patients

The most useful investigations are blood glucose, paracetamol, U&E, and arterial blood gases. Measure paracetamol if there is any possibility of paracetamol poisoning (including all unconscious patients). Record the precise time of the sample on the blood bottle and form and also in the notes.

Reducing absorption of poisons

If a poison has been swallowed it seems logical to try to remove it and reduce absorption from the gut. Activated charcoal may be helpful in some circumstances, but gastric lavage and whole-bowel irrigation are rarely needed, and ipecacuanha is no longer used.

Activated charcoal given within 1 hour reduces absorption of therapeutic doses of many drugs, but there is little evidence of benefit after overdose. It is messy, unpleasant and often causes vomiting, with a risk of aspiration. Do not give charcoal for substances which do not bind to it, such as iron, lithium, ethanol, ethylene glycol, methanol, organophosphates, petrol, acids, and alkalis. Charcoal is useful for drugs which are toxic in small quantities, e.g. theophylline and tricyclic antidepressants. If a dangerous overdose has been taken in the previous hour, give charcoal (adults 50 g, children 1 g/kg, max 50 g, PO or via a gastric tube). Repeated doses are occasionally used, on expert advice, in life-threatening poisoning with drugs such as digoxin, quinine, theophylline, and salicylate.

Gastric lavage used to be done frequently but is now rarely performed. It should only be considered if a patient is deeply unconscious or has taken a life-threatening poison within the previous hour. Do not use lavage for petrol or paraffin compounds or corrosives. Unless there is a good cough reflex a cuffed endotracheal tube is needed to protect the airway. The main value of gastric lavage is to leave activated charcoal in the stomach.

Whole-bowel irrigation using bowel cleansing solution (e.g. KleanPrep®) down a nasogastric tube empties the bowel of solid contents. This is rarely needed and should only be used on expert advice. It might be useful for sustained-release drugs such as iron or lithium, which are not bound to charcoal, or to remove packets of cocaine from body packers.

Ipecacuanha should never be used. In the past it was given frequently, but it does not reduce drug absorption and it may cause prolonged vomiting, aspiration pneumonia, and drowsiness.

Salt solutions may cause fatal hypernatraemia and must never be used as an emetic.

Tricyclic antidepressant poisoning

Common features are tachycardia, dry skin, dry mouth, dilated pupils, urinary retention, jerky limb movements, and drowsiness leading to coma. Unconscious patients often have a divergent squint, increased muscle tone, and extensor plantars. In deep coma there may be muscle flaccidity and respiratory depression needing intermittent positive pressure ventilation. Convulsions may precipitate cardiac arrest. ECG often shows sinus tachycardia with increased PR interval and wide QRS, in a broad complex tachycardia which may be mistaken for ventricular tachycardia.

Treatment is supportive, with intubation and ventilation if necessary. Monitor ECG and check arterial blood gases in unconscious or post-ictal patients. In severe poisoning sodium bicarbonate (adult: 50–100 mL of 8.4%; child: 1 mL/kg) may produce a dramatic improvement in cardiac rhythm and output (by altering protein binding and reducing active free tricyclic drug). Patients recovering from coma often have delirium, hallucinations, jerky limb movements, and dysarthria and need sedation with diazepam.

Paracetamol poisoning

Paracetamol ('acetaminophen' in USA) may cause severe liver damage if 12 g (24 tablets) or >150 mg paracetamol/kg body weight are taken. Liver damage may occur with >75 mg/kg of paracetamol in 'high risk' patients who have alcoholism, malnutrition, or who take anticonvulsants, rifampicin, or St John's Wort. In obese patients (>110 kg) use a weight of 110 kg to calculate the toxic dose and antidote dose.

Record the ingestion time and amount taken as accurately as possible. Take blood (at 4 hours or more after the overdose) for measurement of paracetamol. Use the paracetamol treatment graph (in *British National Formulary* or TOXBASE) to assess risk of liver damage and the need for antidote treatment. If necessary give **acetylcysteine** IV in a loading dose over 15 minutes and an infusion over 20 hours. Acetylcysteine should be given promptly if it is needed: it prevents liver damage if started within 8 hours of the overdose, but later treatment is less effective.

Acetylcysteine may cause an urticarial rash, vomiting, bronchospasm, and hypotension. These usually develop in the first hour of treatment and are dose related. If side effects occur stop the infusion and give an antihistamine (e.g. chlorphenamine) and a bronchodilator. When symptoms have settled, acetylcysteine can be restarted at 50 mg/kg over 4 hours.

Opioid poisoning

The opioids include morphine, diamorphine (heroin), codeine, and related drugs. These are used as analgesics (often combined with paracetamol, as in co-codamol), cough suppressants, and antidiarrhoeal agents. Poisoning is common in heroin addicts, who may have venepuncture marks, thrombosed veins, and a high risk of HIV and hepatitis infection.

Opioid poisoning causes coma, pinpoint pupils, decreased respiratory rate, and sometimes cyanosis, apnoea, convulsions, and hypotension. Respiratory depression may cause death within 1 hour of an overdose. Delayed respiratory depression can occur in poisoning with slow-release drugs, and also with methadone, which has a very long duration of action.

Treatment

Clear and maintain the airway. If breathing appears inadequate, ventilate on oxygen with a bag and mask. Give naloxone to reverse coma and respiratory depression: initial dose for adults is usually 0.8 mg (2 mL) IV, repeated at 2–3 minute intervals if necessary. In known or suspected drug addicts start with smaller doses (0.1 or 0.2 mg) to avoid reversing the opioid completely. If venous access is not available give naloxone IM or intranasally.

Naloxone has a short duration of action and so coma and respiratory depression often recur. Careful observation is essential. Further naloxone is often needed and may be given IM or by IV infusion. Observation is needed for 6 hours after the last dose of naloxone. Dissuade or prevent patients at risk of respiratory depression from leaving hospital: it is best to keep the patient sedated but safe, with constant observation and titration of naloxone dosage, rather than reversing an opioid overdose completely. A heroin addict who insists on leaving hospital could be given naloxone IM, but may still be at risk of fatal respiratory depression.

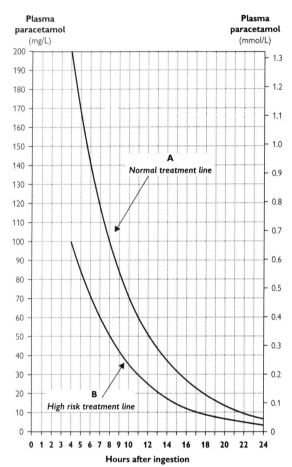

Fig. 33.15 Paracetamol treatment graph. Taken from the *Oxford Handbook of Emergency Medicine* (2006), 3rd edition, p.191, fig 33.14. Reproduced with permission from Oxford University Press.

Seizures

Chapter 13, Epilepsy/seizure, p.448.

A seizure is a sudden excessive disorderly discharge of abnormal electrical impulses to the brain's neurons that causes a temporary alteration in CNS function. Seizures are also known as convulsions or fits. The abnormal stimuli can occur as a result of such varied causes as trauma to the brain, tumours, poisons, hypoxia, high fever in children, and epilepsy. Most seizures are idiopathic (no identifiable cause). In some cases, the patient may recognize that a seizure is imminent (i.e. a warning or aura is present) and they may call out.

Seizures consist of involuntary contractions of many of the muscles in the body and are generally recognized by:
- Sudden unconsciousness
- Rigidity and arching of the back
- Convulsive or sudden violent uncontrollable movements
- Difficulty or cessation in breathing (which can be noisy)
- Blue lips (cyanosis)
- Red and puffy cheeks and face
- Clenching of the jaw
- Biting or chewing of the tongue
- Excessive saliva which may be bloodstained
- Involuntary urination or defecation

The patient is usually unresponsive throughout the seizure but afterwards the muscles relax and the patient gradually regains consciousness. During this period of recovery the patient may be confused and lethargic, and feel embarrassed and vulnerable.

Emergency first aid care

Emergency care is primarily directed towards protecting patients from causing themselves injury during the seizure.
- Remove potentially dangerous objects in the environment.
- Note the time the seizure begins.
- Try to protect the patient's head with soft padding.
- Loosen tight clothing.
- Do not try to move the patient during the attack unless there is immediate danger.
- Do not try to put anything in the patient's mouth or try to restrain the patient's movement.
- Monitor the patient's breathing and vital signs and be prepared to place the patient in the recovery position (See Fig. 33.1) or commence resuscitation.
- Note the duration of the seizure. (Status epilepticus is a seizure that lasts for longer than 30 minutes.)
- Give comfort, support, and reassurance to the patient and their friends, relatives, or other bystanders.
- Call an ambulance if the seizure continues for more than 5 minutes in a known epileptic and immediately if not known to be epileptic.
- Observe for any further attacks.
- Check blood glucose as hypoglycaemia can cause fits.

Fainting (syncope)

A simple faint is a sudden temporary loss of consciousness for a limited period or short duration. It results in a loss of blood flow to the brain and may be caused by low blood pressure or cardiac problems. It can also be a reaction to severe pain, lack of food, exhaustion, stressful circumstances, or pregnancy. Fainting is common in individuals who must stand motionless for long periods such as soldiers on parade. The result is pooling of blood and fluid in the legs. The reduction in effective circulating blood volume results in decreased perfusion to the brain. The patient falls suddenly and appears very pale, cold, and clammy, with a slow pulse.

Emergency nursing and first aid care

- Encourage the patient to lie down.
- Raise the legs to augment venous return.
- Encourage plenty of fresh air.
- Gently sit the patient up again and monitor vital signs.
- Reassure and ask the patient for possible reasons for their faint.
- Assess for fluid replacement.

More severe collapse and syncope

This may be due to a seizure due to a neurological disturbance. The patient may already have a history of seizures. A seizure may be preceded by a warning sign or the patient may cry out. This is followed by tonic/clonic movements of the body, cyanosis, saliva frothing at the mouth, tongue biting, or incontinence (all suggest a generalized seizure). Protect the patient, then put them in the recovery position until full recovery and there is no worry about blockage of the airway.

Severe collapse and syncope may be due to a cardiac event (e.g., cardiac arrhythmia, cardiomyopathy, coronary artery disease) and result in an abrupt onset accompanied by pallor and sweating. Recovery may be rapid with flushing and deep sighing respirations. Other causes include carotid sinus syncope often occurring with shaving or turning the head, concealed internal bleeding (e.g. ruptured spleen or ectopic pregnancy), and pulmonary embolus.

Psychological emergencies

First aid/nursing care

- Assess the patient using the ABCDE system (☐ Administering first aid outside the hospital setting, p.1028). Monitor vital signs and consciousness/responsiveness.
- Maintain a clear airway and position patient in the recovery position if concerned.
- Ask patient if they have any underlying health history which may have caused the problem.

Reactive behaviour in emergencies

Trauma can often cause severe stress and patients vary in their reactions on a continuum from normal to abnormal. They may exhibit unusual, dysfunctional, or even bizarre behaviour. The nurse's role is to intervene to lessen the anxiety and severe discomfort generated by stress and to help affected people cope in more constructive ways. Such approaches are very supportive to the patient.

Normal reactions to trauma

- Numbness, shock, and denial – Give information in small 'doses'. Be patient and willing to repeat things.
- Fear – Support and reassure, use a confident professional approach.
- Depression, apathy, and helplessness linked to loss – Be patient and provide encouragement and reassurance.
- Elation (associated with the relief of being rescued).
- Irritation and anger – Be tolerant as anger may be directed at others and medical staff.
- Guilt – Do not pre-judge; listen empathically.
- Flashbacks (involuntary dramatic replays of events) – Encourage patient to talk about them and reassure that they are normal reactions.
- Cognitive and perceptual disturbances (recall of events may be in slow motion, may have gaps, or may be in the wrong order; patient may feel out of control, helpless, and guilty) – Provide reassurance and encourage verbal expression.
- Hypersensitivity (on guard, overactive, and startled) – Provide calm and confident reassurance.
- Bereavement (not just due to loss of someone, but may be due to loss of function, body part or an object/possession)

Nursing interventions

- Be aware of early stages of shock and disbelief. Later stages include sudden awareness which may involve crying, shouting, and anger; questioning and searching for answers; and guilt.
- Encourage involvement of family and close friends.
- Do not confront. Be honest, empathic, and supportive.
- Encourage ventilation of feelings. Do not be critical, be supportive and listen.

Nursing care of patients with psychological emergencies

Everyone experiences varying degrees of stress in their lives and responses to this stress depend upon previous experience and education. Human contact, security, and a sympathetic ear are the key needs of emotionally disturbed people.

When faced with a patient who is having a psychological emergency, take the following approach:
- Try to ascertain what the crisis is or the cause of the problem.
- Use simple direct communication.
- Be prepared to spend time with the patient.
- Convey a wish to help and a desire to understand.
- Be calm and direct.
- Clearly identify yourself.
- Assess the patient at the scene.
- Encourage the patient to talk about what has happened, but be careful with overactive patients.
- Be interested in the patient's story.
- Support the patient's existing coping skills.
- Maintain a non-judgemental attitude.
- Involve family and significant friends to support the patient.

Acute psychiatric reactions to trauma

Acute stress reaction is defined as a transient disorder of significant severity that develops in an individual without any other apparent mental disorder in response to exceptional physical or mental stress and which usually subsides within hours or days.

Patients display usual signs of shock and disbelief, impaired concentration, and disorientation followed by depression, agitation, anxiety, and social withdrawal.

Panic attack

- Due to sudden severe anxiety
- Unpredictable onset
- Characterized by palpitations, chest pain, profuse sweating, choking, sense of doom, tremor, difficulty breathing, and irresistible urge to run away
- Usually peak within 10 minutes
- Cease when the patient feels safe and secure
- Patients may hyperventilate
- 📖 Chapter 31, Nursing patients with mental health needs, p.983.

Nursing interventions and treatment

- Provide psychological support and reassurance that condition will not last.
- Refer to GP for continuing care and treatment.
- Administer benzodiazepines.
- Hyperventilation in severe cases may need to be treated with re-breathing exercises. 📖 Hyperventilation, p.1041.

Drug abuse

This is use of a drug in excess and for recreational or psychological effect, without regard for its usual medical purposes. Drug dependence is a state in which a person cannot function or suffers extreme discomfort if deprived of the drug.

Signs of drug taking

- Demands analgesia/anti-emetics
- Knows pharmacopoeia well
- Demonstrates erratic behaviour, unexplained absences, mood swings
- Unrousable in the mornings
- Drinks heavily
- Breath smells of acetone or alcohol (solvent abuse)
- Small pupils (opioids), reversed by naloxone
- Needle tracks on arms, legs, between toes, on penis and genitalia
- IV access difficult
- Abscesses and lymphadenopathy in nodes draining injection sites
- Signs of drug-associated illnesses such as endocarditis, AIDS, and hepatitis
- No fixed abode

Common drugs abused

- Marijuana (cannabis)
- Sedatives and tranquillizers (barbiturates)
- Opioids (morphine, heroin)
- Hallucinogens (tranquillizers)
- Stimulants (amphetamines, cocaine)
- Alcohol—most commonly abused drug—treated as a depressant overdose
- Glue, paint thinners, petrol, hair spray, nail polish remover

Nursing interventions

- Use a non-judgemental approach that is calm and reassuring.
- Communicate strict rules of behaviour to the patient.
- Wear gloves and take extra care to avoid needle stick injuries and risk of hepatitis and HIV.
- Observe carefully and monitor vital signs.
- Check airway and breathing.
- Treat changes in body temperature and shock.
- Protect patient from injuring self.
- Take a thorough history, including past medical conditions and hospitalization. Ask direct questions:
  - Do you use any drugs?
  - Have you ever injected drugs?
  - Does your partner use any drugs?
  - Do you share needles?
  - Have you ever had an HIV test?
  - How do you finance your drugs?
  - List drugs used and presented drugs with names of prescriber.

- Inform medical staff of the patient who is withdrawing from alcohol or drugs so that they can be prescribed the appropriate treatment and not suffer adverse side effects.
- Recognize that abusers of cocaine and other drugs may be prone to acts of aggression and violence.
- May need help from security and police.
- Refer to hospital ED if overdose or to GP and community psychiatric nurse.

The patient threatening or attempting suicide

Chapter 31, Suicide and deliberate self-harm, p.995.

Many suicidal patients suffer from depression that is often related to a recent bereavement, loss of self-esteem, prolonged physical illness, or emotional/psychosocial problem with family/friends. Some have a history of alcoholism or drug dependence. Suicide is very common amongst adults in their twenties and thirties.

Ordinary tasks become increasingly difficult. Attention span decreases and fatigue sets in. Patients withdraw from social activities and relationships. May complain of physical illnesses and suffer insomnia and early morning awakening.

A high-suicide-risk patient should not be left alone.

Nursing interventions
- Prevent patient from harming self.
- Remove any possible means of self harm from the patient's environment.
- Demonstrate caring, understanding, and hope that solutions to the patient's problems can be found.
- Be willing to listen and understand.
- Remain accepting and non-judgemental.
- Establish rapport and intervene to preserve the patient's life.
- Involve close family and friends, if appropriate.
- Refer to hospital ED if overdose is suspected, or refer to GP and community psychiatric nurse.

The patient who demonstrates psychotic behaviour

These patients may manifest many of the symptoms of acute anxiety and psychological disequilibria. They can suffer from delusions and can be convinced that others want to harm them, or that peculiar things are happening to their bodies. A few hallucinate, hearing voices that no one else can hear. Confusion, disorganization, vagueness, and memory gaps occur. Patients can be withdrawn or become aggressive and violent.

Nursing interventions

- Be calm and reassuring. Use a firm manner and direct language.
- Talk to the patient, showing concern and a desire to help.
- Do not agree or disagree with the patient's delusions.
- Keep the patient informed.
- Seek the advice of specialist mental health nurse and psychiatrist.
- Encourage the patient to feel cared for and in a safe environment.
- May need referral to an acute psychiatric unit.

Specific female emergencies

These emergencies consist of:
- Accidental injury during pregnancy and miscarriage.
- Deliberate injury such as domestic violence, rape, and ritual female circumcision (genital mutilation).
- Laceration to the vulva region due to falling astride something.
- Vaginal injury following sexual intercourse and sexual abuse resulting from the insertion of a variety of objects into the vaginal tract.

Nursing interventions
- Provide careful and considerate care.
- Monitor vital signs.
- Control bleeding and apply appropriate pads.
- Treat pain.
- Apply cold packs to help reduce swelling.
- Try to alleviate the woman's anxiety and embarrassment. This may include the possibility of pregnancy, sexually transmitted diseases, and HIV.
- Protect privacy and confidentiality.
- Give reassurance and support.
- Encourage expression of feelings and, where appropriate, close involvement of family or friends.
- Perform a careful examination, with consent and chaperone.
- Inform appropriate health care professionals.
- Refer to the police (if the patient agrees).
- If expertise is available, carefully document and record injuries using drawings and diagrams. Involvement of the police surgeon may help in the documentation of injuries and the gaining of information.

Rights of the abuse/assault victim (whatever gender)
- To be treated with dignity and respect.
- To be afforded the same credibility given to victims of other crimes.
- To be asked only questions relevant to their care.
- To be offered a choice in filing assault charges once a report has been made.
- To receive competent and sensitive health care, without parental consent (for minors), if necessary.
- To be given complete and detailed information regarding all medical and legal procedures. Informed consent must be obtained prior to procedures being performed.
- To be given access to counselling, legal advice, and/or psychological support systems.
- To receive medical care and legal advice that is not influenced by prejudices against race, age, sex, class, lifestyle, or occupation.
- To receive strict confidentiality regarding all aspects of the case.
- To be considered a victim of abuse or assault regardless of relationship to the assailant (spouse, sibling, child, significant other, friend).

📖 Chapter 21, Care of the patient suffering from sexual abuse, p.750.
📖 Chapter 29, Nursing the child and adolescent, p.945.

Types of abuse and assault (encountered in the emergency department)

Abuse can be defined as the maltreatment or use of violence against another person.

Child abuse/neglect
The wilful use of bodily harm or actions by a parent, family member, or legal guardian that places a child at risk.

Partner assault
An adult who is physically or emotionally harmed by their spouse or significant other/partner.

Elderly abuse/neglect
The wilful use of bodily harm or actions by a spouse, child, family member, legal guardian, or primary caregiver that places the elderly at risk.

Sexual abuse/assault
The wilful act of sexual relations imposed on a person against his/her will.

Unexpected childbirth

Causes
- Ignoring the estimated, expected delivery time.
- Onset of labour occurs more rapidly than anticipated.
- Expectant mother is involved in an accident that stimulates the premature onset of labour.
- Rapid labour is much more likely in multiparous women than in primips.

Three stages of labour
- First stage – The uterus contracts and baby positions itself for birth.
- Second stage – The baby is born (See Fig. 33.16).
- Third stage – The afterbirth (placenta and umbilical cord) is expelled.

Nursing interventions
- Always call for a midwife, physician, or an ambulance as they have an emergency delivery pack on board.
- Protect the patient from embarrassment.
- Reassure and talk to patient.
- Prepare to receive the baby in a suitable container lined with towels.
- Help the patient to sit or lie on the floor or on a bed, in a position that is comfortable for her. Use plenty of pillows/cushions for support.
- Stay calm. Encourage the patient to breathe deeply or to use any other method that she prefers to cope with the pain and discomfort.
- Massage lower back.
- Maintain good hygiene and a clean environment for baby.
- Wash hands and arms, wear disposable gloves.
- Remove any underclothing that may interfere with the delivery.
- Position the woman on her back, knees bent, and legs spread wide apart.
- Check regularly for the baby's head.
- Once the head emerges, advise the patient to stop pushing and start panting. The baby's shoulders will soon appear.
- Allow the baby to be expelled naturally.
- Check to see if the umbilical cord is wrapped around the baby's neck. Remove if necessary.
- Handle baby carefully.
- Remove mucus from the baby's mouth and nose.
- Elevate the baby's feet and lower the head to help drain the mucus.
- Use cloth or finger to remove mucus.
- If crying is not spontaneous, rub baby's back.
- If baby does not begin to breathe and if in hospital call for neonatal doctors and crash team; perform mouth-to-mouth resuscitation.
- Wrap baby in cloth to keep warm and give to the mother.
- Keep the placenta and umbilical cord intact.
- There is no urgency to cut the cord as this should be done by a midwife or qualified physician.
- When the cord and placenta appear, save them for examination.

- Provide warm water, clean towels, and sanitary pad for the patient. Help her to use them if necessary.
- Check for tears and bleeding. Call for help if necessary.
- Comfort and reassure the patient.

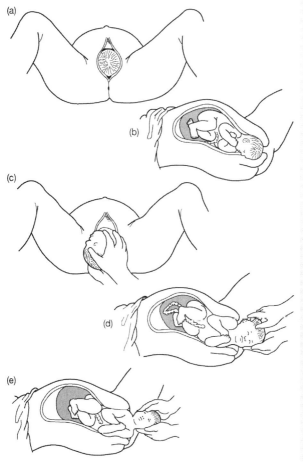

Fig. 33.16 Childbirth sequence.

Care of the patient in the emergency department (ED)

The development of the ED in British hospitals has been a significant step in health care over the past few years. In many ways this has been a response to patient need and the demand for better care and treatment following a medical emergency. The ED is the interface between primary and secondary care. It is often portrayed in the media as exciting and dramatic. Many patients who arrive in the ED are suffering from a very wide variety of health problems and have not seen their local GP. There is now a move to develop specialist EDs linked to major hospitals so that patients can receive the fastest and most efficient expert help.

Caring for patients with medical emergencies requires careful assessment and referral to appropriate services. It is estimated that 15–20% of patients who present to EDs require referral to specialist inpatient medical teams. In some EDs where many GP referrals are seen in the ED, the admission rate is 25%. Patients may be followed up by their GP for care or further medical advice and help. EDs receive referrals from a number of sources, such as NHS Direct, minor injury units, GPs and other smaller hospitals/clinics and care homes.

Priorities of the ED

- To save lives using specialist interventions and resuscitation equipment.
- To provide expert emergency medical and nursing care.
- To provide analgesia and control the patient's pain.
- To listen and respond appropriately to patient's concerns about their urgent health problems.

Characteristics of the ED

- They are concerned with critical life saving decisions.
- The ED staff work closely as a team.
- Most nurses are specially trained in emergency care; some are known as nurse practitioners who 'see and treat' patents with minor injuries, Some are more senior advanced specialists known as nurse consultants.
- Roles within the interdisciplinary team are often blurred.
- Critical decisions are made regarding admission to or discharge from hospital.
- A system of triage is used to sort out and prioritize which patients need attention first.

Key areas of work

- Liaising with the paramedical/ambulance team.
- Caring for patients with minor medical conditions and injuries.
- Caring for critically injured/ill patients following major trauma or acute illness.
- Caring and treating young and old patients who have a whole variety of acute and urgent medical, surgical and trauma conditions.
- Providing major disaster management/care following a major incident such as a train crash or terrorist attack.

- Caring for patients who are suffering from emergency mental health problems and overdoses.
- Caring for patients with drug and alcohol abuse.
- Caring for patients with primary care and social problems due to lack of or difficulty in contacting local GP and social services.

Nursing role within an ED

- Participate in the ED team and play a leading role in helping to assess and treat patients according to their emergency conditions.
- Summon medical attention when it is required immediately.
- Deliver the fundamental aspects of nursing care, monitoring the patient's progress, and maintaining the patient's privacy, respect and dignity.
- Ensure documentation is completed and communications about the patient's condition are transferred and passed on to the appropriate next stage of their care.
- Provide appropriate psychological nursing care to support patients and relatives/friends while they are being treated in the department.
- Contact the patient's close relatives/friends if necessary.
- Coordinate and assess the flow of patients through the department ensuring clinical services such as triage, resuscitation, and care of patients are working efficiently.
- Manage and coordinate the staff and resources of the department in consultation with the senior medical staff.
- Inform security of any potential aggressive incidents involving patients/ visitors or staff.
- Arrange the transfer and discharge of patients from the department including whether the patient needs to return to hospital, continue treatment with their GP, or attend another service.

Emergency nursing

Triage

Because of the wide variety of needs with which patients present in emergency situations and departments, triage systems are used. The word triage is derived from the French word *trier*, meaning 'to pick out or sift'. It is used to identify those patients who are most seriously at risk and who are in need of immediate emergency care.

Triage can take many different forms and operates at a number of different levels, but its overall aim at all times is to give the right patient the right care at the right time in the right place. In pre-hospital situations it is used not only to assign treatment and evacuation but also to determine which hospital the patient goes to, how they get there, and what sort of emergency medical team meets them on arrival. Fig. 33.16 shows a schematic design of patient incoming flow from triage following a disaster.

The principles of triage are fundamentally the same. A descriptive colour coded system is used which indicates the priority of treatment. Key words and colours are as follows:

* *Red* – critical life-threatening immediate casualties.
* *Yellow* – urgent or serious casualties who can wait after initial assessment, e.g. compound fractures, soft tissue injuries, burns less than 40% of whole body.
* *Green* – delayed minimal casualties who are ambulatory and have minor tissue injuries needing general observation, e.g. minor burns, abdominal pain, alcohol intoxication.

A variety of different systems of triage are used in the UK and the rest of the world, depending on the situation. Table 33.4 shows the five category system used in most EDs in the UK.

Table 33.4 A five category system for triage in emergency care

Description	Priority	Colour	Target time
Immediate	1	Red	On arrival
Very urgent	2	Orange	Within 10 min
Urgent	3	Yellow	Within 1 hour
Standard	4	Green	Within 2 hours
Non-urgent	5	Blue	Within 4 hours

Waiting times for triage

* As soon as patients arrive in the ED they are assessed by a specially trained nurse and then, if necessary, by a dedicated trauma team.
* Triage is a dynamic process and may result in patients being re-classified if their condition changes.
* Placement in a particular category does not imply a diagnosis, only the need to be seen by that priority.

- The effect of triage on other patients in non-urgent categories may mean they have to wait longer.
- Nurses should ensure that patients who have long waits are regularly checked and monitored, receive periodic information about what is happening, and receive adequate care and nutrition while they wait.

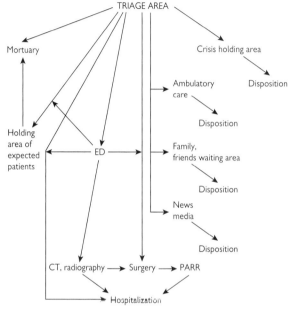

Fig. 33.17 Schematic design of patient incoming flow from triage following a disaster: ED, emergency department; PARR, peri-anaesthesia recovery room. From Selfridge-Thomas J (1995). *The manual of emergency nursing*, Fig. 28.1, Elsevier. Reprinted with permission from Elsevier.

The AMPLE history

The five key pieces of information that must be gathered on all trauma victims are:

- A—allergies
- M—medicines
- P—past medical history
- L—last meal
- E—events leading to the incident

Use of the ABCDE principles in the emergency department

A—airway and cervical spine control

Airway

Talk to the patient and try to rouse them. If the patient replies in a normal voice and gives a logical answer, the airway can be assumed to be patent and the brain adequately perfused. If not, then clear and secure the airway by lifting the chin and thrusting the jaw forwards. Use a guedal airway for unconscious patients without a gag reflex. The airway takes priority over the cervical spine. The patient's airway must be cleared and protected as soon as possible.

Cervical spine

Stabilize the cervical spine immediately if there is any suspicion of spinal injury. Use manual stabilization first with one person in charge. Later use a semi-rigid collar, head blocks or sandbags, and forehead strapping. High flow oxygen needs to be given once the airway is cleared and secured. If possible, attach pulse oximeter. If the patient vomits, turn the whole patient, preferably using a spinal board.

B—breathing
- Examine the chest for life-threatening thoracic conditions, airway obstruction, tension pneumothorax, open chest wound, massive haemothorax, flail chest, and cardiac tamponade.
- Observe and listen for good clear air intake and output.
- Feel for the trachea (to check it is central).
- Observe chest movements (for adequacy and symmetry).
- Check for chest wall tenderness.

C—circulation
- Look for bleeding, especially from long-bone fractures, associated vascular injuries, and soft tissue trauma.
- Use direct pressure to control external haemorrhage. No tourniquets.
- Use splints for fractures and immobilize the patient.
- Trauma victims require large-bore IV access in areas that are not distal to the vascular or bony damage. Once cannulation has been achieved 20 mL of blood is taken for grouping and cross-matching and analysis of plasma electrolytes and FBC. Test with BM stix.

D—disability
- Observe and monitor the patient carefully for any other injuries. Carry out head injury observations such as the Glasgow Coma Score. (May use AVPU, 📖 Administering first aid outside the hospital setting, p.1034.)
- Observe for hypoxia, hypovolaemia, hypoglycaemia (especially in alcoholic and paediatric victims), and raised intracranial pressure by performing blood tests and monitoring oxygen saturation and blood pressure.
- Check pupil responsiveness.

E—exposure

- Protect and keep the patient warm and covered using blankets.
- If there are any other suspected injuries, remove clothing carefully to assess how severe these injuries are.

Nursing care in the emergency department

Charting and recording

- Use the ED's system of reporting and recording information about patients. This should include:
  - Presenting complaint
  - Previous relevant history
  - Current medications
  - Observations
  - Examination findings
  - Investigations performed and their results
  - Possible diagnosis
  - Main nursing problems
  - Medical and nursing treatment given
  - Advice and follow-up arrangements with relevant referrals
- Avoid idiosyncratic abbreviations.
- Always document the name, grade, and speciality of any nurse or doctor who gives you advice or instructions.
- When referring or handing over a patient, always document the time of referral/handover, and use your usual signature.

Team work

All departments work according to a particular system that suits their needs. Nurses are usually allocated according to certain areas and teams. Paediatric patients and their parents/guardians are seen in a separate area, usually by a qualified paediatric nurse.

The staff of an ED includes receptionists, various qualified and specialist nurses and doctors, radiographers, plaster technicians, and specialist on-call nurses such as a psychiatric liaison or a geriatric nurse. In addition, a variety of clinical support staff from within the hospital are involved. There are also many other non-clinical support staff such as security guards, porters, cleaners, and police.

Common therapeutic interventions used in the ED

- Use of the ABCDE principles. 📖 Use of the ABCDE principles in the emergency department, p.1098.
- Focus is on key concerns such as resuscitation, IV fluids, analgesia, antibiotics, insertion of oro/nasogastric tube, urinary catheterization, and chest drains.
- Secondary identification of associated injuries.
- Stabilization and emergency operative intervention.

In-hospital resuscitation

- Start resuscitation immediately.
- Summon help using the emergency call system and the standard number (2222 in the UK).
- Check that the environment is safe for you and the patient.
- Put on gloves.
- Be careful with sharps and follow the organization's local guidelines.
- If a patient is not responding, follow basic life support if adult. 📖 Basic life support, p.1036.
- Check for pulse and regular breathing.
- Identify the patient and get their medical records and any up-to-date information.
- If a patient is monitored and has an arrest that is witnessed, a pre-cordial thump to the chest may be given by an expert practitioner.
- Follow the appropriate algorithm (See Fig. 33.18–33.22).
- Studies have shown that CPR using chest compressions only may be more effective than or as effective as combined ventilation and compression.
- Document any drugs used.

Following resuscitation:
- Monitor patient closely.
- Transfer to high dependency unit, e.g. CCU.
- Support and encourage feedback from all those involved.
- Document outcome and inform relatives.

Hospital life support

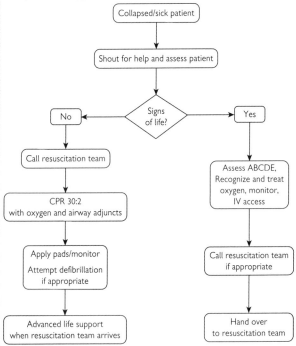

Fig. 33.18 In-hospital resuscitation. Reproduced with kind permission of the Resuscitation Council UK, www.resus.org.uk.

Advanced life support

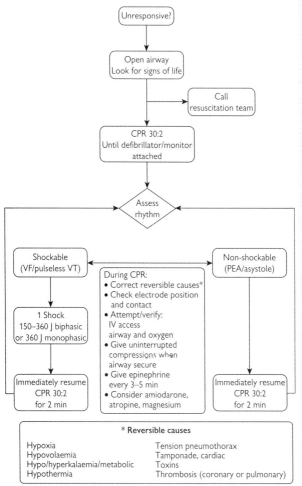

Fig. 33.19 Adult advanced life support. Reproduced with kind permission of the Resuscitation Council UK, www.resus.org.uk.

Automated external defibrillators

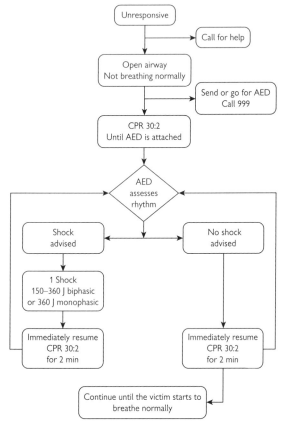

Fig. 33.20 The use of automated external defibrillators (AED). Reproduced with kind permission of the Resuscitation Council UK, www.resus.org.uk.

Tachycardia (with pulse)

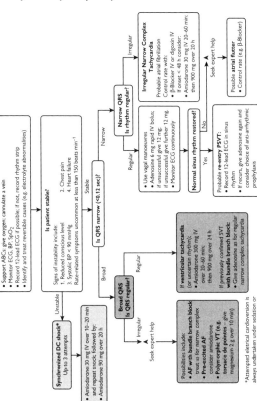

Fig. 33.21 Tachycardia algorithm. Reproduced with kind permission of the Resuscitation Council UK. www.resus.org.uk.

Bradycardia

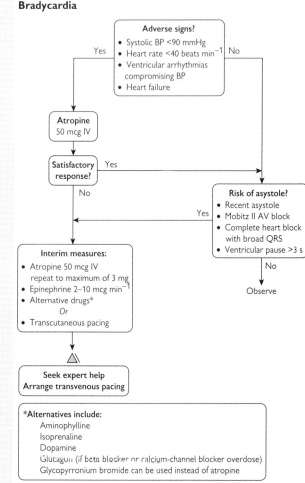

Fig. 33.22 Bradycardia algorithm. Reproduced with kind permission of the Resuscitation Council UK, www. resus.org.uk.

Characteristics of nursing care in the ED

- Coping with a variable throughput of patients of all ages and all types of conditions.
- Caring for patients with acute medical conditions and patients with mental health or social care problems.
- Caring for vulnerable people, especially those who have complex problems such as those who are elderly or who have learning difficulties.
- Treating patients with respect and dignity even though there is a danger that some patients may be labeled as inappropriate attendees or social misfits.
- Involvement in life and death decisions.
- Continually monitoring the patient's length of stay in the ED, thus ensuring that delays in treatment by medical and nursing staff are kept to a minimum.
- Monitoring patients and recording their progress.
- Dealing with unexpected and sudden death, which may lead to individual stress and affect the morale of the staff.
- Coping and being prepared for the risk of violence and unsociable behaviour from patients and their relatives/friends.
- Working as a multidisciplinary team member.

Emergency nursing care—general principles

- Develop a good knowledge of first aid/emergency care and methods of resuscitation.
- Keep up-to-date with knowledge and skills of first aid/emergency care and resuscitation.
- Work as a team member as this is crucial in the ED and at the scene of an incident.
- Take on the leadership role at a situation if there is nobody present who has more experience and knowledge than you have. (Enlist and direct helpers.)
- Always quickly assess an emergency situation.
- Don't put yourself at risk.
- Protect yourself from injury and infection.
- Summon appropriate help as soon as possible.
- Treat the most serious condition first.
- Try to keep calm, logical, and in control.
- Speak and communicate to patients/casualties and try to create an air of confidence.
- Explain what is happening.
- Gather as much information as you can on what happened and the symptoms the patients/casualties have suffered.
- Emergency care and first aid are stressful situations—learn how to cope with these demands and develop coping strategies to suit you and to enable you to be more effective.

Further information

Mental Health First aid

www.communitycare.co.uk

www.redcross.org.uk

www.sja.org.uk

www.firstaid.org.uk

www.firstaidinternational.com.au

The British Association for Immediate Care

www.basics.org.uk/intropage.htm

First Aid Manual (regularly updated)

www.dk.com/firstaidmanual

Emergencies in the clinical environment

Managing adverse incidents

Adverse incidents
This refers to any event that produces unexpected or unwanted effects involving the safety of a person or the loss or damage of property. Incidents may be clinical, health and safety, security, assaults, or accidents.

Near misses
These are unexpected adverse incidents that are prevented and result in no harm.

Serious adverse incidents
These incidents result in death or major permanent harm. They may lead to public concern.

Serial incident
This is a clinical incident that affects multiple patients, e.g. an infected worker, 'rogue staff', incorrect interpretation of specimens.

Management principles (See Fig. 34.1)
- Act to safeguard patients, visitors, and colleagues at all times.
- Remove people from danger.
- Refer to local policy and reporting procedures.
- Report incident to line manager—immediately if serious.
- Report to the patient's physician (if patient is involved).
- Collect statements and retain any evidence securely.
- Identify incidents that are legally notifiable to the Health and Safety Executive under RIDDOR (Reporting of Injuries, Disease and Dangerous Occurrences Regulations); or to the police for assaults of a racial, religious, or physical nature; or to the coroner for unexpected death within 24 hours of admission, operation, or discharge.
- Senior managers will arrange investigations for serious incidents.

Reporting incidents
All incidents should be reported to ensure there is learning from all serious incidents and near misses. Learning should also occur from trends in less serious incidents. All NHS organizations are required to keep a database of incidents, and some should be reported to national organizations such as the National Patient Safety Agency, Health Protection Agency, or Medical Devices Agency. Feedback should be made available to those involved

Further information
Health and Safety Executive: www.hse.gov.uk
National Patient Safety: www.npsa.nhs.uk
Medicines and Healthcare Products Agency: www.mhra.gov.uk

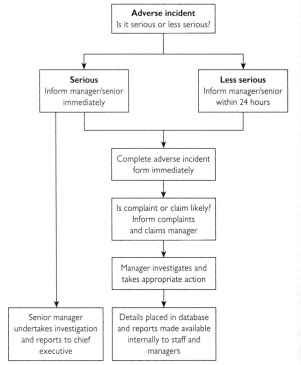

Fig. 34.1 Adverse incident flowchart.

Fire safety

Hospitals are particularly vulnerable to fire because of specialized processes, laboratories, stores, kitchens, gas, and electrical apparatus. All staff have a basic duty to observe fire safety instructions and participate in fire safety training. All health care organizations should have a written fire procedure.

General principles

- Sound the alarm and, if required, contact switchboard to give the exact location.
- If patients are in immediate danger, move them to a safer place, e.g. behind fire doors.
- Close all doors and windows in the immediate area.
- The senior nurse should decide whether evacuation is necessary.
- Go to the designated point when all patients are evacuated. Patients and staff should not re-enter the area.
- Evacuate all ambulant patients first, then non-ambulant patients.
- Take a roll call of all patients, visitors, and staff, and report any missing to the fire service officer.
- Turn off all equipment unless this puts patients in danger.
- Decide whether isolator valves to medical gases need to be turned off.
- Attempt to localize the fire using fire-fighting equipment but only if it is safe to do so.
- Lifts should not be used in the event of a fire.

Information nurses working in an area should know

- The local fire policy and procedure
- Fire alarm sounds and meaning
- The location of fire exits and evacuation routes, alarms, and fire-fighting equipment
- How to use fire-fighting equipment safely
- The evacuation points and how to use evacuation equipment
- Fire-fighting assembly points
- Any particular hazards in their area

Missing and absconding patients

Definitions
Missing patients are those found to be absent from the area with no known reason available to explain their absence.
Absconding patients are those who have wilfully left the clinical areas either secretly or openly.
Absent without leave are those patients who are detained under the Mental Health Act and are absent without authority under Section 17 of the Act.

Characteristics of patients likely to go missing
- History of previous event of being missing or absconding from hospital or home
- History of confusion or dementia
- Withdrawal from alcohol or other substance
- Displays of restlessness, anxiety, agitation, or wandering
- Past or current history of self-harming behaviour

Prevention
- Ensure patients are aware of the need to notify staff if they wish to leave the ward.
- Have a system for recording patients leaving the ward.
- Ensure staff are aware of 'at-risk' patients.
- Consider using seat or door sensor alarms for some patients to indicate when they are mobilizing or leaving the area.
- Provide escorts for 'at-risk' patients attending appointments outside the ward.
- Some patients may have one-to-one observation while on the ward to prevent them absconding.
- Have local policy and procedures for managing missing and absconding patients.

Action if a patient is missing
- Alert security.
- Coordinate a rapid search of the area.
- Ring round other wards and departments.
- Alert senior staff and the responsible physician and inform them of known risks associated with the patient.
- Ask security to check CCTV cameras.
- Gather information about the patient (description and last known movements).
- Inform the patient's relatives and check if patient has returned home.
- Consider police involvement—this will depend on local agreements.
- If found, persuade the patient to return to hospital or to go home.
- In the case of sectioned patients, Section 18 of the Mental Health Act provides power for the return of the patient.
- Report as an adverse incident.

Major incidents

A major incident in the health service is a situation which, because of the number and/or severity of live casualties or its location, requires special arrangements by the Health Service. Incidents arise with little or no warning and may result from road, air, or sea accidents; natural disasters; terrorist or criminal activity; fire; or chemical, biological, or radiation incidents.

Each NHS organization will have its own Major Incident Plan which will link into regional and national plans. Staff should be aware of their own organization's plan. There will be a designated team to coordinate and manage the incident.

The aim of the plan is to:
• save life
• relieve immediate suffering
• minimize long-term effects on health
• protect the health and safety of staff responding to the incident
• ensure rapid and efficient mobilization of services.

The plan ensures that hospitals can be prepared quickly at any time to deal with a large number of casualties. All nursing staff have a role to play in a major incident.
• Know the details of your own procedures (i.e. know what fire exits to use and know the difference between a fire alarm drill and a true fire alarm).
• Have regular updating and practice runs of your local procedure.
• Know the role of your department and how it fits in with the overall procedure working within the hospital.
• Ensure regular checks are made on emergency equipment to ensure it is functioning and stocks are in date.
• Be prepared to be redeployed to areas where you are most needed.
• Be able to direct people to designated areas in the hospital and have a good understanding of the hospital layout.
• Appear calm and confident in your approach to patients and the public.
• Know how you must respond to a call to a major incident when you are off duty.

Medical device failure

Definition

A medical device is any instrument, apparatus, appliance, material, or health care product excluding drugs used for a patient for:

- diagnosis, prevention, monitoring, treatment, or alleviation of disease or compensation for an injury or handicap, e.g. blood gas machine
- investigation, replacement, or modification of the anatomy or a physiological process, e.g. joint prosthesis
- control of conception, e.g. IUD.

Contingency plans should be developed for the event of medical devices failure.

Potential reasons for medical device failures

- Complete power failure and the device has no integrated battery
- Integral or remote battery failure due to drained battery following extensive use of the device
- Software failure—a 'chip' or other component malfunctions
- No disposable equipment to load into the device, e.g. no IV giving sets for infusion pump
- Power-plant or utility failure e.g. electricity, oxygen, air, and suction (📖 Utility failure, p.1116)

Follow local guidelines in the event of medical device failure in order to inform the company concerned.

Further information

The Medical Devices Agency (2000). *Equipped to care—the safe use of medical devices in the 21st century*. MDA, London

Medicine and Health Care Products Regulatory Agency: www.mhra.gov.uk

Utility failure

Possible utility failure in hospitals includes mains electricity (equipment, lighting, and telecommunications), water, and medical gases. Contingency plans for use in the event of such failures to ensure continuity of care for patients should be developed at organization and ward/department levels.

Mains electricity failure

Most hospitals and other health care organizations have back-up generator systems that 'kick in' if the mains power supply fails. The trigger to indicate this is often a brief fluctuation of all lighting. Turn off all non-essential equipment (e.g. kettles, toasters, lights not in use) to prevent generators becoming overloaded. Contingency plans should take account of generator failure.

- Keep electrically operated equipment with integral batteries plugged in where possible to maintain full charge, and check batteries regularly.
- Use additional blankets to keep patients warm.
- Restrict telephone calls and use shared telephones or mobile phones for communicating in an emergency.
- Ensure mechanisms for replacing electronic ordering, e.g. x-ray, laboratory tests.
- Identify manual alternatives, e.g. manual suction, gravity infusion sets, manual sphygmomanometer.
- Keep a supply of batteries, torches, and lamps.

Water failure

This is unlikely. Most hospitals have on-site reservoirs and water can be brought in by tankers. Action to conserve water must be implemented. 📖 Action in the event of water failure, p.1117.

Medical gas failure

Most hospitals have piped medical gases including vacuum, air, oxygen, and nitrous oxide with 'back-up systems' which will switch to bottle if mains supply fails. Contingency plans should include knowing how to access and use portable gas cylinders and battery-operated suction units.

Action in the event of a complete power failure

- Turn off all non-essential equipment to conserve energy, e.g. kettles, toasters, lighting, water boilers.
- Have manual alternative for the devices without an integral or remote battery.
- Ensure batteries are fully charged in case of an event.
- Most establishments will have some form of back-up generator to take over in the event of failure of external power cuts.

Action in the event of utility/plant failure

Have portable suction equipment available and oxygen and air bottles to provide a short-term solution. These require special regulators to connect them to machines by technical personnel.

Action in the event of water failure

- General
  - Turn off all taps securely.
- Toilet provision
  - Ration use of water.
  - Control flushing.
  - Close as many toilets as possible.
- Hygiene
  - Where possible substitute handwashing with hand gels.
- Equipment
  - Use sterile bottled water for devices such as humidifiers and nebulizers.
- Drinking
  - Use bottled water.

Violent and aggressive patients

Definitions

Violence

Any incident in which a member of hospital staff is abused, threatened, or assaulted by a patient in circumstances arising from their employment. This violence may be:

- physical assault with or without a weapon resulting in actual physical harm, e.g. bruising, cuts, or more serious injury
- physical abuse, i.e. attempted assault with or without a weapon which did not result in actual physical harm
- verbal or psychological abuse which may include racial or sexual harassment.

Aggression

Behaviour intended to harm another person or destroy property.

Triggers

- Alcohol or substance misuse or withdrawal
- Mental illness
- Fluid and electrolyte imbalance
- Other clinical reasons, e.g. pain, medications, confusional states
- Anxiety and frustration due to delays in treatment and lack of information

Prevention

- Keep patients informed.
- Communicate effectively and frequently and listen to patients.
- Treat patients politely and with respect.
- Be patient and not abrupt.
- If possible provide space or a quiet environment.
- Check for any previous episodes of violence or aggression.

Actions

- Ensure staff are trained in conflict resolution (which includes key communication skills) and handling violence and aggression.
- Follow local guidelines for handling violence and aggression.
- Do not antagonize difficult patients.
- Assess whether there may be an underlying medical or mental condition.
- Summon medical assistance and, if necessary, security.
- Leave the situation if it is safe to do so. Consider other patients' needs.
- Recognize the individual's rights. 📖 Restraint: rights of the individual, p.1119.
- Consider restraint only as a last resort and in extreme circumstances when safety is endangered. When actions are taken against a patient's will it causes them to lose trust and therefore makes future treatment difficult. Restraint should not be used to administer treatment against the patient's will or to prevent them from withdrawing from treatment or discharging themselves.
- Record and report the incident to senior managers and to the Health and Safety Executive.
- Support other patients and debrief and support staff.

Withholding treatment

This may occur if the violent behaviour:

- prejudices any benefit the patient might receive from care and treatment
- prejudices the safety of staff and other patients
- results in damage to property
- prevents staff from undertaking their duties properly.

Exceptions

- Lack of competency – follow Mental Capacity Act
- Mental illness – determined by psychiatrist
- Patients needing emergency care
- Patients under 16 years of age – if not considered competent to give informed consent. (In these instances, the consent of the parent, guardian or carer would need to be sought.)

Restraint: rights of the individual

- Before imposing any restriction on an individual, their human rights must be considered.
- Patients must not be subjected to any treatment they consider inhumane or degrading, whether physical or psychological.
- Dignity and privacy must be maintained.
- Staff must respect the individual's culture and not discriminate on any grounds.
- Patients have the right to appropriate planned care and treatment.
- Patients have the right to reasonable protection from harm.
- Patients have the right to refuse treatment to the extent permitted by law and to be informed of the consequences of this action.

Violent and aggressive relatives

Definitions
See definition for violent and aggressive patients (📖 Definitions, p.1118).

Triggers
- Delays in treatment of the patient
- Overcrowding, e.g. in waiting areas
- Individual's needs not being met, e.g. lack of information
- Seeing others behave violently
- Abrupt 'off-hand' attitude of staff
- Alcohol or substance misuse

Prevention
- Contact security and keep them aware of the situation.
- Ensure staff are trained in conflict management and managing violent and aggressive people.
- Keep relative(s) informed of what is happening.
- Provide quiet area with access to telephone if possible.
- Use calm and self-controlled manner.
- Do not appear defensive.
- Communicate frequently and apologize for delays.
- Have security alert system in place or personal security alarms.

Actions in the event of verbal abuse
- Advise the individual that the behaviour is unacceptable.
- If safe, leave the scene.
- Contact senior person for advice.
- Record incident and actions.

Actions in the event of violent relatives
- Summon assistance immediately, alert security, or leave the scene if possible.
- Request the individual to leave the premises quietly. The individual becomes a trespasser without consent to be on the premises and can be removed with reasonable force. This should normally be done by security staff.
- Call the police if a serious crime has been or is about to be committed, the situation is out of control, or the individual is drunk and disorderly.

Control of Substances Hazardous to Health (COSHH)

This is a legal framework for controlling the exposure of people to hazardous substances related to work, e.g. micro-organisms, allergens, chemical hazards, and mercury. Employers are required to protect everyone in the workplace against the immediate or delayed risk of such substances.

Common substances

Chemical hazards

Caused by disinfectants, solvents, and cleaning agents, e.g. gluteraldehyde used for decontaminating endoscopes and other equipment that requires rapid turnaround which can cause dermatitis, asthma, and eye irritations. Latex found in gloves and catheters can cause dermatitis.

Microbiological hazards

These include exposure to blood, body fluids, and infected materials.

Mercury spillage

Some instruments containing mercury may still be in use, e.g. thermometers and sphygmomanometers. Mercury evaporates at room temperature, and the vapour is highly toxic by inhalation and can be absorbed through the skin and conjunctiva.

Controls

The nurse should be aware of the controls in place including:

- Policies.
- Safe systems of work, e.g. safe devices to use and procedures to follow. These should be practical and easy to follow.
- The correct personal protective equipment and clothing to use.
- Understanding the risks and consequences of not following procedures.
- Training and instruction to gain the required skills and knowledge.
- Processes in place for reviewing risks and identifying new hazards.
- Support and advice available from health and safety, infection control, and occupational health experts, and from staff-side safety representatives.
- Action to take in the event of exposure and reporting requirements.
- Where records of hazards, risk assessments, controls, and outcomes are kept.
- Incident reporting and monitoring systems to check that the controls are working

Further information

Health and Safety Executive: www.hse.gov.uk

Professional nursing practice

Ethical issues

Ethics

Ethics is the systematic study of the moral principles of self-conduct. In nursing terms this translates to 'not what we *want* to do but what we *ought* to do' for our patients, based on our Professional Code of Conduct, norms, and values.

Ethical dilemmas

Ethical dilemmas occur when situations arise where there is a choice between two or more courses of action. They may occur when:

- Two or more clear moral principles that support mutually inconsistent courses of action apply.
- The problem cannot be solved easily.
- The problem is very perplexing, baffling, or bewildering, causing concern as to which facts and data should be used in making the decision.
- The outcome of the problem may have far-reaching effects.

Ethical frameworks

Ethical frameworks are used to guide ethical decision making. Four of the most commonly used frameworks are:

- *Teleology—utilitarianism:* Decisions are based on what provides the greatest good for the greatest number of people.
- *Deontology—duty-based:* Decisions arise from the intent of the action taken by the decision maker (i.e. a duty to do something or to refrain from doing something).
- *Rights-based:* Decisions are based on the premise that individuals have basic inherent rights that should not be interfered with. Note: rights are different from needs, wants, or desires.
- *Intuitionist framework:* Decisions are made by evaluating each case individually and weighing the relative goals, duties, and rights. The decision maker selects the solution that they believe is right for that particular situation.

Ethical principles

- *Autonomy*—actions are taken that promote self-determination and freedom of choice.
- *Beneficence*—actions are taken in an effort to promote good.
- *Non-maleficence*—actions are taken in an effort to avoid harm.
- *Paternalism*—one individual assumes the right to make decisions for another (may be done for the good of someone, but limits freedom of choice).
- *Utility*—the good of the many outweighs the wants or needs of the individual.
- *Justice*—people are treated fairly; equals are treated equally and unequals are treated according to their differences.
- *Veracity*—obligation to tell the truth.
- *Fidelity*—obligation to keep promises.
- *Confidentiality*—obligation to observe the privacy of another and keep privileged information private.

Ethical decision making

Ethical decision making in nursing and health care has been influenced by various factors over the years:
- Sociocultural changes
- Scientific and medical technological advances
- Legal issues
- An increasing number of older people
- Costs of the National Health Service
- Scarcity of resources
- Politicization of health care
- Greater consumer involvement
- Changes in practice, including the increasing number of nurses working in the independent sector

Overall approach
- Always try to act in the best interests of your patients.
- Make decisions based on ethical principles.
- Recognize that most ethical dilemmas encountered by nurses do not have clear-cut solutions.
- Understand that a collaborative decision-making approach is the best way to solve complex ethical questions.
- Involve all relevant members of the health care team, being aware of confidentiality requirements.
- Consider including members of the clinical governance team to assist you.
- Recognize that joint decision making helps protect the professional nurse from making or participating in unwise or erroneous decisions.

Steps in ethical decision making
- Identify the problem, concern, or question, and determine whether it is an ethical dilemma.
- Gather information to promote clarification of the issue:
  - Self-clarification—Examine personal values, morals, and beliefs as thoroughly as possible.
  - Professional clarification and accountability—Understand the nursing profession's position on the dilemma. Explore NMC guidelines and the Code of Professional Conduct for nurses. Access the NMC Professional Advisory service if necessary. 📖 Chapter 36, The Nursing and Midwifery Council, p.1138.
  - Employer clarification—Understand your employer's guidelines, directives, protocols, rules, and regulations.
  - Public clarification—Consider society's current views of your dilemma and gather any information relating to the dilemma.
  - Patient clarification—Examine the patient and family's view, values, needs, and wishes.
- Consider all possible solutions to the dilemma, regardless of the ethical principles involved.

- Consider who should have access to the patient's information and preserve privacy and confidentiality. Advice may be taken from the hospital's appointed Caldicott guardian ('a senior person responsible for protecting the confidentiality of patient and service-user information and enabling appropriate information-sharing'; Department of Health definition).
- Determine whether the patient needs an advocate to represent them.
- Evaluate the likely outcome of each solution.
- Choose the solution that is in most accord with your personal values and ethical principles. Take into consideration everything else discussed above.
- Communicate with clinical governance structures to ensure that you are protected by your employer's vicarious liability. 📖 Chapter 36, Legal aspects of nursing, p.1134.

Key factors to consider when making an ethical decision are shown in Fig. 35.1.

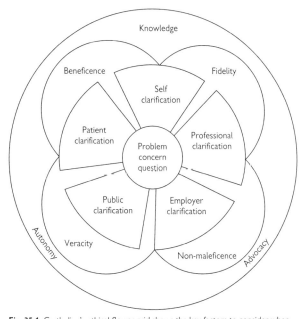

Fig. 35.1 Castledine's ethical flower grid shows the key factors to consider when making an ethical decision in clinical nursing practice. Reproduced from Castledine G (1998). *Writing, documentation and communication for nurses*, p. 58. Quay Books, Mark Allen Publishing.

Nursing codes

The true ethical core of all nursing codes derives from the rights and dignity of the individual—the patient as a person—and this forms the basic criterion of behaviour. Nursing codes:

• Give direction for nursing actions and the form they should take.
• Provide guidance on professional behaviour when at work and when off duty.
• Are concerned with what is done and how it is achieved.
• Are unambiguously explicit and direct.
• Are universal and affect all nurses.

An ethical code for nurses in the UK dates back to July 1983. It was published by the UK Central Council for Nursing and Midwifery. A copy of the code has been enclosed with the registration documents of each nurse being admitted to the Council's Register from 1 July 1983 onwards. The code is regularly updated and reviewed, and the present NMC intends to continue the process. ▣ Chapter 37, The NMC Code: standards of conduct, performance, and ethics for nurses and midwives, p.1152.

The code clearly states the extent of a registered nurse's accountability. It encourages practitioners to assert themselves so that the primacy of the interest of their patients and clients is respected.

The code is now used as the backcloth against which allegations of misconduct in a professional sense are judged. It is regularly referred to in the NMC Professional Conduct hearings and is used in legal courts, employer disciplinary hearings, coroner courts, and by various ombudsmen and investigative health care teams.

Professional codes cannot and do not provide answers to every situation. It is impossible to write a code that provides precise answers for any and every situation. Nurses must evaluate situations carefully, consider their options, and make decisions based on what is reasonable in the circumstances. The nurse must be prepared to justify their decisions and behaviour if called into question. Even after careful consideration and use of their professional judgement, nurses require guidance which should be sought from the regulatory body, currently the Nursing and Midwifery Council. Breaches of the Nursing Code are reported to the Trust's Director of Nursing and/or Senior Trust Management Team (▣ Chapter 37, Managing in the clinical environment, p.1141). If the nurse's behaviour is considered to have been a danger to the public then the NMC will also become involved (▣ Chapter 36, The Nursing and Midwifery Council, p.1138).

Further information

NMC (2008). *The Code*. http://www.nmc-uk.org

Ethical issues in nursing

Rapid advances in technology and science, particularly in biology (genetics) and medical technology, have given rise to ethical dilemmas in health care. Many dilemmas involve critical points in a person's existence such as birth, adjustment to illness, disability, old age, and death. Most ethical issues are further complicated by the legal questions they raise.

Informed consent

Informed consent is permission from a patient to carry out nursing care, special tests, and medical procedures. Written consent should be based on:
- The patient's right of self-determination
- Relevant and appropriate information that the patient understands
- The patient agreeing voluntarily and without coercion or persuasion
- The patient being mentally competent

Right to die and resuscitation

A patient's right to die involves the following issues:
- Whether life-saving measures should be provided or withheld. This should be made clear in the patient's notes and a 'do not resuscitate' form should be completed and available to all of the health care team.
- Whether an older person should be resuscitated.
- Whether life-sustaining methods and occupation of an intensive care bed should be continued.
- Positive euthanasia (i.e. mercy killing). Illegal in the UK.
- Negative euthanasia (i.e. passively allowing a patient to die).
- Living wills or written requests regarding treatment or withdrawal of treatment under certain conditions.
- Who decides and on what criteria to resuscitate a patient.
- What type of nursing care should be provided for patients with a poor prognosis.

Confidentiality

Information recorded in nursing and medical records can be of great help or harm to the patient. Records must be treated with respect. Information should be handled among health professionals with regard for the privacy and dignity of patients.

Ethical dimensions in leadership and management

- What action should nurses follow when there is a conflict between their professional position and that of their employer?
- At what point do the needs of the organization become more important than those of the individual nurse?
- Should quality or cost be the final determinant when selecting the most appropriate method of nursing?
- When should a nurse report an incompetent colleague?
- At what point does understaffing become unsafe?
- Is it ethical for nurses to go on strike?
- What is the best way to create an ethical work environment and a participating ethically based multidisciplinary health care team?

Legal issues

Legal aspects of nursing

The primary purpose of law and legislation is to protect the public, the patient, and the nurse. Laws and legislation define the scope of acceptable practice and protect individual rights. The law is basically the system of rules which a country or a community recognize as a way of regulating the actions of its subjects or members.

Law created by the judicial system is enforced and monitored by the police on behalf of the public. All law is ultimately derived from natural law—the innate human tendency to do good and avoid evil. The law, like many public institutions, is subject to change and can often be subject to interpretation (e.g. translation of EU legislation into UK legislation).

The judicial system attempts to resolve legal controversies over questions of fact regarding what happened at an event or incident. Facts are usually determined by examining evidence presented by lawyers for each side of a controversy, although persons have the right to defend themselves. Facts may be difficult to determine and are open to interpretation, although it is usual for a case to be determined 'beyond reasonable doubt'.

Sometimes nurses act as expert witnesses in legal cases to help establish the facts of a case. Magistrates, or in higher courts juries, must determine what actually happened based on evidence presented to them. When both sides agree on facts, application and interpretation of the law must be determined. A judge or magistrate will then make that decision.

Historically, physicians were the health care professionals most likely to be held liable for nursing care. More recently registered nurses are expected to demonstrate accountability for their own practice. In the UK, employers of the NHS are affected by two forms of liability: vicarious liability and direct liability.

- **Vicarious liability** means that an NHS trust can be deemed responsible for the actions of its employees and its employer's staff. For coverage by vicarious liability, an employee must be working within the framework of their contract of employment and must be working within an area of competence appropriate to their abilities.
- **Direct liability** means that the trust is held accountable in its own right, i.e. the trust itself is at fault if it does something which is its own responsibility.

The law sees all nursing practitioners accountable for their own practice. As a result of increased responsibility in practice, it is advisable that all nurses adhere to prescribed good practice and insure themselves against litigation. The NMC recommends that nurses who are treating or caring for patients in a private capacity should ensure that they have professional indemnity insurance in the event of claims of professional negligence. Of note, students who are gaining practical experience are generally protected from liability as they are working under the supervision of staff who themselves should be covered for liability.

When a patient suffers harm or there is loss of or damage to property, the nurse may be called to account in four different courts or tribunals:

- Professional conduct and competence—NMC (📖 The Nursing and Midwifery Council, p.1138).
- Criminal act—criminal courts
- Civil wrong—civil courts
- Work problem—employment tribunal

Nurses may also appear at a coroner's court if there are questions regarding the death of a patient. They may also be asked to attend a youth or family court (e.g. on behalf of a child).

Acknowledgement

Lynne Rogers

Key legal terms

Duty of care
The nurse owes a duty of care to the patient by virtue of the nurse–patient relationship, the NHS Acts, and Professional Codes of Practice (☐ Chapter 35, Nursing codes, p.1130). Legal principles are used to determine whether this duty of care has failed or whether a nurse should be brought to account. If there is a breach, then the courts will be involved.

Negligence
The nurse should always follow the policies, protocols, procedures, and guidelines set by the NMC, their employer, or other recognized body. If the nurse believes that enacting a policy or protocol may jeopardize the patient's safety and best interest, then they must report and record their decision not to enact the policy or protocol and they must be prepared to justify their actions. Criteria that can be used to determine whether a nurse has been negligent are:
• Was there any reasonable foreseeable risk?
• Was the nurse aware and were knowledge and practice skills up to date?
• Did the nurse make a decision based on balancing the risks?
• What harm has been suffered?

Nurses should be aware of the current legal environment and changes in case law. For example, the well-known 'Bolam test' has been added to recently by a ruling in Chester v Afshar.

Employers
Employers are responsible for providing reasonable resources and staffing levels. Concerns about unreasonable resources or staffing levels should be put in writing to managers.

Whistleblowing
Under the NMC code (☐ The Nursing and Midwifery Council, p.1138), nurses are required to bring hazards and dangers, including incompetence of a nursing colleague, to the attention of management. The NHS publication 'Guidelines for Staff on Relations with the Public and Media' (1993) is available to guide a nurse on proper procedures so that they avoid victimization and fears of reprisal. Each NHS employer has a duty to establish a procedure for employees to raise concerns. Statutory provision was made in the Public Interest Disclosure Act (1998).

Criminal liability
Criminal charges against a nurse or physician are rare, but when they occur they attract a lot of media attention and publicity. Examples are the cases of Beverley Allitt who caused death and injury to children (☐ Further reading, p.1137) and Kevin Cobb who was found guilty of manslaughter of a nurse and who was also convicted of drugging three female patients and raping two of them.

Civil liability

Civil liability gives an individual who alleges to have suffered at the hands of a nurse or from the negligence from an NHS trust the right to sue in the civil courts. Two issues are pursued with civil liability: Is the defendant liable and how much compensation is payable?

Professional liability

When questions arise about the professional conduct or behaviour and competence of a registered nurse, the individual can be referred to the NMC.

Common legal and professional pitfalls in nursing

- Failure to communicate to people
- Verbal abuse and non-verbal threats
- Poor handling and touching without consent
- Lack of consideration of older people
- Alleged abuse of a patient of any age
- Failure to provide the fundamentals of nursing care
- Failure to keep accurate records
- Failure to adhere to legal and professional requirements related to drug administration
- Theft from patients or the employer
- Abuse of authority
- Sleeping on duty
- Sexual harassment or abuse

Common clinical problems

- Medication errors
- Equipment injuries
- Patient falls
- Failure to monitor patients adequately
- Failure to cope with patient's challenging behaviour
- Lack of understanding of patient's psychosocial and spiritual needs

Acknowledgement

Lynne Rogers

Further information

Clothier Report (1994). *Independent inquiry relating to deaths and injuries on the children's ward at Grantham and Kesteven General Hospital.* HMSO, London.

House of Lords. *Opinions of the Lords of Appeal for Judgment in the Cause: Chester (Respondent) v. Afshar (Appellant). [2004] UKHL 41.* http://www.publications.parliament.uk

Bolam v Friern Hospital Management Committee ([1957] 1 WLR 583).

Davies, Nick (1993). *Murder on Ward Four. The Story of Bev Allitt.* Chatto & Windus, London.

The Nursing and Midwifery Council (NMC)

The Nursing and Midwifery Council is the regulatory body for nurses, midwives, and specialist community public health nurses. Its primary aim is to protect the public and maintain an accurate register of practitioners. It is not a nursing union. All professional nurses who practise in the UK must be registered with the NMC. The council sets the standards for education (pre- and post-registration), training, conduct, and performance.

Allegations

A registered nurse's fitness to practice may be questioned for many reasons, including:
- Misconduct
- Lack of competence
- A conviction or caution in a court of law
- Physical or mental ill health
- A finding by any other health or social care regulator or licensing body that a registrant's fitness to practice is impaired
- A fraudulent or incorrect entry in the NMC's register

Anyone has the right to make a complaint to the NMC about a registered nurse. The UK police force and the courts automatically refer nurses to the NMC. Employers and managers should refer a nurse to the NMC if they feel that a nurse is a danger to the public.

The NMC process related to complaints against registered practitioners

Most complaints are firstly processed through the *NMC Investigation Committee*. Once the committee has considered all the available evidence it can:
- close the case,
- refer the case to a conduct hearing, or
- refer the case to a health committee.

In some extreme cases where there is a major concern that a nurse may continue to practise and be a further and immediate danger to the public, the committee can make an interim order and suspend the individual at once from the register.

The Conduct and Competence Committee (CCC)

The Conduct and Competence Committee determines whether allegations against a practitioner warrant them being struck off the register. A panel of at least three people from the same part of the register as the practitioner comprises the committee and will hear the case. The hearing is usually held in public. After hearing a case, the committee can:
- close a case and take no further action;
- find that a practitioner has done wrong but, taking circumstances into consideration, take no further action;
- remove the person from the register;
- suspend the person's registration for a period of time;
- impose conditions of practice; or
- issue a caution which will be for a specified period of up to 5 years.

The Health Committee

The Health Committee meets in private to determine whether physical or mental ill health of a registered nurse impairs their fitness to practise. The committee has the power to remove, suspend, or impose conditions of practice.

Acknowledgement

Lynne Rogers

Common health problems (nurses)

- Alcohol or drug abuse
- Severe stress caused by family and social problems
- Mental health problems such as anxiety, depression, eating disorders
- Failure to recognize or admit to health problems
- Taking non-prescription drugs and addiction

Incompetent practitioner

- Performs work that could be interpreted as misconduct.
- Undertakes work outside their area of knowledge or competence.
- Fails to get things done in a professional, acceptable manner.
- Does not demonstrate safety or understanding of a subject.
- Leaves a practice area while the patient is vulnerable.
- Provides inconsistent care.
- Appears slow and incompetent at tasks.
- Demonstrates poor documentation, reporting, and recording.
- Appears untidy and disorganized or potentially brings the profession into disrepute.
- Manipulates and encourages others to cover for them.

Managing in the clinical environment

Acute staffing problems

Acute staffing problems occur when there are insufficient numbers and/or skill mix of staff to cope with the workload.

Causes
- Higher than usual levels of staff sickness
- Maternity leave
- Other unexpected leave
- Lack of effective management of annual and study leave
- Poor rostering
- Vacancies and failure to recruit to posts at required grade or level
- Unplanned increase in workload, e.g. higher dependency of patients
- Planned increase in workload without adjustment to establishment, e.g. increases in beds or additional outpatient clinics

Prevention
- Agree rules about numbers/skill mix of staff allowed off duty, on study leave, or on annual leave at any time.
- Establish policies to manage sick leave, e.g. follow up every period of sickness with individuals and refer to occupational health if patterns or amount of sickness are untoward.
- Periodically review staffing establishments with senior nurse.
- Agree rules for the use of temporary staff (bank and agency) in specific circumstances.

Immediate action
- Review rosters and agree changes to 'off duties' with individuals if necessary.
- Contact staff who are off duty for possible extra duties, if willing.
- Contact senior nurse for possible redeployment from other areas.
- Contact bank/agency for temporary staff where local policy allows.
- Reprioritize workload and redeploy staff as appropriate.
- Contact senior nurse and request consideration of stopping admissions if additional staff are not available and the situation is unsafe.

Longer-term action
- Establish plan for filling vacancies with senior nurse and recruitment officer.
- Agree ways of providing maternity leave cover, e.g. through fixed-term contract or temporary staff block booking.
- Review staff establishment and skill mix with patient dependency.
- Identify reasons for vacancies (e.g. unpopular speciality, poor management and leadership style, poor team working and reputation) and plan action with senior nurse.

Patients' property

Patients should be encouraged to give non-essential belongings and valuables to relatives or friends on or before admission. They should be informed that hospitals cannot accept responsibility for their property unless it is handed to the ward staff for safekeeping and an official receipt has been obtained. Signed disclaimers may be required by some organizations.

A *patients' property and money book* should be used to record property taken into safe custody for patients who are mentally disordered, confused and/or disorientated, dying in hospital, severely incapacitated, or found to be dead on arrival. Money and valuables should be kept in a secure place, e.g. a safe. Entries in the book should be certified by two staff. When a patient is not able to take responsibility for their clothing, this should be placed in a patient property bag, the contents recorded, and the bag stored according to local policy.

On return of property, a signature by the patient or authorized guardian acknowledging receipt must be obtained and the property checked against the entry in the patients' property and money book.

Property and valuables belonging to deceased patients should only be returned to the next of kin. If valuables are left on the body, this should also be entered into the patients' property and money book stating 'left on body'.

Lost or unclaimed valuables should be retained for 6 months or according to local policy. Other property should be retained for 1 month. Every effort must be made to identify the owner to make arrangements to collect their belongings, indicating that failure to do so after the period will lead to disposal.

Local policies should be followed. The processes related to patients' property are audited regularly by organizations to ensure they are being followed correctly.

Harassment and bullying

Harassment

This is conduct that is unwanted, not reciprocated, and affects the dignity of men and women at work. It may be related to gender, race, colour, language, beliefs, sexuality, national or social origin, or other status. It may be evident in anonymous messages, offensive jokes, written abuse, social isolation, implicit threats, stalking, and other behaviours.

Bullying

This is the misuse of power or position that undermines a person's ability or coerces them into something they do not wish to do and leaves them feeling frightened or powerless. Examples include public criticism, humiliation, persistent criticism, and undermining staff without justification.

Good practice in dealing with bullying and harassment

- All staff should be aware of their personal responsibilities.
- A written policy developed jointly with staff and applicable to all staff in an organization that ensures that staff are treated fairly should be available.
- Processes that ensure early recognition of bullying and harassment and its speedy resolution should be implemented.
- All staff should be properly trained to develop an understanding of the effects of bullying and harassment; expected behaviours; how to recognize and prevent it; what action to take; how to provide support to both the complainant and accused. Specific training for managers undertaking investigations is required to ensure impartiality.
- A risk assessment of bullying and harassment in the workplace should be performed.
- Counselling and support should be provided for staff, e.g. through the occupational health service, a specific staff counselling service, independent counselling, or professional organizations.
- A healthy organizational culture in which all staff treat each other with respect and dignity should be promoted.
- The policy should indicate what action to take if the line manager is perceived as the perpetrator.

Action in the event of bullying and harassment

- Obtain a copy of the organization's harassment and bullying policy.
- Record all incidents.
- Report the incident(s) to the line manager or more senior member of staff.
- Record as an adverse incident.
- Use the organization's whistle-blowing policy or equivalent, if necessary.
- Seek support from colleagues, family, union representative, or counselling service.

Handling complaints

Complaints may pertain to any aspect of the service, e.g. clinical care and treatment, attitude and communication by staff, processes and procedures, access and waiting times, and support services (e.g. transport and hotel service), or even about the way a complaint has been handled.

Precipitating factors

- Care has been or is perceived to be negligent
- Poor communication or attitude of staff
- Lack of information
- Lack of involvement
- Standards have not been met
- Agreed services have not been provided

On receiving complaints

For complaints received in person or by telephone:

- Listen carefully to the nature of the complaint and write down the details of the complaint and complainant.
- Ask the complainant what action they feel should be taken regarding their complaint.
- Give the complainant information, e.g. a complaints leaflet, information and telephone numbers for support services such as PALS (Patient Advice and Liaison Service) and Independent Complaints Advocacy Service (ICAS) or equivalent.
- Resolve the complaint, if possible, and ask the complainant if they are satisfied with the resolution.
- If unable to resolve the complaint, the nurse should immediately contact a more senior colleague for advice on how to proceed and follow local policy.
- Record actions and keep complaints manager informed.
- A statement may be required, which should be limited to the facts alone.

Complaints may be received by letter. These should be passed to the complaints manager and processed according to the organization's policy.

Preventing complaints

- Keep patients and visitors informed about care, treatment, and arrangements affecting them.
- Be available to answer questions and queries.
- Actively seek out concerns before they become complaints.
- Always act in a polite and respectful manner.
- Give explanations when things do not go to plan, e.g. why patients need to wait.
- Seek help from senior colleagues when necessary.
- Apologize when things do not go to plan.
- Do not appear abrupt and defensive.

Fraud and theft

Fraud in the health service may take different forms. Usually it is of low value and opportunistic, but sometimes it is high value and committed by skilled criminals. Collectively, it costs millions of pounds a year that could be spent on patient care.

Examples of fraud

- Prescription fraud
- Submitting claims for work or expenses not earned
- Falsification of documents, e.g. timesheets or travel claims generating fraudulent income
- Accepting gifts as payment in return for placing orders for supplies or drugs
- Patients falsely making claims for benefits or travel expenses
- Theft directly from a patient or member of staff
- Theft from the organization, e.g. equipment, linen

Prevention and detection

All nursing staff should be aware of their responsibilities in creating an anti-fraud culture and of the arrangements in their organization for prevention and detection. This includes:

- having local measures in place for prevention, e.g. processes for signing timesheets, travel allowances, security of prescription pads, etc.
- advising patients on safety of their property and valuables (☐ Patients' property, p.1143)
- implementing processes to detect fraud, e.g. random checks on claims
- knowing the action to take if they suspect fraud or theft
- maintaining confidentiality of information relevant to the investigation of suspected fraud
- contacting the local counter-fraud specialists working for each organization who will investigate fraud
- recognizing that the organization will use appropriate legal action and sanctions and will seek redress in respect of money lost through fraud.

Alcohol and substance misuse by staff

Definition

This is the use of alcohol or other non-prescribed substances that interferes with the individual's health, social functioning, and/or work performance or conduct, and/or endangers colleagues, patients, or visitors.

Selling, possessing, taking, or being under the influence of such substances in the workplace is usually a disciplinary offence and may lead to reports to the registration body of the individual. It may result in removal or suspension from the register.

Signs of staff with problems

- Changes in work performance
- Changes in attendance, sickness, and accident patterns
- Changes in behaviour
- Smell of alcohol
- Drowsiness

Action

- Staff must inform the manager or senior member of staff where there are concerns. Failing to take action may put patients and others at risk as well as the individual. Records will be required of actual events, dates, frequencies, and examples. Concerns raised by colleagues should be kept confidential.
- Further actions by the manager may initially include discussion, counselling, referral to occupational health services and other agencies, monitoring, and review. If this is not effective, disciplinary action may be taken. If there is risk to public protection, disciplinary action would be initiated immediately.

Safeguards

- Individuals should inform managers of any prescribed medicines they are taking that could affect their work performance.
- Individuals should not consume alcohol or non-prescribed medicines that may affect work performance immediately prior to working hours or during working hours and in periods of on-call and standby.
- Individuals with an alcohol problem should request assistance with the abuse from their GP and occupational health department or recognized agencies such as Alcoholics Anonymous and National Drugs helpline.

Accidents and injuries to staff, patients, and visitors

Definition

An accident is an unexpected or unplanned event that causes damage or harm. Approximately 70–75% of accidents in hospital involve patients or visitors and are usually due to slips, trips, and falls. Staff injuries are related to manual handling, physical assault, slips, trips, and falls. About 5% of staff injuries are reportable to the Health and Safety Executive.

Action in the event of accidents, injuries, and dangerous occurrences

Any person involved in or witnessing an accident must:
- Ensure the injured person receives first aid or medical treatment.
- Report the accident to a manager verbally and use reporting systems, e.g. complete an accident or incident form.
- Investigate the circumstance to determine the cause—to include, where relevant, statements from witnesses, reports, photographs, documentation, and training records.
- Take immediate action to make sure the situation is safe and prevent recurrence.
- Report as a Serious Untoward Incident, if necessary, according to local policy.
- Report to the Health and Safety Executive under RIDDOR (Reporting of Injuries, Diseases and Dangerous Occurrences Regulations) if:
  - there is a death or major injury of a member of staff or public or patient, e.g. amputation, loss of sight, unconsciousness
  - an injury to an employee lasts more than 3 days
  - it is a reportable work-related disease
  - it is a dangerous occurrence, e.g. fire.
- Keep detailed and accurate records.
- Inform relatives in the event of a patient, visitor, or staff accident and advise on the outcome of the investigation and the action taken.
- Advise the manager responsible for personal injury and employers' liability claims of the accident and provide a report as required.
- Review further action required to prevent recurrence, e.g. review need for falls prevention programme, awareness raising on needlestick injuries, and manual handling training.
- Review accident trends for wards and department, and plan preventative action for frequent and high-risk accidents.

Poor performance and incompetent practice

This occurs when an individual consistently performs at a standard less than that expected for the qualification and grade and/or who persistently fails to practise at a standard or level agreed within the organization and which is normally maintained by others. It may arise for a number of reasons including:

- the individual is not aware of the standards expected *or*
- has not kept up to date with practice *or*
- takes on responsibilities beyond their capability *or*
- the workload in the clinical area outweighs the resources to provide care.

Poor performance may be identified during appraisal, supervised practice, preceptorship, and clinical supervision, or as a result of several complaints, or as a result of repeated incident reports.

Prevention

- Maintain current registration with the NMC by keeping up with PREP requirements.
- Keep up-to-date personal professional profiles, policies, guidelines, standards, and practices that relate to the area of work.
- Actively participate in appraisal and personal development plans.
- Do not allow staff to undertake duties for which they have not been appropriately trained.
- Identify any areas where updating is required.
- Seek advice from professional organizations (unions) where employers are not willing to support **any** education or training.

Action in the event of poor performance and incompetent practice

- Raise concerns with the individual's line manager, who will investigate and discuss with the individual and make the standards of performance required explicit.
- Develop and implement an action plan to improve skills and knowledge. Include assessment and review periods and ensure accurate feedback is given to the individual.
- Address particular personal circumstances that impact the individual's performance, e.g. through occupational health and counselling.
- Keep accurate records of progress.

Failure to progress may result in further development plans, retraining, redeployment, external help and support, or disciplinary action.

Safe practice in employment of nurses

Bogus staff may try to gain employment or attempt to work with a team of health care professionals. Action should be taken to safeguard and promote the interests of patients and the organization, justify public trust and confidence, and uphold and enhance the good standing and reputation of the professions. Senior members of the organization and line managers have responsibility for ensuring that relevant policy is developed and implemented. All staff hold responsibility to protect patients and staff by following established policies.

Pre-employment screening for each individual

- *Health screen* by occupational health department, which includes checks on sickness records
- *Registration*—all RN registration must be checked directly with NMC for registration and any ongoing investigations
- *Additional qualifications*—original certificates should be checked
- *References*—including one from previous employer (manager not colleague)
- *Criminal Records Bureau* checks

During employment

Regular checks to ensure currency of registration and occupational health checks to keep up-to-date with required immunizations or for specific problems, e.g. hepatitis B, TB, hepatitis C.

Temporary staff (bank and agency)

- Only use sources agreed by the organization.
- Keep records of requests for temporary staff and check individual against this.
- Check photographic identity against individual.
- Do not accept substitutes without checking with supplier.
- Do not accept staff who have not been requested.
- Use the organization's systems for induction and checking competence.
- Report concerns to line manager immediately.

Organizational safeguards

- Verify initial supply of uniforms and perform checks for collection of laundry (where available) to ensure no unauthorized use.
- All staff must wear photographic identity at all times.
- Check new or unfamiliar staff against ID (all staff and volunteers).
- Report any suspicions to line manager immediately.
- Ensure any alert notices are stored securely and checked when new or unfamiliar staff commence on the ward.

Equipment

Report all adverse incidents involving equipment, including failure of an alarm, as this may indicate individuals tampering with equipment.

Reporting unfitness to practise

All registered nurses are personally accountable for their practice to the NMC, the regulatory body. The purpose of the NMC is to protect the public's health from registrants whose fitness to practise is impaired and whose situation cannot be managed locally.

Fitness to practise

This may be impaired by misconduct, lack of competence, a conviction or caution, or a health condition. 📖 Poor performance and incompetent practice, Common examples of unfitness to practise, pp.1149; 1153.

The NMC Code: Standards of conduct, performance, and ethics for nurses and midwives

This is used as a benchmark for judging professional misconduct and was last published in 2008. The code states that:

'The people in your care must be able to trust you with their health and wellbeing. To justify that trust, you must:

- make the care of people your first concern, treating them as individuals and respecting their dignity
- work with others to protect and promote the health and wellbeing of those in your care, their families and carers, and the wider community
- provide a high standard of practice and care at all times
- be open and honest, act with integrity and uphold the reputation of your profession.

As a professional, you are personally accountable for actions and omissions in your practice and must always be able to justify your decisions. You must always act lawfully, whether those laws relate to your professional practice or personal life. Failure to comply with this Code may bring your fitness to practise into question and endanger your registration.'

The Code should be considered together with the Nursing and Midwifery Council's rules, standards, guidance and advice available from the NMC website.

Most allegations of unfitness to practise are dealt with locally through the organization's professional structures led by the most senior nurse. When a nurse witnesses an event or suspects an individual is unfit to practise they should:

- Take action to ensure the safety and well-being of patients.
- Report to the senior nurse responsible.
- Provide a clear account of the alleged incident and a brief description of the context or circumstances.
- Provide a witness statement.
- Preserve any evidence.
- Follow local guidelines or policies.
- If all else fails, the person has been well supported, and has followed instructions but is still having difficulties, report to the NMC.

Further information

NMC (2008). *The Code:* www.nmc.uk.org

Common examples of unfitness to practise

Misconduct
- Physical or verbal abuse
- Theft
- Deliberate failure to deliver adequate care
- Deliberate failure to keep proper records

Lack of competence
- Persistent inability to correctly calculate, administer, and record the administration or disposal of medicines
- Persistent inability to properly identify care needs and plan and deliver appropriate care

Conviction or caution
- Theft
- Fraud
- Dishonest activities
- Violence
- Sexual offences
- Accessing and downloading child pornography
- Illegally dealing or importing drugs

Health
- Alcohol or drug dependence
- Untreated serious mental illness

Managing the press and media

Good relationships with the media are important. If journalists fail to obtain a response then they may use 'back door' methods to get a story which may mean hassle for staff and distress for patients, and a misleading story.

Principles

- Most organizations will have procedures for dealing with the press and these should be followed.
- Front-line staff are not usually asked to handle press inquiries but may be asked for information by a senior member of staff.
- Wherever possible nurses should never give information to the media. However, if you are the delegated spokesperson for the health care organization in which you are employed you must:
  - Remember patient confidentiality is paramount—staff should not be bullied into giving information.
  - Never give a patient's name.
  - Never talk about the patient's treatment or give details of their illness or injury.
  - If the patient is capable of making a decision, his/her written consent must be obtained before passing on personal information. This includes celebrities and public figures.
- If a patient is incapable of making a decision, consult with the relatives and also consider whether giving information is in the best interests of the patient, e.g. correcting misleading or damaging speculation.
- Obtain as much information from the journalist as possible including what they have been told and what questions they want answered.
- Check the journalist's deadline.
- Seek help and advice from senior managers and, where necessary, the legal team especially if the information is sensitive, complex, or potentially damaging. There are usually arrangements for contacting senior staff outside office hours.
- Senior staff may seek advice from solicitors.
- Get back to the journalist at the agreed time even though you may not be able to provide information they want.
- The duty of confidence to the patient is paramount.
- Never promise anything to a member of the press.
- Always check that any statement (verbal or written) offered to a journalist has been agreed by the management/organization/communications/media department of the employing organization.

Sharps injuries

Sharps injuries can result in infections with blood-borne viruses such as hepatitis B and C, and HIV. Always follow local policy.

Prevention

- Avoid the use of sharps where possible.
- Avoid passing sharps from hand to hand.
- Each individual using sharps is responsible for safe disposal in approved containers.
- Train to heighten awareness and reinforce good practice.

Safe disposal of sharps

- Dispose of sharps immediately after use.
- Do not resheathe needles unless there is a safe means, e.g. capping device.
- Discard the entire needle and syringe. Needle should not be disconnected, bent, or broken.
- Keep sharps containers in areas where sharps are being used, e.g. treatment room, nurses' bases, dirty utility rooms, etc.
- Use portable sharps containers in the community and at patient's bedside.
- Ensure sharps containers are of an adequate capacity; emptied when three-quarters full or weekly; labelled with ward or department of origin; and securely closed for removal.
- Removal of containers must be done by designated staff wearing suitable protective clothing.

Management of sharp injuries

- First aid measures include washing the wound and making it bleed under running water. Exposed mucous membranes and conjunctiva should be irrigated copiously with water.
- Further advice should be obtained from occupational health or from the emergency department depending on local policy. Further advice can be obtained from Infection Prevention and Control Team.
- Report to line manager and complete an adverse incident form. The injury may need to be reported to the Health and Safety Executive under RIDDOR if there is significant occupational exposure of a blood-borne virus. (📖 Accidents and injuries to staff, patients, and visitors, p.1148).
- Retain the sharp item if known and identify the source patient on which it was used if possible. Blood samples may be collected from the patient and staff member if they consent. Post-exposure prophylaxis may be required.

Items to be discarded in approved sharps containers

- Needles, lancets, scalpel blades
- Syringes
- Glass vials, broken glass, slides
- Biopsy needles
- Disposable razors
- Intravascular guide wires
- IV giving sets, cannulae
- Arterial blood sample packs
- Other disposable sharps

The nurse's role in coordinating care

Multidisciplinary team work

The nurse plays a key role in coordinating care and ensuring continuity for the patient while in hospital, on admission, and after discharge into the community.

Team members

Team members comprise all public and private health care and social care professionals who come into contact with the patient.

- Therapists (physiotherapists, occupational therapists, chiropodists, etc.)
- Technicians (phlebotomists, ECG, etc.)
- Nurses
- Physicians
- Midwives
- Pharmacists
- Radiographers
- Social workers
- Clinical managers
- Matron
- Community staff from both health and social care

Sometimes people from voluntary groups (e.g. Age Concern, Citizens' Advice Bureaux and expert patients) play a part along with family and friends.

Problems in multidisciplinary working

These problems are often caused by a lack of or poor communication.

- Lack of referrals causes poor access to care if staff are unaware of the roles of each member of the team.
- Late referral results in lack of time to assess needs and provide treatment, education, or planning for discharge, and may lead to delay in discharge.
- Inappropriate referrals lead to time-wasting and frustration.
- Team members feel undervalued if they are not given the opportunity to use their special skills and are stressed when they have little time to carry out care.
- Patients and families can become frustrated and confused if they receive conflicting or repetitive information or if there is no coordinated approach.

Methods of enhancing the team approach

- Understand the roles and expertise of other disciplines as well as the roles of other nurses within primary and secondary care —find out what they do, shadow team members, observe them.
- Communicate effectively—hold multidisciplinary team meetings across primary and secondary care to agree pathways of care, guidelines, protocols, and processes as well as care of individuals.
- Work in collaboration, e.g. in clinical audit or developing patient information materials.
- Have a common goal and positive attitude toward the contribution of other team members.
- Share teaching and learning events—learn from each other and learn together.
- Consider whether social events will assist team development.

Benefits

- Improves continuity of care.
- Identifies clear areas of responsibility.
- Breaks down barriers between professional groups resulting in mutual respect and recognition of expertise.
- Develops commitment and involvement of staff and better staff development.
- Improves the quality of care and patient and staff satisfaction.
- Many universities now engage in multidisciplinary shared learning (www.commonlearning.net/newsletters/newgeneration).

Characteristics of an effective team

- *Mutual respect*—members should feel they can contribute to the team, be willing to challenge and be challenged, and be able to criticize constructively for the patient's best interest.
- *Clarity*—about goals for the team and individual patients and who is responsible for what aspects of care delivery and management.
- *Flexible*—and adaptable to meet the changing needs of patients or circumstances.
- *Creative and innovative*—to identify new ways of working to improve services.
- *Open*—demonstrate a willingness to look at new ideas without being obstructive.
- *Decisive*—act in a purposeful way to move ideas forward quickly.
- *Supportive*—willingness to assist and help when there are difficulties.
- *Able to manage conflict*—willingness to moderate, conciliate, or arbitrate for the team to continue effectively.
- *Being assertive,* but not aggressive, to ensure the best care and treatment is delivered to the patient.
- *Patient partnership*—the patient or the advocate should be included in partnership with any decisions in respect of their care.

Admission

Patients and their families' first impressions are often lasting impressions of their experiences. A welcoming approach from professional staff, efficient processes and good communication, and a clean and tidy environment are essential.

Routes of admission
- Routine planned admission
- Emergency
- Direct GP referral following a domiciliary visit
- From outpatients
- Patient's self-referral through emergency department

Initial assessment and action
- Determine urgency and priority by simple observation, respiratory rate and pattern, temperature, blood pressure, oxygen saturation levels, general appearance, pallor, pain, and any immediate risks or dangers (pressure damage, haemorrhage, dehydration). Use head-to-toe assessment man to assist in assessment (See Fig. 38.1).
- Identify any immediate worries, e.g. dependants at home.
- Identify any anxiety and undue stress.
- Use assessment tools available in the organization. Document findings clearly and implement immediate and preventative measures.

A more detailed assessment is carried out later. 📖 Chapter 3, Individualizing nursing care practice, p.27.

Important information
Explain the things that are important to patients and visitors including location of toilets, washing facilities, use of locker, patient call systems, who is who, daily events on ward (e.g. meal times), visiting hours, local guidelines, and rounds. Provide information on the patient's condition, care, tests, and expected length of stay. Check what they want to know and provide information materials.

Communication
- Use aids if necessary, e.g. interpreters, audio tapes, pictures, large print, sign language to enhance communication.
- Use plain English and avoid technical jargon.
- Be available to answer questions, repeat explanations, listen, and check understanding.
- Involve the family if the patient is agreeable.

📖 Chapter 3, Interviewing tips and communication skills, p.34.

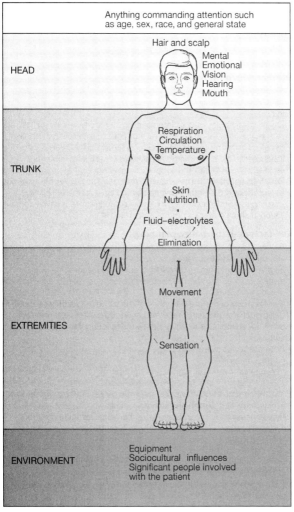

Fig. 38.1 Assessment Man. Reprinted with permission from McFarlane J and Castledine G (1982). *A guide to the practice of nursing using the nursing process,* Elsevier, London.

Discharge planning

Purpose
The purpose of a discharge plan is to ensure the continuity of care from one environment to another.

Discharge problems
- Premature discharge—due to demand on hospital beds and pressure to achieve set waiting time targets. Services in community may not be in place.
- Delayed discharge—due to internal hospital delays (waiting for test results, medication, or late referrals) or patients and relatives making decisions about future care or due to external delays—delays in assessments and putting in place packages of care in community settings by local health and social care providers.
- Poorly managed discharge—patients and their families' wishes have not been considered or if they have not been kept informed of plans.
- Discharge against medical advice—may result in services having to be set up at short notice or not being provided at all.

Key factors in discharge planning
- Ensure the patient has information about the diagnosis, care, treatment, and services planned in the community.
- Involve relevant primary care staff in discharge planning.
- Involve patients and their families in decisions and take account of their needs and wishes.
- Take account of the patient's physical, social, and psychological needs.
- Begin discharge planning pre-admission in some cases (e.g. planned surgery if adaptations or equipment are needed); otherwise on admission.
- Promote self-care and encourage patient to take responsibility and control of decisions.
- In conjunction with the patient and the next-of-kin, determine who will care for patient if unable to provide self-care.
- Involve community staff with complex discharges—undertake relevant assessments (e.g. Bartel) and identify patients who require additional health, housing, or social support (e.g. homeless, continuing disability, financial problems) and refer to relevant agencies. Where relevant in the most complex cases this should be undertaken in conjunction with the community matron.
- Involve multidisciplinary team but with one person identified as coordinator or lead.
- Follow a clear pathway and use a checklist to ensure all areas are covered (See Table 38.1).
- Refer early to multidisciplinary team, e.g. therapists, dietitian to ensure all areas are covered, and maintain links with primary care staff to ensure package of care is relevant and in place prior to discharge.
- Ensure appropriate transport arrangements are made, with patient accompanied, if necessary.

- Ensure discharge summaries are provided to relevant professionals which have been agreed with the patient where relevant.
- Ensure patient has the necessary equipment, drugs, and information including written details of support provided and a point of contact.

Table 38.1 Discharge checklist: an example

Check	Tick when complete	Signature	Comments
Discharge details			
Planned date and time of discharge			
Patient informed			
Relative/carer informed			
Information			
Diagnosis, care, treatment in hospital explained/written information given			
Care treatment and services planned explained/written. Patient's discharge information given			
Relevant health education and leaflets			
Contact number for support/advice			
Comments/suggestion/complaints forms			
Local self-help groups			
Charging for any care services			
Benefits and how to apply for them			
Support for carers			
Appointments/referrals			
GP/practice nurse			
Community nurse/district nurse			
Follow-up outpatients			
Other			
Medications and equipment			
Medication and TTOs explained			
Information leaflets given			
Dressings and wound care explained			
Dressings supplied			
Equipment demonstrated and action to take if breakdown occurs			
Venflon removed			
Letters			
Discharge medical summary for GP			
Discharge nursing summary			
Transport			
Other			

Common laboratory tests and their interpretation

Introduction

Laboratories offer an extensive and ever-growing repertoire of tests. Nurses should become familiar with tests that are frequently requested in their area. It is always prudent to seek the advice of the laboratory when results do not seem appropriate in the clinical context. This chapter describes the commonest laboratory tests used and the causes of abnormal results. Reference ranges can vary among laboratories and it is important to always check reference ranges with the local laboratory. Grossly abnormal results, which need urgent attention, are normally telephoned to the requester or the nurse in charge.

Renal profile (U&E)

Urea (reference range: 2.5–6.5 mmol/l)

Urea is the major end-product of protein metabolism. It is synthesized in the liver and excreted by the kidneys. It is measured as part of the renal profile but creatinine provides a better index of renal function.

Causes of high urea
- Renal failure
- Dehydration
- High protein intake
- Gastrointestinal bleeding (due to catabolism of retained blood)

Causes of low urea
- Starvation

Creatinine (reference range: 60–120 µmol//l)

Creatinine is a waste product of muscle metabolism. It is produced at a constant rate and is excreted in the urine. Its measurement in serum is used as a test of renal function, but the glomerular filtration rate (GFR) must fall to about half the normal value before serum creatinine is increased. For this reason, most laboratories in the UK now calculate GFR on all samples sent for creatinine measurement. This estimated **GFR (eGFR)** is usually based on serum creatinine concentration, age, sex, and race. Normal GFR is approximately 100 mL/min/1.73 m^2. The five stages of chronic kidney disease (CKD) are mainly based on measured or eGFR.

Causes of high creatinine
- Renal failure (acute or chronic)

Causes of low creatinine
- Young age
- Severe muscle wasting

Sodium (reference range: 135–145 mmol/l)

Sodium (Na^+) is the major extracellular cation and its plasma concentration is the determinant of extracellular fluid osmolality and volume. Sodium is usually measured as part of a renal profile and its abnormalities can be related to abnormal water or sodium homeostasis.

Hyponatraemia (low blood sodium) is relatively common in hospitalized patients but is often mild and asymptomatic. When severe (<120 mmol/l), it may cause confusion, disorientation, ataxia, and coma. *Hypernatraemia (high blood sodium)* is less common and is usually due to dehydration.

Causes of hypernatraemia
- Dehydration
- Diabetes insipidus
- Excessive salt intake (oral or parenteral)
- Spurious: contamination (e.g. blood collected from an arm with an IV infusion running)

Causes of hyponatraemia
- Salt loss
  - GI (diarrhoea and vomiting)
  - Renal (diuretics, adrenal failure)
  - Skin (burns)
- Water overload
  - Oedematous states (cirrhosis, CCF)
  - Renal failure (acute or chronic)
  - Inappropriate IV fluid regimen
  - Psychogenic polydipsia
  - Syndrome of inappropriate anti-diuretic hormone (SIADH)
- Spurious: contamination (e.g. blood collected from an arm with an IV infusion running)
- Diuretics

Potassium (reference range: 3.8–5.2 mmol/l)

Potassium (K^+) is the major intracellular ion but its plasma concentration has a major effect on the excitability of nerve and muscle membranes. It is measured as part of the renal profile. *In vitro* haemolysis can be caused by strong aspiration of blood using large needles, specimen collection with a syringe, and subsequent splitting of the sample into blood tubes or shaking the blood in the tube too vigorously.

Hypokalaemia (low blood potassium) causes muscle weakness, cardiac dysrhythmias, constipation, thirst, polyuria, and intestinal pseudo-obstruction. *Hyperkalaemia (high blood potassium)* is often clinically silent, but at concentrations >6.5 mmol/l there is an increased risk of cardiac arrest. Haemolysis and delay in separating cells from serum can cause falsely high results.

Causes of hyperkalaemia
- Renal failure
- Potassium-sparing diuretics
- Acidosis (except renal tubular acidosis)
- Addison's disease
- Hypoaldosteronism
- Pseudo-hyperkalaemia:
  - Haemolysis, delay in separation of cells from serum

Causes of hypokalaemia
- GI loss: diarrhoea, vomiting, laxatives
- Renal loss: thiazides and loop diuretics
- Dextrose infusions
- Alkalosis of any cause
- Cushing's syndrome
- Primary hyperaldosteronism

Liver profile (LFT)

Albumin (reference range: 35–50 g/l)

Albumin (Alb) is synthesized solely in the liver and is the major plasma protein. It is the most important determinant of plasma oncotic pressure (osmotic pressure due to protein) and therefore the distribution of fluid between the vascular and interstitial spaces. It is also involved in the transport of numerous substances including bilirubin, calcium, hormones, metals, and drugs.

Causes of low albumin	*Causes of high albumin*
• Poor nutrition	• Dehydration
• Chronic liver disease	
• Hypercatabolic states (sepsis, malignancy)	
• Loss from gut (Crohn's disease, ulcerative colitis)	
• Loss from kidneys (nephrotic syndrome)	
• Overhydration (iatrogenic: inappropriate IV fluids)	

Alkaline phosphatase (reference range: 25–120 IU/l)

Alkaline phosphatase (ALP) is mainly present in the liver and bone. Therefore increased plasma activity occurs in liver and bone diseases. When the origin of high ALP is in doubt, a high GGT (📖 Gamma-glutamyltransferase, p.1174) may suggest a liver origin, whereas an abnormal serum calcium may indicate a bony origin. In children, ALP is normally up to 3 times the adult range.

Causes of high ALP	*Causes of low ALP*
• Bone disease	• Low levels are uncommon and are rarely of any consequence
• Bone tumours (secondary or primary)	
• Fractures (healing)	
• Osteomalacia and rickets	
• Osteomyelitis	
• Paget's disease of bone	
• Primary hyperparathyroidism	
• Renal osteodystrophy	
• Pregnancy	
• Liver disease	
• Biliary obstruction	
• Cholangitis	
• Cirrhosis	
• Hepatic tumours (secondary or primary)	

Alanine aminotransferase (reference range: 0–45 IU/l)

Alanine aminotransferase (ALT) is widely distributed in body tissues but is present in high amounts in the liver. It is released into the circulation when there is cell damage as in hepatitis.

Causes of high ALT

- Cirrhosis
- Cholestasis
- Hepatic congestion (congestive cardiac failure), also shock
- Hepatocellular damage (e.g. viral hepatitis, paracetamol overdose)

Causes of low ALT

- Low levels are uncommon and are rarely of any consequence

Aspartate aminotransferase (reference range: 0–55 IU/l)

Aspartate aminotransferase (AST) is widely distributed in body tissues, particularly in the liver, striated muscle (skeletal and cardiac), red cells, brain, kidneys, and lung. Haemolyzed samples can give erroneous results.

Causes of high AST

- Liver disease: hepatocellular damage
  (e.g. viral hepatitis, paracetamol overdose),
  cirrhosis, cholestasis, and hepatic congestion (congestive cardiac failure). Elevations up to 1–2 times the upper limit of reference range can occur with excessive alcohol intake, obesity, diabetes mellitus, and as side effects of many common drugs
- Myocardial infarction: levels rise 12–18 hours after the onset of chest pain and may remain elevated for 3 days
- Skeletal muscle: myositis, rhabdomyolysis, and myopathy

Causes of low AST

- Low levels are uncommon and are rarely of any consequence

Bilirubin (reference range: 0–22 μmol/l)

Bilirubin is the end-product of haem (a complex pigment containing iron) degradation. It is a yellow-orange pigment that is normally metabolized in the liver and then excreted into the bile. Jaundice usually only becomes apparent when serum bilirubin is at least 2–3 times the upper normal value.

Causes of high bilirubin
- Biliary obstruction
- Cirrhosis (advanced)
- Hepatitis (not initially)
- Hepatic metastases
- Pancreatic carcinoma
- Congestive cardiac failure
- Drug reactions
- Gilbert's disease
- Haemolytic conditions

Causes of low bilirubin
- None

Gamma-glutamyltransferase (reference range: <58 IU/l)

Gamma-glutamyltransferase (GGT) is an enzyme that is mainly present in the liver. High GGT can occur in all types of liver disease but it is particularly useful as an indicator of excessive alcohol consumption.

Causes of high GGT
- Hepatitis
- Cholestatic liver disease
- Excessive alcohol consumption
- Drugs: anticonvulsants, amitriptyline, warfarin
- Fatty liver (diabetes mellitus, obesity)

Causes of low GGT
- None

Bone profile

Calcium (reference range: 2.20–2.60 mmol/l)

Calcium has a vital role in many physiological and biochemical processes as well as in the structure of bone. Serum calcium is an important determinant of the excitability of nerve and muscle cells.

Approximately 50% of calcium in the blood is bound to proteins (mainly albumin) and about 50% is unbound or ionized. It is the ionized fraction that is physiologically active. Most laboratories measure total calcium but some report corrected calcium (if albumin is abnormal).

Hypercalcaemia is often discovered incidentally. It can cause abdominal pain, constipation, thirst, and polyuria. *Hypocalcaemia* can cause paraesthesiae, muscle cramps, spasm, and rarely convulsions.

Causes of high calcium
- Malignancy (with or without metastases)
- Primary hyperparathyroidism
- Dehydration (if albumin is increased)
- Thiazide diuretics (mild)
- Sarcoidosis
- Vitamin D intoxication

Causes of low calcium
- Vitamin D deficiency (rickets or osteomalacia)
- Chronic renal failure
- Hypoparathyroidism
- Thyroid surgery
- Pancreatitis

Phosphate (reference range: 0.8–1.4 mmol/l)

Phosphate is usually measured with calcium and alkaline phosphatase as part of a bone profile. It is an essential precursor of high-energy phosphate compounds (e.g. ATP) and a component of nucleic acids, phospholipids, and bone. Severe hypophosphataemia can cause muscle weakness.

Causes of high phosphate
- Renal failure
- Bone tumours (especially metastatic)

Causes of low phosphate
- Starvation or malnutrition
- Dextrose infusions
- Alcohol withdrawal
- Hyperparathyroidism
- Renal tubular disease

Alkaline phosphatase (ALP)

📖 Alkaline phosphatase, p.1172.

Blood gases

Arterial blood gas analysis typically measures:
- pH (a measure of acidity or alkalinity of the blood)
- PCO_2 (partial pressure of carbon dioxide)
- PO_2 (partial pressure of oxygen)
- Base excess (the loss of buffer base to neutralize acid)
- SaO_2 (oxygen saturation)
- HCO_3 or bicarbonate (derived)

Reference ranges

pH	7.35–7.45
PCO_2	4.7–6.0 kPa
PO_2	10.6–13.3 kPa
Base excess	±3 mmol/l
SaO_2	>94%
HCO_3	22–30 mmol/l

Sample:
Whole arterial blood (heparinized)

Causes of low pH (acidosis)
- Metabolic acidosis
  - Lactic acidosis
  - Diabetic ketoacidosis
  - Renal failure
  - Renal tubular acidosis
  - Severe diarrhoea (loss of bicarbonate)
  - Drugs: salicylates
  - Ethanol, ethylene glycol, or methanol
- Respiratory acidosis
  - Lung disease (emphysema, asthma, COPD)
  - Neuromuscular (Guillain–Barré syndrome)
  - CNS disease (trauma, infection, tumours)
  - Drugs: sedatives, anaesthetics

Causes of high pH (alkalosis)
- Metabolic alkalosis
  - Vomiting
  - Hypokalaemia
  - Mineralocorticoid excess (e.g. Cushing's syndrome)
- Respiratory alkalosis
  - Lung disease (pneumonia, asthma, tumours, embolism)
  - Septicaemia (gram negative)
  - Liver failure
  - Drugs: salicylates
  - Hysterical over-breathing

Cardiac tests

Cholesterol (optimal levels: total cholesterol <4.0 mmol/l and LDL-C <2.0 mmol/l)

Cholesterol circulates in the blood and is incorporated into particles called lipoproteins. The two principal lipoproteins that contain cholesterol are low-density lipoprotein (LDL) and high-density lipoprotein (HDL). High LDL levels are associated with high risk of cardiovascular disease (CVD), whereas HDL levels are inversely correlated with CVD (i.e. HDL is protective).

High serum cholesterol (due to an excess in LDL) is an important risk factor for atherosclerosis and there is strong evidence that lowering serum cholesterol reduces the risk of CVD and stroke.

Reference ranges should not be used for cholesterol because CVD risk exists within a wide range of concentrations seen in healthy individuals. The optimal lipid targets in people with established CVD, people with diabetes, and those asymptomatic individuals at high CVD risk ≥ 20%, are total cholesterol and LDL-C <4.0 mmol/l and <2.0 mmol/l, respectively.

Fasting is not strictly necessary if only total cholesterol is required. Overnight fasting is necessary if a full lipid profile is required. In patients with suspected myocardial infarction, cholesterol should be measured within 24 hours of admission. After 24 hours and for the following 3 months, cholesterol may be falsely low.

Triglycerides are usually measured as part of the full lipid profile. After an overnight fast, triglycerides are normally ≤ 1.7 mmol/l. Mild or moderate hypertriglyceridaemia (1.7–10 mmol/l) is often secondary to obesity, poorly-controlled diabetes, excessive alcohol intake, renal disease, liver disease, or medications such as diuretics and oral contraceptives. Severe hypertriglyceridaemia (>10.0 mmol/l) is usually associated with rare genetic conditions and can lead to acute pancreatitis. The association of hypertriglyceridaemia with CHD is complex.

Causes of high cholesterol
- Familial
- Acquired: hypothyroidism, liver disease, renal failure, nephritic syndrome, diabetes mellitus, excess alcohol

Causes of low cholesterol
- Acute or chronic illness of any type

Troponins: cardiac troponin I (cTnI) and T (cTnT)

Troponins (I, T, and C) are components of the muscle contractile structure. Assays have been developed for the detection of cardiac-specific forms of troponin: cardiac troponin I (cTnI) and cardiac troponin T (cTnT). These assays are sensitive and specific markers of myocardial injury.

After the onset of acute myocardial infarction, blood levels of troponins start to rise at 4–6 hours and peak at about 18–24 hours. They remain elevated in the serum for 6–10 days. Troponins are not 'early markers' of cardiac damage. A negative value on blood collected less than 12 hours after onset of chest pain does not exclude cardiac damage.

Reference ranges for cTnI:

<0.1 ng/mL	Negative
0.1–0.25 ng/mL	Intermediate
>0.25 ng/mL	Positive

Causes of high troponins
- Acute myocardial infarction
- Myocarditis
- Congestive cardiac failure
- Unstable angina
- Chest trauma
- Cardiac surgery

Hormones

Cortisol (reference range: 200–600 nmol/l)

Cortisol is a hormone secreted by the adrenal gland and is involved in mediating the body's response to stress, maintenance of blood pressure, and fluid balance.

Serum cortisol shows a diurnal variation with a peak at 9.00 a.m. and a trough at around midnight. Plasma concentrations are increased by stress from any cause (including surgery and infection).

There is a wide variation in normal serum cortisol between individuals as evidenced by the large reference range and therefore measuring a random cortisol is often unhelpful. However, a cortisol value <100 nmol/l is strongly suggestive of hypoadrenalism. Cortisol should not be measured in patients taking steroids since steroids in pharmacological doses suppress endogenous cortisol production and may also interfere with the cortisol assay.

Causes of high cortisol
- Stress from any cause
- Cushing's syndrome

Causes of low cortisol
- Primary hypoadrenalism
  - Autoimmune (Addison's disease)
  - Infiltration (e.g. TB, amyloidosis, metastases)
  - Haemorrhage (e.g. meningococcal meningitis)
  - Congenital adrenal hyperplasia
  - Trauma
  - Adrenoleukodystrophy
  - Drugs (e.g. etomidate, ketoconazole, metyrapone)
- Secondary hypoadrenalism
  - Pituitary disease
  - Long-term use of synthetic steroids

Prolactin

Serum prolactin (PRL) is raised physiologically during pregnancy and lactation. The physiological role of prolactin in non-lactating women and men is unknown.

Causes of high prolactin
- Pregnancy, lactation
- Prolactin-secreting adenoma
- Pituitary tumours
- Primary hypothyroidism
- Drugs (e.g. anti-emetics and antipsychotics)
- Renal failure
- Macroprolactin

Causes of low prolactin
- Hypopituitarism

Reproductive hormones (gonadotrophins, testosterone, and oestradiol)

The gonadotrophins (luteinizing hormone [LH] and follicle-stimulating hormone [FSH]) are released from the pituitary gland after stimulation by hypothalamic gonadotrophin-releasing hormone (GnRH). In the male, LH stimulates testosterone secretion and FSH controls spermatogenesis. In the female, FSH stimulates ovarian follicular development and therefore oestradiol secretion, whereas LH stimulates ovulation at mid-cycle. In primary gonadal failure, testosterone or oestradiol is low and gonadotrophins are high, whereas in secondary gonadal failure, all levels are low.

Thyroid function tests (TFT)

The thyroid gland produces thyroxine (T_4) and tri-iodothyronine (T_3). This production is regulated by thyrotropin or thyroid-stimulating hormone (TSH) produced by the pituitary gland. T_4 and T_3 are extensively protein bound in the plasma but only the free hormones are physiologically active. Most laboratories now measure the free hormone concentrations (FT_4 and FT_3) in addition to TSH.

Many laboratories measure serum TSH as a first-line test and other tests (FT_4, FT_3, or both) are only added if TSH is abnormal. In *primary hypothyroidism*, TSH is typically high and FT_4 is low. In mild or early disease, TSH may be elevated but FT_4 may be normal or low normal. In *secondary hypothyroidism* (secondary to pituitary failure), FT_4 is low and TSH is also low or inappropriately normal. In *hyperthyroidism*, TSH is suppressed and both FT_4 and FT_3 are high.

Reference ranges

TSH	0.3–4.0 mIU/l
FT_4	9.8–19.8 pmol/l
FT_3	3.0–6.9 pmol/l

Reference ranges may vary between laboratories.

Tumour markers

Tumour markers are substances secreted into body fluids or expressed on cell surfaces that are characteristic of the presence of a tumour. Generally, tumour markers are of potential value in diagnosis, prognosis, and assessing the response to treatment. In practice, however, the number of tumour markers of proven value in the management of malignancy is small. The commonly performed tumour markers are alpha-fetoprotein (AFP), ovarian marker (CA 125), carcino-embryonic antigen (CEA), human chorionic gonadotrophin (HCG), and prostate-specific antigen (PSA).

General points

- No serum marker in current use is specific for malignancy.
- Generally, serum marker levels are rarely elevated in patients with early malignancy.
- Very few markers have absolute organ specificity.
- Most tumour markers do not have sufficient sensitivity or specificity to make their measurements reliable in the diagnosis or exclusion of cancer.
- Requesting multiple markers (AFP, CEA, HCG, and CA 125) in an attempt to identify an unknown primary cancer is rarely of use.

Some of the tumour markers currently in use are listed below:

Tumour markers	Cancers	Also elevated in:
AFP	Liver and germ cell cancer of ovaries or testes	Pregnancy, hepatitis
CA 15–3	Breast, lung, and ovarian	Benign breast conditions
CA 19–9	Pancreas, bowel, and bile ducts	Pancreatitis and inflammatory bowel disease
CA-125	Ovarian	Endometriosis and peritonitis
CEA	Bowel, lung, thyroid, pancreatic, liver, cervical, and bladder	Hepatitis, COPD, pancreatitis, and cigarette smokers
HCG	Testicular and gestational trophoblastic	Pregnancy and testicular failure
PSA	Prostate	Benign prostatic hypertrophy and prostatitis

Miscellaneous tests

C-reactive protein (reference range: <5.0 mg/l)

C-reactive protein (CRP) is a marker of inflammation and infection. Its measurement is useful in the management of patients with inflammatory diseases, such as rheumatoid arthritis or Crohn's disease, when it can provide an early indication of an exacerbation (increase) or a response to treatment (decrease).

It rises within 6–12 hours and peaks at about 48 hours following the onset of inflammation or infection. Very high CRP concentrations are usually associated with bacterial infection. CRP can be suppressed by salicylates, steroids, or NSAIDs.

Creatine kinase (reference ranges: <190 IU/l in men and <170 IU/l in women)

Creatine kinase (CK) is an enzyme that is present in high concentrations in skeletal muscle (CK-MM isoenzyme) and cardiac muscle (CK-MB isoenzyme). Its major use is in the diagnosis and management of muscle disease. Its use in the investigation of chest pain has now been superseded by cardiac troponins.

CK activity may be raised immediately after exercise and reaches a peak after 1–2 days. The more severe the exercise the higher the increase in CK. The effect on CK is more pronounced in subjects who do not exercise regularly. Afro-Caribbeans (particularly males) have up to twice the CK level found in Caucasians. Asians have intermediate values.

Causes of high CK
- Myopathy and muscular dystrophies
- Muscle injury (trauma, surgery, exercise)
- Myositis (viral, alcoholic)
- Myocardial damage (MI, cardioversion)
- CNS: stroke, meningitis, head injury
- Pulmonary or intestinal infarction
- Others: hypothyroidism, sepsis, shock, and acute psychosis

Glucose (reference range: 4.5–5.2 mmol/l)

In healthy subjects, blood glucose concentration is maintained within relatively narrow limits through a tightly controlled balance between glucose production and glucose utilization. After an overnight fast, blood glucose is usually between 4.5 and 5.2 mmol/l. After meals, glucose levels increase, but typical meals will not raise glucose above 10.0 mmol/l and normal levels are usually restored within 2–4 hours.

In stress due to injury or infection, the concentrations of various hormones (catecholamines, cortisol, glucagons, and growth hormone) increase causing insulin resistance and consequently raised blood glucose levels.

Diabetes mellitus can be diagnosed if fasting plasma glucose is ≥7.0 mmol/l or random glucose is ≤11.1 mmol/l in a patient with symptoms of diabetes, or possibly in a patient without symptoms. Diabetes should never be diagnosed on the basis of glycosuria alone.

Causes of high blood glucose
- Diabetes mellitus
- Impaired glucose tolerance
- Severe stress

Causes of low blood glucose
- Tumours: insulinoma, non-islet cell tumours
- Endocrine deficiencies: Addison's disease, hypopituitarism
- Drugs: insulin, sulphonylureas, quinine, salicylates, beta-blockers
- Autoimmune hypoglycaemia (rare)

Lactate dehydrogenase (reference range: 0–550 IU/L)

Lactate dehydrogenase (LDH) is an enzyme found in the cells of many body tissues, including the heart, liver, kidneys, skeletal muscle, brain, red blood cells, and lungs. The main use of measuring serum LDH has been in the monitoring of some types of cancer, particularly haematological cancers, such as lymphoma and leukaemia.

Causes of high LDH
- Haemolytic anaemias
- Haematological cancers (lymphoma or leukaemia)
- Kidney disease
- Liver disease
- Muscular dystrophy
- Myocardial infarction
- Pancreatitis (acute)
- Stroke

Causes of low LDH
- Uncommon and of no consequences

Uric acid (reference ranges: 200–500 µmol/l in men and 200–400 µmol/l in women)

Uric acid (urate) is the end-product of nucleic acid metabolism (cell nuclei). Uric acid is excreted in urine and increases in serum uric acid may be caused by either increased production or decreased excretion. High uric acid concentrations can predispose to gout due to deposition of urate crystals in joints.

Causes of high uric acid	*Causes of low uric acid*
• Renal failure	• Hypo-uricaemia is uncommon and is of no clinical consequence
• Gout	
• Certain cancers or chemotherapy	
• Pre-eclampsia	
• Starvation	
• Diabetic ketoacidosis	
• Trauma	
• Drugs: thiazide diuretics	

Urinalysis

Dipstick testing of urine is useful in screening for certain disorders and in identifying a need for further investigations. Tests for protein, pH, blood, leucocytes, glucose, bilirubin, urobilinogen, ketones, and specific gravity are available. The number of tests on each stick depends on the brand and type used.

Bilirubin
• A positive test indicates an elevation of conjugated bilirubin in the plasma that is indicative of hepatobiliary disease.
• A positive test may precede clinical jaundice.

Blood
• The presence of blood in urine should always be investigated further (provided that contamination, e.g. with menstrual bleeding, can be excluded).
• A positive test may indicate haematuria or myoglobinuria and therefore should be sent to microbiology for microscopic examination.
• Causes of a positive test include renal disease, urinary tract infection or tumours, renal stones, and rhabdomyolysis (muscle breakdown).

Glucose
• Glycosuria indicates either diabetes or a low renal threshold for glucose.
• A positive test in a non-diabetic patient should always be followed by measurement of blood glucose.
• The diagnosis of diabetes should never be made solely on the finding of a positive urine dipstick.

pH
• Knowledge of urine pH is rarely of diagnostic value.
• A high urine pH (>7.5) may result in a falsely low result for protein.

Ketones
• Testing for ketones is useful in patients with diabetes mellitus, as ketonuria in a patient with type 1 (insulin-dependent) diabetes suggests a developing ketoacidosis.
• Ketonuria can also occur in non-diabetic patients who are losing weight.

Leucocytes
- The test is useful as a screening test for urinary tract infection.
- A positive test should be followed by urine microscopy and culture.

Protein
- The test detects albumin at concentrations as low as 200 mg/l.
- Proteinuria can occur in renal disease and urinary tract infections, or can be an incidental finding.
- A positive test should always be followed up.

Urobilinogen
- The presence or absence of urobilinogen is of little diagnostic significance.

Haematology

Full blood count (FBC)

Laboratories rely on automated counters to provide information on hae-moglobin concentration (Hb), red blood cell count (RBC), mean corpus-cular volume (MCV), and white blood cell count (WBC). Other red cell indices such as packed cell volume (PCV), mean corpuscular haemoglobin (MCH), and mean corpuscular haemoglobin concentration (MCHC) are derived.

Automated counters recognize leucocytes as nucleated cells, and differentials (neutrophils, lymphocytes, monocytes, and eosinophils) are obtained on the basis of relative nuclear size to the cell, nuclear complexity, and the presence of cytoplasmic granules.

Reference ranges

	Men	Women	(Unit)
Hb	14.0–18.0	12.0–16.0	(g/dl)
RBC	4.5–6.0	4.2–5.4	($\times 10^{12}$/l)
WBC	4.0–11.0	4.0–11.0	($\times 10^{9}$/l)
Platelets	150–400	150–400	($\times 10^{9}$/l)

Sample: Whole blood (EDTA)
Reference ranges depend on age and sex.

Red blood cells are highly specialized cells that are filled with haemo-globin, and have a life span of approximately 120 days. Haemoglobin is a unique oxygen-binding molecule for the efficient uptake of oxygen in the high partial pressure environment of the lungs, avidly retaining it while circulating in the arterial vasculature and releasing it when the appropriate pressures are reached in the capillary bed.

Anaemia, a decrease in the number of red cells, can be due to decreased red cell production, increased destruction, or blood loss. Polycythaemia, an increase in circulating red blood cells, can be due to an increase in red cell mass or a decrease in plasma volume.

Causes of low Hb and RBC
- Anaemia of any cause
- Iron, vitamin B_{12}, or folate deficiency
- Haemodilution (e.g. excessive IV fluids, pregnancy)
- Haemorrhage
- Haemolysis
- Chronic renal failure
- Chronic liver disease

Causes of high Hb and RBC
- Polycythaemia
- Haemoconcentration (dehydration)
- COPD
- Smoking
- Pre-eclampsia

Useful tips
- Smokers typically have elevated haemoglobin levels in response to chronic low-grade carbon monoxide poisoning and other respiratory ailments. Because of the carbon monoxide binding, these patients may still be functionally anaemic even though their haemoglobin levels appear higher than normal.
- During the initial phase of acute haemorrhage, haemoglobin levels do not change very much. After several hours, as extracellular fluid is mobilized and IV fluids are given, haemoglobin levels go down because of the dilutional effects.

White blood cells (WBC)

White blood cells (WBCs) are produced in the bone marrow, lymph nodes, spleen, and thymus. They fight infection and foreign bodies and help distribute antibodies throughout the body. Unused, a white blood cell lives for 2–3 weeks and then disintegrates.

Causes of high WBC
- Infection
- Haemorrhage
- Trauma
- Some malignancies
- Exposure to toxic substances
- Renal failure
- Drugs, e.g. quinine, epinephrine
- Chronic inflammatory conditions
- Stress reaction
- Exercise, heat, and cold
- Anaesthesia
- Cigarette smoking

Causes of low WBC
- Viral infections
- Bone marrow depression, secondary to:
  - Drugs, e.g. analgesics, antibiotics, antihistamines, anticonvulsants, anti-inflammatory drugs, anti-thyroid drugs, barbiturates, chemotherapy, and diuretics
  - Arsenic and heavy metal exposure
  - Radiation exposure

Platelets

Platelets are formed primarily in the bone marrow. They are released into the blood stream where they normally live for about a week. Platelets assist in clotting, coagulation, and maintaining vascular integrity.

Causes of increased platelets (thrombocytosis)
- Infection
- Inflammation or trauma
- Cancer
- Bleeding
- Regular athletic activity and high altitudes

Causes of decreased platelets (thrombocytopenia)
- Haemorrhage
- Infection
- Liver disease
- Disseminated intravascular coagulopathy (DIC)
- Severe pre-eclampsia

- HELLP syndrome (haemolysis, elevated liver enzymes, low platelets)
- Allergic reactions
- Drugs, e.g. NSAIDs, diuretics
- Alcohol excess
- Bone marrow suppression
- Idiopathic thrombocytopenic purpura (ITP)
- Haemolytic uraemic syndrome (HUS)

Useful tips
- Abnormal bleeding due to low platelet counts does not normally occur until platelets fall below 50×10^9/l.
- Aspirin affects platelet function, causing abnormal bleeding despite a normal platelet count.
- After discontinuation of aspirin, platelet function will be regained within 7 days.
- Platelet count may be falsely low because of 'clumping'.

Erythrocyte sedimentation rate (ESR)
ESR is the speed at which non-clotted RBCs settle to the bottom of a test tube. Increased rates of RBC settling are caused by changes in plasma proteins following tissue damage or during inflammation.

Reference ranges		
	Men	Women
	0–5 mm/hour	0–7 mm/hour
Sample:	Whole blood (EDTA or citrated)	

Causes of high ESR
- Inflammation or infection (due to increase in plasma proteins)
- Chronic disease (due to increase in IgG)
- Pregnancy (due to raised fibrinogen)
- Elderly (due to reduced plasma albumin)

Coagulation screen
The coagulation screen is usually requested for patients with bleeding or who bruise easily. The coagulation screen includes prothrombin time (PT) and activated partial thromboplastin time (APTT or PTTK).

Reference ranges	
PT	10–13 seconds
APTT (PTTK)	25–35 seconds
Sample:	Whole blood (citrated)

Prothrombin time (PT)

PT is a measure of how long it takes the blood to clot. At least a dozen blood-clotting factors are needed for blood to clot normally. PT is an important coagulation test because it measures the presence and activity of five different vitamin-K-dependent clotting factors (factors I, II, V, VII and X).

Causes of prolonged PT
- Liver disease
- Vitamin K deficiency (secondary to malabsorption)
- Warfarin therapy
- Factor I, II, V, VII, or X deficiency

Activated partial thromboplastin time (APPT)

APPT (PTTK) is a functional measure of the intrinsic pathway of coagulation activation.

Causes of prolonged APPT
- Liver disease
- Deficiency of one or more of the clotting factors
- Presence of inhibitors, e.g. lupus anticoagulant (in systemic lupus erythematosus, neoplasia)
- Heparin therapy

International normalized ratio (INR)

Because normal values may vary from one laboratory to another, a method of standardizing prothrombin time results, called the INR, has been used. The INR is a prothrombin time ratio (normal/control) that has been corrected for the type of thromboplastin used. This method of expression ensures that INR results are equivalent both over time and between laboratories.

The INR is used to monitor patients who are on anticoagulant therapy (warfarin). In most of these patients, the INR is usually kept at 2–3 to prevent blood clots from forming. For patients with mechanical prosthetic heart valves or recurrent thromembolic disease, a higher INR of 3–4.5 is recommended.

Blood transfusion

Where possible, patients who are likely to need a blood transfusion should receive the NBS leaflet 'Receiving a Blood Transfusion: A Leaflet for Patients and their Relatives'.

A cross-match involves the incubation of the patient's serum with donor RBCs; if no reaction occurs, the donor unit is labelled and reserved exclusively for the identified patient for up to 72 hours. An alternative method of ensuring the availability of blood for elective surgery is the Group & Save (G&S) technique, whereby the patient's serum is incubated with pooled RBCs containing all common RBC antigens; if no reaction occurs the patient can safely have any ABO-and Rhesus-compatible blood 'off the shelf'. If the G&S is performed pre-operatively, blood can be provided rapidly on request. This method avoids the ordering of blood destined not to be transfused and ensures the efficient use of blood.

Obtaining blood specimens for cross-match

- The blood specimen should be obtained using the approved procedure.
- Blood should be collected into a plain cross-match bottle.
- Patient details should be handwritten on the cross-match form and all questions on the form must be answered.
- All details should be checked with the patient's notes and the patient's wristband, and, if possible, confirmed by the patient.
- The specimen should be labelled with the patient's name, unit number, date of birth, and address.
- The specimen should be dated, timed, and signed immediately after collection.
- Blood should not be collected from an arm with an IV infusion *in situ*.
- All high-risk specimens must have self-adhesive biohazard labels attached and be packed in a sealable plastic specimen bag.

Collecting blood products from the blood bank refrigerator

- When blood or platelet bags are removed from the blood bank, the person removing the bags should check the patient's details from the prescription sheet or patient's notes against the bag removed and must *sign*, *date*, *and time* the laboratory copy, which is kept in the blood bank. The white form is kept with the patient's notes where it will ultimately be filed following completion of the transfusion.
- Units of blood or platelets must be taken and used in the order stated on the form.
- Only one unit of blood per patient should normally be removed from the blood bank refrigerator at any one time. In cases of massive blood loss where more units are needed, they should be transported in an appropriate container which will be supplied by the blood bank on request.
- Check the patient's details carefully prior to starting the transfusion: numerous errors still occur from giving the wrong blood to the wrong patient.
- Transport boxes are only suitable for storage of blood for a maximum of 2 hours.
- Unused units must be returned to the issue refrigerator as soon as possible with the time of return documented on the blue copy of the cross-match form.
- The total transfusion episode, from signing out of the issue refrigerator to completion of the transfusion, must be less than 5 hours.
- If the decision to transfuse is cancelled and the blood is returned within 30 minutes of removal, record the date and time of return on the blue copy of the cross-match form. If the unit has been out of the issue refrigerator for 30 minutes or longer, *do not return* to the issue refrigerator. Contact blood bank staff for advice.

Microbiology

- Specimens for microbiological tests must be transported in robust and leak-proof containers.
- Specimens must be placed individually in self-sealing plastic bags.
- Specimens from patients suspected of having hepatitis B or HIV infection must be securely packaged and the request form and specimen should bear 'Danger of Infection' labels.

Urine culture and sensitivity

Urine is normally sterile. However, in the process of collecting the urine, some contamination from skin bacteria is frequent. For that reason, up to 10 000 colonies of bacteria/mL are considered normal and only >100 000 colonies/mL represents urinary tract infection.

Before a 'mid-stream' urine sample is taken, the urethral meatus should be carefully cleaned with soap and water or wipe. In catherized patients, samples should be aspirated from the tubing, not taken from the collection bag. A report stating 'heavy mixed growth' means that two or more types of organisms have been cultured. As true mixed infections are extremely rare, it is likely that either the culture was contaminated when taken or there was a delay in culture which led to overgrowth of some organisms.

Sensitivity refers to the antibiotics tested to be effective in stopping the bacteria. While clinical response will generally follow therapy guided by sensitivity testing, the response can be variable.

Indications for urine microscopy, culture, and sensitivity
- Cystitis
- Pyelonephritis
- Prostatitis
- Suspected urinary tract infection in children
- Assessment of unwell patients who are permanently catheterized
- Suspected TB
- Immunocompromised patients
- Pregnancy (on booking/first presentation)

Throat culture

Throat culture may be obtained for nearly any micro-organism, but is usually performed to detect streptococcal infection. The throat swab must be taken with reasonable pressure against the fauces and tonsils and placed in a tube of transport medium.

Indications for a throat swab
- Severe sore throat
- Acute cervical lymphadenopathy
- Oral ulceration (herpetic, gingivitis)
- Screening for carriage of MRSA

Blood culture

Particular care must be taken to avoid skin bacterial contamination when blood cultures are drawn. The skin should be cleaned for 30 seconds with isopropyl alcohol and allowed to dry. After the blood is drawn, the needle should be replaced with a fresh sterile needle before injecting the blood into the culture bottle.

Indications for blood culture
- High fever or rigor
- Fever of unknown origin
- Immunocompromised patients or indwelling Hickman line
- Diabetic patients with cellulitis or infected foot ulcer
- Pneumonia, especially post-influenzal
- Abdominal sepsis
- Pyelonephritis

Stool culture

Stool normally has a large number of various organisms present. Stool should be passed directly into a collection jar or a bedpan. A sample can be separated with a tongue blade and placed into a specimen container.

Stool cultures are used to identify viruses, parasites, and other pathogenic micro-organisms. The routine culture can identify *Shigella*, *Salmonella*, *Campylobacter*, and *E. coli* 0157.

Indications for stool microscopy and culture
- Significant diarrhoea of any cause
- Diarrhoea in a patient who has returned from abroad in the previous month
- Diarrhoea in immunocompromised patients
- Diarrhoea with significant systemic symptoms

Cerebrospinal fluid (CSF)

CSF is normally sterile, colourless, and clear. It contains most of the same constituents as blood, but generally in lower concentrations. In bacterial meningitis, CSF is cloudy, WBCs are primarily neutrophils, and CSF glucose is generally decreased. In non-bacterial meningitis CSF is clear and CSF glucose is normal or decreased.

Reference ranges
Glucose	60–80% of plasma glucose
WBC	0–5/mm^3
RBC	<1/mm^3
Protein	<0.4 g/l
Sample: CSF	

Causes of yellow CSF
- Previous subarachnoid bleeding
- Severe jaundice
- High concentrations of protein (>1.5 g/l)

Causes of bloody CSF
- Bloody tap
- Subarachnoid or cerebral haemorrhage
- At least 400 RBC/μl must be present before CSF is visibly bloody

Causes of cloudy CSF
- Infection (bacterial or other micro-organisms)
- Increased WBC or RBC count

Hepatitis serology

Hepatitis serology for hepatitis A, B, and C is indicated in all patients with jaundice and in certain high-risk patients.

Hepatitis A
- Transmitted by the faecal/oral route.
- Affects children and young adults more often.
- Not associated with chronic hepatitis or a carrier status.
- Has an incubation period of 2–6 weeks.
- Hepatitis A IgM will be elevated from 6–14 weeks after infection.

Hepatitis B
- Transmitted parenterally (drug injection or blood transfusion).
- 10% of patients become carriers.
- Has an incubation period of 6–26 weeks.
- Hepatitis B surface antigen (HbsAg) appears in the serum 4–12 weeks after infection.
- Hepatitis B core antibody appears within 6–14 weeks.
- Hepatitis B surface antibody appears 4–10 months after infection, indicating clinical recovery and immunity to the virus.

Hepatitis C
- Transmitted parenterally (drug injection, needlestick injury, or blood transfusion).
- 80% of persons have no signs or symptoms.
- Associated with high rates of chronic hepatitis with progression to cirrhosis.
- Persons at risk of hepatitis C might also be at risk for infection with hepatitis B virus or HIV.
- Antibodies (anti-HCV) are generally detectable approximately 6–8 weeks after exposure.
- HCV-RNA tests are usually positive within 1–2 weeks of exposure and indicate active infection.
- Viral load or quantitative tests measure the number of viral RNA particles and are often used to determine the response to treatment.

HIV
- Carried in certain body fluids including blood, semen, vaginal secretions, and breast milk.

- Transmitted through sexual contact, needlestick injury, and during birth or breastfeeding.
- HIV infects and destroys white blood cells called CD4$^+$ T cells, which are cells of the immune system that protect against infections.
- Acquired immune deficiency syndrome (AIDS) develops when the body succumbs to opportunistic infections or cancers that take advantage of the body's lowered defences.
- HIV antibodies generally appear within 3 months after infection with HIV, but may take up to 6 months in some persons.

MRSA

- *Staphylococcus aureus*, often referred to simply as 'staph', is commonly carried in the skin or in the nose of healthy people.
- Occasionally, staph can cause infections but most of these are minor (e.g. boils) and most can be treated with antibiotics. However, staph can cause serious infections, such as surgical wound infections and pneumonia.
- Over the past 50 years, treatment of staph infections has become more difficult because staph bacteria have become resistant to various antibiotics, including the commonly used penicillin-related antibiotics. These resistant bacteria are called MRSA.
- MRSA infection occurs more commonly among persons in hospitals and health care facilities. It usually develops in hospitalized patients who are elderly or very sick or who have an open wound (e.g. bedsore) or a tube (e.g. urinary catheter or IV catheter).
- MRSA can spread among people having close contact with infected people (📖 Chapter 20, Nursing patients with infectious diseases, p.695). It is almost always spread by direct physical contact, and not through the air. Spread may also occur indirectly by touching objects (e.g. towels, sheets, wound dressings) contaminated by the infected skin.

Screening patients or staff for MRSA carriage

- When: staff (before starting work) or patients (on admission/ pre-admission to hospital) if either staff or patient has been in a health care facility (nursing homes) in the previous 6 months, where cross-transmission may have occurred. Screening may also occur as part of an outbreak investigation in conjunction with the Infection Control Officer.
- How: one nasal swab (both anterior nares), one swab from the perineum, and swabs from any skin lesions, surgical wounds, or catheter sites.

Clostridium difficile

- *C. difficile* is carried as part of the normal gut flora in very young children.
- In adults, particularly those who are elderly or very sick and have previously received antibiotics, it can cause a severe diarrhoeal illness.
- *C. difficile* can be spread by direct physical contact and also by contact with contaminated hospital equipment (e.g. commodes).
- The *C. difficile* toxin test detects toxin A and/or B in a fresh or frozen stool sample and has high sensitivity and specificity.

Appendices

Height and weight conversions

Height conversion

To convert a patient's height from inches to centimetres, multiply the number of inches by 2.54. To convert a patient's height from centimetres to inches, multiply the number of centimetres by 0.394.

Imperial (ft and inches)	Inches	Metric (cm)
4'8"	56	142
4'9"	57	144.5
4'10"	58	147
4'11"	59	150
5'	60	152.5
5'1"	61	155
5'2"	62	157.5
5'3"	63	160
5'4"	64	162.5
5'5"	65	165
5'6"	66	167.5
5'7"	67	170
5'8"	68	172.5
5'9"	69	175
5'10"	70	177.5
5'11"	71	180
6'	72	183
6'1"	73	185.5
6'2"	74	188
6'3"	75	190.5

Approximate weight conversions

kg	st	lb	kg	st	lb	kg	st	lb	kg	st	lb
0.5		1	44	6	13	83	13	1	122	19	3
1		2	45	7	1	84	13	3	123	19	6
1.5		3	46	7	3	85	13	6	124	19	7
2		4	47	7	6	86	13	7	125	19	10
2.5		6	48	7	8	87	13	10	126	19	11
3		7	49	7	10	88	13	11	127	20	0
3.5		8	50	7	13	89	14	0	128	20	1
4		9	51	8	0	90	14	3	129	20	5
4.5		10	52	8	3	91	14	4	130	20	7
5		11	53	8	4	92	14	7	131	20	8
5.5		12	54	8	7	93	14	8	132	20	11
6		13	55	8	10	94	14	11	133	20	13
			56	8	11	95	14	13	134	21	1
10	1	8	57	9	0	96	15	1	135	21	3
15	2	6	58	9	1	97	15	4	136	21	6
20	3	1	59	9	4	98	15	6	137	21	8
21	3	4	60	9	6	99	15	8	138	21	10
22	3	7	61	9	8	100	15	10	139	21	13
23	3	8	62	9	11	101	15	13	140	22	0
24	3	11	63	9	13	102	16	1	141	22	3
25	3	13	64	10	1	103	16	3	142	22	5
26	4	1	65	10	3	104	16	6	143	22	7
27	4	3	66	10	6	105	16	7	144	22	10
28	4	6	67	10	7	106	16	10	145	22	11
29	4	8	68	10	10	107	16	11	146	23	0
30	4	10	69	10	13	108	17	0	147	23	1
31	4	13	70	11	0	109	17	3	148	23	5
32	5	0	71	11	3	110	17	5	149	23	6
33	5	3	72	11	4	111	17	7	150	23	8
34	5	6	73	11	7	112	17	8	151	23	11
35	5	7	74	11	8	113	17	11	152	23	13
36	5	10	75	11	11	114	17	13	153	24	1
37	5	11	76	12	0	115	18	1	154	24	3
38	6	0	77	12	1	116	18	5	155	24	6
39	6	1	78	12	5	117	18	6	156	24	7
40	6	3	79	12	6	118	18	8	157	24	10
41	6	7	80	12	8	119	18	10	158	24	13
42	6	8	81	12	10	120	18	13	159	25	0
43	6	11	82	12	13	121	19	0	160	25	3

Adult immunization schedule

The immunization schedule below is recommended for adults older than age 18.

Vaccine	Timing and considerations
Hepatitis A for those at risk	Two doses 6–12 months apart to provide long-term protection; first dose 4 weeks before departure to endemic countries
Hepatitis B if never had initial series	Three doses: second dose at least 1 month after first; third dose 5 months after first dose
Measles, mumps, and rubella	Two doses 1 month apart if born after 1957 and immunity cannot be proved; contraindicated in pregnancy, cancer, immunosuppression, and HIV infection
Tetanus–diphtheria if never had initial series	Three doses: second dose 1 month after first, third dose 6–12 months after second; booster for all patients every 10 years
Varicella-zoster	Two doses for susceptible adults who have not had chickenpox; second dose 1 month after first; contraindicated in pregnancy, cancer, immunosuppression, and HIV infection
Influenza	Annually before influenza season (September to December in the UK), especially for those aged 65 and older, those with heart or lung disease, diabetes, or other chronic conditions, and those who work or live with high-risk individuals
Pneumococcal	One dose at age 65; also recommended for persons with chronic disease (see indications for influenza) and those with kidney disorders or sickle cell anaemia; possibly a repeat dose 5 years later for those at highest risk; may be given at any time of the year

Mental assessment

Each question scores one mark

1 Age
2 Time (to nearest hour)
3 Address for recall at end (e.g. 42 West Street)
4 What year is it?
5 Name of institution
6 Recognition of two persons
7 Date of birth (day and month)
8 Year of First World War
9 Name of present monarch
10 Count backwards from 20 to 1

A score of 6 or below is likely to indicate impaired cognition

Reproduced with permission from Hodkinson HM (1972). Evaluation of a mental test score for assessment of mental impairment in the elderly. *Age and Ageing*, **1**, 233–8.

Human skeleton

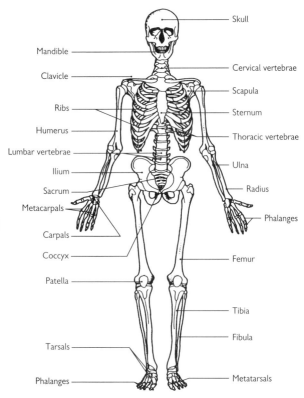

The skeleton

The Bristol stool chart

Type 1		Separate hard lumps, like nuts (hard to pass)
Type 2		Sausage-shaped but lumpy
Type 3		Like a sausage but with cracks on its surface
Type 4		Like a sausage or snake, smooth and soft
Type 5		Soft blobs with clear-cut edges (passed easily)
Type 6		Fluffy pieces with ragged edges, a mushy stool
Type 7		Watery, no solid pieces ENTIRELY LIQUID

Reproduced by kind permission of Dr KW Heaton, Reader in Medicine at the University of Bristol.

Management of constipation

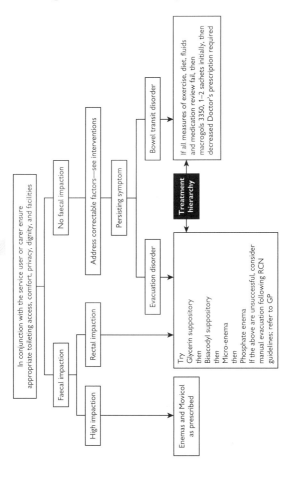

In conjunction with the service user or carer ensure appropriate toileting access, comfort, privacy, dignity, and facilities

Faecal impaction

No faecal impaction

High impaction

Rectal impaction

Address correctable factors—see interventions

Persisting symptom

Evacuation disorder

Bowel transit disorder

Treatment hierarchy

Enemas and Movicol as prescribed

Try
Glycerin suppository
then
Bisacodyl suppository
then
Micro-enema
then
Phosphate enema
If the above are unsuccessful, consider manual evacuation following RCN guidelines; refer to GP

If all measures of exercise, diet, fluids and medication review fail, then macrogols 3350, 1–2 sachets initially, then decreased Doctor's prescription required

With thanks to Sussex Health Care

Bony prominences that are main sites of pressure sores

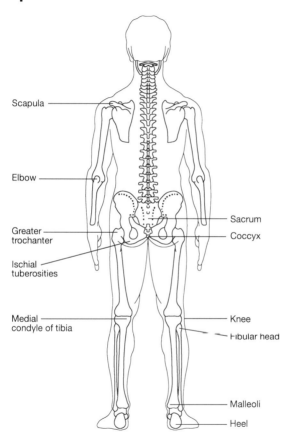

Assessing stages of skin ulceration

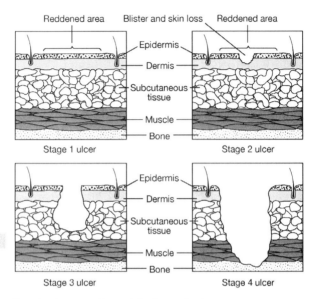

Stage 1: ulcer presents as a defined area of redness.
Stage 2: superficial ulcer with some skin loss, blister appearance, and a
shallow crater.
Stage 3: full-thickness skin loss, damage to subcutaneous tissue, and
deep crater.
Stage 4: full-thickness skin loss, damage extends to muscle and bone
with tunnelling and sinus.

PQRST mnemonic for pain

P = provokes/point   What provokes or exacerbates the pain? What
                           helps relieve it? Point to area of pain.

Q = quality   What does it feel like? Which words describe it?
                           Sharp? Dull? Stabbing? Burning? Crushing? Aching?

R = radiation/relief   Does it radiate? Where to? What relieves it?

S = severity   Rate the pain on a scale of 1–10 or 1–3 where
                           1 = no pain.

T = time   When did it start? What brings it on?
                           How long does it last?

T = treatment   What helps and what are you using to treat it?

Eye chart

He moved
N. 48

all the brightest gems
N. 24

faster and faster towards the
N.18

ever-growing bucket of lost hopes;
had there been just one more year
N. 14

of peace the battalion would have made
a floating system of perpetual drainage.
N. 12

A silent fall of immense snow came near oily
remains of the recently eaten supper on the table.
N. 10

We drove on in our old sunless walnut. Presently
classical eggs ticked in the new afternoon shadows.
N. 8

We were instructed by my cousin Jasper not to exercise by country
house visiting unless accompanied by thirteen geese or gangsters.
N. 6

The modern American did not prevail over the pair of redundant bronze puppies.
The worn-out principle is a bad omen which I am never glad to ransom in August.
N. 5

Record the smallest type (eg N.12 left eye, N.6 right eye, spectacles worn) or object accurately read or named at 30cm

Reprinted from Longmore and Wilkinson, *Oxford Handbook of Clinical Medicine 6e*, p.63.
Reproduced with permission from Oxford University Press.

Dermatome chart

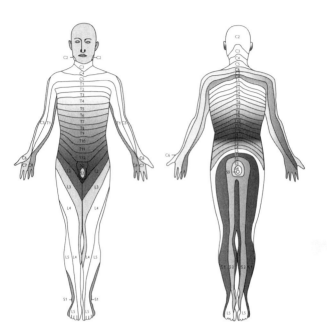

An abridged form of the NMC Code

The people in your care must be able to trust you with their health and wellbeing. To justify that trust, you must:

1. Make the care of people your first concern, treating them as individuals and respecting their dignity.

   This includes; treating people as individuals, respecting people's dignity and confidentiality, acting as an advocate, collaborating with those in your care, ensuring you gain consent, maintaining clear professional and sexual boundaries, and refusing gifts, favours, or hospitality.

2. Work with others to protect and promote the health and wellbeing of those in your care, their families and carers, and the wider community.

   This includes; sharing information with your colleagues, working effectively as part of a team, delegating effectively, managing risk, and informing someone in authority if you experience problems that prevent you working within the Code or other agreed standards.

3. Provide a high standard of practice and care at all times.

   This includes; using the best available evidence, using complementary or alternative therapies carefully, keeping your skills and knowledge up to date, working within your competence, and keeping clear and accurate records, clearly and legibly signed, dated, and timed.

4. Be open and honest, act with integrity and uphold the reputation of your profession.

   This includes; acting with integrity, adhering to the laws of the country you are practising in, dealing with problems, acting promptly, cooperating with internal and external investigations, being impartial, and upholding the reputation of your profession by not using your professional status to promote causes that are not related to health.

5. The NMC recommends that all registered nurses have professional indemnity insurance. This is in the interests of clients, patients, and registrants in the event of claims of professional negligence. Whilst employers have vicarious liability for the negligent acts and /or omissions of their employees, such cover does not normally extend to activities undertaken outside the registrant's employment.

Full NMC code can be found at www.nmc-uk.org

Contact

Nursing and Midwifery Council
23 Portland Place
London
W1B 1PZ

020 7333 9333
advice@nmc-uk.org
www.nmc-uk.org

Malnutrition Universal Screening Tool (MUST)

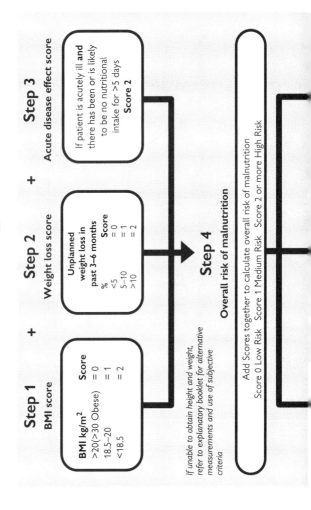

Step 1
BMI score

BMI kg/m²	Score
>20(>30 Obese)	= 0
18.5–20	= 1
<18.5	= 2

If unable to obtain height and weight, refer to explanatory booklet for alternative measurements and use of subjective criteria

+

Step 2
Weight loss score

Unplanned weight loss in past 3–6 months	Score
%	
<5	= 0
5–10	= 1
>10	= 2

+

Step 3
Acute disease effect score

If patient is acutely ill **and** there has been or is likely to be no nutritional intake for >5 days
Score 2

Step 4
Overall risk of malnutrition

Add Scores together to calculate overall risk of malnutrition
Score 0 Low Risk   Score 1 Medium Risk   Score 2 or more High Risk

Step 5
Management guidelines

0
Low Risk
Routine clinical care

- Repeat screening
  Hospital – weekly
  Care Homes – monthly
  Community – annually
  for special groups
  e.g. those >75 yrs

1
Medium Risk
Observe

- Document dietary intake
  for 3 days if subject in
  hospital or care home
- If improved or adequate
  intake – little clinical
  concern; if no improvement –
  clinical concern – follow
  local policy
- Repeat screening
  Hospital – weekly
  Care Home – at least monthly
  Community – at least every
  2–3 months

2 or more
High Risk
Treat*

- Refer to dietitian, Nutritional
  Support Team or implement
  local policy
- Improve and increase
  overall nutritional intake
- Monitor and review care plan
  Hospital – weekly
  Care Home – monthly
  Community – monthly

*Unless detrimental or no benefit
is expected from nutritional
support, e.g. imminent death.

All risk categories:

- Treat underlying condition and provide help and
  advice on food choices, eating and drinking when
  necessary.
- Record malnutrition risk category.
- Record need for special diets and follow local policy.

Obesity:

- Record presence of obesity. For those with
  underlying conditions, these are generally
  controlled before the treatment of obesity.

Re-assess subjects identified at risk as they move through care settings

BMI score

Step 1 – BMI score (& BMI)

Height (feet and inches)

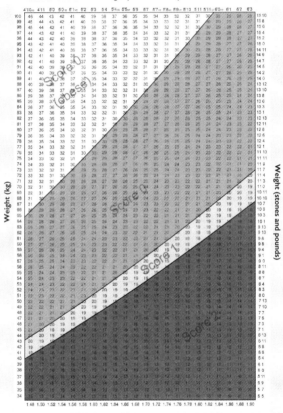

Note: The black lines denote the exact cut off points (30, 20 and 18.5 kg/m²), figures on the chart have been rounded to the nearest whole number.

Index

Note: Subjects are indexed in their expanded form. A list of abbreviations is given on pp. xxxv–xx